Endoscopic Cardiac Surgery

Springer Nature More Media App

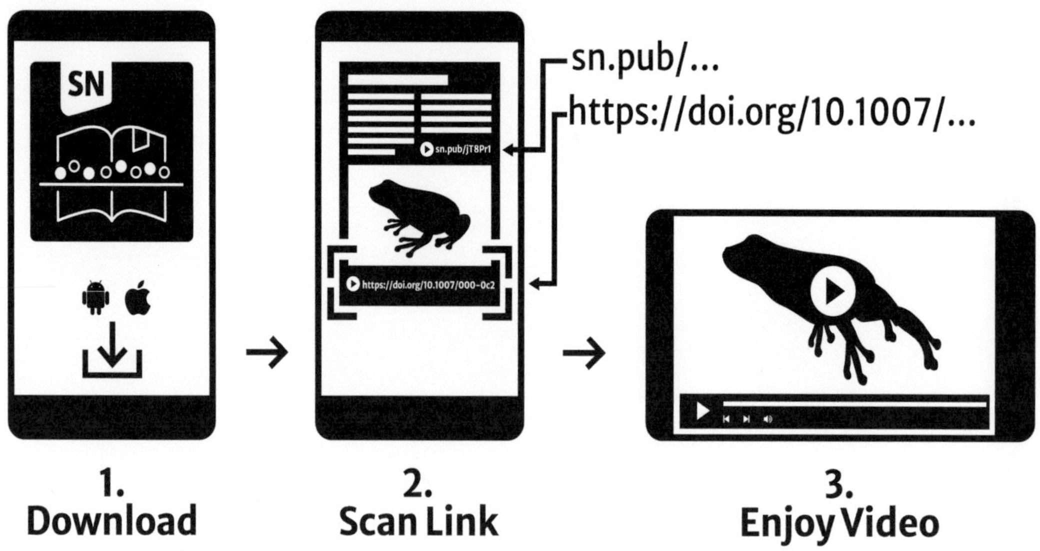

Support: customerservice@springernature.com

Joseph Zacharias

Editor

Endoscopic Cardiac Surgery

Tips, Tricks and Traps

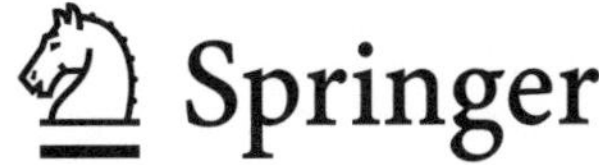

Editor
Joseph Zacharias
Lancashire Cardiac Centre
Victoria Hospital
Blackpool, UK

ISBN 978-3-031-21106-5   ISBN 978-3-031-21104-1   (eBook)
https://doi.org/10.1007/978-3-031-21104-1

This Springer imprint is published by the registered company Springer Nature Switzerland AG
The registered company address is: Gewerbestrasse 11, 6330 Cham, Switzerland

Foreword

Medicine is all about care, Cardiac Surgery is about care and ... dare!

The first pioneers in the middle of the twentieth century epitomised this adage. Hundreds of cardiac surgeons all over the world took advantage of their pioneering and panache. More so, it allowed them to thrive on a stream of patients that badly needed this daring surgery to survive, whatever it meant in terms of invasiveness.

Some thought that the "midstream flow" with surgery through a classical mid-sternotomy access would never come to an end.

But then, a new era of possible treatments for cardiac disease came up with a variety of different treatment options for:

Revascularisation (*Bypass vs. PCI*)
Aortic Valve Procedures (*AVR vs. TAVI*)
Mitral Valve Procedures (*MVRepair vs. MitraClip*)
Aortic Diseases (*Operation vs. Stent*)
Electrophysiology (*Thoracoscopic Ablation vs. PVI*).

Not only did we see a great number of interventional cardiologists put a lot of effort into the improvement of all these catheter-based techniques, but also the industry poured lots of money into the creation of start-ups to venture brand new techniques that particularly challenged the surgical techniques with one adage: perfect cosmetics, virtually no pain and immediate reha-bilitation, particularly for a growing number of older and more frail patients, for which surgery remained pretty invasive.

In the twentieth century, the saying was: no pain without gain.

In the twenty-first century, it became: whatever gain, but certainly without pain.

As a result, the number of coronary artery bypass grafting, and aortic valve procedures decreased.

A number of pioneering surgeons realised that in one area, namely the reconstructive surgery of the mitral valve, there wasn't a lot of competition with the excellent results of the repair techniques that surgeons had devel-oped over two decades as it is the best treatment that one can offer to younger patients with a failing degenerative mitral valve apparatus. There was one big improvement to be made though: our impact on the patients in terms of invasiveness had to be way better.

In the late nineties, many techniques were developed to do much less invasive cardiac interventions but … with all the respect of the high long-term quality of a pure surgical repair. It led to complete endoscopic surgery with obvious advantages versus the standard median sternotomy techniques:

> *Less trauma and pain*
> *Less blood-air interface*
> *Less sequestration of white cells in the lungs*
> *Less blood loss*
> *Less wound infections*
> *Shorter rehabilitations and*
> *Way easier redo-surgeries.*

As these efforts were heavily criticised in the beginning by conservative surgeons, it took ten years for younger surgeons to realise that this was the way to go to *compete with or—even better—"complete" catheter-based techniques.*

The faith of totally endoscopic surgery was born: do not touch or harm the bony structure of the thoracic cavity as it was the only way to result in reduced intensive care unit and hospital length of stay postoperatively; patients are monitored overnight in the intensive care unit. Chest tubes can be removed after 24–36 h.

It was a lot about "daring" though as we were not allowed to offer mediocre results let alone more risk than before.

With many lessons learned from the pioneers, a growing number of young surgeons adapted very well to these disruptive gestures, performing remarkably well, keeping in mind these gold rules:

> *Create Your Team: failing to prepare is preparing to fail*
> *Seldinger Cannulation is crucial for ECC installment*
> *Be extremely meticulous with Myocardial Preservation*
> *Surgery remains exposure, even more so in small access surgery*
> *Practice endoscopic Surgery and Shafted Instruments Skills.*

The true non-rib spreading technique limits scar, discomfort and physiologic responses of the intervention, ensures a two weeks rehab-period and comes very close to the "puncture-hole, no pain, no rehab qualities" of percutaneous gestures but with a long-term repair-for-life result in a very high percentage.

The Credo is, an excellent mitral valve repair is pure gold for a patient, but always go for it with minimally invasive techniques that can compete with or be a complement for the interventional cardiologist.

In conclusion, totally endoscopic surgery is a great asset for the surgeon in times where trans-catheter techniques become widely adopted and are often the first choice for the patient of the twenty-first century.

This book is a very remarkable document for all cardiac surgeons who want to become less invasive and it should be first-class inspiration for young surgeons: a must read and a professional companion for the rest of their careers.

Hugo Baron Vanermen
Founder and Head of the Cardiac
Surgery Department (1980 > 2013)
OLVZ-Aalst
Aalst, Belgium

Endoscopic Mitral Valve Surgeon and former
consultant for MICS
@ Klinik Im Park, Zurich, Switzerland
@ Clinica St-Anna, Catanzaro, Italia
@ Institut Mutualiste Montsouris, Paris, France
@ LUMC, Leiden, the Netherlands
@ UCL, St Luc, Woluwe, Belgium
@ AZ, VUB, Brussels, Belgium
@ European Hospital, Roma, Italia
@ Policlinico di Monza, Italia

Preface

There are more books being published every year today, and than can be read by a particular individual. Why then did SpringerNature decide to embark on this one? That would be a very good question to try and answer right at the start. Surgeons are a lot like Chefs. We often have a similar recipe but add our own individual touch to make each procedure slightly different and unique. The finished product may be similar but there are always subtle variations in how we achieve the final result. Of course like chefs, we are influenced by the culture we are working within and societal constraints of what is funded and accepted. Herein lies the big challenge for all those who would like to see surgery standardised. Even though we are making progress on this front, we in cardiac surgery are a while away from getting there. This book was put together to mirror a "cookbook" rather than a "textbook" of techniques in a new emerging and exciting subspecialty of cardiac surgery!

On this background of variation, the introduction of endoscopic techniques within cardiac surgery has been a challenge across the globe and even though it is widely recognised as potentially the least invasive way of achieving good long-term results in cardiac pathology, the reality of introducing this into practise, making it safe and reproducible in the hands of a critical mass of surgeons, has been elusive. The reasons for this may be multifactorial, but need to be considered in order to overcome.

The first obvious reason is the already excellent results that a sternotomy approach brings to deal with a diverse set of cardiac pathology and as these techniques have been around for over 50 years, there is an excellent training program in many countries to get young surgeons from beginners to a fully trained cardiac surgeon which takes from 3 to 8 years depending on the country and exposure available. Over the past 30 years, there has also been a genuine hope that trans-catheter procedures will provide an alternative, and these procedures have been funded and adopted widely in many health systems to varying degrees of success. There is now an increasing acceptance that trans-catheter procedures and conventional cardiac surgery are in a "positive sum" game rather than a "zero sum" game as previously envisioned by some. As we cardiac surgeons are increasingly getting involved with patients who are asymptomatic or old and frail, there is a need for a less invasive incision than a sternotomy.

An endoscope has revolutionised many sub-specialities of surgery, and its time to do so in cardiac surgery is ripe. I believe this, because we are now increasingly supported by not only improved images both preoperatively with computerised tomography scanning and trans oesophageal echocardiography but also intra-operative imaging with better endoscopic equipment and depth perception of three-dimensional cameras. Despite these adjuncts, the gradual shift away from sternotomy is a big move for surgeons and teams. This has to be achieved in an era of a lack of tolerance for learning curves and increased public scrutiny of surgeons and teams. All surgical change needs a combination of "will and skill". The cycle of change classically follows 5 stages and the first three are pre-contemplation, contemplation and preparation. I hope for many this book helps at one of these stages.We as authors also hope that this has a place for surgeons who enjoy the details seen in operative videos and also other clinicians who would like a better understanding of the beautiful anatomy within the heart that these videos capture.

The unique feature of this book was the embedded videos created especially for this project, which hopefully helps to explain concepts more easily than pictures or text. So the hope is that this book will be different and useful to you readers. This book would not have been possible without the support of Grant Weston and Antony Joseph from SpringerNature who have backed the procedure through a global pandemic to make it into a reality.

I have to thank the exceptional line-up of authors who selflessly gave up their time for this new project. Despite work pressures and new challenges, these remarkable individuals have contributed their wisdom and I encourage readers to directly contact them as I know they have so much more to share and give, which could not be captured in these pages.

This book has tried to distil the experiences of many clinicians who have successfully navigated the cycle of change and are now well established in the last two stages, of action and maintenance. There are many ways to establish an endoscopic cardiac surgery program, and I do hope as a reader you consider this book as a starting point on a journey of serious contemplation. As my mentor, Dr. Vanerman often, quoted Victor Hugo saying, "nothing is more powerful than an idea whose time has come!", has the time come for endoscopic cardiac surgery? That reality is in the hands of all you readers. We need to see the partnership between a pill, a saw and a catheter increased to include an endoscope in the armamentarium of clinicians involved in the fight against heart disease around the world.

Blackpool, UK   Joseph Zacharias

The original version of the book was revised: ESM link and videos has been updated for chapters 1, 2, 3, 5, 6, 9, 11, 14, 19. The correction to the book is available at https://doi.org/10.1007/978-3-031-21104-1_25

Contents

Operative Planning for Safe Endoscopic Mitral Valve Surgery

Luca Aerts and Peyman Sardari Nia

Abstract

The increasing interest in minimally invasive approaches has induced fast expansion of minimally invasive mitral valve surgery (MIMVS) over the past two decades. However, MIMVS is not included in the most recent valvular heart disease guidelines due to the lack of convincing data supporting this approach. Due to the different techniques applied by individual surgeons and centers, there has been no scientific nor expertise-based consensus developed regarding standardization in MIMVS and consequently its absolute contra-indications. Therefore, a change of mindset is required to shift the focus from the superiority of a procedure toward which particular patients have the greatest benefit from specific surgical approaches. In light of personalized medicine, we have developed a standard procedural planning to ensure a standard approach to patients undergoing MIMVS.

Supplementary Information The online version contains supplementary material available at https://doi.org/10.1007/978-3-031-21104-1_1. The videos can be accessed individually by clicking the DOI link in the accompanying figure caption or by scanning this link with the SN More Media App.

L. Aerts (✉) · P. Sardari Nia
Department of Cardiothoracic Surgery, Maastricht University Medical Center, Maastricht, the Netherlands
e-mail: lucaaerts@hotmail.com

Keywords

Mitral valve repair · Minimally invasive surgery · Preoperative planning · Three-dimensional imaging · Computed tomography (CT)

1 Introduction

The increasing interest in minimally invasive approaches has induced fast expansion of minimally invasive mitral valve surgery (MIMVS) over the past two decades. However, MIMVS is not included in the most recent valvular disease guidelines due to the lack of convincing data favoring this approach [1–3].

Several studies, including meta-analyses and single-center retrospective studies, demonstrate reduced blood loss, ventilation time and postoperative pain as well as shorter intensive care unit admission and overall hospital stay in comparison to conventional surgery [6–8]. However, increased cardiopulmonary bypass (CPB) and clamping times were also reported.

Additionally, the level of complexity and its steep learning curve contributes to the reticence of interested surgeons to put their hands to the plow and start, persevere and fine-tune such comprehensive surgery [4, 5].

Due to the different techniques applied by individual surgeons and centers, there has been

J. Zacharias (ed.), *Endoscopic Cardiac Surgery*,
https://doi.org/10.1007/978-3-031-21104-1_1

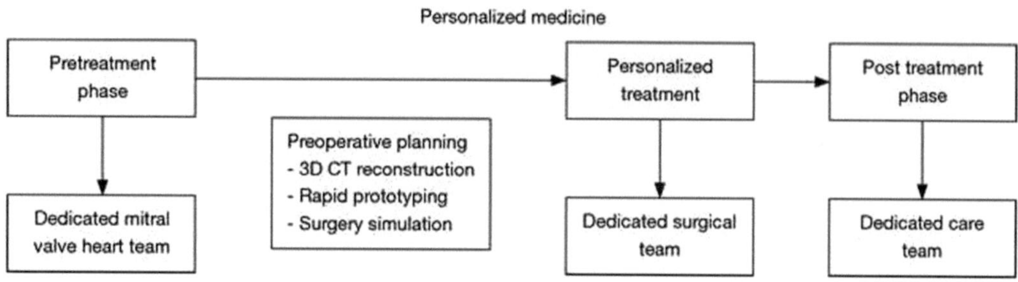

Fig. 1 Concept of personalized medicine. 3D, three-dimensional; CT, computed tomography. *Reprinted from Interactive CardioVascular and Thoracic Surgery, Volume 24, Issue 2, Sardari Nia P, Heuts S, Daemen J, Luyten P, Vainer J, Hoorntje J, Cheriex E, Maessen J, Preoperative planning with three-dimensional reconstruction of patient's anatomy, rapid prototyping and simulation for endoscopic mitral valve repair, 163–168, 2017 with permission from Elsevier [27]*

no scientific nor expertise-based consensus developed regarding standardization in MIMVS and consequently its absolute contra-indications. There is great variability in technical strategies in terms of access, vision, perfusion techniques and conditioning [9].

Therefore, a change of mindset is required to shift the focus from the superiority of a particular procedure toward which patients have the greatest benefit from a specific surgical approach. Careful patient selection and extensive preoperative planning is mandatory for MIMVS and accentuating the advantages of this approach, leading to less conversions and reducing peri- and postoperative complications.

In light of personalized medicine, we have developed a standard preoperative procedural planning to ensure personalized treatment (Fig. 1).

2 Teamwork Approach

In cardiac surgery, teamwork and communication are the key to success. It is well established that failures in coordinated teamwork contribute to avoidable harm and inefficiency in the surgical field. Complex procedures, such as MIMVS, are even more in need of a dedicated team to minimize these failures.

In our center, all patients referred for a mitral valve procedure are discussed in our weekly mitral valve heart team, consisting of interventional cardiologists, imaging cardiologists and cardiothoracic surgeons with expertise in the mitral valve. After careful consideration, the patients are allocated to their designated treatment [10].

We have shown in a recent retrospective cohort that patients treated by a dedicated mitral heart team have superior survival compared to patients treated by a nonspecialist heart team. Between July 2009 and December 2014, a total of 504 patients with mitral valve pathologies were discussed in the general heart team. This team consisted of two members: a specialized cardiothoracic surgeon and an interventional cardiologist. If they concluded that additional imaging was required, patients would be discussed a second time by this team after substantial imaging was acquired.

Additionally, 641 patients were presented in a dedicated mitral valve heart team in a four-year time period from December 2014 to December 2018. This larger team consisted of dedicated mitral valve surgeons (>25 mitral valve procedures per year), interventional and imaging cardiologists, both specialized in mitral valve pathology. As for the general heart team, when required, further investigation was obtained in order to make a final decision.

When comparing the results of both multidisciplinary teams, these are in favor of the dedicated mitral valve heart team in our clinic. The 5-year survival probability was 0.70 (95% confidence interval (CI) 0.66 – 0.74) for the general heart team in comparison to 0.74 (95% CI 0.68 – 0.79, P = 0.040) for the dedicated mitral valve heart team. A subgroup of cases was identified where the advice of the team was not followed and compared to the patients when it was followed. The adjusted relative risk of mortality was reduced by 61% (hazard ratio 0.39, 95% CI 0.25 – 0.62, P < 0.001) when following the advice of the dedicated mitral valve heart team and reduced by 43% (HR 0.57, 95% CI 0.37 – 0.87, P = 0.010) when following the advice of the general heart team. These results were independent of the baseline characteristics, the mitral valve pathology and the allocated treatment [11].

3 Procedural Planning

All patients with an indication for mitral valve surgery in our center are subjected to standard procedural planning to identify comorbidities and anatomical variations. Relative contra-indications are identified and taken into consideration during the preoperative process (Table 1).

3.1 Electrocardiography

At the first outpatient visit, our patients are screened for the presence of atrial fibrillation (AF) or ventricular dys-synchrony. If AF is detected by electrocardiography, the patient will be reviewed in our rhythm heart team, composed of rhythm surgeons and electrophysiologists. During this consultation, the team decides whether a concomitant surgical ablation will be performed according to the most recent guidelines [12].

3.2 Chest X-ray

The second step in the workup process is radiography. The standardly performed chest X-ray is evaluated for anomalous thoracic anatomy, acute or chronic pulmonary pathology and the position of the diaphragm, with a special interest in the right hemi-diaphragm. Additional diagnostic modalities can be opted for during the screening pathway, or a pulmonologist can be consulted for further evaluation.

3.3 Echocardiography

When referring a patient to our center, the cardiologist is usually sending a transthoracic echocardiography (TTE) performed at their own hospital in advance. During the multidisciplinary meeting, all the echocardiographic images will be analyzed by a dedicated mitral heart team including an imaging cardiologist with expertise in mitral valve pathology.

To date, TTE is the golden standard for the evaluation of mitral valve disease. The mechanism of mitral regurgitation (MR) is identified by valve morphology, color jet flow, vena contracta

Table 1 Relative contra-indications for MIMVS in our center. BMI: body mass index; MIMVS: Minimally Invasive Mitral Valve Surgery

Relative contra-indications for MIMVS at the beginning of the learning curve
Significant mitral annular calcification
More than grade I + aortic valve regurgitation
Extensive aortic dilatation
Morbidly obese and extremely muscular patients
Large chest with a distance between the MV annulus and right-sided chest wall of more than 25 cm
Extensive pulmonary adhesions
Extensive abdominal aortic atherosclerosis or peripheral arterial diameters <7 mm
High BMI

width, pulmonary vein flow, time-velocity integral of mitral inflow, effective orifice regurgitant orifice and regurgitant volume [13]. The severity of MR is determined multifactorial, rather than by solely one parameter.

For example, a small jet reaching just above the mitral valve annulus is classified as 'non-severe', but can be potentially misinterpreted by increased pressure in the left atrium [14]. On the other hand, patients with Barlow's disease (extensive myxomatous valve disease) can conceal signs of severe MR due to 'mitral valve disjunction'. This physiological phenomenon is characterized by a total displacement of the mitral valve into the left atrium, without a large flow jet presented on echocardiography [15, 16].

Additionally, TTE gives a global overview of cardiac function and other valvular abnormality. Preoperatively we are specifically interested in the mitral valve; we evaluate left and right ventricular function, pulmonary artery pressure and concomitant aortic and tricuspid regurgitation. Right ventricular dysfunction has been proven to be a substantiate predictor for postoperative mortality [17].

According to recent guidelines, tricuspid repair during the same procedure is advocated when there is a tricuspid annular dilatation of >40 mm regardless of the severity of tricuspid regurgitation. This is associated with a better outcome of mitral valve surgery [18].

If repair is possible on grounds of the TTE images, the patient will need transesophageal echocardiography (TEE). TEE is superior to TTE regarding the identification of the localization and mechanism of the mitral valve prolapse that is used to envision the repair strategy [19]. Furthermore, the TEE is a resourceful modality when predicting the exact ring size of the mitral valve annulus. By measuring the anterior mitral leaflet length and intercommissural distance, the required ring size can be calculated [20].

By using dedicated software, three-dimensional printing of the mitral valve can be used to visualize the anatomy and pathology of an individual valve (Video 1). This will be discussed in another chapter.

3.4 Coronary Angiography

All patients who meet the criteria for MIMVS will undergo a coronary angiography (CAG) mainly to exclude subclinical coronary artery disease (CAD) requiring sequential coronary artery grafting (CABG). Secondly, CAG is used to preoperatively strategize the procedure by investigating the patient's coronary anatomy. The CAG is evaluated to identify potential impediments, such as mitral annular calcification and the circumflex artery (RCx) trajectory and to determine the dominance of the cardiac vascular system. In a left dominant coronary system, RCx runs closer to the mitral valve annulus [22].

One of the most dangerous but uncommon complications of mitral valve surgery is accidental (partial) occlusion of the RCx [23, 24]. This presents itself postoperatively with reduced ventricular function and ischemia-like features, due to either kinking of the artery toward the mitral valve or a fully obliterated lumen of the artery by annular sutures (Fig. 2, Video 2).

3.5 Computed Tomography

Computed Tomography (CT) plays a major role in the preoperative process. MIMVS is accomplished by peripheral cannulation due to the keyhole approach. For this reason, an electrocardiography-triggered computed tomography angiography is made to visualize the aortic root and ascending aorta, followed by a high pitch spiral computed tomography angiography to visualize the aortic arch down to the femoral bifurcation. Relative contra-indications such as calcification, dilatation and stenosis in the trajectory of the peripheral arteries will be traced to minimize the risk of vessel wall damage and consequently stroke peri- and postoperative (Fig. 3, Video 3).

With the help of three-dimensional reconstructing nowadays, we can create a three-dimensional reconstruction of each individual patient's anatomy preoperatively. Using this technology, we get insight into the visuospatial relations between anatomic structures to enhance

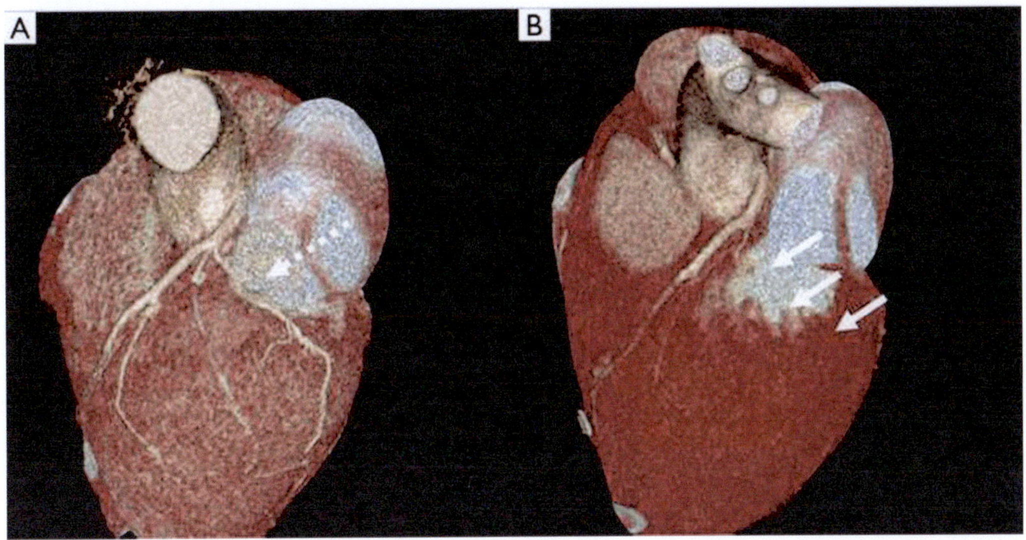

Fig. 2 Contrast-enhanced cardiac CT in a patient with postoperative iatrogenic occlusion of the RCx after mitral valve repair. **A** Preoperative CT revealing an intact RCx (dotted arrow) and **B** postoperative CT 3 months after mitral valve repair showing a fully obliterated RCx (arrows) due to annular sutures. CT, computed tomography; RCx, circumflex artery. *Reprinted with permission from The Journal of Visualized Surgery,* https://doi.org/10.21037/jovs.2018.09.07 [21]

Fig. 3 Reconstruction of the iliofemoral vessels and aorta based on CT images for simulation of arterial cannula introduction and advancement. **A** A 21 Ch arterial cannula can safely be introduced in the right femoral artery while **B** the right femoral artery has an insufficient luminal diameter for a 23 Ch cannula. *Reprinted with permission from The Journal of Visualized Surgery,* https://doi.org/10.21037/jovs.2018.09.07 [21]

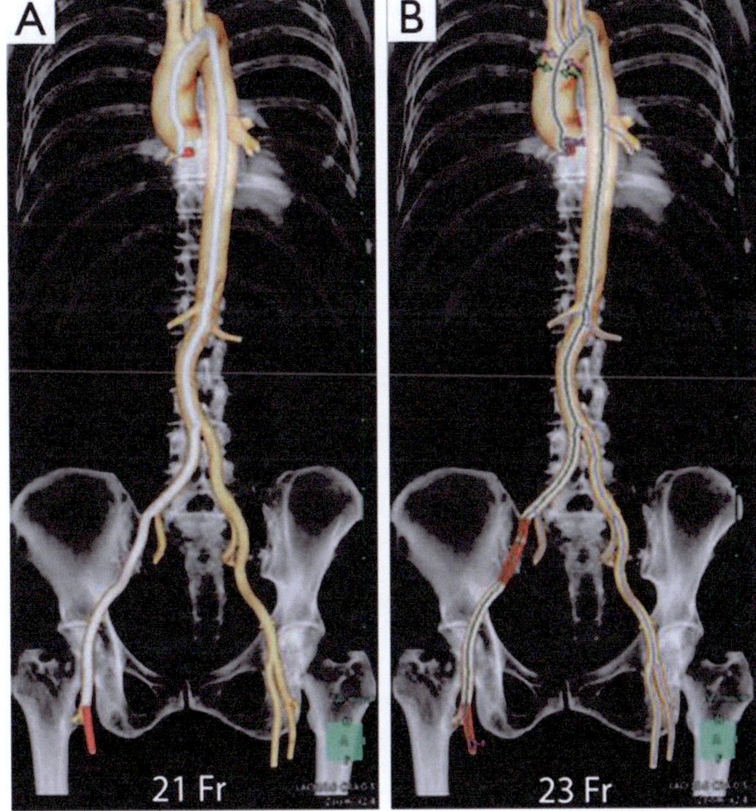

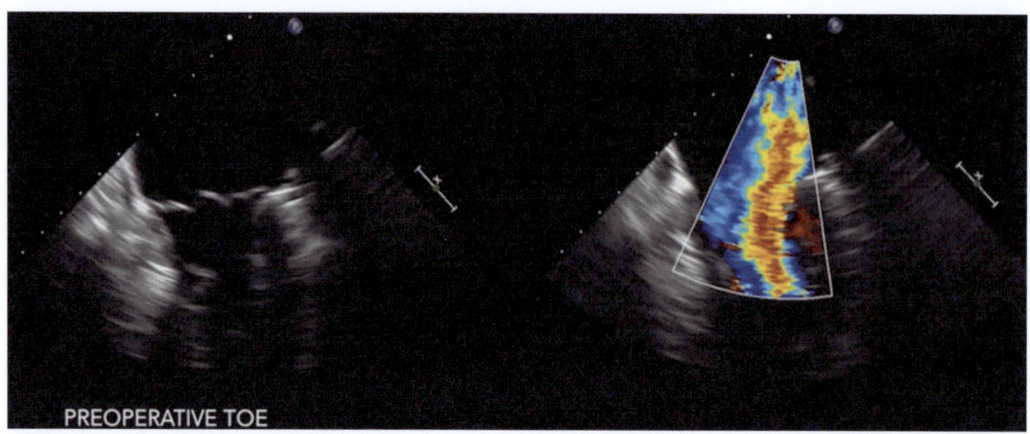

Video 1 Mitral valve repair for posterior leaflet prolapse. Available online: http://www.asvide.com/article/view/32378. *Reprinted with permission from The Journal of Visualized Surgery,* https://doi.org/10.21037/jovs.2018.09.07 [25] (▶ https://doi.org/10.1007/000-a6j)

surgical intervention and analyze the procedure layer by layer to enhance safety, efficacy and reproducibility.

Approximately 30% of patients referred to our clinic for minimally invasive aortic or mitral valve surgery workup have anatomic variations based on three-dimensional reconstruction based on CT-imaging. The following features can be seen: severe calcification of the abdominal aorta or the pericardium, iliofemoral vessel tortuosity and aortic elongation [26]. This does not mean these patients cannot be accepted for a minimally invasive approach, but it requires a modified approach and change in strategy.

To illustrate the full trajectory of a patient, a case is presented:

Mitral valve repair for posterior leaflet prolapse

A 64-year-old man visited the outpatient clinic with progressive dyspnea. There was no medical history and no use of medication. TTE was performed to evaluate overall cardiac function. This imaging technique showed a left ventricular function of 68%, left ventricle diastolic diameter of 52 mm, left ventricle systolic diameter of 32 mm and mitral regurgitation classified as 'severe' with an effective regurgitant orifice of 0.53 cm^2. There were no other valvular pathologies. TEE was added to the diagnostic pathway and clarified the mechanism of regurgitation. There was a P2 segment prolapse of the posterior leaflet.

The mitral valve heart team decided to accept the patient for MIMVS. A CT scan was performed, and no contra-indications were found. To determine the preoperative strategy, a three-dimensional printed mitral model was reconstructed. Using a simulation model, this three-dimensional model was implanted and it was determined preoperatively to use 3 pairs of neochordae and a stabilizing ring (See Video 1).

4 Future Perspectives

The ultimate aim is to strive for the best outcomes in mitral valve surgery by putting an excessive focus on the prevention of adverse events. Adverse events should not form any barrier in developing a programme, but should be a trigger to improve and excel. Measurement is fundamental to evolve, and the process, structure and outcome are helpful resources to achieve this (See Videos 2, 3 and 4).

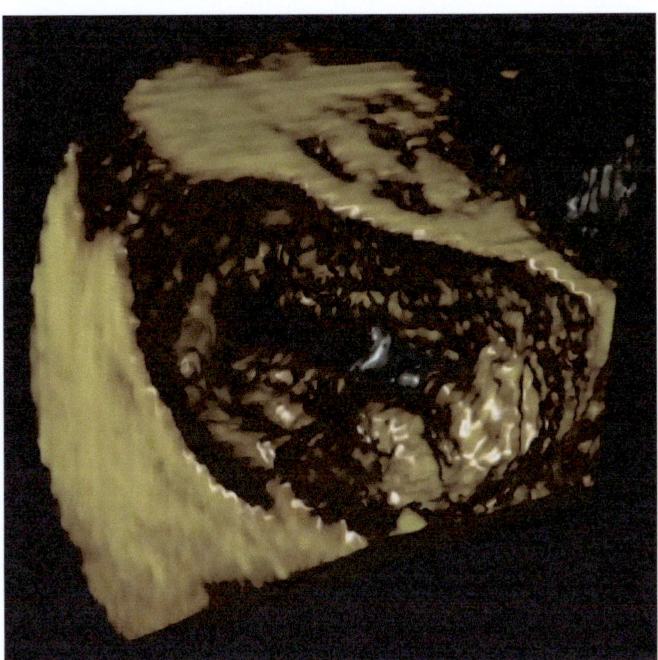

Video 2 Three-dimensional mitral valve reconstruction based on TEE images. The model can be stopped at any moment during the cardiac cycle for optimal assessment of valvular pathology. TEE: transesophageal echocardiography. Available online: http://www.asvide.com/article/view/27630. *Reprinted with permission from The Journal of Visualized Surgery,* https://doi.org/10.21037/jovs.2018.09.07 [21] (▶ https://doi.org/10.1007/000-a6h)

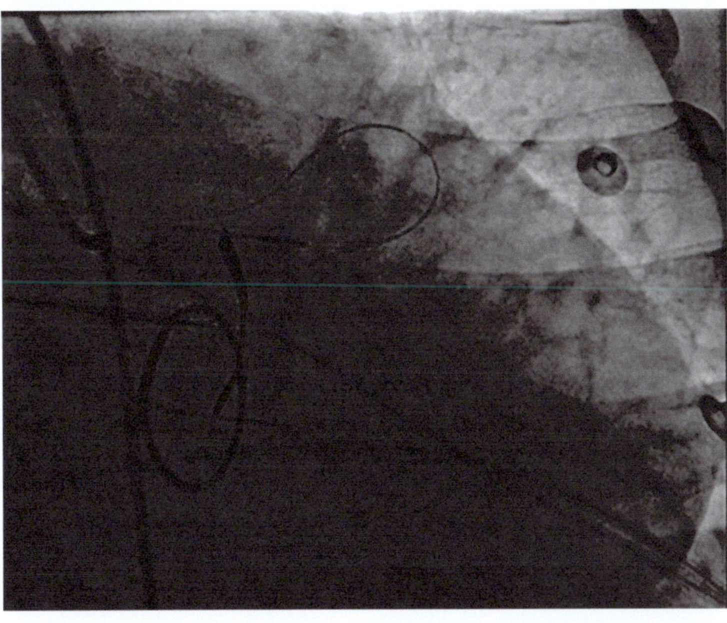

Video 3 Direct postoperative invasive coronary angiography after mitral valve repair, revealing an iatrogenic total occlusion of the proximal RCx. RCx: circumflex artery. Available online: http://www.asvide.com/article/view/27631. *Reprinted with permission from The Journal of Visualized Surgery,* https://doi.org/10.21037/jovs.2018.09.07 [21] (▶ https://doi.org/10.1007/000-a6g)

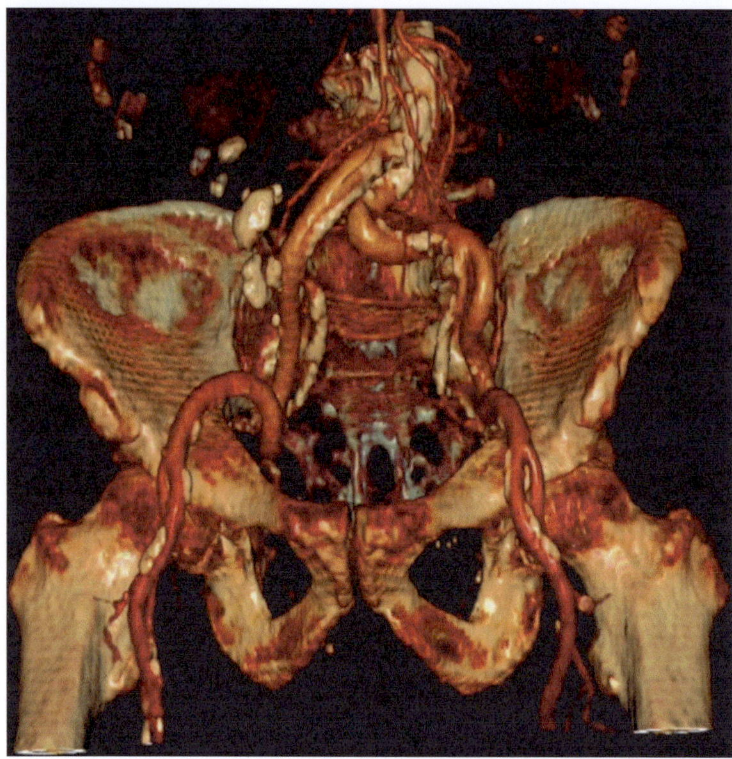

Video 4 Three-dimensional anatomical reconstruction of the abdominal aorta and peripheral vessels revealing extensive calcification and tortuosity of the iliofemoral vessels CPB, cardiopulmonary bypass. Available online: http://www.asvide.com/article/view/27632. *Reprinted with permission from The Journal of Visualized Surgery,* https://doi.org/10.21037/jovs.2018.09.07 [21] (▶ https://doi.org/10.1007/000-a6k)

References

1. Gammie JS, Zhao Y, Peterson ED, O'Brien SM, Rankin JS, Griffith BP. J. Maxwell Chamberlain Memorial Paper for adult cardiac surgery. Less-invasive mitral valve operations: trends and outcomes from the society of thoracic surgeons adult cardiac surgery database. Ann Thorac Surg. 2010; 90 (5):1401–8, 1410.e1; discussion 1408–10.

2. Baumgartner H, Falk V, Bax JJ, De Bonis M, Hamm C, Holm PJ, Iung B, Lancellotti P, Lansac E, Rodriguez Muñoz D, Rosenhek R, Sjögren J, Tornos Mas P, Vahanian A, Walther T, Wendler O, Windecker S, Zamorano JL. ESC Scientific Document Group. 2017 ESC/EACTS Guidelines for the management of valvular heart disease. Eur Heart J. 2017; 38(36):2739–91.

3. American College of Cardiology Foundation, American Heart Association Task Force on Practice Guidelines, American Association for Thoracic Surgery, American College of Radiology, American Stroke Association, Society of Cardiovascular Anesthesiologists, Williams, DM. 2010 ACCF/AHA/ AATS/ACR/ASA/SCA/SCAI/SIR/STS/SVM guidelines for the diagnosis and management of patients with thoracic aortic disease. J Am College Cardiol 2010; 55(14):e27–e129.

4. Holzhey DM, et al. Learning minimally invasive mitral valve surgery: a cumulative sum sequential probability analysis of 3895 operations from a single high-volume center. Circulation 2013; 128.5:483–91.

5. Loulmet DF, et al. Less invasive techniques for mitral valve surgery. The J Thor Cardiovasc Surg 1998; 115.4:772–9.

6. Dogan S, et al. Minimally invasive port access versus conventional mitral valve surgery: prospective randomized study The Ann Thor Surg 2005; 79.2:492–8.

7. Sündermann SH, et al. Mitral valve surgery: right lateral minithoracotomy or sternotomy? A systematic review and meta-analysis. The J Thor Cardiovasc Surg 2014; 148.5:1989–95.

8. Modi P, Hassan A, Chitwood Jr WR. Minimally invasive mitral valve surgery: a systematic review and meta-analysis. Eur J Cardio-Thor Surg 2008; 34.5:943–52.

9. Misfeld M, et al. Cross-sectional survey on minimally invasive mitral valve surgery. Ann Cardiothor Surg 2013; 2.6:733.

10. Heuts S, et al. Multidisciplinary decision-making in mitral valve disease: the mitral valve heart team. Netherlands Heart J 2019; 27.4:176–84.

11. Sardari Nia P, Olsthoorn JR, Heuts S, van Kuijk SMJ, Vainer J, Streukens S, Schalla S, Segers P, Barenbrug P, Crijns HJGM, Maessen JG. Effect of a dedicated mitral heart team compared to a general heart team on survival: a retrospective, comparative, non-randomized interventional cohort study based on prospectively registered data. Eur J Cardiothorac Surg. 2021; 60(2):263–73.

12. Calkins H, et al. 2017 HRS/EHRA/ECAS/APHRS/ SOLAECE expert consensus statement on catheter and surgical ablation of atrial fibrillation. Ep Europace 2018; 20.1:e1–e160.

13. Lancellotti P, et al. Recommendations for the echocardiographic assessment of native valvular regurgitation: an executive summary from the European Association of Cardiovascular Imaging. Eur Heart J–Cardiovasc Imaging 2013; 14.7:611–44.

14. McCully RB, Enriquez-Sarano M, Tajik AJ, Seward JB. Overestimation of severity of ischemic/ functional mitral regurgitation by color Doppler jet area. The Am J Cardiol 1994; 74(8):790–3.

15. Enriquez-Sarano M. Mitral annular disjunction: the forgotten component of myxomatous mitral valve disease 2017; 1434–6.

16. Luyten P, Heuts S, Cheriex E, Olsthoorn JR, Crijns HJGM, Winkens B, Roos-Hesselink JW, Sardari Nia P, Schalla S. Mitral prolapsing volume is associated with increased cardiac dimensions in patients with mitral annular disjunction. Neth Heart J. 2021 May 4.

17. Haddad F, Denault AY, Couture P, Cartier R, Pellerin M, Levesque S, Lambert J, Tardif JC. Right ventricular myocardial performance index predicts perioperative mortality or circulatory failure in high-risk valvular surgery. J Am Soc Echocardiogr. 2007; 20(9):1065–72.

18. Chikwe J, Itagaki S, Anyanwu A, Adams DH. Impact of concomitant tricuspid annuloplasty on tricuspid regurgitation, right ventricular function, and pulmonary artery hypertension after repair of mitral valve prolapse. J Am Coll Cardiol. 2015;65 (18):1931–8.

19. Chandra S, Salgo IS, Sugeng L, Weinert L, Tsang W, Takeuchi M, Spencer KT, O'Connor A, Cardinale M, Settlemier S, Mor-Avi V, Lang RM. Characterization of degenerative mitral valve disease using morphologic analysis of real-time three-dimensional echocardiographic images: objective insight into complexity and planning of mitral valve repair. Circulation: Cardiovasc Imaging 2011; 4(1):24–32.

20. Ender J, Eibel S, Mukherjee C, Mathioudakis D, Borger MA, Jacobs S, Mohr FW, Falk V. Prediction of the annuloplasty ring size in patients undergoing mitral valve repair using real-time three-dimensional transoesophageal echocardiography. Eur J Echocardiogr. 2011; 12(6):445–53.

21. Heuts S, Olsthoorn J, Maessen J, Nia PS. Planning minimally invasive mitral valve surgery. J Vis Surg. 2018;2018(4):212–22.

22. Virmani R, Chun PK, Parker J, McAllister HA Jr. Suture obliteration of the circumflex coronary artery in three patients undergoing mitral valve operation. Role of left dominant or codominant coronary artery. J Thorac Cardiovasc Surg. 1982; 84(5):773–8.

23. Hiltrop N, Bennett J, Desmet W. Circumflex coronary artery injury after mitral valve surgery: a report of four cases and comprehensive review of the literature. Catheter Cardiovasc Interv. 2017;89:78–92.

24. Tavilla G, Pacini D. Damage to the circumflex coronary artery during mitral valve repair with sliding leaflet technique. Ann Thorac Surg. 1998;66:2091–3.

25. Olsthoorn JR, Heuts S, Daemen J, Maessen J, Nia PS. Clinical implications of three-dimensional mitral valve modelling, printing and simulation in mitral valve surgery. J Visualized Surg 2019; https://doi.org/10.21037/jovs.2019.05.01.

26. Heuts S, Maessen JG, Nia PS. Preoperative planning of left-sided valve surgery with 3D computed tomography reconstruction models: sternotomy or a minimally invasive approach? Interact Cardiovasc Thorac Surg 2016; 22.5:587–93.

27. Nia PS, Heuts S, Daemen J, Luyten P, Vainer J, Hoorntje J, Cheriex E, Maessen J. Preoperative planning with three-dimensional reconstruction of patient's anatomy, rapid prototyping and simulation for endoscopic mitral valve repair. Interact Cardiovasc Thorac Surg. 2017; 24(2):163–8.

Anaesthesia for Endoscopic Cardiac Surgery

Andrew Knowles and Palanikumar Saravanan

Abstract

The origins of cardiac surgery involved a thoracotomy approach. The sternotomy was noted to be a relatively pain free incision. As surgeons move away from sternotomy there is a crucial role played by anaesthesia in the pre, intra and post operative optimisation of the patient. Safe endoscopic surgery requires safe and progressive anaesthesia techniques. We have summarised in this article our experience of anaesthesia and pain control options that are used in our hospital which were picked up from many visits and discussions with other experienced teams.

Keywords

Cardiac anaesthesia · Endoscopic cardiac surgery · Enhanced recovery · Postoperative pain control

Supplementary Information The online version contains supplementary material available at https://doi.org/10.1007/978-3-031-21104-1_2. The videos can be accessed individually by clicking the DOI link in the accompanying figure caption or by scanning this link with the SN More Media App.

A. Knowles (✉) · P. Saravanan
Department of Cardiothoracic Anaesthesia,
Lancashire Cardiac Centre, Blackpool, England
e-mail: Dr.knowles@nhs.net

1 Introduction

Delivery of anaesthesia for endoscopic cardiac surgery (ECS) is a demanding subspecialty combining aspects of both cardiac and thoracic anaesthesia together with the skills to perform and interpret perioperative transoesophageal echocardiography (TOE).

The authors' experience of over 450 minimally invasive cases has been based on a single surgeon's experience in a low volume centre, the learning curve and aspects of which have been detailed by Kirmani et al. [1]. This has spanned decreasing size of thoracotomy incisions, the adoption of endoscopic techniques and use of an intraaortic occlusion balloon or endo balloon (Intraclude Edwards Irvine CA USA) (Fig. 1). Insertion of perfusion cannulas into the internal jugular vein and the use of balloon occlusion techniques of the SVC in re- do cases have brought new challenges to the role of anaesthetists.

The use of transoesophageal echocardiography is a prerequisite for the safe conduct of endoscopic cardiac surgery and requires knowledge of probe manipulation and views over and above those used in standard cardiac surgery.

We have now incorporated a day of surgery admission and enhanced recovery programme for our patients undergoing endoscopic surgery which have led to improved quality of postoperative recovery and shorter length of hospital stay.

J. Zacharias (ed.), *Endoscopic Cardiac Surgery*,
https://doi.org/10.1007/978-3-031-21104-1_2

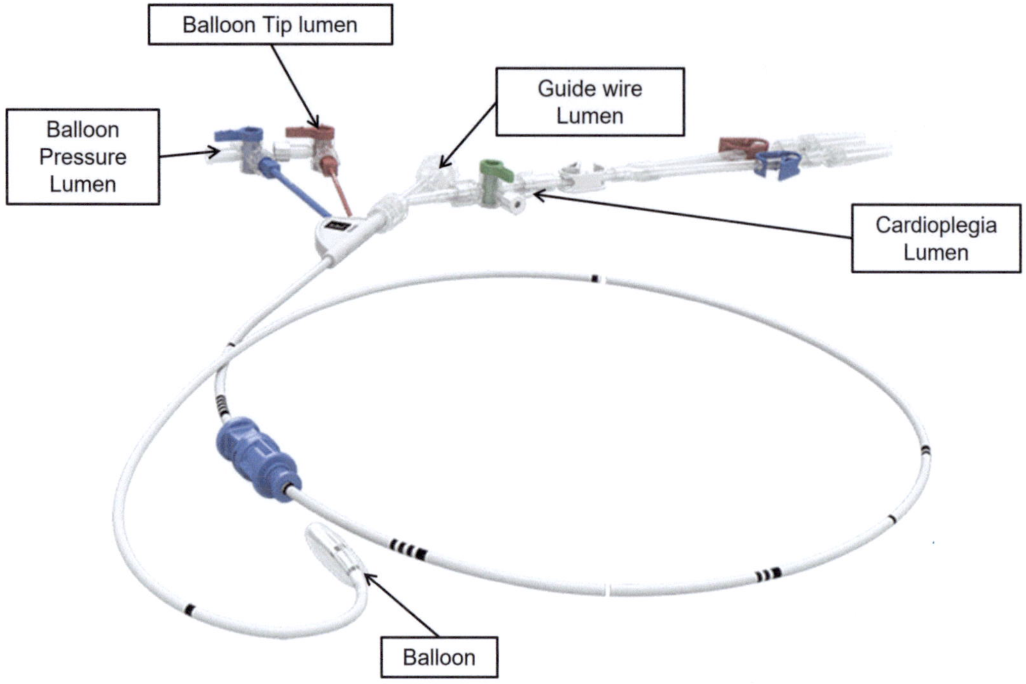

Fig. 1 Endo balloon (Intraclude Edwards Irvine CA USA)

In order to develop a successful programme, the anaesthetist must also work effectively with all the dedicated team members—surgical, perfusion and nursing/theatre practitioners involved in minimally invasive and endoscopic cardiac surgery. While the learning curve and success of the programme improves with cumulative experience, a wide variation is seen between different organisations (Pisano et al. [2]).

However, all patients will reap some benefits from the differing advantages of minimally invasive surgery namely quicker post-operative mobilisation and rehabilitation, reduced blood transfusion requirements and improved cosmesis.

The safe conduct of ECS begins with thorough multidisciplinary preoperative assessment involving surgeons, anaesthetists and radiologists.

2　Preoperative Assessment

The scope of ECS—mitral, tricuspid, atrial septal, myxoma, ventricular septal and re-do procedures presents in a diverse mix of patients in terms of sex, age, frailty and comorbidities varying from essentially fit asymptomatic patients to the very sickest redo patients.

2.1　Cardiovascular

A routine history, examination of the cardiovascular system must focus on the biventricular function, valvular pathology and any other structural cardiac defects.

Imaging review of echocardiography, coronary and aortofemoral angiography is required.

CT angiogram is now routinely performed in assessing suitability of these patients and will provide information on coronary arteries, thoracolumbar aortic pathologies, and femoral vessels.

2.2 Respiratory

Airway assessment, respiratory review and review of respiratory function tests are required for suitability of both anaesthesia and single lung ventilation. Respiratory review includes any obvious anatomical abnormalities such as kyphosis or scoliosis which may make the positioning and surgical access difficult. History suggestive of previous lung pathology such as pleurisy, pneumothorax or pneumonia or previous heart surgery may indicate pleural adhesions and difficult surgical access.

2.3 Gastrointestinal

Any contraindications to TOE must be excluded as it plays a major role in positioning the cannulas and safe conduct of surgery.

2.4 Assessment of Frailty

The boundaries for offering minimal access surgery have been stretched and it is important to assess the frailty of the elderly patients when indicated. We use a Frailty Toolset described by Afilalo et al. [3]. (Hb%, Serum creatinine, Serum albumin and ability to rise from chair) (Fig. 2).

3 Patient Set Up, Positioning and Monitoring

The anaesthetic set up depends on the surgical technique. The surgical approach and technique vary between the surgeons and depending on the procedure performed.

The surgical technique may involve, using cardioplegia delivered by endo balloon or chitwood clamp or beating heart with no cardioplegia. Drainage cannula in the neck may be used routinely by some surgeons especially while establishing the program or for specific surgical procedures involving right side of the heart. A balloon device to occlude the Superior Vena Cava (SVC) can be used in redo procedures. The set up for anaesthesia provision and lines insertion vary depending on the above.

4 Standard Set Up for These Procedures

1. Standard ECG leads and pulse oximetry
2. Large bore peripheral venous access
3. Left upper limb arterial line
4. Intubation with a single lumen endotracheal tube, followed by positioning of a bronchial blocker into the right main bronchus under bronchoscopic view. The merits of bronchial blocker versus double lumen tube are discussed below.
5. A central venous cannula placed in the right internal jugular vein (IJV). A pulmonary artery (PA) catheter introducer may also be placed in the right internal jugular vein for

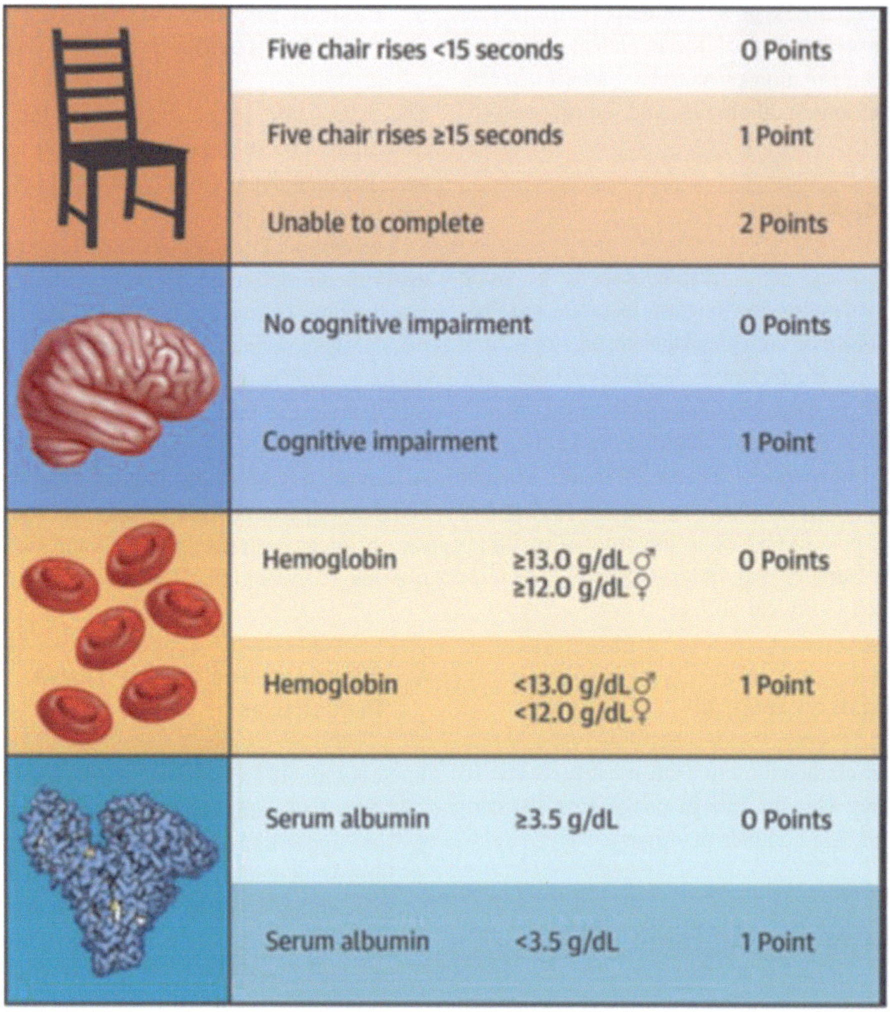

EFT Score	1-Year Mortality	
	TAVR	SAVR
0-1	6%	3%
2	15%	7%
3	28%	16%
4	30%	38%
5	65%	50%

Fig. 2 Frailty Toolset described by Afilalo

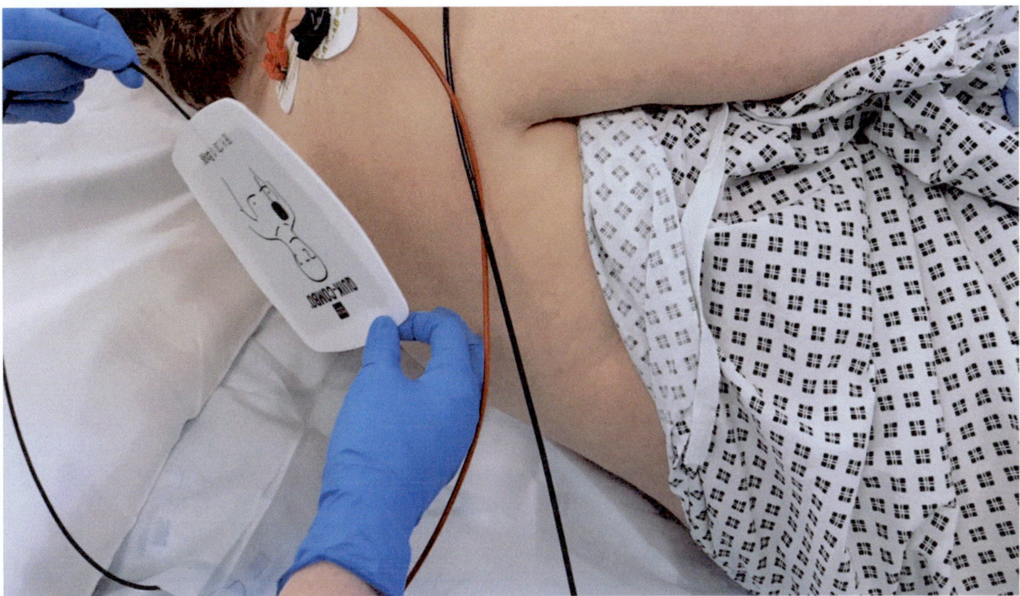

Video 1 Application of external defibrillation pads (▶ https://doi.org/10.1007/000-a6w)

additional wide bore venous access or if insertion of pulmonary artery catheter is required. This cannulation may be combined with the insertion of a venous drainage cannula as discussed below.

6. Transoesophageal echocardiography probe
7. Cerebral oximetry sensors applied across the frontal bones with BIS sensor.
8. Nasopharyngeal temperature probe to facilitate rewarming.
9. External defibrillation pads attached to the right posterior and left lateral chest walls (Video 1).

5 Additional Set Up in Specific Cases

5.1 Use of Endo Balloon

a. Right upper limb arterial line if endo balloon is used. Comparison of the two arterial lines will demonstrate whether distal migration of the balloon to the level of the innominate artery has occurred. The drop in pressure in right arterial line compared to the left is clearly seen when the traces are displayed together on the monitor.

b. Additional pressure monitoring line to monitor the pressures in femoral arterial cannula and tip of the endo balloon. It is required to monitor the arterial pressure initially from the femoral bypass cannula and then from the tip of an endo balloon. On balloon inflation the proximal aortic pressure will be seen to fall from the level of retrograde arterial bypass pressure at the point of complete aortic occlusion

c. Urinary catheter with temperature probe. Patient cooling may be prolonged due to the longer length of procedures, especially in the early phase of surgical programs. Urinary temperature facilitates the correct rate of rewarming when combined with a nasopharyngeal temperature probe (Fig. 4).

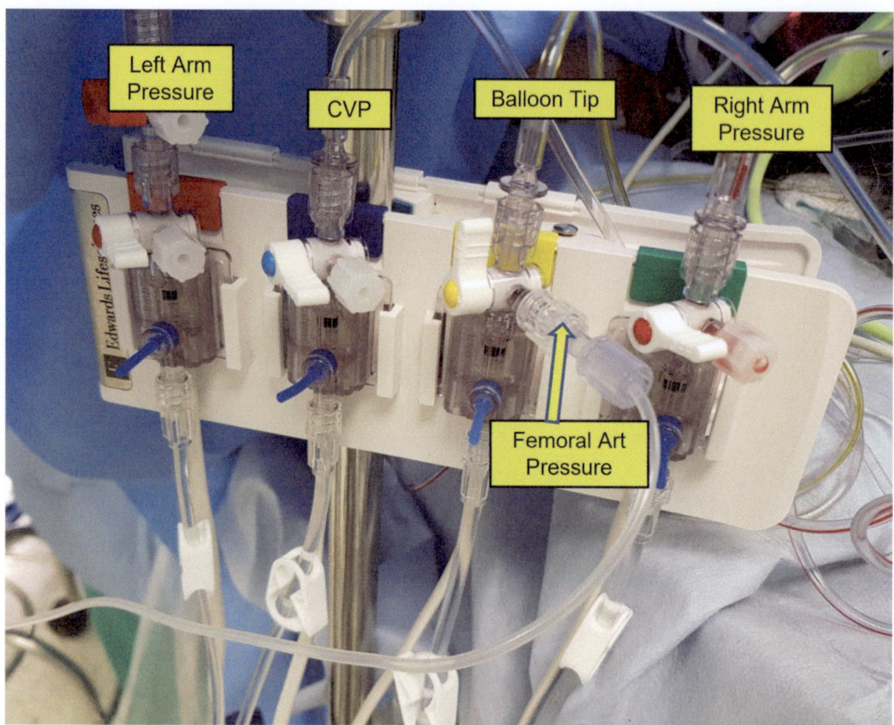

Fig. 3 Pressure monitoring transducers

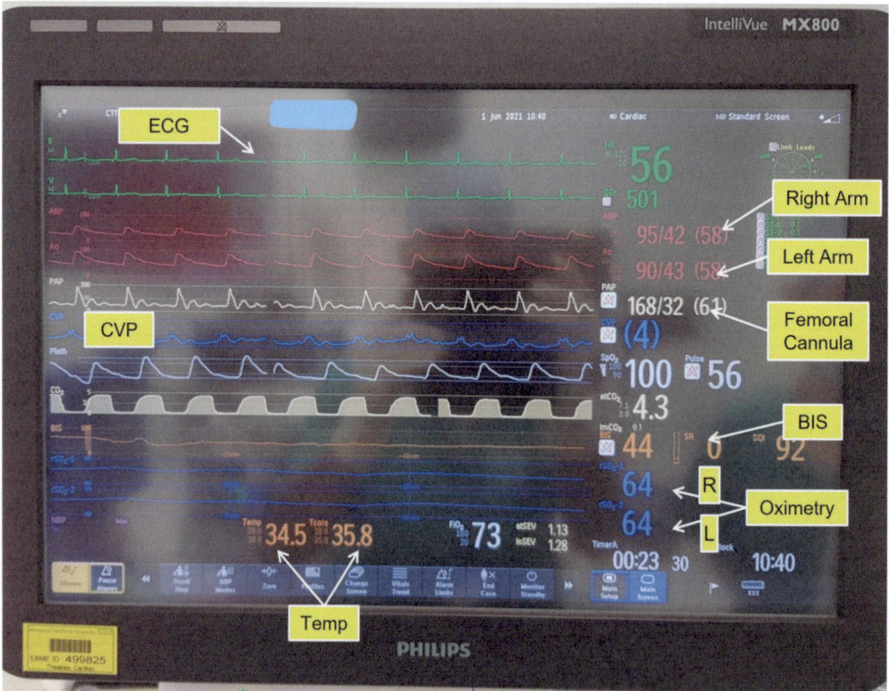

Fig. 4 Anaesthetic monitor pre-cardiopulmonary ypass

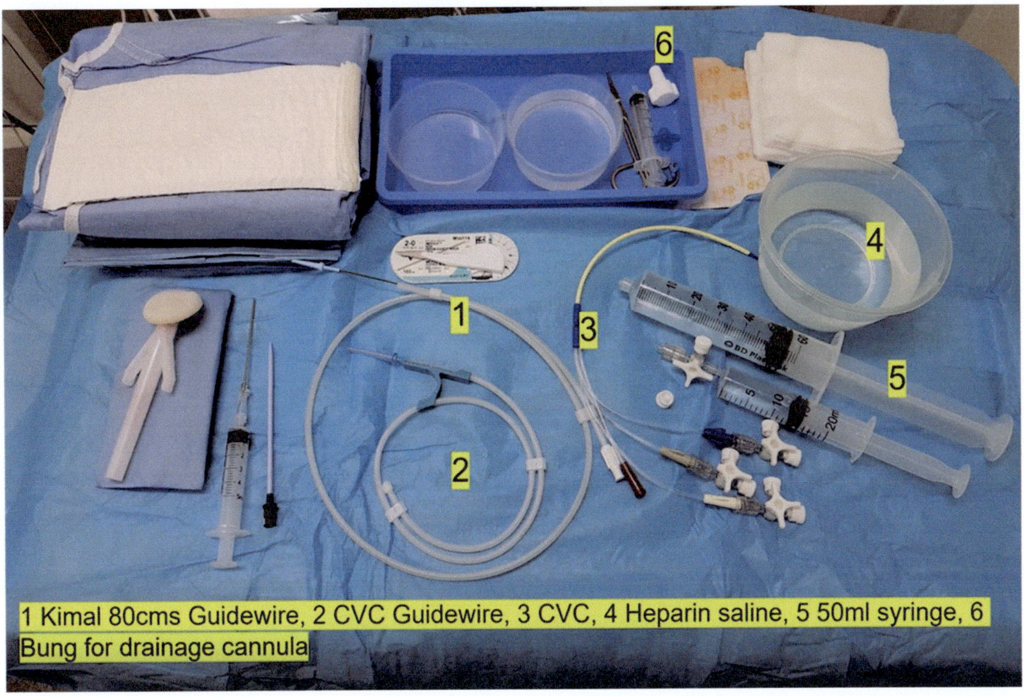

Video 2 Set up for insertion of CVC and SVC drainage cannula (▶ https://doi.org/10.1007/000-a6r)

5.2 Right Heart Procedures

a. Drainage cannula of appropriate size added to the right IJV cannula setup. This may be used sometimes in left heart procedures to facilitate venous drainage in patients who are over approximately 75–80 kgs (Video 2).

5.3 Redo Procedures

a. Either two drainage cannulae used separately or large drainage cannula (21Fr) is used with an Edwards Intraclude introducer with a Y connection. This is to facilitate insertion of Fogarty catheter for SVC isolation. (Video 3).

b. Pacing PA catheter insertion guided by TOE to facilitate pacing postoperatively.

6 Induction of Anaesthesia

The key points to consider at induction of anaesthesia are the presence of impaired ventricular performance, the increased drug circulation time in the presence of valvular lesions or

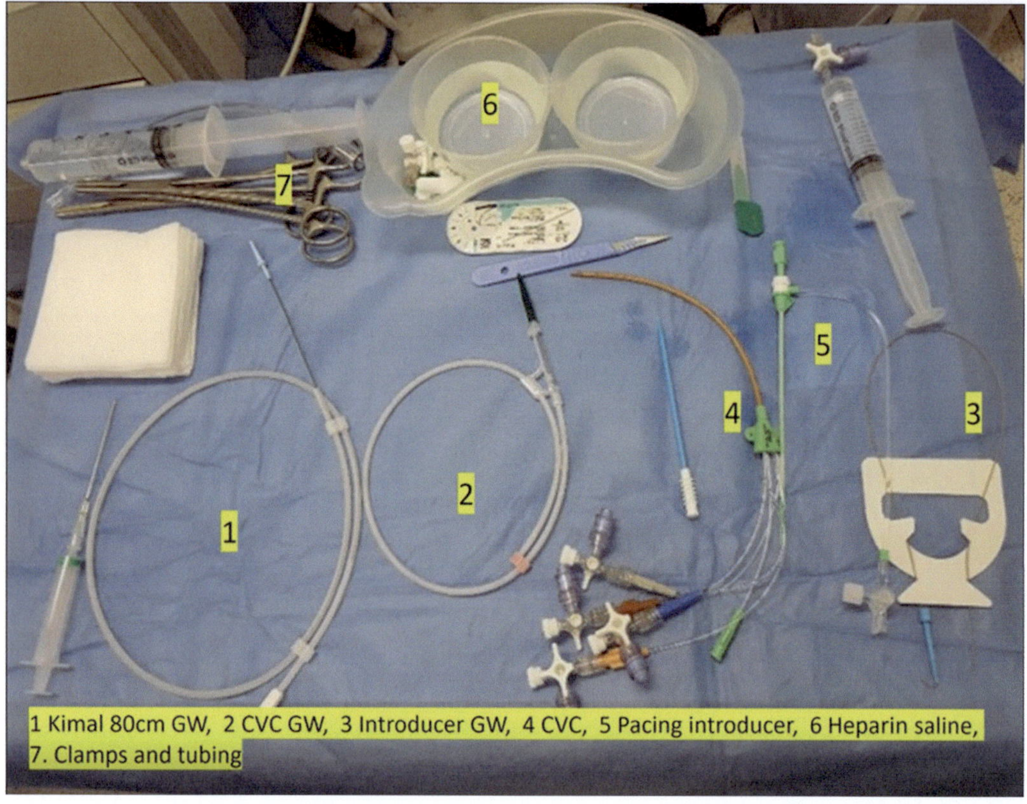

Video 3 Set up for insertion of CVC, SVC drainage cannula and Pacing PA catheter introducer
(▶ https://doi.org/10.1007/000-a72)

arrythmias and the requirement to keep the oesophagus and stomach free of gas to facilitate TOE views. There must be thorough preoxygenation, caution in the speed of delivery of the induction agents, meticulous technique in hand ventilation to prevent air entry into the oesophagus and intubation once complete muscle relaxation has been achieved to prevent coughing and interruption in venous return.

7 Intubation—Single Lumen Tube (SLT) Plus Bronchial Blocker (BB) Versus Double Lumen Tube (DLT)

The use of either a double lumen tube or bronchial blocker to facilitate single lung ventilation to allow access via a thoracic incision has been debated in both cardiac and thoracic anaesthesia [4, 5]. Whilst either technique is valid it is the authors' preference to use a single lumen tube together with bronchial blocker. This is based on

1. Less compression at glottic opening with SLT plus TOE probe compared to DLT and probe.
2. No need for tube change at end of procedure with SLT.

The results of the trial by Knoll et al. show that the risk for airway complications may increase when using a DLT instead of a BB to achieve one-lung ventilation [4]. The intubation performed with video laryngoscopy will aid in minimising and identifying injury to glottis (Videos 4 and 5). The insertion of BB is performed under vision using flexible bronchoscopy to avoid the tip getting caught in the Murphy's

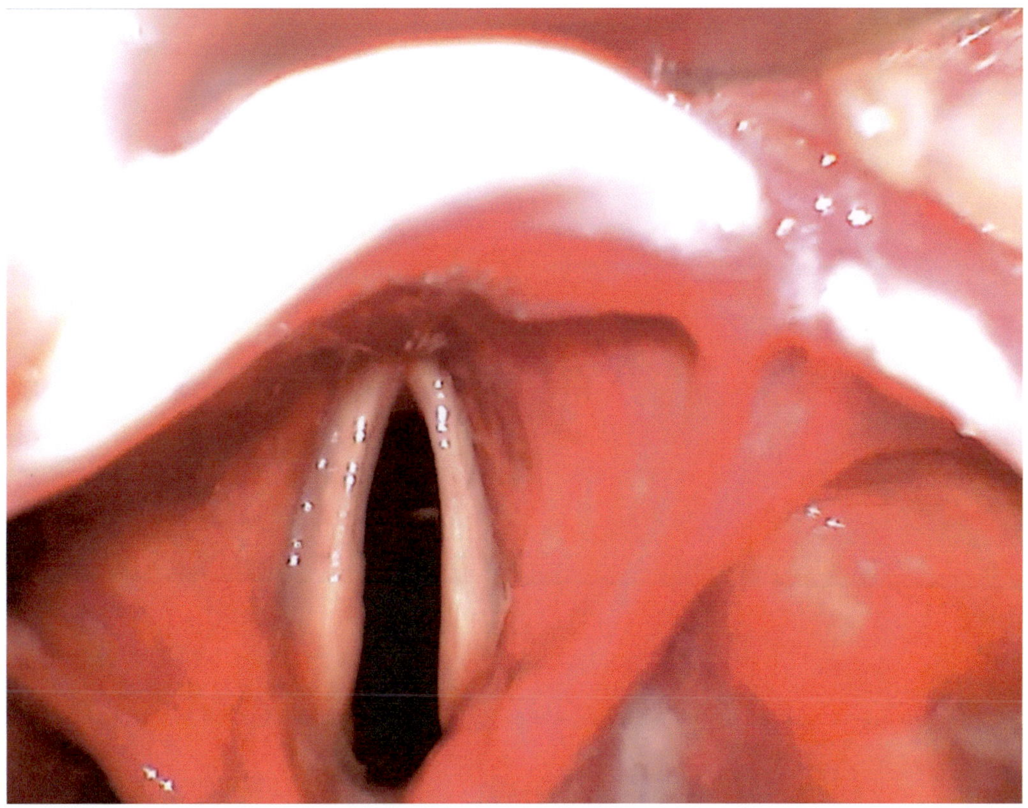

Video 4 Video Laryngoscopy (▶ https://doi.org/10.1007/000-a6x)

eye and broken. If DLT is used, its position in left main bronchus is confirmed using flexible bronchoscopy.

8 Cerebral Oximetry

The use of cerebral oximetry in cardiac surgery has been much debated and usually in relation to post-operative cognitive dysfunction [6, 7]. However in endoscopic cardiac surgery it is a vital monitor

a. To confirm the adequacy of venous drainage with or without neck cannula,
b. A marker of perfusion with retrograde peripheral bypass and
c. An adjunct to the two arterial lines system of monitoring the position of an endo balloon (intra aortic occlusion balloon).

The right arm pressure and right cerebral oximetry are set to display above the respective left side measurements for standardisation and ease of visual identification during placement of endo balloon.

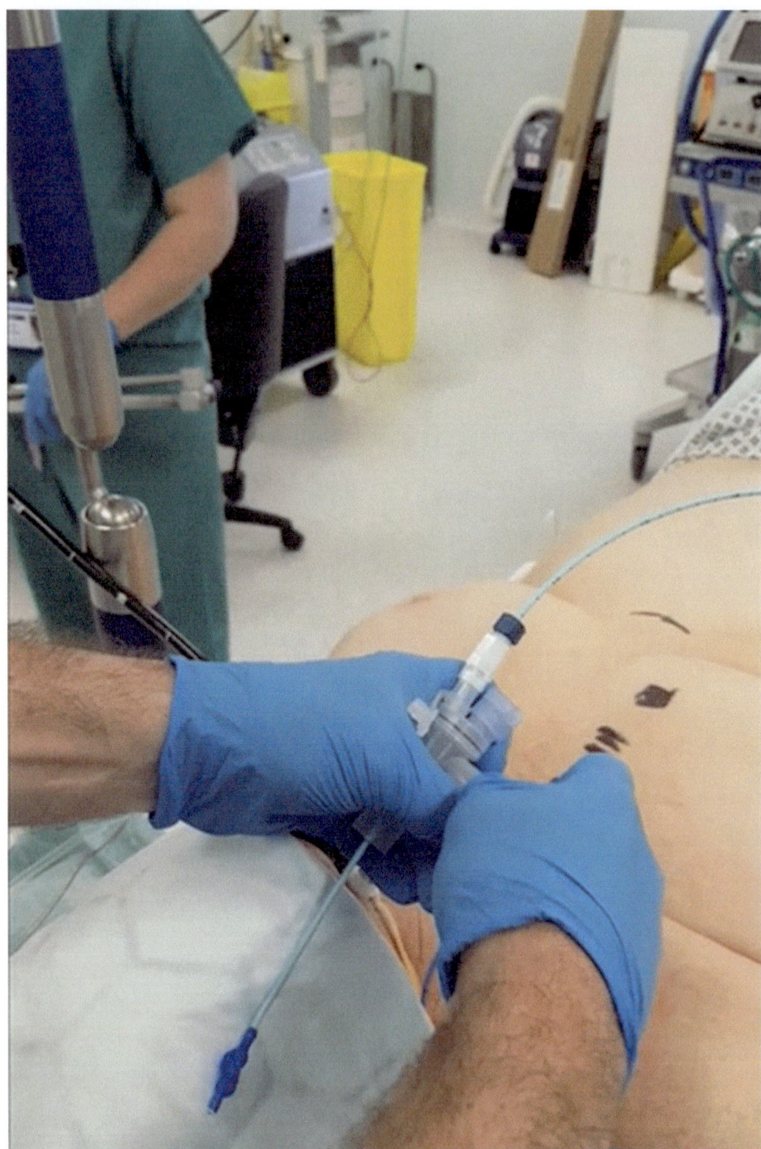

Video 5 Insertion of bronchial blocker (▶ https://doi.org/10.1007/000-a6p)

9 Transoesophageal Echocardiography

After induction of anaesthesia, TOE is performed and reviewed. This serves us a final check and confirmation to rule out echocardiographic contraindications to perform aspects of minimal access surgery. These include, significant aortic valve regurgitation, ascending aorta diameter more than 4cms, significant and/or mobile atheroma in descending and/or ascending thoracic aorta and complicated mitral valve disease. The details of TOE are discussed elsewhere (Chap. 3).

Guidelines for performing a comprehensive echocardiographic examination is described by Hahn et al. [8]. A thorough step wise initial assessment based on standard views is mandatory followed by dynamic monitoring of line insertion, establishment of cardiopulmonary bypass (CPB), intra aortic occlusion balloon positioning, cardioplegia delivery, de-airing and separation from bypass and the assessment of the specific surgery, ventricular performance and aortic integrity.

10 Jugular Vein Cannulation

Additional venous drainage may be required via the SVC. In our practice this is utilised in patients over 75–80 kg or in those undergoing right heart surgery. Following a perfusion strategy discussion, a 15F, 17F or 19F cannula (Medtronic Biomedicus) is inserted via a percutaneous technique (Videos 6, 7 and 8). Cannulation is performed under TOE guidance. The TOE probe and machine are set up so that the anaesthetist can perform the cannulation with minimal additional help.

It is the authors' preference to insert this cannula alongside a central line into the right IJV thereby avoiding the, albeit rare complication of vascular injury on the left side when one lung (left) ventilation is to be utilised. The case of a persistent left superior vena cava may be an exception to this rule.

The procedure commences with ultrasound examination of the internal jugular vein to ensure adequacy of calibre to accommodate the number and size of cannulae required for the case which is generally more than 1 cm in diameter. A Kimal 80 cm Guide wire insertion (Fig. 5) is performed under ultrasound guidance and then correct passage into the SVC confirmed on TOE. Prior to cannula insertion a dose of 5000u heparin is administered.

In left side heart surgery, the tip of the cannula is positioned at the junction of the right atrium and SVC. In right side surgery the cannula is withdrawn into the SVC to allow for snaring of the vena cava. In the case of re-do surgery a Fogarty balloon is used to achieve caval occlusion instead of an external venous snare. Positioning of the cannula is confirmed by TOE.

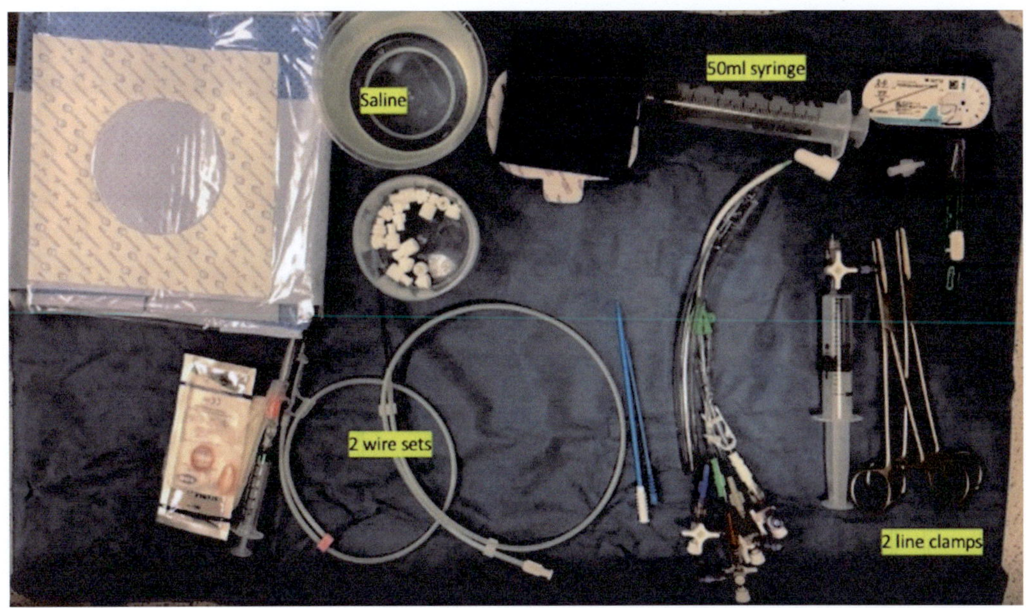

Video 6 SVC cannulation 1 (▶ https://doi.org/10.1007/000-a6s)

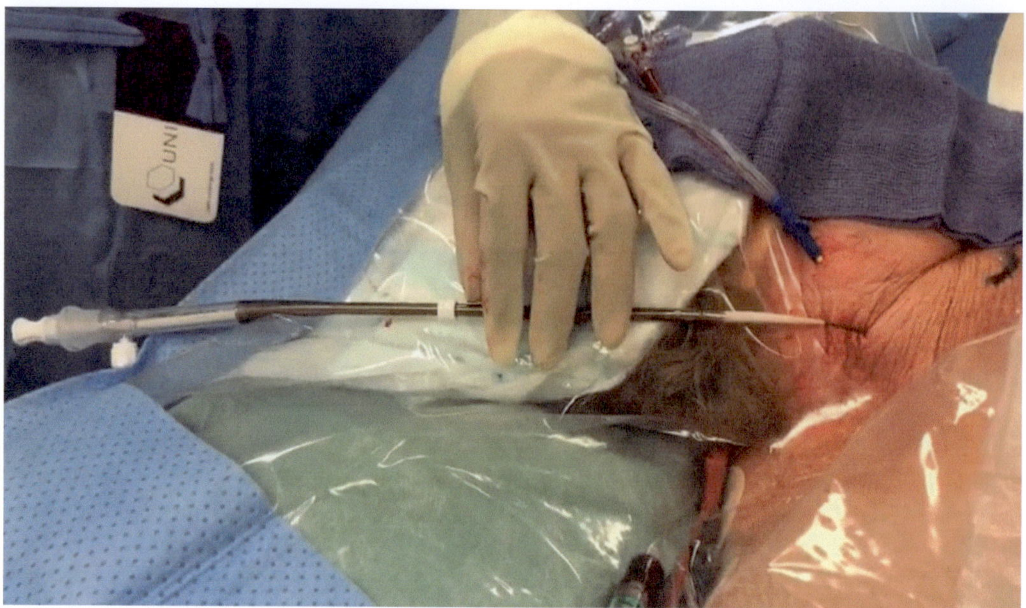

Video 7 SVC cannulation 2 (▶ https://doi.org/10.1007/000-a6m)

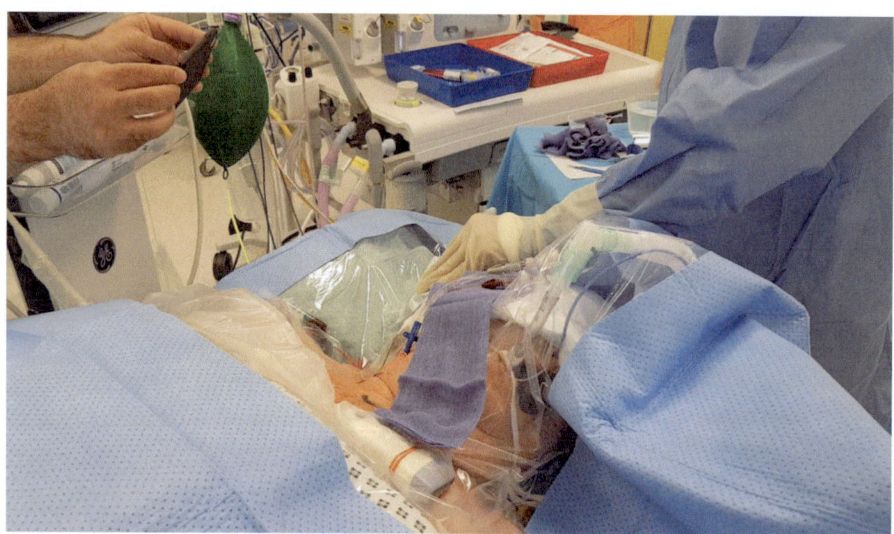

Video 8 SVC cannulation 3 (▶ https://doi.org/10.1007/000-a6n)

11 Jugular Vein Cannulation in Redo Right Heart Surgery

In redo surgery ability of to snare the vena cava to facilitate right heart surgery may be lost due to tissue adhesions. In order to prevent air entering the venous drainage cannula and to create a bloodless field it is our strategy in such cases to occlude the SVC opening by means of a Fogarty balloon inserted via a cannula in the right IJV [9]. The inferior caval opening is occluded by surgical swabs placed under vision.

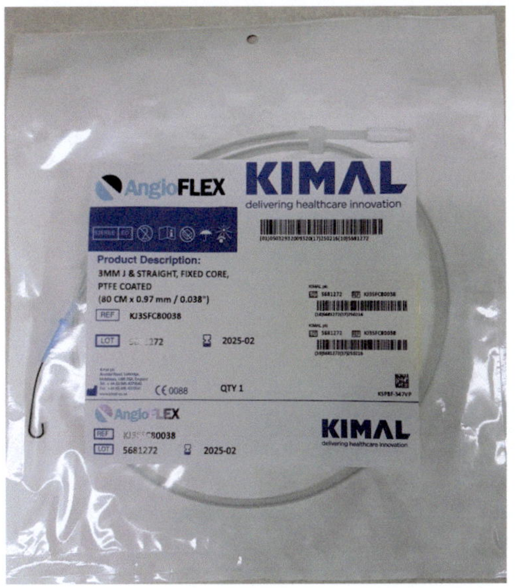

Fig. 5 Kimal 80 cm guidewire

An 8F Fogarty balloon is inserted via a haemostatic valve in Edwards Intraclude introducer attached to a 19F or 21 Fr Medtronic Biomedicus cannula (Video 9). This is inserted either alongside a separate venous drainage cannula (Fig. 6) or through a Y introducer as previously described (Fig. 7). In such cases there is dilatation of the right heart due to tricuspid regurgitation which leads to an enlarged SVC which allows sufficient calibre for multiple cannulae insertion. Adequacy of venous drainage is confirmed by the perfusionist together with adequacy of cerebral oximetry.

A pacing catheter introducer is also inserted in most redo cases in view of anticipated difficulties in placing epicardial pacing wires because of right ventricular adhesions to chest wall (Fig. 8).

12 Patient Positioning

The patient is placed supine upon the operating table with an inflatable bag under the right side of the chest (Video 10). On inflation of the bag care must be taken to support the head and neck in a neutral position, particularly in the elderly, with a head ring and padding (Fig. 9). The arms are placed at the side of the patient with padding to protect the ulnar nerve at the elbow. The right arm may require to be placed away from the body in order to facilitate surgical access (Video 11).

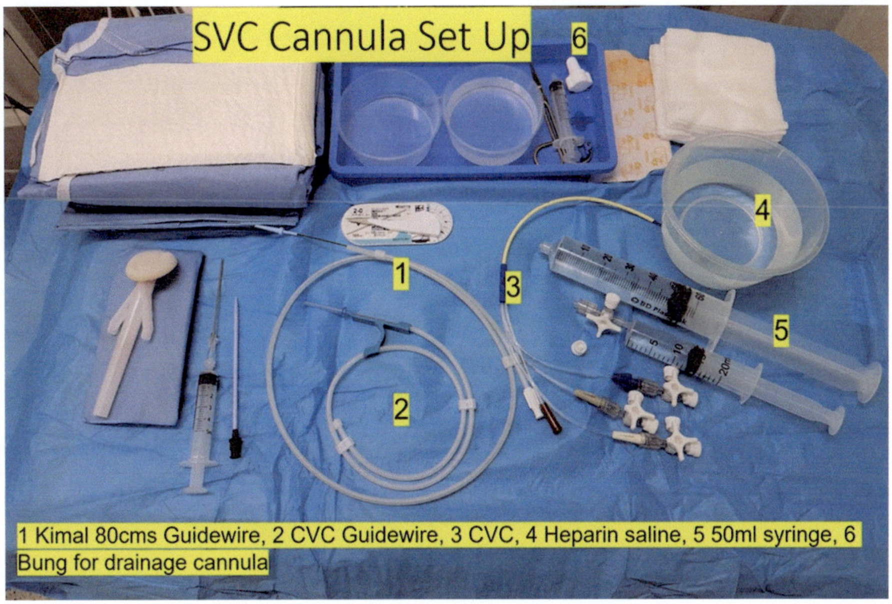

Video 9 SVC cannulation in re-do surgery (▶ https://doi.org/10.1007/000-a6t)

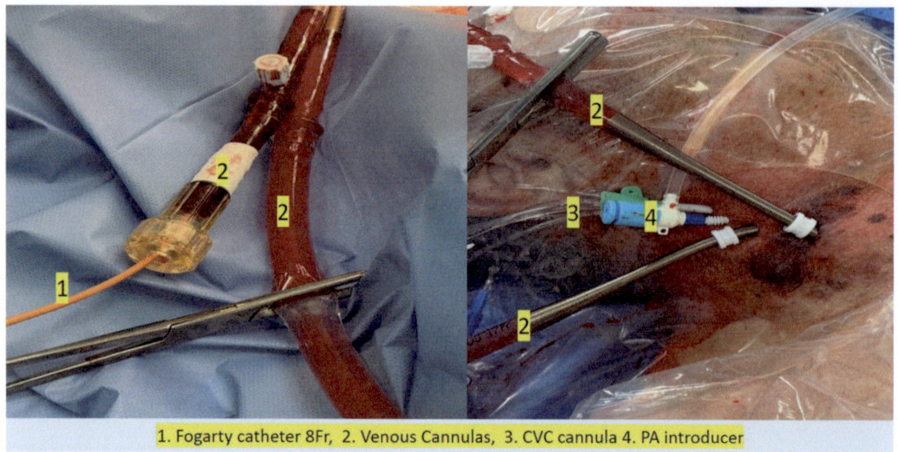

Fig. 6 Fogarty balloon catheter inserted via Edwards Intraclude introducer and separate venous drainage catheter

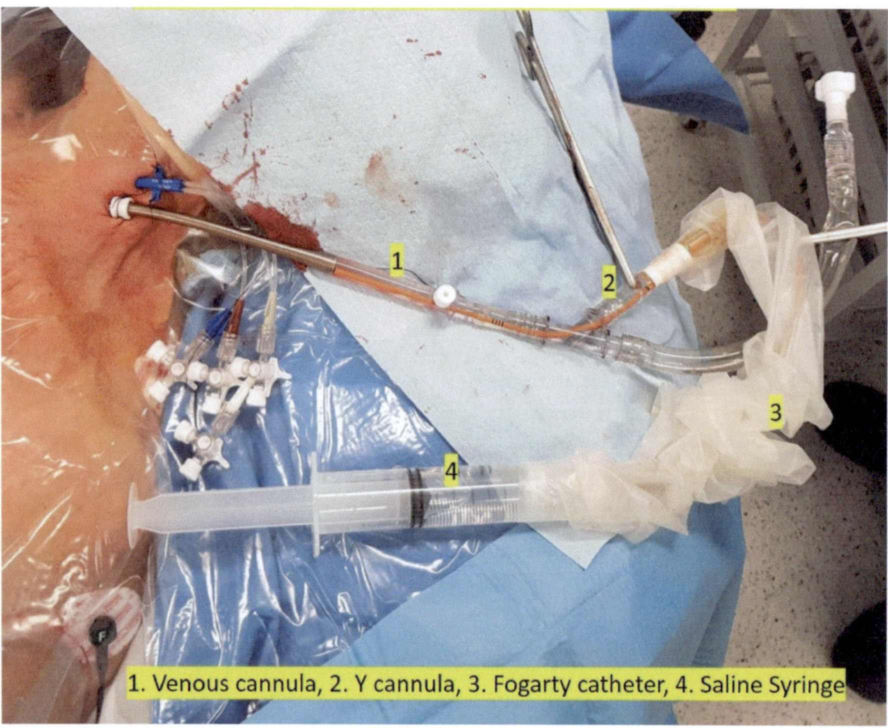

Fig. 7 Fogarty balloon inserted via Y-piece and via single 21Fr venous drainage catheter

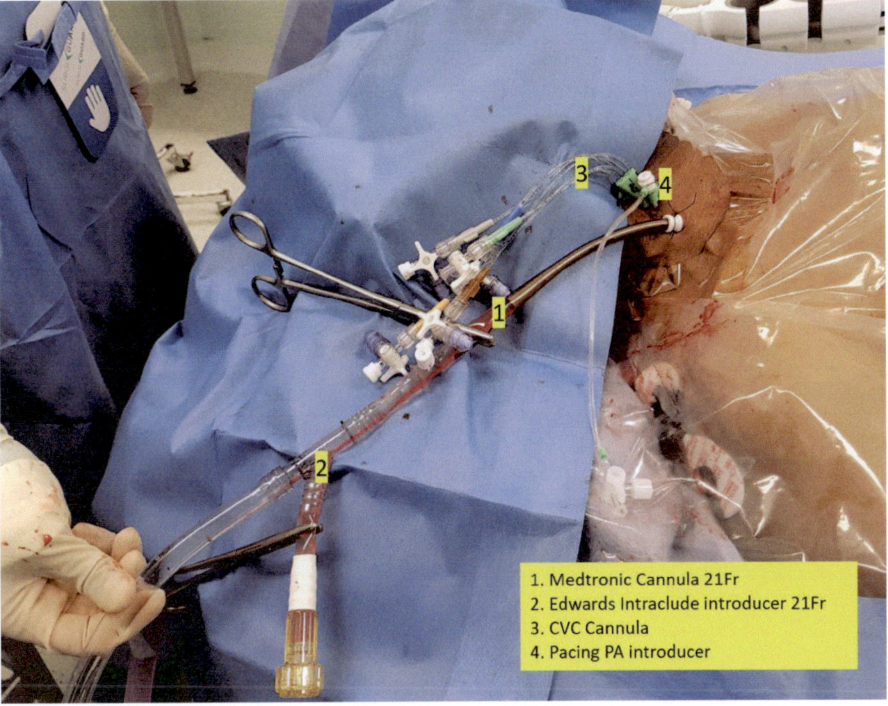

Fig. 8 CVC, Pacing PA introducer and 21Fr SVC drainage cannula with Y-piece

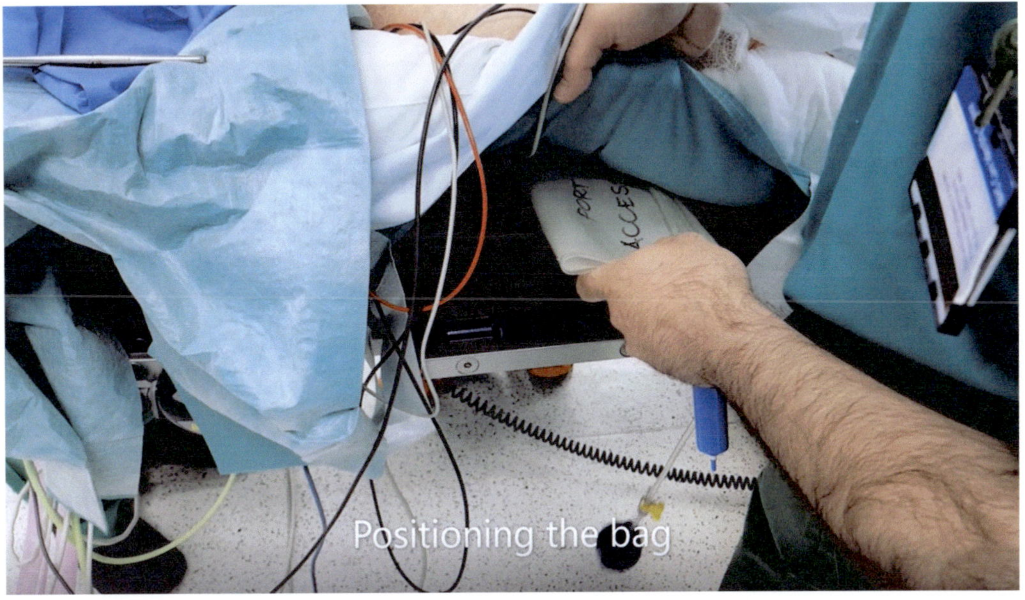

Video 10 Positioning inflatable bag under right chest (▶ https://doi.org/10.1007/000-a73)

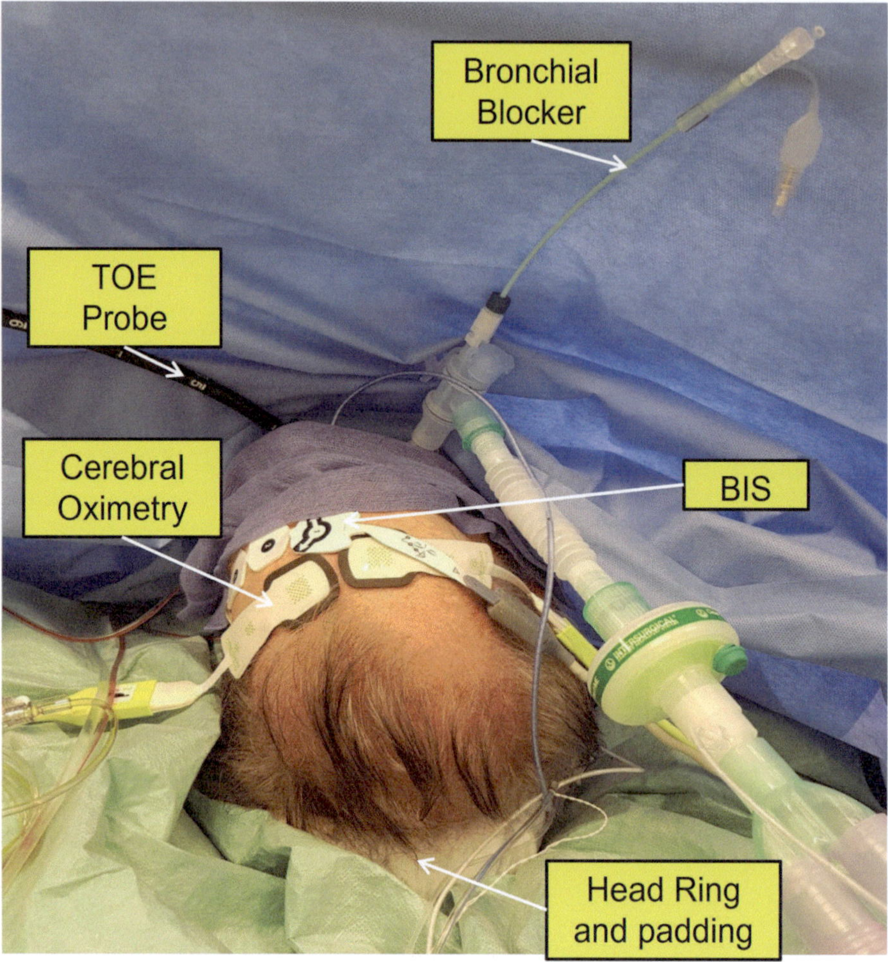

Fig. 9 Head ring and padding for support following right chest bag inflation

The defibrillator pads should be connected and checked whether they are working by obtaining ECG trace from paddles and the default current setting (Fig. 10).

13 Start of Surgery

After timeout to go through routine pre incision checks, usually a groin is opened first to assess vascular access. If additional surgical expertise is present, both groin and chest may be opened at the same time. Additional analgesia may be required in the form of intravenous opioids. The authors prefer ventilating patients on pressure controlled ventilation on 100% O2 to facilitate lung collapse during chest opening (Fig. 11). Inspiratory pressures are adjusted to achieve adequate tidal volumes. Pre bypass blood tests usually include arterial blood gases, near patient clotting tests such as INR, thromboelastography or platelet function test as appropriate. The authors also use HMS Plus haemostasis management system (Medtronic) for heparin and protamine dosing.

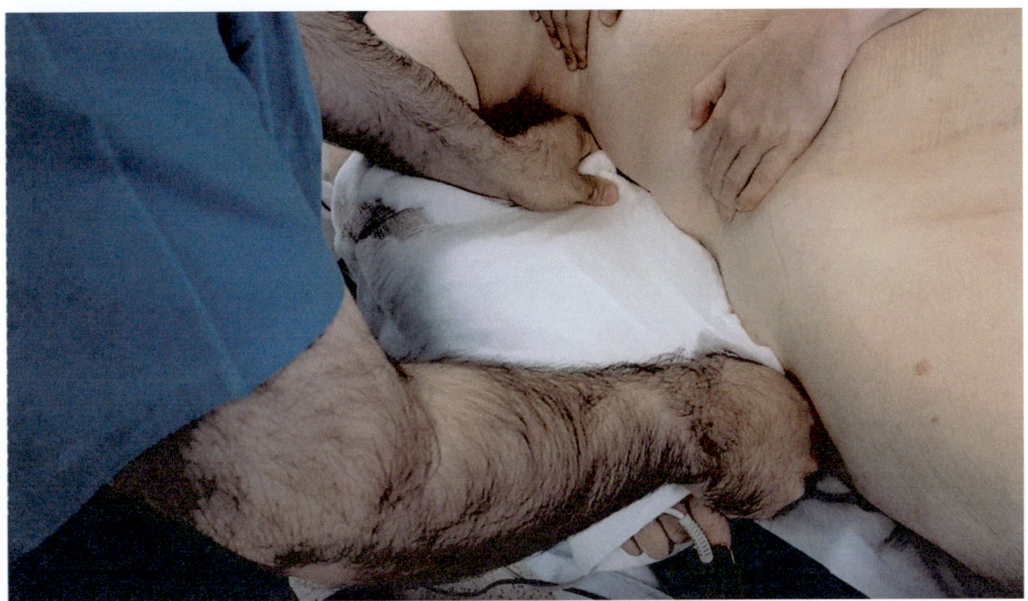

Video 11 Positioning of right arm away from the trunk (▶ https://doi.org/10.1007/000-a71)

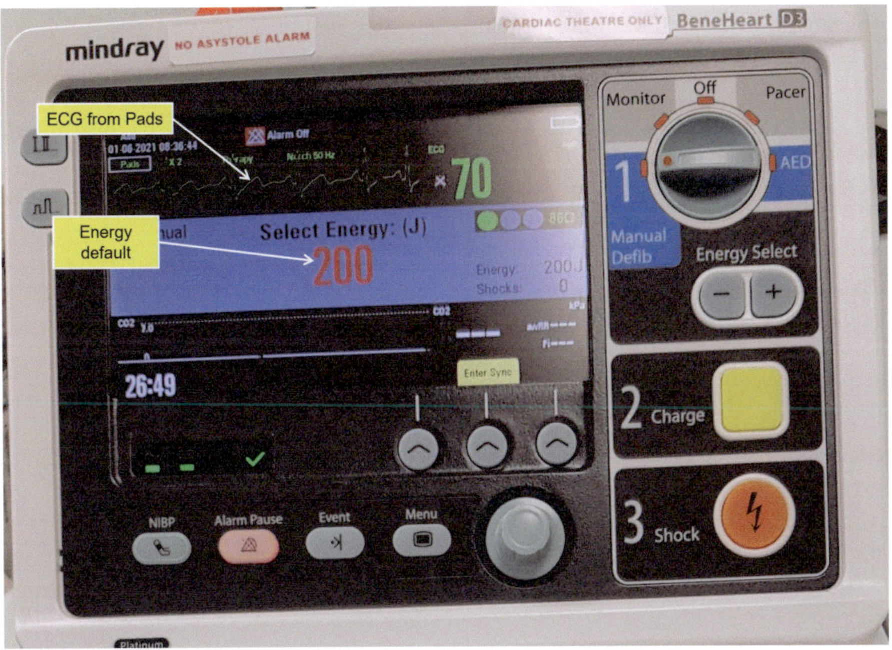

Fig. 10 Display from external defibrillation pads

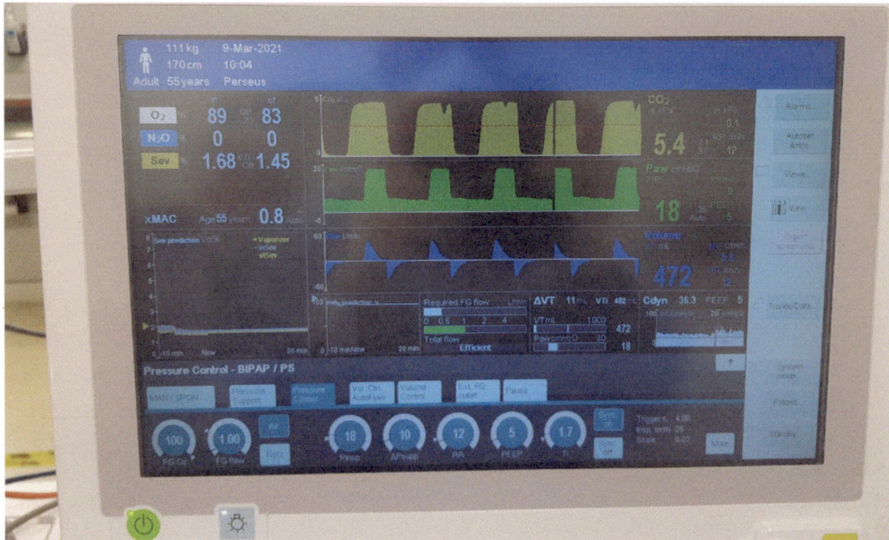

Fig. 11 Ventilatory settings prior to one-lung ventilation

One lung ventilation should be initiated prior to chest opening. While no special technique is required when DLT is used, additional steps as described by Yoo et al. are required with BB [9].

14 One Lung Ventilation with Use of Bronchial Blocker

1. Confirmation of anatomy in lower trachea, showing RUL bronchus
2. BB balloon inflated in right main bronchus

To achieve good lung deflation the following steps are used (Video 12) [10]
1. Ventilation of both lungs with 100% oxygen prior to balloon inflation
2. The ventilator is stopped and expiratory valve is fully open allowing time for the End tidal CO2 (EtCO2) trace to disappear indicating complete exhalation of gases.
3. The balloon is inflated in the right main bronchus under direct vision with bronchoscope.

4. If the lung collapse is found to be unsatisfactory upon chest opening, the steps are repeated.
5. To repeat the steps, once the chest cavity is open the ventilator should be stopped, the balloon deflated and SLT disconnected from the circuit to allow raid deflation of the right lung which can be observed via the camera to display satisfactory collapse
6. The balloon is the reinflated under vision in the right main bronchus, circuit reconnected and single lung ventilation commenced with FiO2 adjusted as required.

15 Prebypass Management

Heparin is administered prior to placement of peripheral cannulas. Once the activated clotting time (ACT) of 480 s is achieved indicating full anticoagulation, the peripheral cannulas are placed in femoral vessels for bypass under TOE guidance. The venous cannula is inserted first followed by arterial cannula. The pressure in the

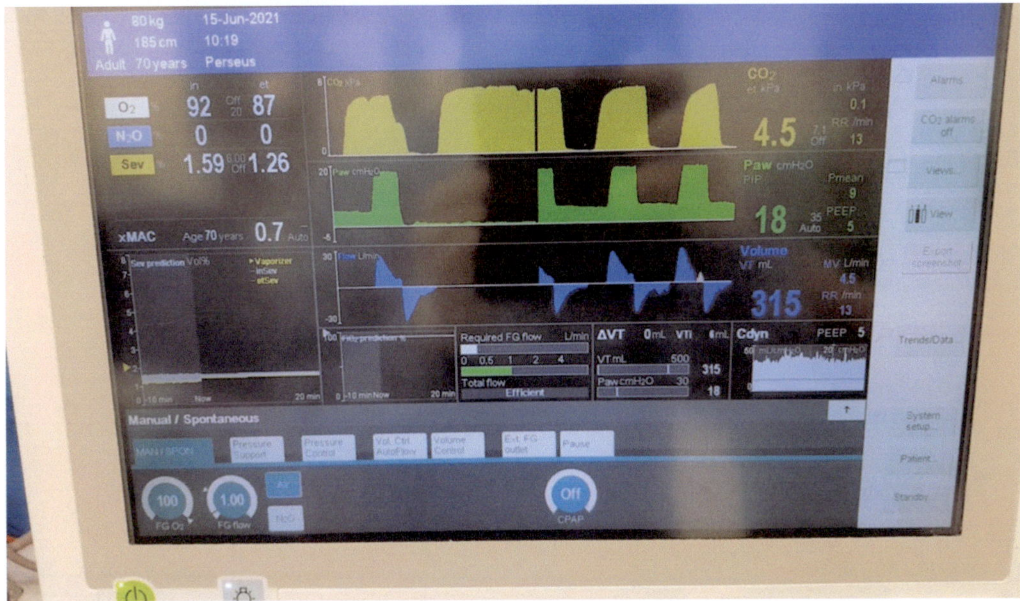

Video 12 Inflation of bronchial blocker (▶ https://doi.org/10.1007/000-a6y)

arterial cannula is measured through a transducer. Good trace and mean pressure in line with arm pressures will indicate good position of femoral arterial cannula (Fig. 12).

Following this the endo balloon and guide wire will be inserted through the y connection in the arterial cannula under TOE guidance. The endo balloon is positioned in the ascending aorta at the level of pulmonary artery. The cardiopulmonary bypass is initiated and descending thoracic aorta is monitored using TOE guidance. Once bypass is established the three arterial wave forms (Left arm, Right arm and Femoral) should read similar mean arterial pressures (Fig. 13).

16 Cardioplegia Delivery

The ascending aorta is clamped using either the endo balloon or chitwood clamp. In some cases, beating heart technique is employed. In these cases, Esmolol is used as a bolus of 0.5 mg/kg followed by an infusion of 100mcg/kg/hr and adjusted accordingly to maintain bradycardia. This is stopped at the time of rewarming.

Chitwood clamp is used in a similar fashion to aortic cross clamp.

When the endo balloon is used as a method for cardioplegia the following steps are observed. Communication between the surgeon, anaesthetist, perfusionist and the scrub staff is paramount at this stage to maintain safety and achieve best results (Video 13).

1. The tip of the endo balloon is connected to the pressure transducer that is used to monitor the femoral pressure through a manometer line. This will read similar mean pressures as arm pressures.

2. The balloon is then inflated with 'n' mls of saline (where n was the measured aortic diameter in mm). During inflation of the balloon there is a potential movement of the balloon distally blocking right innominate artery. This will be identified by fall in right arm pressure followed by right cerebral saturation after a delay.

3. When the balloon is nearly inflated to the size of ascending aorta (approximately 15–20mls of saline), adenosine is administered at a dose of 250 µg/kg through the distal lumen of the

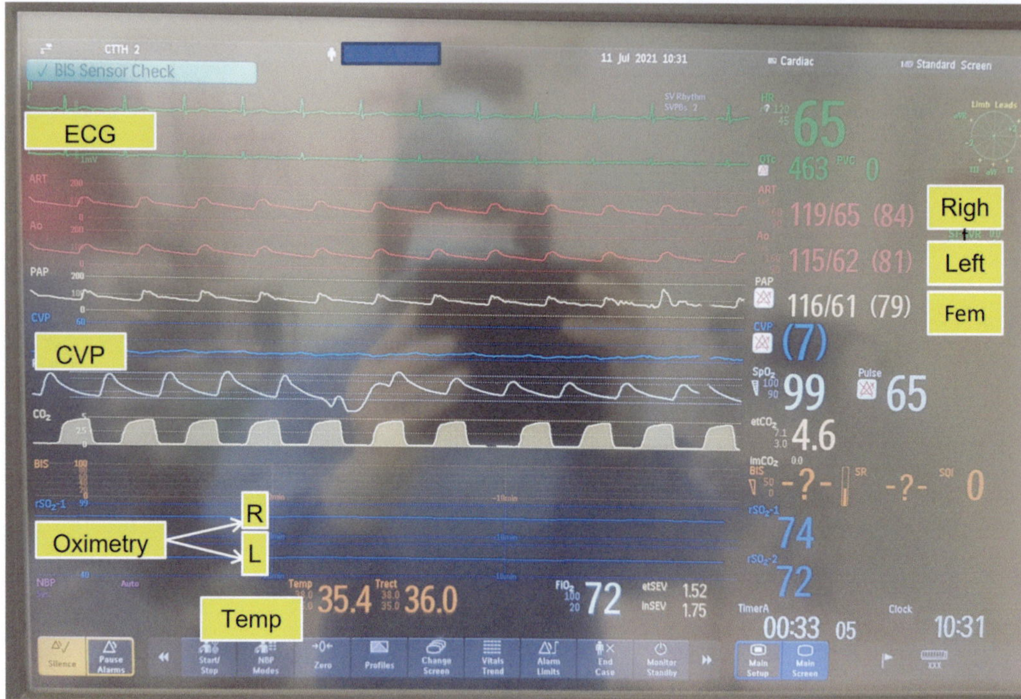

Fig. 12 Pressure traces following insertion of femoral cannula

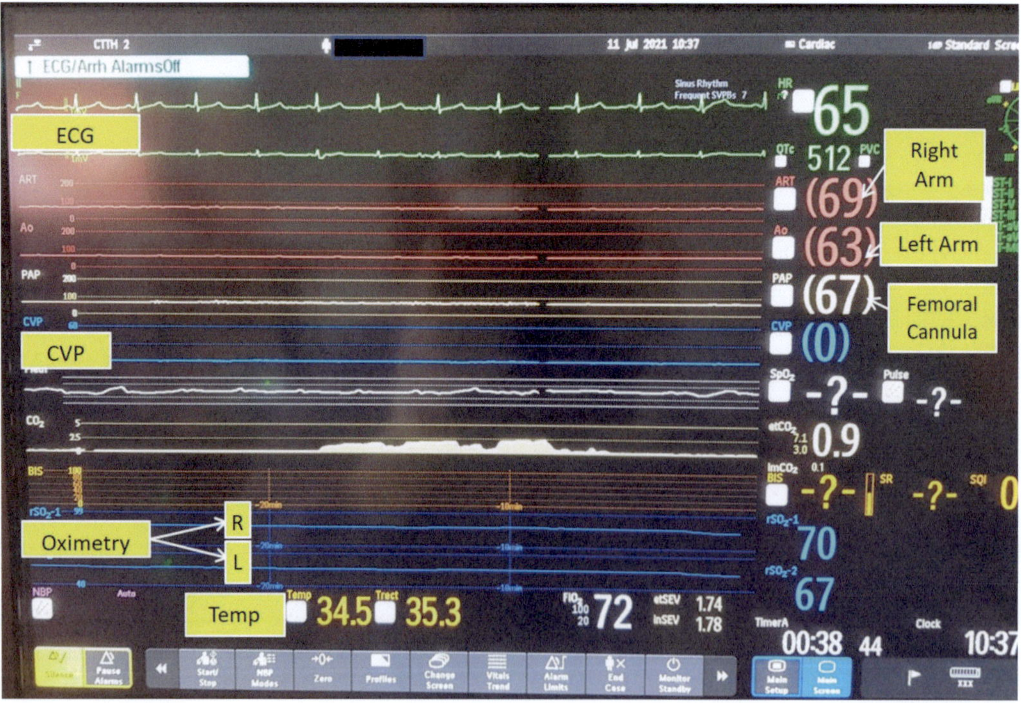

Fig. 13 Pressure traces following onset of cardiopulmonary bypass

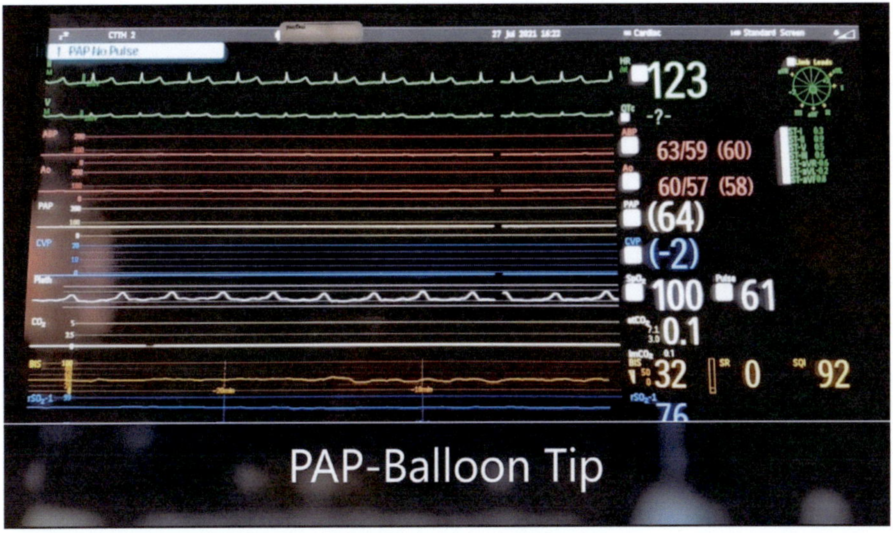

Video 13 Endoclamp balloon inflation (▶ https://doi.org/10.1007/000-a6z)

endo balloon directly into the partially occluded aortic root causing cardiac standstill to allow accurate landing of the balloon. This prevents ventricular ejection and allowing the full balloon inflation to occur without movement of the balloon.

4. When the balloon is inflated to the required diameter, a drop in the pressure of the endo balloon manometry line is seen indicating occlusion of the ascending aorta and isolation from CPB pressure in the distal aorta.

5. Cardioplegia is administered through the balloon which will maintain asystole and facilitate surgery. The balloon tip pressure can be seen to rise during cardioplegia administration.

6. The whole procedure is performed under TOE guidance with monitoring of arm and balloon tip pressures while maintaining good communication.

17   Management During CPB

The management of patients on bypass is similar to sternotomy. Management of anticoagulation, gas exchange, temperature and flows follow the same line as in patients having cardiac procedures with sternotomy. The variations in management include,

1. The patients are filtered on bypass to maintain neutral fluid balance while using crystalloid cardioplegia through endo balloon (Fig. 14).

2. The acid base balance is corrected using Insulin infusions all through CPB and Sodium bicarbonate boluses during rewarming as required.

3. Cerebral oximetry is used as a guide for venous drainage and perfusion in addition to standard monitoring during bypass.

18   Separation from Cardiopulmonary Bypass

1. Endo balloon is deflated under TOE guidance and deairing is performed through the tip of balloon.

2. TOE is used to assess the success of the surgical procedure.

3. Separation from CPB is optimally achieved with the resumption of two lung ventilation rather than single lung ventilation to allow for optimal oxygenation, normocarbia and lower pulmonary vascular resistance. Therefore, surgical haemostasis must be ensured before the view is obscured by complete inflation of the right lung.

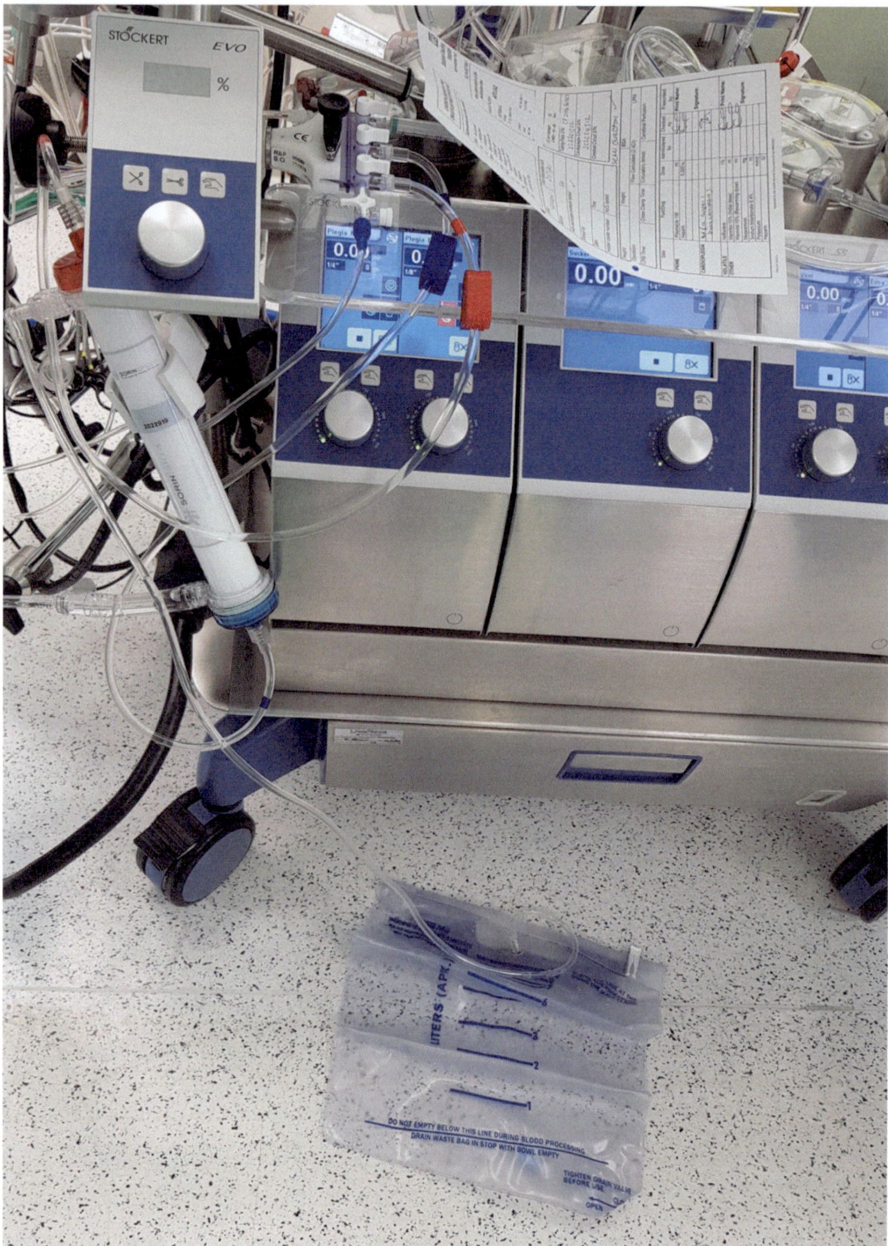

Fig. 14 Haemofilter added to cardiopulmonary bypass circuit

4. The use of TOE on separation from CPB is key in assessing right ventricular performance on resumption of volume loading, the effect of any residual air entering the right coronary artery and subsequently following protamine administration. Left ventricular performance is analysed in the standard way followed by assessment of the surgical procedure.

19 Cerebral Oximetry

The use of cerebral oximetry in cardiac surgery has been much debated and usually in relation to post-operative cognitive dysfunction [7, 8]. However in endoscopic cardiac surgery it is a vital monitor
1. To confirm the adequacy of venous drainage with or without neck cannula,
2. A marker of perfusion with peripheral bypass and
3. An adjunct to the two arterial lines system for monitoring the position of an endo balloon.

The right arm pressure and right cerebral oximetry are set to display above the respective left side measurements for standardisation and ease of visual identification during placement of endo balloon.

20 Removal of Jugular Venous Drainage Cannula

Following the administration of protamine, the cannula is clamped proximal to the side port which is then opened to allow drainage of blood in the lines back to the perfusionist (Video 14). After correcting any coagulation abnormalities, the patient is placed in a slight Trendelenburg position to avoid air embolism and the venous cannula withdrawn (Video 15) using a cannula removal kit

(Fig. 15). Digital pressure is applied for usually up to 10 min. Once haemostasis is achieved, wound closure strips and an occlusive dressing are applied to the insertion site (Video 16).

21 Postoperative Care

These patients are managed postoperatively in the cardiac intensive care in our unit. The postoperative management is similar to sternotomy patients [11] and includes early extubating, analgesia and management of complications.

21.1 Analgesia

Analgesia postoperatively is achieved by multimodal approach. Smaller chest incisions and lack of rib spreading techniques make it easier to control postoperative pain. Paravertebral nerve blocks with continuous infusion through a catheter is an option. After a bolus of 0.25% bupivacaine and placement of catheter an infusion of 0.25% bupivacaine can be used. It is usually performed after induction of anaesthesia and prior to surgical incision (Video https://www.nysora.com/techniques/neuraxial-and-perineuraxial-techniques/thoracic-lumbar-paravertebral-block/). Intercostal nerve blocks after protamine can be performed by surgeons with thoracic experience using up to 30mls of 0.25% bupivacaine with 3–4 mls in each space from 3rd to 8th spaces combined with wound infiltration. Smaller chest incision can make it difficult but on the other hand larger incisions are the ones which would require this. The regional analgesia methods are often supplemented with regular paracetamol and Gabapentin along with opioids as required. In authors experience Gabapentinoids are particularly helpful for pain associated with drains. Prompt drain removal helps in better pain management and mobilisation.

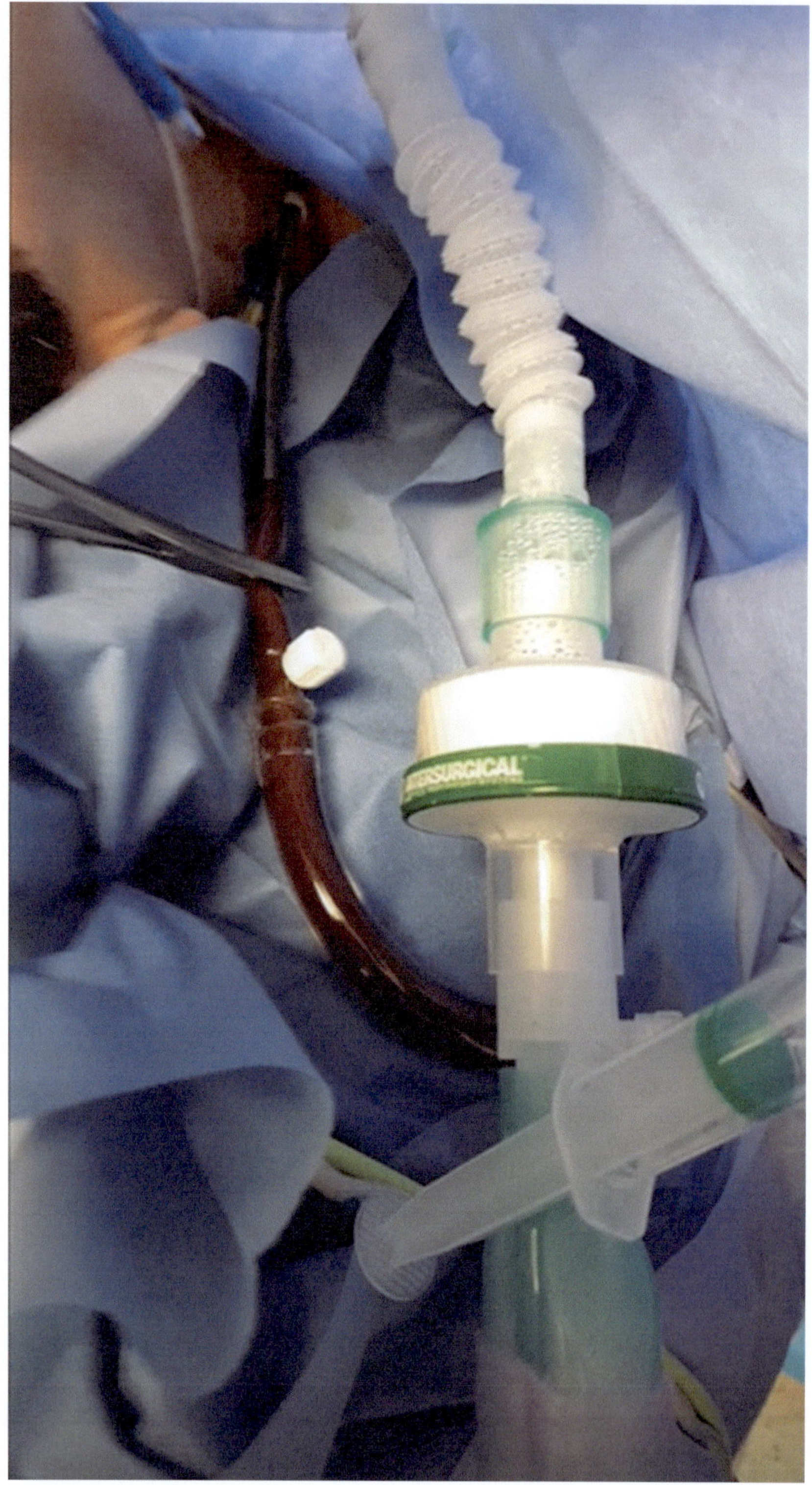

Video 14 Clamping and returning of blood via venous drainage cannula (▶ https://doi.org/10.1007/000-a6q)

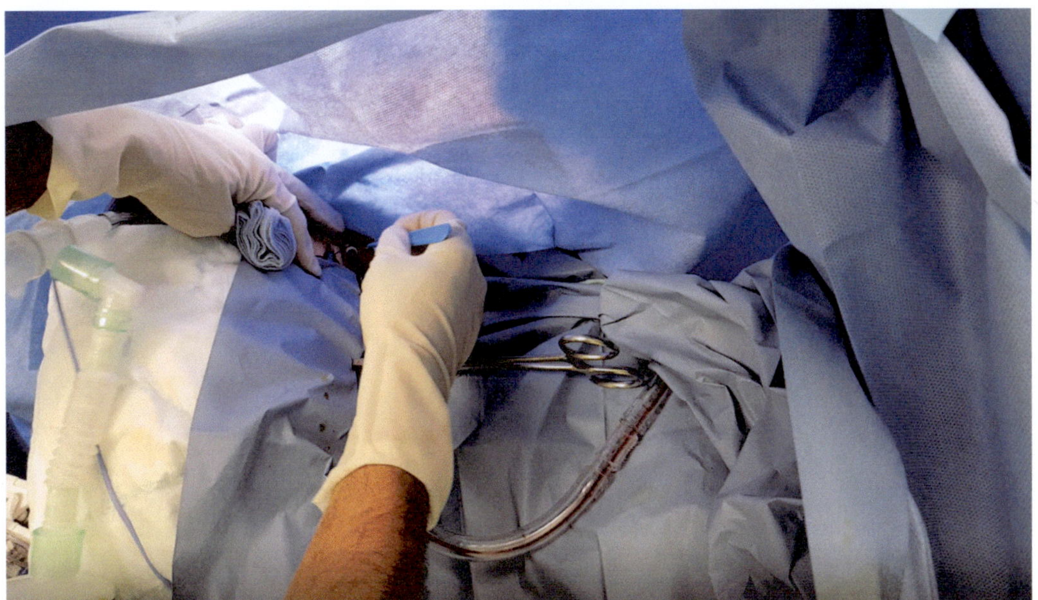

Video 15 Removal of venous drainage cannula (▶ https://doi.org/10.1007/000-a70)

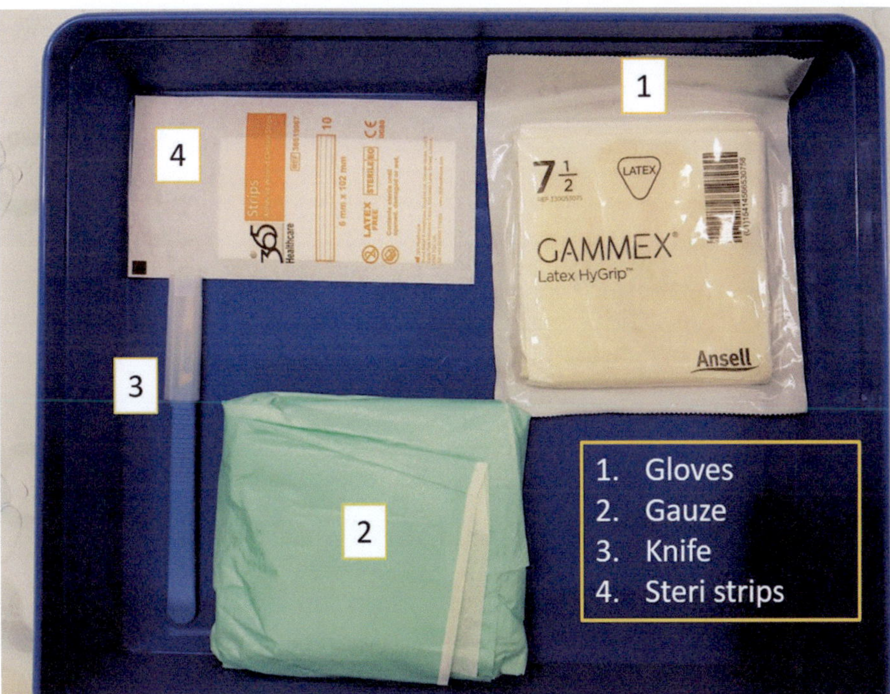

Fig. 15 Venous cannula removal kit

                                                            A. Knowles and P. Saravanan

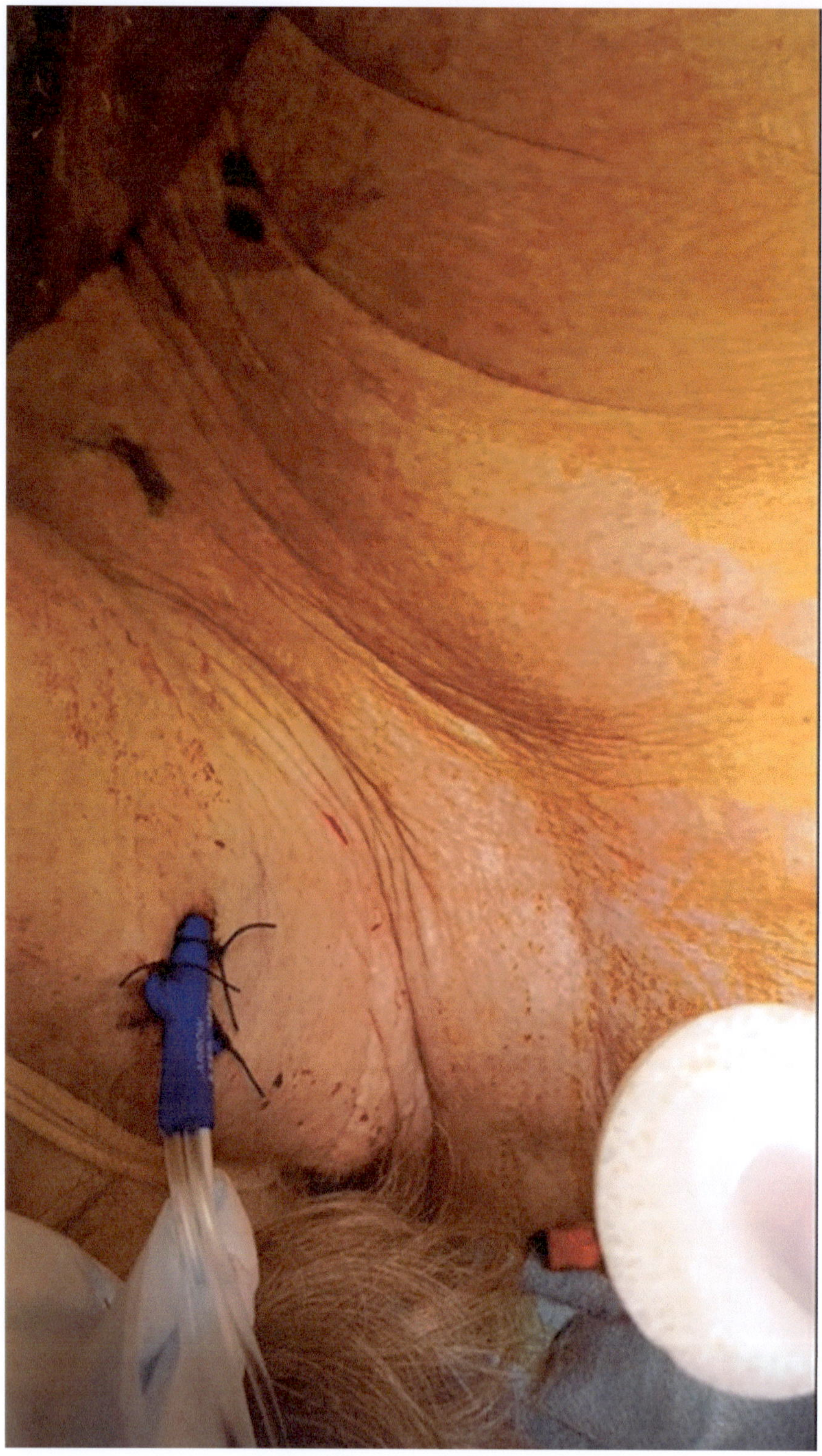

Video 16 Dressing of cannulation site (▶ https://doi.org/10.1007/000-a6v)

22 Pulmonary Oedema

Unilateral pulmonary oedema (UPE) of the unventilated right lung has been reported from centres performing minimal access surgery around the world with an incidence of 0.6 to 20% [11–14]. Bilateral pulmonary oedema is reported as well. The etiology of this problem is unclear. These seem to have occurred more frequently during the initial stages of setting up the program. Various theories have been proposed. COPD, renal dysfunction, prolonged bypass times, transfusion, right ventricular dysfunction and injury to pulmonary veins are some of the causes stipulated and associated mortality can be high. The authors had two incidences of pulmonary oedema both of which recovered by 48 h. There are multiple reports of UPE from UK centres and five patients have needed extra corporeal membrane oxygenation (ECMO) support. A number of measures have been proposed to minimise the risk. These include

1. Choosing surgically straightforward cases at the beginning of the program to minimise bypass times
2. Neck cannula for every patient during the start of the program to improve the drainage and surgical access
3. One lung ventilation strategy with pressure controlled ventilation with the driving pressures of 15cms of water or less.
4. Fluid restrictive strategy intraoperatively with routinely filtering on bypass
5. Use of centrifugal pumps
6. Use of steroids perioperatively

Treatment includes lung protective ventilation, identifying and treating potential surgical causes, steroids and ECMO if ventilatory support fails.

22.1 Bleeding and Re-exploration

Bleeding is usually less common after minimal access procedure. Use of endoballoon and avoiding incision on aorta are some of the proposed factors. Bleeding can occur from the chest wound due to injury to intercostal artery or from chest wall due to preexisting adhesions. Initial management of bleeding is similar to post sternotomy patients [15]. Postoperative chest x-ray or ultrasound will help in diagnosing chest collection. If exploration is required, it can be performed by video assisted thoracoscopic technique. In an emergency, the chest needs to be reopened via sternotomy. Electric saw to facilitate immediate chest opening in cardiac ITU in the rare event of cardiac tamponade is required and should be part of the emergency reopening tray (Fig. 16).

22.2 Pacing After Surgery

Epicardial pacing wires are placed under vision to facilitate pacing if required. Occasionally the wires may need to be placed rather than stitched on the inferior surface of the heart due to difficult access. Higher threshold may be needed to achieve capture in these circumstances. This more often is the case following redo surgeries because of adhesions posing difficulty in placing the wires. We use transvenous pacing catheters in cases with anticipated difficulty (Fig. 17). Other options include isoprenaline infusion or transvenous pacing wire insertion by cardiologist.

22.3 Haemodynamic Instability

Abnormal pacing if the wires are not stitched to right ventricle or occlusion or impingement of circumflex artery are some of the potential causes for haemodynamic instability after minimal access surgery. Pacing can be switched off if there is an underlying rhythm. If there is no underlying rhythm or severe bradycardia, transcutaneous pacing and isoprenaline infusion can be used while transvenous pacing is established.

Circumflex artery occlusion or impingement is a rare complication following mitral valve surgery and can cause haemodynamic instability. Usually this would have been identified intraoperatively during TOE assessment as poor function of lateral wall of left ventricle associated

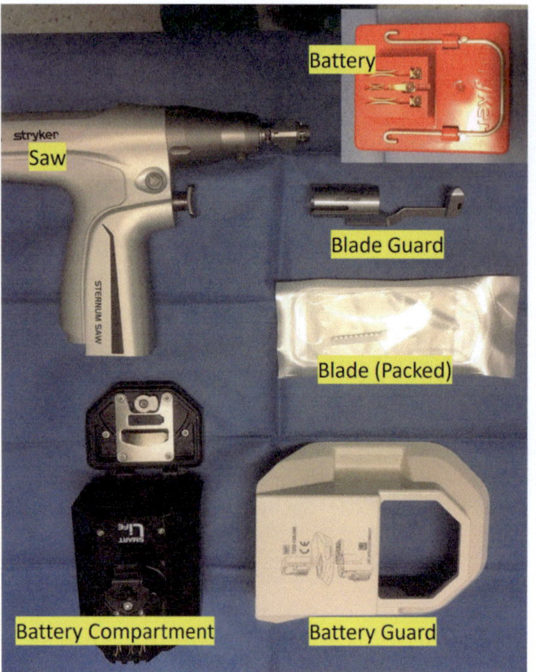
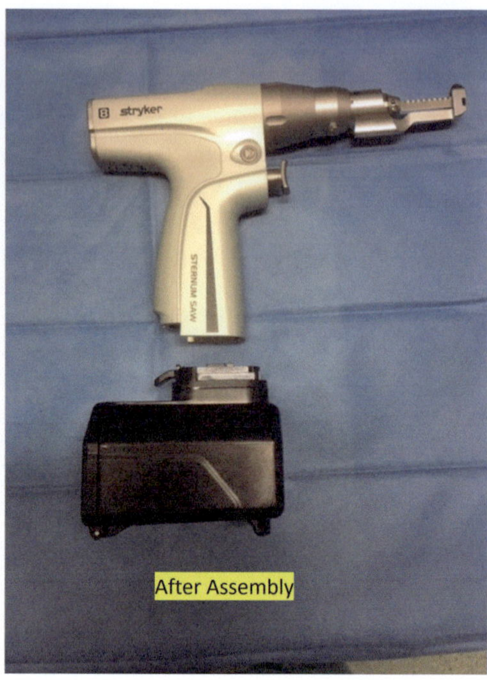

Fig. 16 Emergency sternotomy equipment

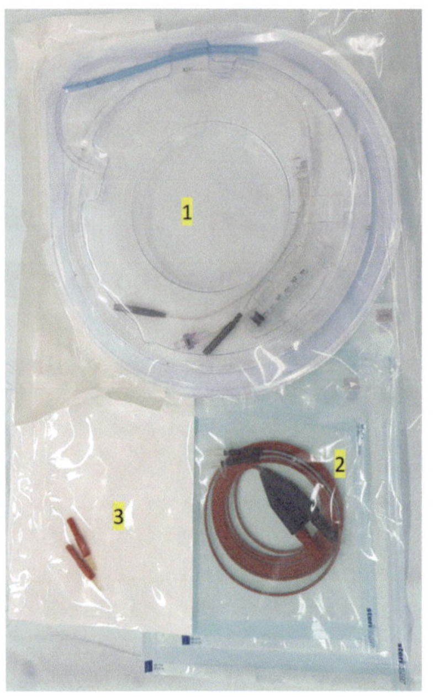

Pacing PA Set Up
1. Pacing PA
2. Extension Cable
3. Connector

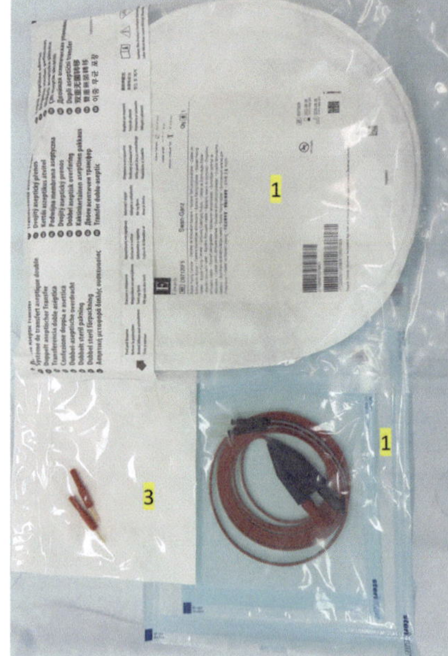

Fig. 17 Pacing PA catheter and attachments

with ECG changes. The patient may need to be taken to catheter lab for emergency angiogram and stent placement. Emergency reoperation with circumflex artery grafting may be required if the resultant impingement has caused complete occlusion and loss of blood flow resulting in failure to wean off bypass.

23 Enhanced Recovery

In the authors institution we use a combination of day of surgery admission together with an enhanced recovery after surgery (ERAS) programme to improve outcomes.

Our enhanced recovery programme is based on the following principles:
1. Established Patient pathway and diary
2. Early mobilisation and twice daily physiotherapy
3. Twice daily Enhanced recovery nurse visit
4. ERAS daily targets discussed and set
5. Discharge discussions from outset
6. Care tailored for each patient
7. Post discharge support and hospital point of contact
8. Nurse, doctor, patient and family education.

The programme resulted in 55–66% mobilised within 6 h and a reduced length of hospital stay of 1–1.5 days compared to non- ERAS in minimally invasive cardiac surgery.

The results of this were highlighted by the Getting it right first time (GIRFT) study in cardiothoracic Surgery in 2018 [16].

- Core recommendation—"more efficient bed management by ensuring surgery on day of admission is delivered routinely leading to reduced delays and time in hospital"
- Good practice case study—Blackpool Teaching Hospitals—same day admission (SDA)
  - 61% SDA at the same time maintaining one of lowest average rate of post op length of stay, average readmission rate and below average complication rate—day of surgery admission does not cause problems later in patient stay
  - Same day admission plus improved length of stay plus reduced cancellations results in reduced costs

Results of our same day admission programme were presented at Association of Cardiothoracic Anaesthetists meeting in 2015 [17]. We presented a 95% patient satisfaction rating together with no increased mortality or morbidity in same day admission program in cardiac surgery.

References

1. Kirmani B, Knowles A, Saravanan P et al. Establishing minimally invasive cardiac surgery in a low-volume mitral surgery centre.Ann R Coll Surg Eng 2021;000:1–8
2. Pisano GP, Bohmer RMJ, Edmondson AC. Organizational differences in rates of learning: evidence from the adoption of minimally invasive cardiac surgcry. Manag Sci 2001; 47:752 68.
3. Afilalo J, Lauck S, Kim H, et al. Frailty in older adults undergoing aortic valve replacement. The Frailty AVR Study. JACC 2017; 70(6):689–700.
4. Knoll H, Ziegeler S, Schreiber JW, et al. Airway injuries after one-lung ventilation: a comparison between double-lumen tube and endobronchial blocker: a randomized, prospective, controlled trial. Anesthesiology. 2006;105:471–7.
5. Clayton-Smith A, Bennet K, Alston RP, et al. A comparison of the efficacy and adverse effects of double lumen tubes and bronchial blockers in thoracic surgery. JCVA. 2015;29(4):955–66.
6. Green DW, Kunst G. Cerebral oximetry and its role in adult cardiac, non-cardiac surgery and resuscitation from cardiac arrest. Anaesthesia. 2017;72 (S1):48–57.
7. Deschamps A, Hall R, Grocott H, et al. Cerebral oximetry monitoring to maintain cerebral oxygen saturation during high-risk cardiac surgery: a randomised controlled feasibility trail. Anesthesiology. 2016;124:826–36.
8. Hahn RT, Abraham T, Adams MS, et al. Guidelines for performing a comprehensive echocardiographic examination: Recommendations from the American society of Echocardiography and the Society of Cardiovascular Anaesthesiologists. J Am Soc Echocardiogr. 2013;26:921–64.
9. Simpson W, Knowles A, Zacharias J, Heggie A, Saravanan P. Role of transesophageal echocardiography in minimally invasive redo surgery of the tricuspid valve—a case series. SCTS—ACTA joint annual meeting. Manchester, 25–27th March 2015.

10. Yoo JY, Kim DH, Choi H, Kim K, Chae YJ, Park SY. Disconnection technique with a bronchial blocker for improving lung deflation: a comparison with a double lumen tube and bronchial blocker without disconnection. JCVA. 2014;28(4):904–7.
11. Irisawa Y, Hiraoka A, Totsugawa T, et al. Re-expansion pulmonary oedema after minimally invasive cardiac surgery with right mini thoracotomy. Eur J Cardiothorac Surg. 2016;49:500–5.
12. Rennera J, Lorenzena U, Borzikowskyb C, et al. Unilateral pulmonary oedema after minimally invasive mitral valve surgery: a single-centre experience. Eur J Cardiothorac Surg. 2018;53:764–70.
13. Puehler T, Friedrich C, Georg G, et al. Outcome of unilateral Pulmonary Edema after minimal-invasive mitral valve surgery: 10-year follow-up. J Clin Med. 2021;10:2411. https://doi.org/10.3390/jcm10112411.
14. Vohra HA, Salmasi MY, Chien L, et al. On behalf of the British and Irish Society for Minimally Invasive Cardiac Surgery. BISMICS consensus statement: implementing a safe minimally invasive mitral programme in the UK healthcare setting. Open Heart 2020; 7:e001259. https://doi.org/10.1136/openhrt-2020-001259
15. Mackie S, Saravanan P. Postoperative care of the adult cardiac surgical patient. Anaesthesia Intensive Care Med. 2021;22(5):279–85.
16. Richens D. Cardiothoracic surgery. Getting it right first time (GIRFT) programme, National specialty report. NHS Improvement March 2018. Accessed on line 04 August 2021. https://gettingitrightfirsttime.co.uk/wp-content/uploads/2018/04/GIRFT-Cardiothoracic-Report-1.pdf.
17. Williams B, Zacharias J, McAlea B, Saravanan P. Same day admission for cardiac surgery. Safety and outcomes. SCTS—ACTA joint annual meeting. Manchester, 25–27th March 2015.

Further Readings

Parnell A, Prince M. Anaesthesia for minimally invasive cardiac surgery. BJA Education. 2018;18(10):323–30.
Vishwas M, Jha AK, Kapoor PM. Anesthetic challenges in minimally invasive cardiac surgery: are we moving in a right direction? Ann Card Anaesth 2016; 19 (3):489–97.

Transoesophageal Echocardiography for Safe Endoscopic Cardiac Surgery

Palanikumar Saravanan and Andrew Knowles

Abstract

The safe practice of Endoscopic cardiac surgery is linked with the provision of good Trans oesophageal images during every stage of the procedure. One of the reasons for the slow uptake is likely to be the sporadic availability of expert TOE operators in a cardiac surgery theatre. The authors have an experience of over a decade of developments in this field and play a very important role is the provision of this service. This chapter tries to give the reader a overview of what is required and what is possible with a particular focus on the critical role of the TOE operator in the endoscopic cardiac surgery team.

Supplementary Information The online version contains supplementary material available at https://doi.org/10.1007/978-3-031-21104-1_3. The videos can be accessed individually by clicking the DOI link in the accompanying figure caption or by scanning this link with the SN More Media App.

P. Saravanan (✉) · A. Knowles
Department of Cardiothoracic Anaesthesia,
Lancashire Cardiac Centre, Blackpool, England
e-mail: Dr.saravanan@nhs.net

Keywords

TOE · Safe conduct of surgery · Quality control in endoscopic cardiac surgery

Transoesophageal echocardiography (TOE) is essential for the safe conduct of endoscopic cardiac surgery. With limited direct surgical access into the chest cavity, it allows review and confirmation of surgical pathology, aids the placement of various cannulae and has a vital role in diagnosing and troubleshooting problems during the procedure. It is usually performed by cardiac anaesthetists in UK though some centres around the world will have dedicated cardiologists for this purpose [1].

It is mandatory in the preoperative assessment to exclude any contraindications for TOE probe insertion.

Full informed consent from the patient must detail possible trauma to lips, teeth, pharyngeal structures and the risk of oesophageal perforation which may vary from approximately 1 in 1000 to 1in 10000 cases [2].

Insertion of a well lubricated TOE probe is ideally performed with direct or video laryngoscopy. This may be augmented with anterior traction on the mandible to open up the oropharynx and laryngopharynx.

Space for the TOE machine may be limited with a number of anaesthetic equipment (Fibreoptic bronchoscopy, Video laryngoscopy,

J. Zacharias (ed.), *Endoscopic Cardiac Surgery*,
https://doi.org/10.1007/978-3-031-21104-1_3

Cerebral oximetry and Defibrillator), surgical equipment (3D stack and multiple trays needed for insertion of cannulas) and number of personnel in theatre (cardiologist and anaesthetic assistants). Arranging the work space to accommodate the devices and personnel will help in efficient and continuous use of TOE that is required for these procedures. The TOE screen should be clearly visible to anaesthetists, surgeons and scrub nurse. The authors use a monitor to display FOB and Video Laryngoscopy in one device and the cerebral oximetry is slaved to anaesthetic monitor. The defibrillator is placed over and forms part of anaesthetic machine.

Some procedures performed by an endoscopic approach (Video 1).

1. Left heart procedures
   a. Mitral valve repair and replacement
   b. Left Ventricular myomectomy
   c. Left atrial myxoma.

2. Right heart procedures
   a. Tricuspid valve repair and replacement
   b. Closure of Atrial septal defect or patent foramen ovale
   c. Closure of Ventricular septal defect
   d. Right atrial or ventricular mass lesions.

3. Others as combined procedures
   a. LA appendage clipping
   b. Atrial fibrillation ablation.

Timing of TOE:

The authors routinely perform TOE immediately after induction of anaesthesia and intubation. This will provide confirmation of the pathologies, review of ventricular performance and suitability of the patient's anatomy to undergo endoscopic procedures. If any supporting or new evidence found at this stage, endoscopic approach has to be abandoned and sternotomy is

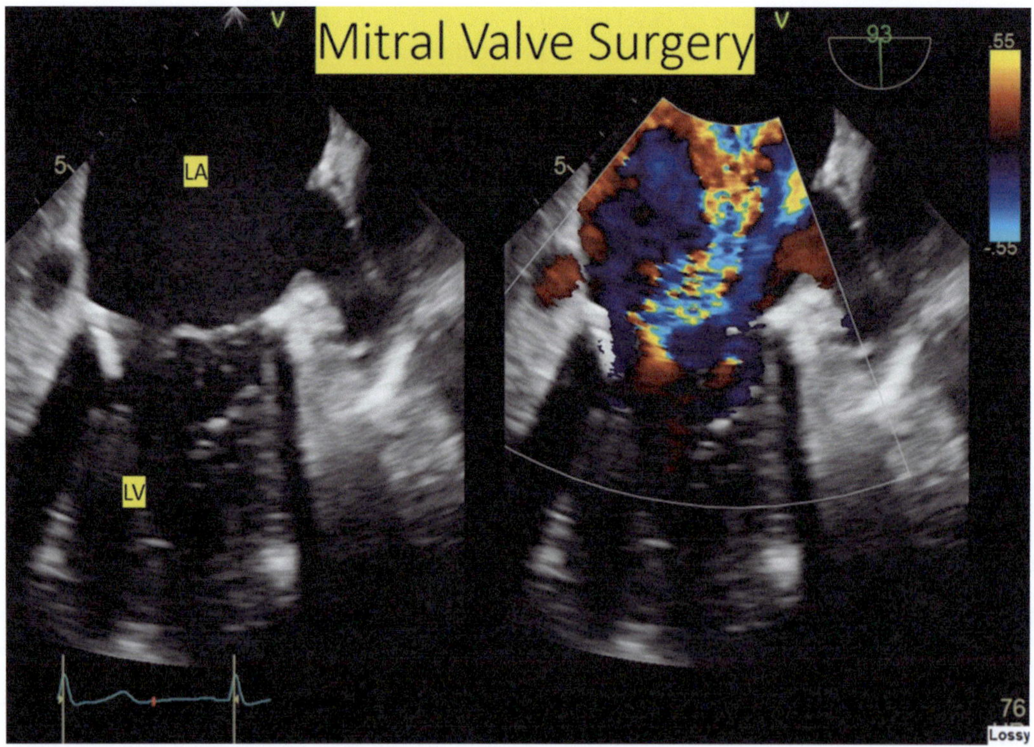

Video 1 Some procedures performed by minimal access (▶ https://doi.org/10.1007/000-a79)

performed. This will prevent unnecessary insertion of right arm arterial line for monitoring in the use of Endo Balloon device or a neck cannula when indicated. This is important in health care systems where there may be a long wait from the time surgical decision is made to patient arrival in theatre. Some surgeons and some centres perform TOE after anaesthesia and lines insertion are complete and prior to start of surgery. This can be safely done in those centres where the patient has a recent preoperative Echocardiogram and when the surgical preference is to use other forms of aortic occlusion.

Standard TOE assessment during endoscopic surgery using both 2D and 3D scanning:

1. Routine cardiac surgery standard views to assess anatomy, physiology and pathology
2. Dynamic assessment of arterial and venous wire and cannula insertion
3. Safe establishment of cardiopulmonary bypass flow
4. Endo balloon (intra aortic occlusion balloon) positioning, inflation and cardioplegia delivery
5. Assessment of de-airing
6. Separation from cardiopulmonary bypass (CPB) and assessment of ventricular performance
7. Assessment of surgical procedures
8. Confirmation of aortic integrity post bypass and endo balloon usage.

TOE assessment specific for endoscopic surgery in addition to the routine cardiac surgery standard views includes:

1. Aortic Valve: Mid oesophageal Long axis (ME LAX) and short axis (ME SAX) views and Deep Transgastric (DTG) view

Aortic Valve is assessed for its leaflet integrity and any degree of regurgitation. Any regurgitation must be carefully assessed due to the risk of ventricular distension during administration of cardioplegia. A grading more than mild may well preclude use of an Endo balloon. The vena contracta measurement in DTG view and flow reversal pattern in descending thoracic aorta (DTA) is helpful in decision making.

2. Ascending aorta (AA): ME LAX view, Upper oesophageal (UE) views

In the ME LAX view reducing the angle closer to 90 and pulling the probe back will give a clear view of AA. In the UE AA view, using 90 degrees or using X plane or Biplane views will provide good assessment of a long segment of AA.

In some patients these views may not provide satisfactory assessment and we find the views are better after positioning of the patient. Presence of severe atheromatous disease or mobile atheroma will preclude endoballoon use.

AA diameter of less than 40mm at the level of the pulmonary artery is generally required for endo balloon usage.

3. Aortic arch & descending thoracic aorta (DTA): ME and UE views

DTA can be seen well upon rotating the probe towards the left (posterior) in ME views. Keeping DTA in view, pulling the probe back will help in assessing the entire length of it. Using X plane or Biplane views will help in viewing longitudinal section of DTA alongside the cross section. If the TOE machine do not provide this facility, 90 degree angle is used and probe pulled back. When the proximal part of DTA is reached, the probe needs to rotated towards right (anterior) to follow the arch. Ability to obtain these views are important for placement of Endo balloon. Presence of intraluminal pathology and/or atheroma will preclude use of retrograde bypass and passage of Endo Balloon. Certainly atheroma of Katz grade 4 and 5 in DTA would be a contraindication for retrograde bypass or guidewire and endoballoon catheter passage.

Routine preoperative aorto femoral CT scan can also identify this problem (Video 2).

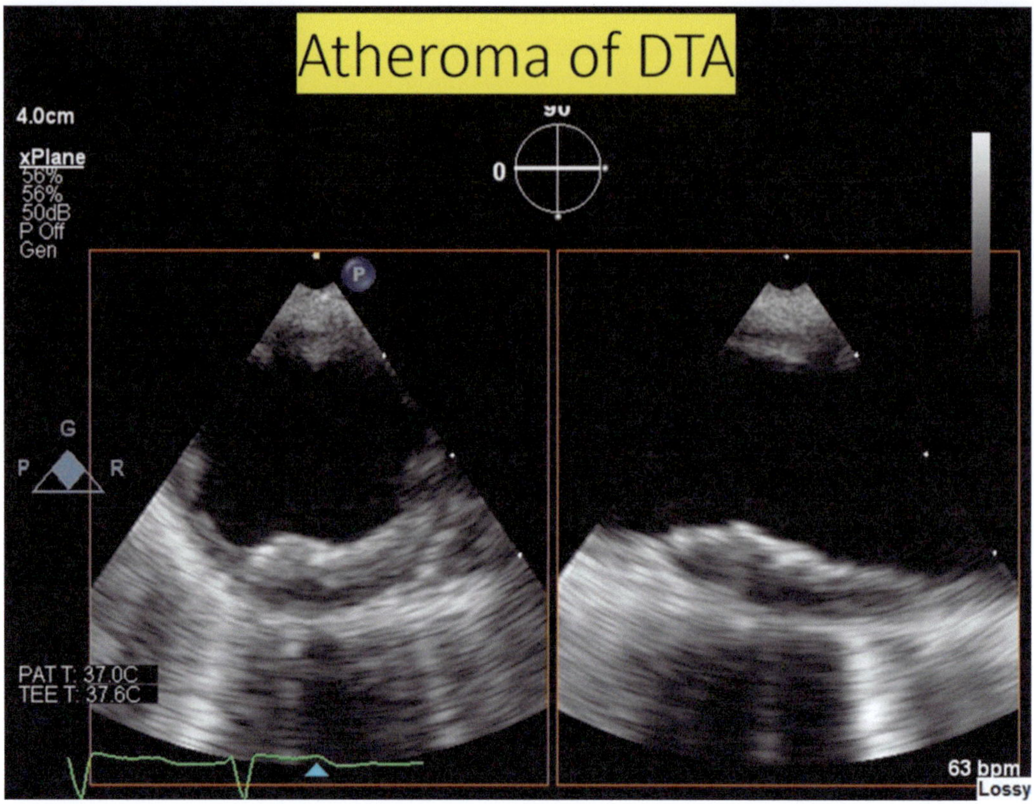

Video 2 Pre bypass TOE (▶ https://doi.org/10.1007/000-a78)

1 Standard Assessment of Surgical Pathology and Other Structures

Mitral Valve: All standard views and 3D views

Assessment of mitral valve which includes leaflet pathology, mechanism of regurgitation, annular diameter and length of anterior leaflet assists in valve repair planning. 3D echo can be used if available to provide supporting information. During the initial stages of setting up an endoscopic program the prolonged nature of surgery should be considered before undertaking complex mitral surgery. Any abnormal and significant calcification in mitral annulus may also make surgery by endoscopic approach difficult even in experienced hands.

Left ventricle: ME and TG views

Overall performance, presence of regional wall motion abnormalities, degree of dilatation and hypertrophy of left ventricle is assessed using all the standard views.

Right ventricle: ME and TG views

Overall performance, degree of dilatation is assessed using the standard views. Presence of dilated and impaired right ventricle necessitates robust plans for myocardial protection strategies and postoperative management.

Tricuspid Valve: All standard views, ME coronary sinus view

Tricuspid valve is assessed using standard views. Annular diameter is measured at the level of coronary sinus. A diameter greater than 40 mm with or without significant regurgitation is usually considered for annuloplasty surgery.

Cannulation of the superior vena cava via the internal jugular vein under TOE control will be required as part of bicaval cannulation to facilitate tricuspid surgery.

Atria: All standard views

Assessment of degree of dilatation, left atrial appendage for thrombus is performed in patients scheduled for AF ablation and/or clipping of LA appendage.

Integrity of interatrial septum is assessed and presence of any PFO or ASD can make the insertion and placement of femoral venous cannulation tricky. The area of defect needs to be continuously monitored to avoid the guidewire in left atrium during IVC cannula insertion.

Superior vena cava (SVC): (Bicaval view, upper oesophageal AA view)

Suitability of diameter for placement of drainage cannulae and Fogarty balloon in tricuspid or re-do surgery is probably best seen in the bicaval view.

The circumflex artery blood flow: (two and four chamber view)

Attempts are made to look for circumflex artery blood flow in the two chamber view where it can be usually seen as a small circular structure at the anterior mitral annulus or along its length in the 4 chamber view. Probe can be tilted and angle decreased or increased to view this as a tubular structure. Colour flow Doppler is utilised to view blood flow.

Pericardial and Pleural spaces: All Standard views and DTA views

Any fluid collections in pleural spaces need to be noted. The effusion on left pleura will impair the ability to safely achieve one lung ventilation while effusion on right which may be associated with adhesions can make surgical access difficult due to failure of lung to collapse and increase the risk of bleeding postoperatively.

Conduct of surgery
SVC cannulation: Bicaval view

Initially jugular venous guidewire insertion is performed under ultrasound control. Guidewire passing down the SVC must be confirmed and therefore rule out passage of the wire into the arm. Attempts should be made to pass the guidewire into inferior vena cava (IVC) to avoid arrhythmias. After insertion, the cannula is positioned at the right atrial SVC junction or within the SVC if caval snaring is to be undertaken.

Femoral Venous Cannulation: Bicaval view, TG IVC view

A bicaval view is obtained for guidewire and cannula positioning. The angle of the probe may need to decreased to 80 to 90 degrees to visualise the guidewire as well as small left and right manipulations to keep the thin guidewire in the ultrasound beam. This view is used to ensure initial wire passage into the SVC and not into the right ventricle via the tricuspid valve or into the right atrial appendage both of which may be perforated by the drainage cannula following an abnormal wire passage.

In presence of an ASD or PFO, additional precautions are taken to identify and avoid the wire in left atrium. This is in the form of continuous monitoring of the wire position with surgical manoeuvres. A cross sectional view of SVC along with the bicaval view increases sensitivity. This can be obtained in different TOE machines as X plane view or Biplane view.

Femoral arterial Cannulation: Short/long axis of descending aorta

The DTA views are obtained as described in standard assessment. This is to confirm passage of the guidewire into the descending aorta and which should be clearly seen moving freely within the lumen. Every effort is made to see the J tip as confirmation. Longitudinal view of DTA alongside the cross sectional view increases the sensitivity (Video 3).

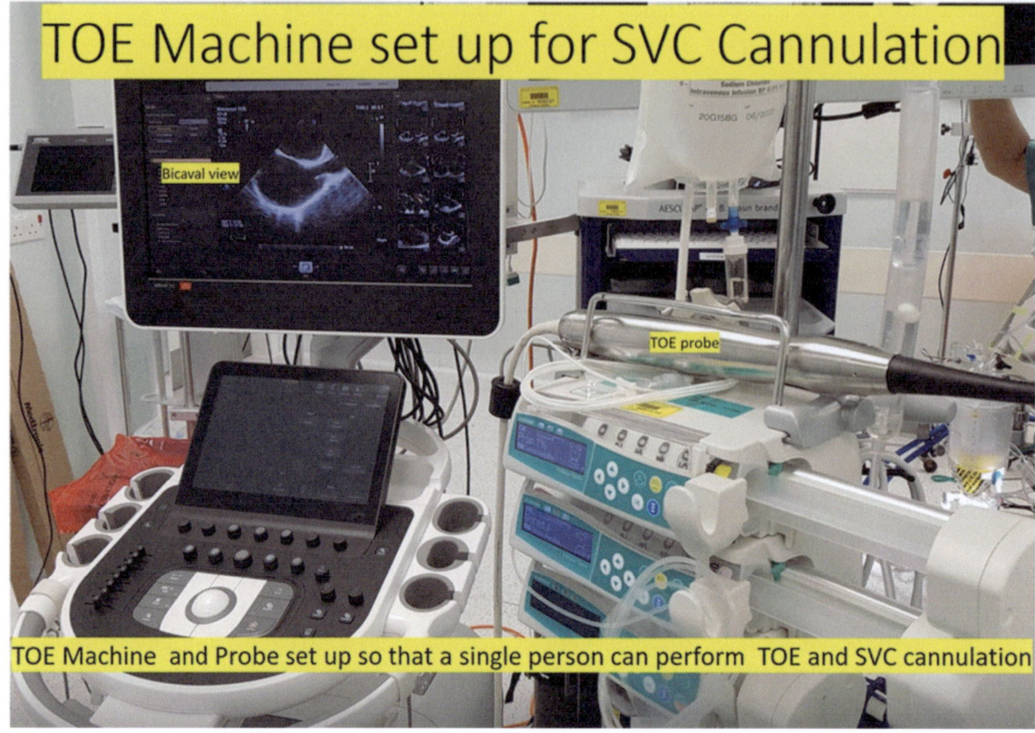

Video 3 TOE for cannulations (▶ https://doi.org/10.1007/000-a75)

Placement of Endo aortic occlusion balloon —DTA views, ME LAX view of aortic valve and ascending aorta

The guidewire of the Endo Balloon is visualised in the descending thoracic aorta similar to guidewire of femoral arterial cannula and followed up into arch and then ascending aorta. The X-plane or biplane view is used to increase the sensitivity. Continuous wire passage via the descending, arch and into the ascending aorta must be confirmed. Erroneous passage into the arch vessels may result in vascular spasm within that vessel. The left subclavian artery is most likely to be affected and is indicated by drop in left arm pressure.

Following correct position of the wire within the ascending aorta the balloon catheter is advanced to be positioned at the level of the main pulmonary artery. During the passage of the balloon through the guidewire, the AA is monitored for continuous presence of J tip of the guidewire till balloon tip is visualised. The balloon tip is positioned at the level of pulmonary artery (Video 4).

Commencement of cardiopulmonary bypass: DTA views

Monitoring DTA during commencement of CPB allows confirmation of safe retrograde flow and absence of aortic dissection. The artefacts due to the mixing of forward flow from myocardial contraction and retrograde bypass flow may be visualised and should not be mistaken for aortic dissection.

If the arterial line pressures are reported as high on commencement of bypass, the patient is weaned off bypass, ventilation resumed and contralateral femoral artery is also cannulated using TOE guidance. During this time, the presence of Endo Balloon in DTA should be taken into account while visualising guidewire. Attempts are then remade to commence bypass via both femoral arterial cannulae.

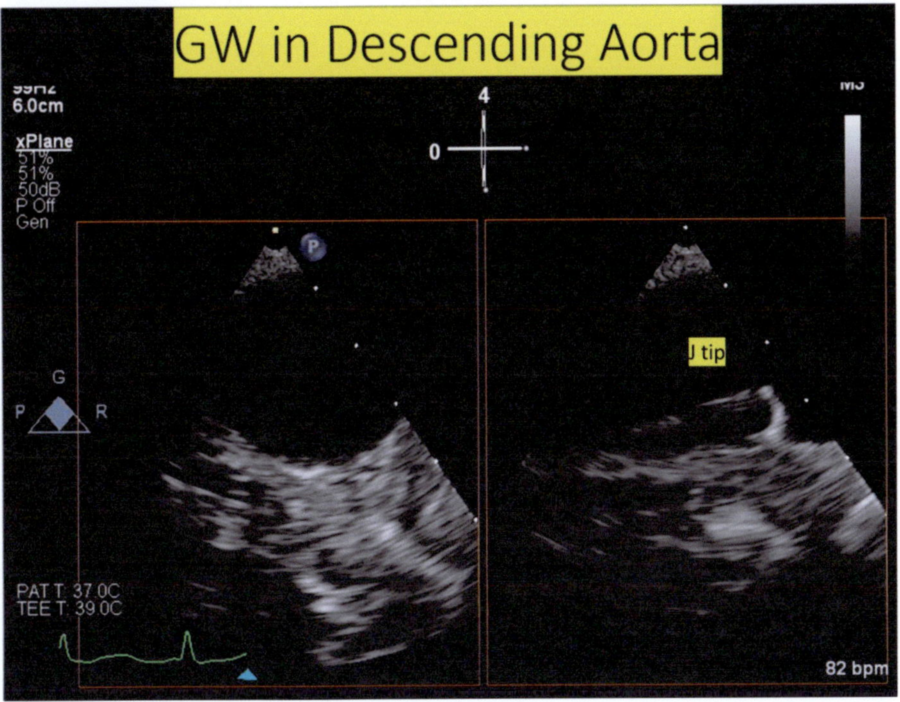

Video 4 TOE for Endo Balloon (▶ https://doi.org/10.1007/000-a76)

Balloon inflation: ME LAX of aortic valve and ascending aorta

The Endo Balloon is placed under direct TOE guidance into the ascending aorta at the level of the pulmonary artery. To occlude the ascending aorta, it is inflated with approximately n mls of saline (where n was the measured aortic diameter in millimetres). At approximately 15–20 ml of inflation, 250 µg/kg of adenosine is administered through the distal lumen of the intra-aortic balloon directly into the partially occluded aortic root causing cardiac standstill to allow accurate landing of the balloon. This prevents ventricular ejection and allowing the full balloon inflation to occur without movement of the balloon. Once the balloon is inflated to the required diameter a drop in the pressure of the endoballoon manometry line is seen indicating occlusion of the ascending aorta and isolation from CPB pressure in the distal aorta.

Delivery of cardioplegia—Long axis of aortic valve and ascending aorta

Delivery of cardioplegia into the aortic root should be visible with flow from the balloon or cardioplegia cannula, pressurisation of the root, competence of the aortic valve and flow seen into the right coronary artery.

Inflation of Fogarty catheter in Redo procedures: Bicaval view

In patients undergoing redo tricuspid valve procedures external snaring of the SVC may not be possible and therefore a Fogarty catheter is used to occlude the SVC opening from inside the right atrium. We use a Fogarty balloon which can be inflated up to 48 mls. The inflation can be visualized in the bicaval view. The SVC drainage cannula is pulled back to lie approximately 3–4 cm above the junction of RA/SVC junction. Adequate drainage is the confirmed by the

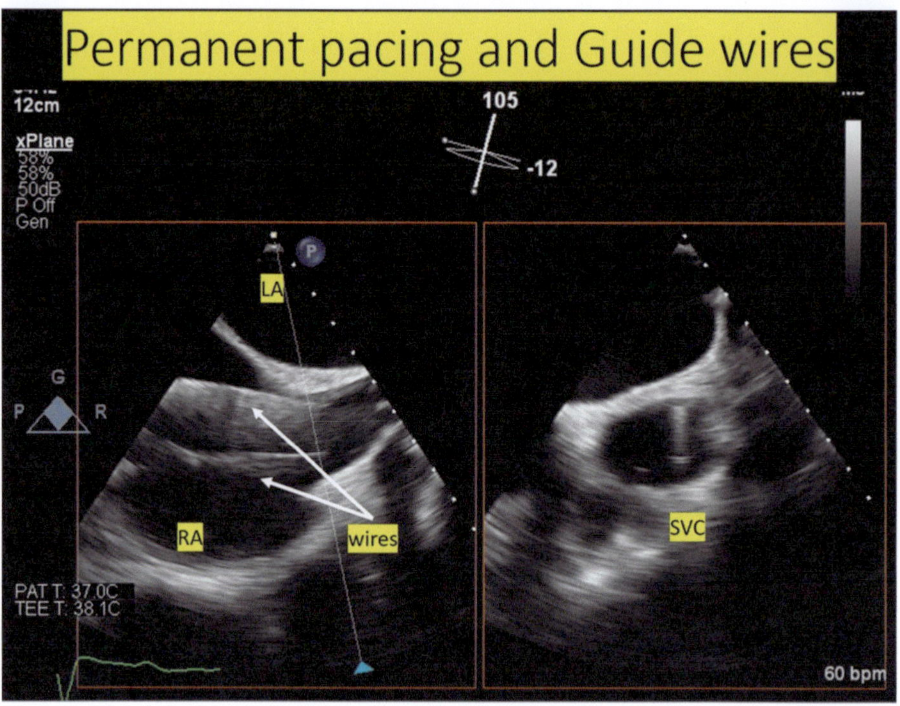

Video 5 TOE specific to redo surgery (▶ https://doi.org/10.1007/000-a74)

perfusionist and also in cerebral oximetry readings (Video 5).

Deflation of Balloon and deairing: ME LAX view

Balloon is deflated under vision, aortic integrity confirmed and positioned close to aortic valve to aid deairing.

Following CPB: All standard views

Assessment of biventricular function is mandatory as separation from CPB occurs.

Then assessment of the surgical procedure is confirmed using all relevant standard views. The views used will depend on the procedure performed.

AA is examined to confirm aortic integrity.

Following mitral valve surgery, the coaptation length, valve gradient, presence of Systolic anterior motion (SAM) and circumflex artery flow are routinely checked.

The Aortic valve integrity is assessed especially following Endo Balloon use. Right coronary artery flow is assessed following tricuspid valve surgery.

In contrast to sternotomy cardiac surgery the right ventricle is only visible by TOE and therefore this must be assessed during protamine delivery (Video 6).

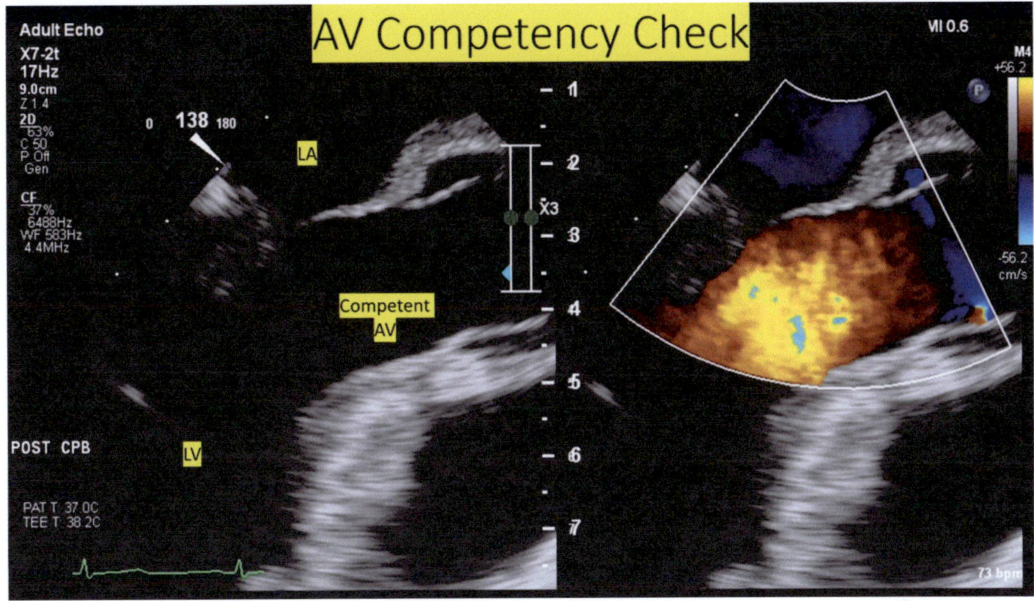

Video 6 TOE post bypass (▶ https://doi.org/10.1007/000-a77)

References

1. Hahn RT, Abraham T, Adams MS, et al. Guidelines for performing a comprehensive echocardiographic examination: Recommendations from the American society of Echocardiography and the Society of cardiovascular anaesthesiologists. J Am Soc Echocardiogr. 2013;26:921–64.

2. Purza R, Ghosh S, Walker C, Hiebert B, Koley L, Mackenzie S, et al. Transesophageal echocardiography complications in adult cardiac surgery: a retrospective cohort study. Ann Thorac Surg. 2017;103:795–803.

Endoscopic Conduit Harvesting: Best Practice Training Guidelines

Bhuvaneswari Krishnamoorthy
and Jared Blackmore

Abstract

The great saphenous vein remains the most commonly used conduit for non-left anterior descending coronary artery bypass graft surgery. The aim of this chapter is to define the best practice training standards for use of the Endoscopic Vein Harvesting (EVH) technique during coronary artery bypass surgery. This chapter has been collated by an international multidisciplinary panel of advanced practice providers, surgeons, cardiologists and anaesthetists with common interests and expertise in caring for patients with coronary artery disease. These proposed training standards have been developed using current best evidence and from experiences of those most closely involved in the process, with proposals receiving approval for recommendation by consensus. A total of 11 criteria for best training practice were defined including recommendations on patient selection, surgical training, ultrasound vein scanning, heparinisation, diathermy settings, CO_2 insufflation and setting, training/volume threshold, harvesting with minimal surrounding tissues, use of pressure-controlled syringe for vein disten-sion and the need for regular audit. The team agrees that EVH is a standard practice in USA, however in the rest of the world there still remains a reticence about EVH due to concerns about the quality of the vein and cost of equipment. There are lots of differences in harvesting practices between USA and the rest of the world due to there being no documented and accepted standards of EVH best practice. The main aim of writing this chapter was to produce a resource to which all EVH trainee practitioners can refer. We hope it will provide the first set of standards and promote safe practice by surgical colleagues to ensure high quality conduits are retrieved and prevent harm to the patient during training.

Keywords

Endoscopic conduit harvesting · Best practice guidelines · Standardisation

1 Introduction

Coronary Artery Bypass Grafting (CABG) remains the gold standard surgical procedure to relieve the symptoms and provide long term prognosis in multivessel coronary artery disease [1]. In spite of evidence that multiple arterial grafts provide better long-term patency rate [2, 3], the Greater Saphenous Vein (GSV) is the

B. Krishnamoorthy (✉) · J. Blackmore
The University of Salford and Manchester Foundation Trust, Manchester, England, UK
e-mail: b.bibleraaj@salford.ac.uk

© The Author(s), under exclusive license to Springer Nature Switzerland AG 2023
J. Zacharias (ed.), *Endoscopic Cardiac Surgery*,
https://doi.org/10.1007/978-3-031-21104-1_4

most commonly used supplementary conduit with the left internal thoracic artery grafted to the left anterior descending coronary artery, with more than 90% of coronary bypass surgery conducted with GSV [4–6]. Open vein harvesting has been the standard technique for harvesting GSV conduits for bypass surgery since 1950. However, open vein harvesting is associated with a high incidence of postoperative leg wound complications and morbidity [7]. In an attempt to reduce postoperative pain, lower wound complication rates and improve patient satisfaction, the Endoscopic Vein Harvesting (EVH) technique was developed and introduced to clinical practice in mid-1990 [8, 9]. In the USA, approximately 90% of CABG patients receive EVH as a standard of care but in other parts of the world there is still significant practice variability and debate about the quality of the conduit and long-term patency when using the EVH approach [7, 10–13].

The International Society for Minimally Invasive Cardiothoracic Surgery (ISMICS) 2017 consensus statement recommends that EVH should be the standard of care (class I, level B), to reduce the wound related complications (class I, level A), to improve patient satisfaction and postoperative pain (class I, level A), to reduce the postoperative length of stay and outpatient wound management resources (class I, level A) and the quality of conduit harvested (class IIa, level B-R) [14]. Furthermore, the ISMICS panel concluded that the rigorously analysed, high quality evidence demonstrates no increase in major adverse cardiac events or decrease in graft patency for endoscopically harvested saphenous vein [14]. Unfortunately, this consensus statement has failed to allay the fears of non EVH users regarding the quality of harvested vein and long-term patency rates [15, 16].

Over the past 10 years multiple publications have looked at medium- and long-term outcomes of patients who have had endoscopic vein harvesting against open vein harvesting [17–19]. No long-term registry has shown adverse outcomes among patients with EVH against OVH. Despite this there remain concerns of graft patency in a subgroup analysis of a Randomised Control Trial (RCT) ([20] which have raised some questions that can only be answered by an adequately powered RCT looking at graft patency over time. As most patients and funders are more interested in quality of life and survival among patients this trial may never be funded, and we may have to continue to rely on real world registry data. If EVH surgery is to become routine standard of care for CABG surgery, the harvesting technique should be exposed to close scrutiny to safeguard that the highest standards of practice are achieved.

The delivery of surgical care in modern healthcare systems is rapidly evolving into a multidisciplinary approach with increased involvement of more specialised staff for each point of intervention in order to provide best possible care to all service users [21]. To design, understand and set the best practice standards for endoscopic vein harvesting, we have utilised a multidisciplinary team approach. Due to the paucity of proposed standards in cardiac surgery for vein harvesting, this best practice training standards chapter was produced using the existing best practice model for mitral valve repair as a template [21].

2 Methods

The training standards were developed and assessed using all the data assembled from the existing literature followed by discussion by a group of multidisciplinary panel members to achieve an agreement. The panel members were selected for their expertise in EVH harvesting, bypass surgery and caring for CABG patients. The following questions were asked to set proposed standards of EVH practice:

1. What institutional and local criteria are required to achieve best EVH practice during training?
2. Are there any local guidelines for EVH best practice?
3. What clinical outcomes are expected after leg vein harvesting surgery?

4. Is it feasible to define training standards for best practice for EVH by a multidisciplinary panel agreement?
5. Are there any identifiable criteria for selecting EVH as the vein harvesting technique or can the EVH be applied universally to all patients?
6. Do we need to monitor trainees in order to minimise/avoid damage that may have an impact on the quality of the vein?
7. Is it possible to set a threshold for training requirements and caseload volume for best practice?

3 Results

To develop best surgical training standard guidelines, it is vital that initial criteria proposals are set out by experienced surgical colleagues and practitioners. A total of 10 recommendations were made by the panel from their experience of what was required to retrieve a vein conduit of quality equal to that achieved with the current standard open vein harvesting technique. These key recommendations involved:

- Patient selection
- Surgical training
- Ultrasound scanning of the GSV before surgery
- Heparinisation
- Diathermy settings
- CO_2 insufflation and setting
- Training and volume threshold
- Harvesting with minimal surrounding tissue
- Use of a pressure-controlled syringe
- Use of vacuum suction leg drain
- Auditing routine practice to benchmark against other hospitals.

3.1 Patient Selection

The panel believes that there should be a criterion for selecting patients both during and following successful completion of the EVH training period. Patients with conditions such as diabetes mellitus, peripheral vascular disease and diseased veins (previous incidence of superficial thrombophlebitis) may be predisposed to accelerated myointimal proliferation which leads to luminal narrowing and early occlusion of the vein graft [22, 23].

Patients with varicose veins have vein walls that are thin and inelastic and consequently have high risk of rupture compared to normal veins [24]. Similarly, patients with thin legs and/or superficial veins have the possibility of more thin hair line branches. This poses a higher risk for avlusion at the base of the vein branch during EVH [20]. Any trauma during harvesting in these patients with co-morbidities is likely to accelerate vein stenosis in the long-term. Indeed, any damage to the fragile thin GSV endothelium appears to be a key promotor for the development and progress of vein graft disease, stenosis and complete failure [25].

3.2 Contraindications for EVH and Rationale

- EVH should not be performed by novice practitioners during ongoing ischemia necessitating an emergency CABG due to the duration of vein harvest and risk for conduit damage. However, if the practitioner is experienced and has shown the ability to expeditiously harvest a quality conduit, it would be appropriate to utilise EVH during an emergency CABG.
- Superficial GSV (<1/2 cm below the skin) should be avoided due to spatial limitations for the operator between the skin and vein. The EVH cannula shaft external diameter is a further consideration, being approximately 1.5 cm (Maquet Vasoview Hemopro™) or greater from some other companies. It is important not to insert the scope forcefully as this may damage the adventitial layer of the vein which causes localised bruising and haematoma inside the layers of the vein [26]. This additional trauma caused by the

harvesters can accelerate the natural progression of graft degeneration leading to early graft occlusion.

- Varicose veins are thin-walled vessels characterised by a loss of elasticity and the presence of numerous vein bulbs. This is associated with a high risk of rupture during harvesting when compared to normal veins [27]. There are many factors that can significantly affect graft patency in CABG surgery. However, patients with saphenofemoral incompetency or thrombophlebitis of superficial veins can increase the risk of poor graft quality and subsequently affect its patency. Many histological studies have illustrated that the varicose veins have intimal hypertrophy, subendothelial fibrosis, luminal dilation and wall thickening [27–30]. These varicose veins have persistent venous hypertension, chronic inflammation and genetic variations that alter the vessel wall of the GSV. As such, it is good practice to avoid harvesting these veins by EVH. Experienced practitioners can harvest the patients with minimal varicose veins with maximum care.

- Patients with small or thin legs (<7.5 cm diameter at the lower calf) determined via an ultrasound scan [31] should not have veins harvested using the EVH technique. These veins tend to have more superficial hair line branches which are highly likely to be torn from the base of the vein during harvesting. However, some argue that performing fasciotomy on these patients can open up the space between the skin and the vein yet still there remains a high risk of vein bruising and vein/branch tear [22, 26]. Again, it is important for the EVH trainee practitioner to assess the situation carefully and take decision to harvest suitable conduit for the surgery.

4 Ideal Patients for EVH Training

It is the opinion of the panel that novice practitioners should avoid the most technically challenging patients (those with venous co-morbidities, BMI above 35, peripheral vascular disease and muscular patients) during their training period. By doing so, novice practitioners can focus on implementing their learned skills and obtaining good quality veins for CABG surgery without unnecessary stress. For at least their first 25 cases, novice trainees should harvest veins from patients with good quality veins as confirmed by ultrasound. The trainees should be taught gradually, initially harvesting one length of vein starting with few dissections and few branches. Only once proficient with a single length of good quality vein should the practitioner moved to two or more lengths of vein. The final stage of training should incorporate more complex cases such as female patients and obese patients. This way, novice practitioners can accelerate their learning curve [22, 32, 33] rather than struggling with difficult cases early on, which can impact upon the practitioner's confidence. It can potentially reduce the perception that EVH technique is responsible for poor quality veins with worse long-term outcomes.

4.1 Surgical Training for EVH

Training modalities vary depending on region and country. In the UK, the previous standard requirement was an in-house training which led to a diploma in cardiothoracic surgery. These practitioners were then trained in-house on how to assist and perform open vein harvesting. However, in 2014 the Department of Health in UK published a Surgical Care Practitioner (SCP) curriculum, which made a Masters in Surgical Practice a recognised academic national qualification for all SCPs. This way the SCPs undergo rigorous academic and speciality training for two years in a UK academic institute which covers the pre, intra and postoperative care pathway of a patient. For international EVH practitioners, they should follow their local academic/institutional training programme. In the USA and other parts of the world, these surgical team members can be referred to as Physician Assistants, Surgical Assistants, Certified Registered Nurse First Assistants or Nurse Practitioners depending on the training.

In-house training of practitioners to perform specific jobs is no longer common practice. It is vital for members of the surgical team to be educated to a consistently higher level of skill and knowledge to deliver high quality patient care. The practitioners who work in a surgical team should have basic knowledge and understanding of the anatomy and pathophysiology of a disease condition, its differential diagnosis and management pathway. Importantly, practitioners must also be comfortable working as part of a large multidisciplinary team.

During training, junior surgeons and junior practitioners should be exposed to the standard open vein harvesting of 10 cases (depends upon individual manual dexterity) to gain knowledge of vein harvesting and the importance of vein preservation for conduit surgery. Exposing trainees too soon to EVH can yield poor quality vein conduits. This is because the EVH technique requires good hand-eye co-ordination with psychomotor technical skills to operate the EVH equipment [22]. Many studies have concluded that experienced practitioners obtain good quality veins due to the skills they acquired during their prolonged experience [22, 34]. It is important to have a standardised and structured training curriculum for the EVH trainees to accumulate the skills and the theoretical knowledge required to obtain the best quality vein conduit [31, 35]. The panel believes that the length of skin incision for harvesting the vein is in itself not as important as preserving its integrity and obtaining better quality of conduit, which is vital for the patient to ensure graft patency for a number of years to come [36]. However, this can be argued by the high volume EVH centres across the world that they teach their practitioners only EVH not traditional open vein harvesting technique. It should be considered as a local preference and these centres should collect their local data to compare the quality of the vein with experienced practitioners.

4.2 Structured Training

The quality of the vein harvested by novice practitioners remains questionable due to their lack of familiarity with the EVH technique and lack of endoscopic skills [37]. It is important to devise a structured training curriculum to improve the theoretical and practical knowledge of the novice EVH practitioners [26]. The departments can devise their own style of teaching method using Manchester Endoscopic Learning Tool (MELT) [26] training model to guide their trainees through EVH (Fig. 1). Minimising vein trauma can improve the surgeons' confidence with the endoscopic procedures and also provides good quality veins as conduits for the patient. The inexperience of the novice practitioners can increase the risk of vein trauma and denudation of the endothelium which gradually leads to vein graft failure [26, 38]. Furthermore, appropriate teaching of novice trainers will help alleviate the stress of learning. Competency based e-learning theoretical modules that continually reinforce the importance of vein preservation, provide anatomy and physiology knowledge, and walk through the steps of the EVH surgical procedure should form the core of the initial training.

5 E-Learning Theoretical Module

As we are in the twenty-first century with wide access to technologies for teaching purposes, it is vital that we take advantage of this and utilise the e-learning platform for teaching the EVH technique outside of the theatre. It is not possible for the trainer to transfer all knowledge to the trainee within the theatre environment. Learning within the theatre can be very difficult and creating a conducive environment is important for the trainee to learn in a stress-free environment [39].

There is no currently available e-learning based module or accredited programme for EVH. The EVH equipment has been modified many times by the surgical companies to obtain improved quality veins. It is vital that the EVH product companies spend time and effort on producing these educational tools in order to ensure the best possible trainee experience, which may allow an acceleration of the learning curve and reduce the incidence of poor-quality conduit during the learning phase.

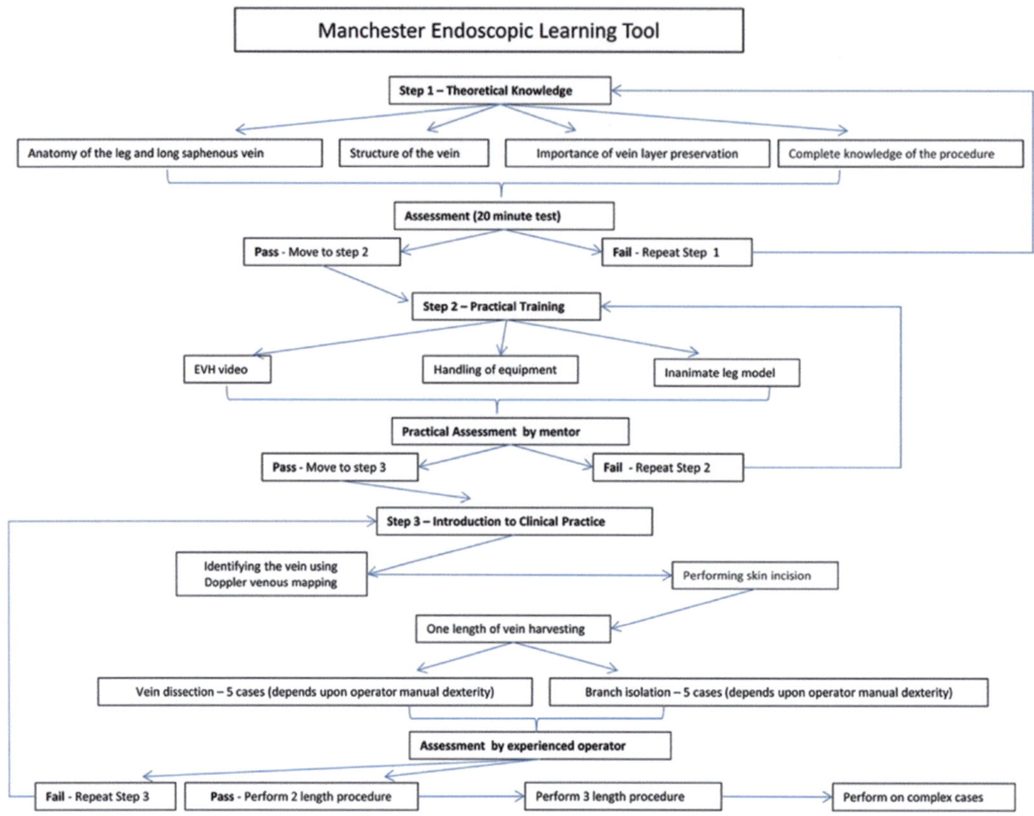

Fig. 1 This schematic diagram illustrating an overview of the MELT [26] training regimen

6   Vein Doppler Ultrasound Mapping

Traditionally, ultrasound vein assessment is carried out for cardiac surgery patients with varicosities clinical indications of potentially poor vein conduits and history of vascular diseases [16]. However, the recent UK National Institute of Clinical Excellence 2014 guidelines rightly insist that all patients who undergo vein harvesting for CABG surgery should undergo ultrasound mapping to identify the quality, size, depth (Fig. 2), placements (Fig. 3) and anatomical variations of the GSV. The use of ultrasound by the anaesthetist for insertion of the central venous line has become mandatory and it is readily available with low cost to the theatre department. The use of these machines for GSV assessment prior to vein harvesting can therefore help the EVH practitioner to understand the depth of the vein and where to make the skin incision. It can also identify the size of the vein and any abnormalities. GSV anatomical variations can range from 20 to 40%, which can be easily detected by the ultrasound guided scan and this helps the practitioner to plan the surgical technique and pick the appropriate leg [40].

Studies have demonstrated that the scanning of veins prior to coronary surgery minimises unnecessary surgical skin incisions, reduces the risk of postoperative wound complications, particularly in female, obese and diabetic patients, and allows accurate prediction of the anatomy and size of the harvested veins. They have also concluded that the use of ultrasound by the practitioners/surgeons in theatre prior to surgery or the day before surgery is feasible, simple, and reduces the surgical harvest

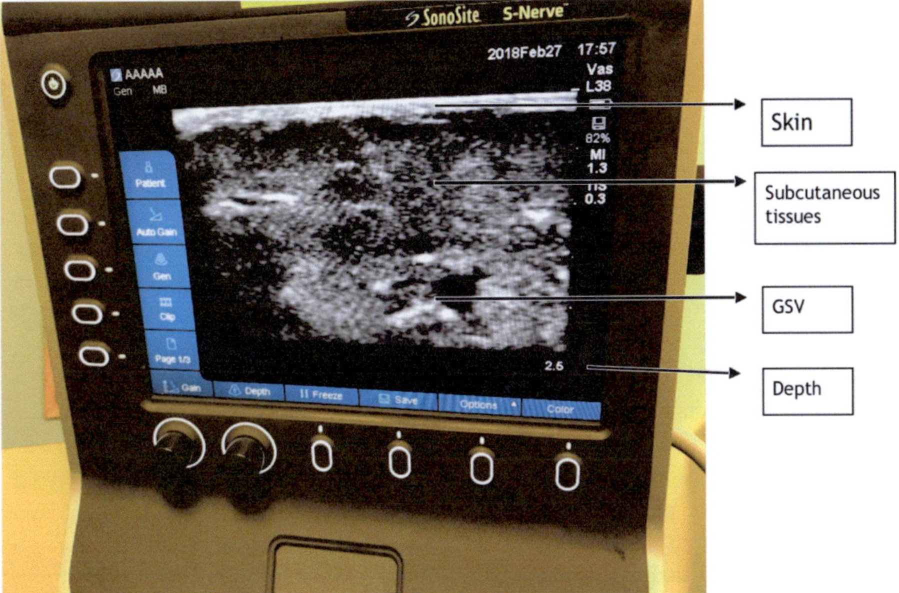

Fig. 2 Illustrates the vein doppler scan with the long saphenous vein on the transverse section

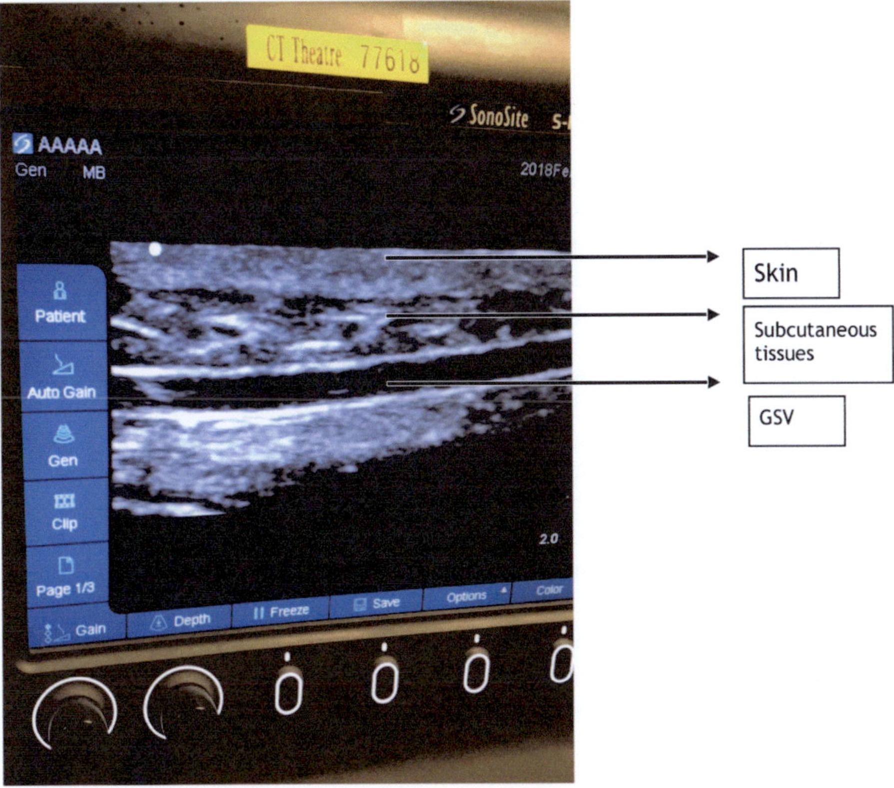

Fig. 3 Illustrates the longitudinal vein doppler scan of the long saphenous vein

time, is cost effective and diminishes postoperative morbidity [16, 40–43].

The use of a vascular lab scientist to scan each and every cardiac surgery patient can be very expensive, and as such this needs to be audited and a cost analysis performed. In order to minimise the cost impact of scanning each patient, the SCPs who are trained to work as part of the surgical team in cardiac theatres should take the role of routine ultrasound scanning of the veins if no additional co-morbidities are present. This will also be beneficial in reducing the pressure and workload of the vascular scientist. However, this panel suggests that the patients with severe varicosities, peripheral vascular disease and clinical signs of poor vein conduits need to be sent to the vascular department for detailed scanning including radial artery perfusion scanning. There should be a national protocol/guideline on how to scan, when to scan and when to refer the patient to the vascular department in order to prevent increased costs and unnecessary delays in most patients.

Importantly, there are no accredited vein mapping courses for SCPs in Great Britain to teach the basic theoretical knowledge, hands on practical skills and competency curriculum which need to be devised as a matter of urgency. It is important to teach practitioners these skills in a structured competency-based curriculum for patient and practitioner safety. We believe that in-house training on how to scan needs to be stopped and an agreed curriculum developed to deliver a high standard educational programme.

7 Importance of Heparinisation Prior to EVH Technique

All EVH surgical patients need to be heparinised as part of the best surgical practice. The veins taken by endoscopic surgery are at high risk of developing micro intraluminal clots inside the vein lumen [44]. Studies performed without pre-heparinisation have demonstrated a nonsignificant trend towards reduced patency of the harvested GSV, which may be due to intraluminal clot formation [45, 46]. The heparin should be

given intravenous once the vein is identified and at least five minutes before starting the vein dissection. According to Brown et al., pre-heparinisation did not change blood loss or transfusion requirements but the experience of this panel is different. The use of 5000 units' heparin for all patients without exclusion can increase blood loss during sternotomy and internal mammary artery harvesting. Each panel members have experience of at least 1000 cases of EVH, with some members having performed over 3000 cases. Our recommendation would be to provide a lower (2500 units) dose to patients who have been receiving antiplatelet medications until the day before surgery to avoid risk of bleeding and haematoma formation. Patients who have stopped the use of anticoagulants as part of normal local practice seven days prior to the surgery should be administered 5000 IU of heparin systemically to avoid intraluminal clots in the harvested vein [31, 35, 44].

7.1 Diathermy Settings

Most surgical procedures use diathermy, which is the process of using electricity to produce cauterisation burn at the point of contact [47]. In the infancy of endoscopic surgery, bipolar diathermy was considered as an accurate control of the electric current by limiting the thermal spread into the surrounding tissues. However, the new latest technologies such as the Harmonic Scalpel™ (Ethicon, Endo-surgery, Cincinnati, Ohio, USA) and Ligasure™ (Valleylab, Boulder, Colorado, USA) are better than the traditional bipolar diathermy for many endoscopic surgeries [48, 49]. The Hemopro™ diathermy system has the same effect as Harmonic Scalpel™, which has a generator, an ultrasonic transducer and an instrument. This system produces ultrasonic energy which directly controls the bleeding through the process of coaptive coagulation which allows cut-and seal without thermal spread [24]. In contrast, the Ligasure utilises a mixture of pressure and current to melt the collagen and elastin comprised within the blood vessel walls and then seals the vessels [24].

In the EVH surgical procedure, the bipolar and Hemopro diathermy systems are used. From the introduction of EVH equipment in the mid-1990s, there are many instances in the literature of surgeons concerned about the intimal electrocautery damage mainly due to thermal spread into the intima. If we look at the different equipment available between1990 and now, company product research has evolved to make single handed equipment instead of multiple different items. This is a significant improvement as it minimises the risk of damage to the vein due to repeated insertion of multiple instruments to harvest the vein endoscopically.

The bipolar diathermy EVH system requires the application of electrosurgical energy which is always controlled by a foot switch. The harvester needs to be very careful especially on EVH technique to make sure that there is enough length left on the side branches from the base of the vein to avoid any damage caused during cauterisation. Leaving at least 1 cm branch length from the base of the vein will prevent thermal spread to the main conduit. However, there has been no study performed to evaluate the extent of the thermal spread from the bipolar cautery tip to the base of the vein in patient samples. A porcine study comparing the spread of heat on monopolar, bipolar, harmonic scalpel and ligasure concluded that there is no change of temperature more than 1 cm from the tip of the instrument [47]. Until more definitive data is collected from thermal studies on the vein, the panel believe that it is best practice to keep more than 1 cm distance from the base of the vein branch to avoid heat and thermal spread.

Intriguingly, only one company (Getinge™) [50] has mentioned that their equipment uses in-line instrumentation with strategies to mitigate thermal spread by using Hemopro 2 technology which seals the vein with cut in a single step. Their Hemopro 2 simultaneous cut-and-seal technology virtually eliminates the thermal spread beyond the device. There is also a safety system inbuilt so that the Hemopro 2 system does not produce any heat or shorten branches which

consequently preserves the integrity of the harvested vein [51]. However, there is no histological study to determine the effect of thermal spread on harvested veins.

From the collective panel, who have the experience of performing more than 5000 EVH procedures, the recommendation is to set the Hemopro diathermy between 2 and 2.5 [31] in order to avoid any burning and cause minimal damage to the small/thin hairline branches. The use of Hemopro 2 until release of resistance followed by visual confirmation of branch and/or connective tissue ligation is significantly better practice than pulling or intermittent diathermy use. The Getinge™ EVH user manual [50] recommendation of setting at 3 and above is too much for any GSV branches unless you have a duplicate GSV with diameter greater more than 0.4 cm on the ultrasound. The other companies using bipolar diathermy for EVH recommends around 15 W to 30 W [52]. However, in order to reduce the thermal damage to the vein, 10 W might be better.

This area needs to be explored in more depth as a multicentre randomised control trial to determine the optimal device and settings for future use.

7.2 CO$_2$ Settings and Insufflation

Most of the EVH systems utilise CO_2 insufflation (open or closed tunnel) as a method to create a subcutaneous tunnel for tissue dissection and for clear visualisation [35, 53]. The insufflation helps to create a subcutaneous tunnel which directly facilitates the harvesting of the GSV without working close to the vessel. The insufflated CO_2 is normally absorbed by the blood stream and eliminated by the lungs [54]. However, the insufflation can cause CO_2 embolism and hypercarbia via absorption through an injured GSV. If the CO_2 enters directly into the blood stream, it can result in the stimulation of the sympathetic nervous system [35, 52]. These life-threatening events are very rare in cardiac surgery due to careful monitoring by the transoesophageal echo (TOE), end-tidal carbon dioxide (EtCO_2) and haemodynamic monitoring as a gold standard [55].

Studies in the literature have reported CO_2 embolism occurrence if the company recommendation of 12 to 15 mmHg pressure are used on the tunnel [35, 54, 56]. However, the current recommendation from the Getinge White paper is that the harvesters should set their pressure setting to as low as possible to avoid any complications. However, there is no mention of recommended numbers.

From the panel experience, the pressure setting should be kept to 10 mmHg [31, 35] and the flow setting at 3 L of CO_2 per minute. Moreover, making the skin incision longer by a few millimetres, will avoid having a tight fit of the sealing port. This way, the flow of CO_2 is not going to create a tight tunnel and also compress the GSV on the port site. Many practitioners do not inflate the sealing port to avoid any damage to the vein on the entry site which is also best practice. However, in obese patients, creating the tunnel and keeping the subcutaneous tissue away from the vein is important for clear visualisation and minimising the damage to the vein.

Many cardiac surgeons worry about the acidic environment and the damage to the endothelium with CO_2 insufflation. The optimal pH for endothelial cell viability ranges between pH 7.3 and 7.4 and below this points the acidic environment can damage vessel viability [22, 35, 57]. A study comparing the absorption of CO_2 and endothelial integrity has shown no statistical difference in conduit integrity but there was a drop in pH in the vein harvested by an experienced practitioner [35]. During the learning curve period, the novice practitioner is likely to take a longer time to harvest the GSV and this prolonged CO_2 exposure can create an acidic environment. Improved training of the novice practitioner with a structured programme and teaching them the importance of acidosis and vein preservation can reduce the time of harvesting and improve the quality of the vein.

8 Harvesting the Vein with Surrounding Tissues During EVH

The panel believes that harvesting the vein with minimal surrounding tissues (Fig. 4) during EVH is preferable to complete stripping of the adjacent tissues and adventitia, which can lead to destruction of the vasa-vasorum of the GSV and intimal damage [22]. Dissecting the vein with surrounding tissue can protect the small vein tributaries and avoid a number of small branch avulsions at the base which can cause endothelial damage. Endothelial damage caused during vein harvesting can induce diminished release of nitric oxide, smooth muscle proliferation and finally intimal hyperplasia [22, 58]. Small avulsions must be sutured, which can increase cardiopulmonary bypass and surgical time. Also, these veins are not histologically analysed or followed up over the long-term, so it is unclear how well they perform compared to vessels without avulsions. As such, the panel recommends harvesting the vein with a layer of surrounding tissue in order to avoid any tearing of the vein and yielding a conduit of equal quality to that obtained with open vein harvesting.

9 Volume Thresholds and Learning Curve

9.1 Trainee Volume Threshold

No recommended consensus is available to confirm how many open or EVH cases need to be done by the novice practitioner to become an expert. There is little data available, especially for EVH, assessing the outcome associated with

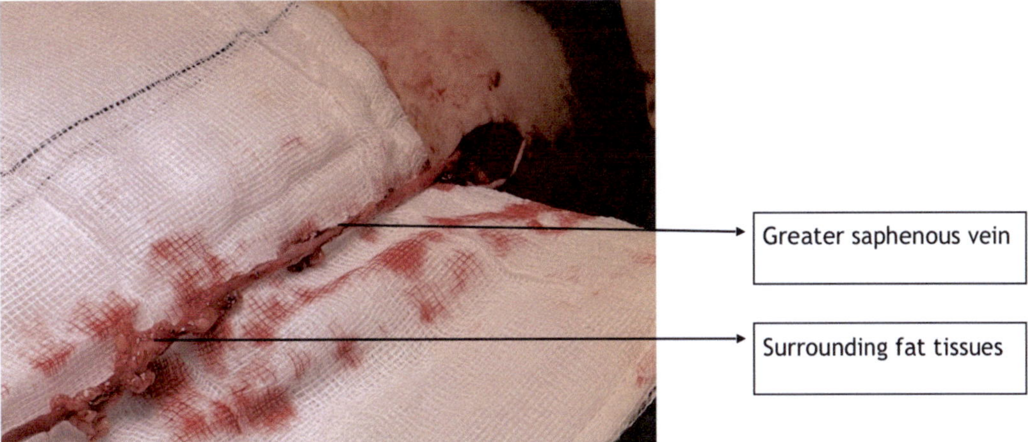

Fig. 4 This figure illustrates the GSV with minimal surrounding tissues

these practitioners. However, some studies suggest that the learning curve for EVH can vary from 20 to 50 cases [26, 33]. Every practitioner has their own rate at which they can acquire new skills and as such the learning curve is likely to be quite variable across a training cohort. Thus, it is important to allow these practitioners to have regular exposure and input to EVH cases in order to promote their acquisition of skills necessary to perform independently. This is particularly important for developing adequate hand eye co-ordination and familiarity with the intricacies of the EVH equipment. Regular audits must be performed to evaluate their clinical outcomes and determine where further guidance may be required to ensure optimal performance. In the recently published REGROUP trial, a minimum experience with 100 EVH cases was required in order to participate as a GSV harvester in any research or audit study [11].

Novice practitioners should be asked to do at least 10 (depends upon the manual dexterity) open vein harvesting cases in order to familiarise themselves with the surgical techniques, anatomical course of the vein and how to avoid any complications prior to attempting EVH. The consensus is that for EVH the trainee should be performing at least 25 cases with gradually increasing complexity. Undertaking competency-based e-learning EVH training rather than in-house training should be encouraged.

9.2 Competency Volume Threshold for Experienced Practitioners

Other surgical areas have suggested volume and outcome thresholds for the surgeons [21, 59–61] yet there is absence of substantial evidence in the literature for EVH practitioners. The practitioners or surgeons who are undertaking EVH should be performing more than 50 cases per year in order to maintain their skills in clinical practice. This continual exposure to the technique should ensure familiarity and build practitioner confidence, which may translate into better quality conduits and improved outcomes for CABG surgery. Volume of cases by practitioners need to be recorded on a local or national database and monitored to ensure the highest quality of outcomes is achieved.

9.3 Continuous Professional Development

The relevant practitioner associations and societies should provide further training, which could involve simulation-based courses held annually in order to train practitioners on endoscopic surgical skills. These are currently not included in their national curriculum for cardiothoracic surgery. An annual update and training on new technology will improve their evidence-based learning and also assist them in continuous professional development.

10 Use of Pressure-Controlled Syringe

Intraoperative over-distension or unregulated pressure applied to the vein can induce graft injury, neointimal hyperplasia and graft failure [62, 63]. Intraluminal pressures can go above 600 mmHg with manual handheld syringe distension [64–66]. Studies have concluded that pressure below 100 mmHg is sufficient to allow assessment of the conduit with no damage to the endothelium, whereas pressures greater than 140 mmHg can damage the intima of the vein [63, 67, 68]. The panel also recommends the use of pressure-controlled syringes as a standard of care in CABG surgery to avoid manual over distension of the vein during vein preparation, which should reduce the endothelial damage at this stage. Importantly, there currently remains no standardised recommendation for the amount of pressure to set for vein distension during preparation.

11 Use of Closed Vacuum Suction Drain on the Leg

The EVH technique requires the formation of a tunnel in the leg to harvest the GSV. It is known that this has the potential to cause haematoma formation and bruising of the donor leg after GSV harvesting. A randomised study has concluded that the insertion of vacuum drains in EVH patients reduces haematoma formation, postoperative pain, reduces the need for administration of antibiotics and improves patient satisfaction with better cosmetic appearance [69]. Many surgeons do not like drains due to the high volume of blood collected in the drain bottle as a result of being fully heparinised during the bypass time period. The insertion of a vacuum drain and bandaging the leg with Gamgee pad should be performed immediately but the drain system should be unlocked 20 min after heparin reversal (protamine administration) in order to prevent unnecessary blood loss. The drain can be removed on the first postoperative day to prevent any drain related infection and colonisation of bacteria.

12 Avoiding Potential Complications

Many studies have demonstrated the odds of wound complications are reduced significantly by up to 71% with EVH compared to OVH [14]. However, during the learning curve, the selection of patients and careful dissection is important to avoid complications such as compartment syndrome [70], necrotising fasciitis [71], pneumoperitoneum [72] and scrotal distension [73]. These are the only four reported case studies; however, we believe there are more than these four cases and that many of these complications are treated locally and not reported.

- The patients who had a scrotal distension had a history of inguinal hernia repair or weakness of the muscular wall. It is vital for the novice practitioner to obtain a detailed history of these patients before selecting them for EVH with CO_2 insufflation. The same applies for the pneumoperitoneum patient. Careful dissection is required, especially on the thigh and teaching the novice practitioner to not go above the femoral triangle and stop the dissection close to the groin crease can avoid causing pneumoperitoneum and other related complications.
- The compartment syndrome and necrotising fasciitis can be avoided by not performing fasciotomy for thin/superficial vein patients and staying on the GSV plane without creating any unnecessary pockets or pseudo-tunnels. Careful ultrasound scanning by the practitioner who is going to perform the EVH

procedure to understand the complete anatomy and the course of the vein is important. Staying within the EVH rules of dissection is important [50]. This involves anterior, posterior and lateral dissections rather than random dissection, which can lead to the unnecessary creation of pseudo-tunnels. Going into the muscular plane can potentially cause unwanted complications in EVH.

13 Audit

The practitioners or surgeons who are routinely carrying out endoscopic vein harvesting should subject their results to regular audit which should include the full short-term and long-term outcomes of these EVH patients. There should be a system locally or nationally such as a registry where all the EVH patients can be entered and monitored for any morbidity and mortality related to myocardial infarction, recurrent angina or death. Maintaining these types of vital data can support the cardiac surgeons, EVH practitioners, cardiologists, guideline makers and finally patients to choose their surgical technique according to the clinical evidence from their local hospital.

This data can help in patient selection and in determining or ruling out graft patency issues directly related to EVH technique. Such data can also improve our understanding of what variables impact the quality of the conduits harvested by novice and expert EVH practitioners. In addition to all vital patient data, the audit registry should compile important variables such as the number of veins, harvesting time, experience of the practitioner, surgical technique, quality of the vein before surgery (any scan reports), predisposing vein related factors (vein diseases etc.) and quality of the harvested vein. These cardiac surgery registries should be combined with the other registries to get accurate data and it should be presented to the wider multidisciplinary community to obtain wide support.

14 Discussion

It is an under appreciated fact that conduit harvesting is a crucial aspect of coronary surgery, despite it being considered to be a junior doctors/practitioner's job. If the quality of the vein is not good, then it has a direct impact on the outcome of that patient. Therefore, it is vital to train these practitioners to the highest possible level using competency-based training and provide them with continuous professional development opportunities and education to maintain and advance their surgical skills.

Graft failure in CABG surgery is multifactorial and most of the patients have re-occurrence of symptoms or require coronary reinterventions within 15 postoperative years [74, 75]. However, poor quality harvested conduits (whether EVH or OVH) is one modifiable risk factor that contributes to early graft failure. When EVH is performed correctly, it is associated with significant benefits, although there are also some practical difficulties to its use. The aim of this panel in proposing these EVH best practice standards is to highlight the best practice and minimise the effect of factors associated with surgical technique that could predispose to early graft failure due to intimal proliferation [36].

This document has demonstrated that it is possible to define the best practice standards for processes and outcomes for EVH by consensus of a multidisciplinary group of clinicians and practitioners. We are not aware of any existing best practice standards for EVH but there are training manuals and video clips which do not insist on factors which have been mentioned by this panel.

The proposed standards in this document are based on the current literature, from which there are many good systematic reviews, a limited number of randomised controlled trials, meta-analysis, as well as cohort/retrospective studies alongside strong recommendation from ISMICS class B evidence for EVH use.

This document has given many options for the regular EVH practitioners to audit their current practice and benchmark it against other national and international standards.

This proposed best practice standards document has used current evidence but still there are a number of unknown factors that are yet to be optimised. These include vein distension pressures, inexperience vs experienced practitioners, volume threshold on both trainees and experienced harvesters and the effect of thermal spread on the EVH vein with bipolar and Hemopro diathermy. These factors require further evaluation in future studies before our recommendations can be updated. Finally, there remains no validated competency based EVH training programme, which must be produced, evaluated and implemented into common practice.

15 Conclusion

Whilst EVH is adopted as a standard of care in United States with approximately 90% usage in CABG procedures [11], other centres worldwide have a much lower rate of use. This is due to a lack of appropriately trained personnel, learning curves and the institutional cost of implementation [76]. However, the benefits that can be achieved with EVH suggest that it is important to utilise this technique whenever it is feasible. To minimise concern, it is vital that the training provided to practitioners is of high quality. More investment in producing a structured training programme is required. This must ensure that the trainee receives one-to-one training and regular practice on a daily/weekly basis, with incremental advances in the input of the trainee to the case. Most studies have concluded that there is no difference between OVH and EVH if it is performed by an expert practitioner.

All endoscopic procedures are reliant on adequate training as this involves a shift of the surgeon from looking at the field of surgery to a larger high-definition magnified view on a large screen. This shift needs to be managed and audited in order to avoid any compromise in outcomes during this transition period. This document is a first attempt at trying to establish a set of standards that should be matched to achieve a safe and smooth shift. We believe that today there is less of an appetite to accept learning curves and all attempts should be made to avoid their impact in introducing new technology into the NHS. The strength of this document is that this is a consensus document based on best available literature put together by individuals who have been involved in introducing this technology over the past decade safely in NHS organisations. To achieve wider dissemination, we believe this best practice document will help new centres and surgeons to be confident that they are able to access this comprehensive document.

It is time to reform the training of these novice practitioners to have a structured learning curve of EVH to obtain good quality veins to provide best care for our patients.

16 Competing Interests

BK has been an international EVH trainer for the Sorin EVH Company and worked on an e-learning platform as an EVH consultant for Getinge company. She is also a NIHR postdoctoral fellow exploring the use of structured based training programme for all EVH users. She holds a clinical post as a surgical care practitioner at Manchester Foundation trust and professor of Surgical Practice at the University of Salford.

JZ: None related to this document.

Acknowledgements I would like to acknowledge all the experts who have given their expert advice for this chapter are Prof. Simon Ray (Manchester Foundation Trust hospital, Manchester, UK), Mr. Simon Kendall (South Teesside university hospital, Teesside, UK), Mr. Heyman Luckraz (American Dubai hospital, Dubai, UAE), Prof. Marco A Zenati (Harvard Medical School, Boston, MA), Dr. Keith Allen (St. Luke's Mid America Heart Institute, Kansas City, MO) and Mr. Jared Blackmore (Miami Valley Hospital, Dayton, OH).

References

1. Salsano A, Mariscalco G, Santini F. Endoscopic saphenous vein harvesting and surgical site infections after coronary artery bypass surgery. Ann Transl Med. 2018;6(Suppl 1):S37.
2. Dimitrova KR, Hoffman DM, Geller CM, Dincheva G, Ko W, Tranbaugh RF. Arterial grafts protect the native coronary vessels from atherosclerotic disease progression. Ann Thorac Surg. 2012;94 (2):475–81.
3. Locker C, Schaff HV, Dearani JA, Joyce LD, Park SJ, Burkhart HM, et al. Multiple arterial grafts improve late survival of patients undergoing coronary artery bypass graft surgery: analysis of 8622 patients with multivessel disease. Circulation. 2012;126(9):1023–30.
4. Alexander JH, Smith PK. Coronary-artery bypass grafting. N Engl J Med. 2016;374(20):1954–64.
5. Head SJ, Milojevic M, Taggart DP, Puskas JD. Current practice of state-of-the-art surgical coronary revascularization. Circulation. 2017;136(14):1331–45.
6. Verma S, Mazer CD. Open or endoscopic vein harvesting for coronary-artery bypass grafting. N Engl J Med. 2019;380(2):189–91.
7. Sastry P, Rivinius R, Harvey R, Parker RA, Rahm AK, Thomas D, et al. The influence of endoscopic vein harvesting on outcomes after coronary bypass grafting: a meta-analysis of 267,525 patients. Eur J Cardiothorac Surg. 2013;44(6):980–9.
8. Allen KB, Griffith GL, Heimansohn DA, Robison RJ, Matheny RG, Schier JJ, et al. Endoscopic versus traditional saphenous vein harvesting: a prospective, randomized trial. Ann Thorac Surg. 1998;66(1):26–31; discussion -2.
9. Lumsden AB, Eaves FF 3rd, Ofenloch JC, Jordan WD. Subcutaneous, video-assisted saphenous vein harvest: report of the first 30 cases. Cardiovasc Surg. 1996;4(6):771–6.
10. Accord R, Maessen J. Endoscopic vein harvesting for coronary bypass grafting: a blessing or a trojan horse? Cardiol Res Pract. 2011;2011: 813512.
11. Zenati MA, Bhatt DL, Bakaeen FG, Stock EM, Biswas K, Gaziano JM, et al. Randomized trial of endoscopic or open vein-graft harvesting for coronary-artery bypass. N Engl J Med. 2019;380(2):132–41.
12. Raja SG, Sarang Z. Endoscopic vein harvesting: technique, outcomes, concerns & controversies. J Thorac Dis. 2013;5(Suppl 6):S630–7.
13. Kodia K, Patel S, Weber MP, Luc JGY, Choi JH, Maynes EJ, et al. Graft patency after open versus endoscopic saphenous vein harvest in coronary artery bypass grafting surgery: a systematic review and meta-analysis. Ann Cardiothorac Surg. 2018;7 (5):586–97.
14. Ferdinand FD, MacDonald JK, Balkhy HH, Bisleri G, Hwang HY, Northrup P, et al. Endoscopic conduit harvest in coronary artery bypass grafting surgery: an ISMICS systematic review and consensus conference statements. Innovations (Phila). 2017;12(5):301–19.
15. Lopes RD, Hafley GE, Allen KB, Ferguson TB, Peterson ED, Harrington RA, et al. Endoscopic versus open vein-graft harvesting in coronary-artery bypass surgery. N Engl J Med. 2009;361(3):235–44.
16. Aguirre V, Connolly C, Stuklis R, Cullen H, Viana F, Worthington M. Surgeon's focussed ultrasound examination of the long saphenous vein reduces surgical time and wound complications. Heart Lung Circ. 2019;28(11):1735–9.
17. Grant SW, Grayson AD, Zacharias J, Dalrymple-Hay MJ, Waterworth PD, Bridgewater B. What is the impact of endoscopic vein harvesting on clinical outcomes following coronary artery bypass graft surgery? Heart. 2012;98(1):60–4.
18. Ouzounian M, Ali IS. Endoscopic versus open saphenous vein harvest technique in the randomized on/off bypass (ROOBY) trial. J Thorac Cardiovasc Surg. 2011;142(3):724–5; author reply 5.
19. Allen KB, Heimansohn DA, Robison RJ, Schier JJ, Griffith GL, Fitzgerald EB. Influence of endoscopic versus traditional saphenectomy on event-free survival: five-year follow-up of a prospective randomized trial. Heart Surg Forum. 2003;6(6):E143–5.
20. Zenati MA, Shroyer AL, Collins JF, Hattler B, Ota T, Almassi GH, et al. Impact of endoscopic versus open saphenous vein harvest technique on late coronary artery bypass grafting patient outcomes in the ROOBY (Randomized On/Off Bypass) Trial. J Thorac Cardiovasc Surg. 2011;141(2):338–44.
21. Bridgewater B, Hooper T, Munsch C, Hunter S, von Oppell U, Livesey S, et al. Mitral repair best practice: proposed standards. Heart. 2006;92(7):939–44.
22. Krishnamoorthy B, Critchley WR, Venkateswaran RV, Barnard J, Caress A, Fildes JE, et al. A comprehensive review on learning curve associated problems in endoscopic vein harvesting and the requirement for a standardised training programme. J Cardiothorac Surg. 2016;11:45.
23. Francis SE, Holt CM, Taylor T, Gadsdon P, Angelini GD. Heparin and neointimal thickening in an organ culture of human saphenous vein. Atherosclerosis. 1992;93(1–2):155–6.
24. Koch C, Friedrich T, Metternich F, Tannapfel A, Reimann HP, Eichfeld U. Determination of temperature elevation in tissue during the application of the harmonic scalpel. Ultrasound Med Biol. 2003;29 (2):301–9.
25. Caliskan E, Sandner S, Misfeld M, Aramendi J, Salzberg SP, Choi YH, et al. A novel endothelial damage inhibitor for the treatment of vascular conduits in coronary artery bypass grafting: protocol and rationale for the European, multicentre, prospective, observational DuraGraft registry. J Cardiothorac Surg. 2019;14(1):174.
26. Krishnamoorthy B, Critchley WR, Bhinda P, Crockett J, John A, Bridgewater BJ, et al. Does the introduction of a comprehensive structured training

programme for endoscopic vein harvesting improve conduit quality? A multicentre pilot study. Interact Cardiovasc Thorac Surg. 2015;20(2):186–93.

27. Oklu R, Habito R, Mayr M, Deipolyi AR, Albadawi H, Hesketh R, et al. Pathogenesis of varicose veins. J Vasc Interv Radiol. 2012;23(1):33–9; quiz 40.

28. Wali MA, Dewan M, Eid RA. Histopathological changes in the wall of varicose veins. Int Angiol. 2003;22(2):188–93.

29. Elsharawy MA, Naim MM, Abdelmaguid EM, Al-Mulhim AA. Role of saphenous vein wall in the pathogenesis of primary varicose veins. Interact Cardiovasc Thorac Surg. 2007;6(2):219–24.

30. Travers JP, Brookes CE, Evans J, Baker DM, Kent C, Makin GS, et al. Assessment of wall structure and composition of varicose veins with reference to collagen, elastin and smooth muscle content. Eur J Vasc Endovasc Surg. 1996;11(2):230–7.

31. Krishnamoorthy B, Critchley WR, Thompson AJ, Payne K, Morris J, Venkateswaran RV, et al. Study comparing vein integrity and clinical outcomes in open vein harvesting and 2 types of endoscopic vein harvesting for coronary artery bypass grafting: the VICO randomized clinical trial (vein integrity and clinical outcomes). Circulation. 2017;136(18):1688–702.

32. Howie DW, Beck M, Costi K, Pannach SM, Ganz R. Mentoring in complex surgery: minimising the learning curve complications from peri-acetabular osteotomy. Int Orthop. 2012;36(5):921–5.

33. Chiu KM, Chen CL, Chu SH, Lin TY. Endoscopic harvest of saphenous vein: a lesson learned from 1,348 cases. Surg Endosc. 2008;22(1):183–7.

34. Dangel M, Lowe B, Pfeiffer S, Gulielmos V. Schuler S [A comparative study of minimal invasive harvesting of vena saphena magna segments]. Langenbecks Arch Chir Suppl Kongressbd. 1998;115:1305–7.

35. Krishnamoorthy B, Critchley WR, Nair J, Malagon I, Carey J, Barnard JB, et al. Randomized study comparing the effect of carbon dioxide insufflation on veins using 2 types of endoscopic and open vein harvesting. Innovations (Phila). 2017;12(5):320–8.

36. Sabik JF 3rd, Blackstone EH, Gillinov AM, Smedira NG, Lytle BW. Occurrence and risk factors for reintervention after coronary artery bypass grafting. Circulation. 2006;114(1 Suppl):I454–60.

37. Souza DS, Dashwood MR, Tsui JC, Filbey D, Bodin L, Johansson B, et al. Improved patency in vein grafts harvested with surrounding tissue: results of a randomized study using three harvesting techniques. Ann Thorac Surg. 2002;73(4):1189–95.

38. Kiani S, Poston R. Is endoscopic harvesting bad for saphenous vein graft patency in coronary surgery? Curr Opin Cardiol. 2011;26(6):518–22.

39. Robinson WP, Doucet DR, Simons JP, Wyman A, Aiello FA, Arous E, et al. An intensive vascular surgical skills and simulation course for vascular trainees improves procedural knowledge and self-rated procedural competence. J Vasc Surg. 2017;65 (3):907–15 e3.

40. Luckraz H, Lowe J, Pugh N, Azzu AA. Pre-operative long saphenous vein mapping predicts vein anatomy and quality leading to improved post-operative leg morbidity. Interact Cardiovasc Thorac Surg. 2008;7 (2):188–91; discussion 91.

41. Lopes FC, Oliveira OWB, Moreira DG, Santos MAD, Oliveira JLR, Cruz CB, et al. Use of Doppler ultrasound for saphenous vein mapping to obtain grafts for coronary artery bypass grafting. Braz J Cardiovasc Surg. 2018;33(2):189–93.

42. Noritomi DT, Zigaib R, Ranzani OT, Teich V. Evaluation of cost-effectiveness from the funding body's point of view of ultrasound-guided central venous catheter insertion compared with the conventional technique. Rev Bras Ter Intensiva. 2016;28 (1):62–9.

43. Matera JT, Egerton-Warburton D, Meek R. Ultrasound guidance for central venous catheter placement in Australasian emergency departments: potential barriers to more widespread use. Emerg Med Australas. 2010;22(6):514–23.

44. Brown EN, Kon ZN, Tran R, Burris NS, Gu J, Laird P, et al. Strategies to reduce intraluminal clot formation in endoscopically harvested saphenous veins. J Thorac Cardiovasc Surg. 2007;134(5):1259–65.

45. Perrault LP, Jeanmart H, Bilodeau L, Lesperance J, Tanguay JF, Bouchard D, et al. Early quantitative coronary angiography of saphenous vein grafts for coronary artery bypass grafting harvested by means of open versus endoscopic saphenectomy: a prospective randomized trial. J Thorac Cardiovasc Surg. 2004;127(5):1402–7.

46. Burris N, Schwartz K, Brown J, Kwon M, Pierson R 3rd, Griffith B, et al. Incidence of residual clot strands in saphenous vein grafts after endoscopic harvest. Innovations (Phila). 2006;1(6):323–7.

47. Sutton PA, Awad S, Perkins AC, Lobo DN. Comparison of lateral thermal spread using monopolar and bipolar diathermy, the Harmonic Scalpel and the Ligasure. Br J Surg. 2010;97(3):428–33.

48. Liang J, Xing H, Chang Y. Thermal damage width and hemostatic effect of bipolar electrocoagulation, LigaSure, and Ultracision techniques on goat mesenteric vessels and optimal power for bipolar electrocoagulation. BMC Surg. 2019;19(1):147.

49. Kunde D, Welch C. Ultracision in gynaecological laparoscopic surgery. J Obstet Gynaecol. 2003;23 (4):347–52.

50. Getinge, inventor endoscopic vessel harvesting: using advancement and best practices to enhance conduit quality. 2018.

51. Zingaro C, Cefarelli M, Berretta P, Matteucci S, Pierri M, Di Eusanio M. Endoscopic vein-graft harvesting in coronary artery bypass surgery: tips and tricks. Multimed Man Cardiothorac Surg. 2019.

52. Zingaro C, Pierri MD, Massi F, Matteucci ML, Capestro F, D'Alfonso A, et al. Absorption of carbon

dioxide during endoscopic vein harvest. Interact Cardiovasc Thorac Surg. 2012;15(4):661–4.

53. Maslow AM, Schwartz CS, Bert A, Hurlburt P, Gough J, Stearns G, et al. Endovascular vein harvest: systemic carbon dioxide absorption. J Cardiothorac Vasc Anesth. 2006;20(3):347–52.

54. Crozier TA. Anesthesiologic aspects of minimally invasive surgery. Zentralbl Chir. 1993;118(10):573–81.

55. Standards for Basic Anesthetic Monitoring. American Society of Anesthesiologists 2005.

56. Chavanon O, Tremblay I, Delay D, Bouveret A, Blain R, Perrault LP. Carbon dioxide embolism during endoscopic saphenectomy for coronary artery bypass surgery. J Thorac Cardiovasc Surg. 1999;118 (3):557–8.

57. Rousou LJ, Taylor KB, Lu XG, Healey N, Crittenden MD, Khuri SF, et al. Saphenous vein conduits harvested by endoscopic technique exhibit structural and functional damage. Ann Thorac Surg. 2009;87 (1):62–70.

58. Sepehripour AH, Jarral OA, Shipolini AR, McCormack DJ. Does a "no-touch" technique result in better vein patency? Interact Cardiovasc Thorac Surg. 2011;13(6):626–30.

59. Hannan EL, Wu C, Ryan TJ, Bennett E, Culliford AT, Gold JP, et al. Do hospitals and surgeons with higher coronary artery bypass graft surgery volumes still have lower risk-adjusted mortality rates? Circulation. 2003;108(7):795–801.

60. Bridgewater B, Grayson AD, Jackson M, Brooks N, Grotte GJ, Keenan DJ, et al. Surgeon specific mortality in adult cardiac surgery: comparison between crude and risk stratified data. BMJ. 2003;327(7405):13–7.

61. Dimick JB, Cowan JA Jr, Stanley JC, Henke PK, Pronovost PJ, Upchurch GR Jr. Surgeon specialty and provider volumes are related to outcome of intact abdominal aortic aneurysm repair in the United States. J Vasc Surg. 2003;38(4):739–44.

62. Tineli RA, Viaro F, Dalio MB, Reis GS, Basseto S, Vicente WV, et al. Mechanical forces and human saphenous veins: coronary artery bypass graft implications. Rev Bras Cir Cardiovasc. 2007;22(1):87–95.

63. Angelini GD, Breckenridge IM, Psaila JV, Williams HM, Henderson AH, Newby AC. Preparation of human saphenous vein for coronary artery bypass grafting impairs its capacity to produce prostacyclin. Cardiovasc Res. 1987;21(1):28–33.

64. Zhao J, Andreasen JJ, Yang J, Rasmussen BS, Liao D, Gregersen H. Manual pressure distension of the human saphenous vein changes its biomechanical properties-implication for coronary artery bypass grafting. J Biomech. 2007;40(10):2268–76.

65. Okon EB, Millar MJ, Crowley CM, Bashir JG, Cook RC, Hsiang YN, et al. Effect of moderate pressure distention on the human saphenous vein vasomotor function. Ann Thorac Surg. 2004;77 (1):108–14; discussion 14–5.

66. Wise ES, Brophy CM. The case for endothelial preservation via pressure-regulated distension in the preparation of autologous saphenous vein conduits in cardiac and peripheral bypass operations. Front Surg. 2016;3:54.

67. Li FD, Eagle S, Brophy C, Hocking KM, Osgood M, Komalavilas P, et al. Pressure control during preparation of saphenous veins. JAMA Surg. 2014;149 (7):655–62.

68. Wise ES, Hocking KM, Feldman D, Komalavilas P, Cheung-Flynn J, Brophy CM. An optimized preparation technique for saphenous vein graft. Am Surg. 2015;81(7):E274–6.

69. Krishnamoorthy B, Al-Fagih OS, Madi MI, Najam O, Waterworth PD, Fildes JE, et al. Closed suction drainage improves clinical outcome in patients undergoing endoscopic vein harvesting for coronary artery bypass grafting. Ann Thorac Surg. 2012;93(4):1201–5.

70. Kolli A, Au JT, Lee DC, Klinoff N, Ko W. Compartment syndrome after endoscopic harvest of the great saphenous vein during coronary artery bypass grafting. Ann Thorac Surg. 2010;89(1):271–3.

71. Lihav B, Yakoub D, Kasabian A. Necrotizing fasciitis following endoscopic harvesting of the greater saphenous vein for coronary artery bypass graft. JSLS. 2011;15(1):90–5.

72. Lehmann A, Lang J, Weisse U, Boldt J. Pneumoperitoneum secondary to endoscopic harvest of saphenous vein graft. Ann Thorac Surg. 2000;69(6):1937–8.

73. Najam O, Krishnamoorthy B, Kadir I, Karagounis AP, Waterworth P, Fildes JE, et al. Scrotal distension after endoscopic harvesting of the saphenous vein in patients with inguinal hernia. Ann Thorac Surg. 2011;92(2):733–5.

74. Sergeant P, Lesaffre E, Flameng W, Suy R, Blackstone E. The return of clinically evident ischemia after coronary artery bypass grafting. Eur J Cardiothorac Surg. 1991;5(9):447–57.

75. Sergeant P, Blackstone E, Meyns B, Stockman B, Jashari R. First cardiological or cardiosurgical reintervention for ischemic heart disease after primary coronary artery bypass grafting. Eur J Cardiothorac Surg. 1998;14(5):480–7.

76. Hameed I, Naik A, Gaudino M. Commentary on: endoscopic vein harvesting for coronary artery bypass grafting in the UK: what we believe and what we do: a Commentary on the article "use of endoscopic vein harvesting (EVH) during coronary artery bypass grafting in United Kingdom: the EVH survey". Int J Surg. 2019;69:146–151. Int J Surg. 2019;70:103

Endoscopic Cardiac Surgery—Tips, Tricks and Traps; Endoscopic Vessel Harvesting for Coronary Artery Revascularization Surgery with a Non Sealed Reusable System

Fabrizio Rosati, Saurabh Gupta, and Gianluigi Bisleri

Abstract

Minimally invasive radial artery and saphenous vein graft harvesting gained popularity in the last decade as they showed to be safe and effective approaches associated with comparable results in terms of graft quality and long-term patency over conventional "open" techniques. Moreover, endoscopic harvesting technique provides clear advantages in terms of reduction in wound infections, neurological disturbances, pain, and patient satisfaction. This approach can be safely performed after adequate training and should be adopted as a standard of care.

Supplementary Information The online version contains supplementary material available at https://doi.org/10.1007/978-3-031-21104-1_5. The videos can be accessed individually by clicking the DOI link in the accompanying figure caption or by scanning this link with the SN More Media App.

F. Rosati
Division of Cardiac Surgery, Spedali Civili Di Brescia, University of Brescia, Brescia, Italy

S. Gupta
Division of Cardiac Surgery, Department of Surgery, McMaster University, Hamilton, ON, Canada

G. Bisleri (✉)
Division of Cardiac Surgery, St. Michael's Hospital, University of Toronto, Toronto, ON, Canada
e-mail: gianluigi.bisleri@utoronto.ca

Keywords

Revascularization surgery · Coronary artery bypass surgery · Graft harvesting · Minimally invasive cardiac surgery · Endoscopic graft harvesting · Endoscopic radial artery harvesting · Endoscopic saphenous vein harvesting · Non-sealed system · Grafts procurement

1 Introduction and Background

Endoscopic techniques for radial artery (RA) and saphenous vein graft (SVG) harvesting during coronary artery bypass surgery (CABG) are becoming well-established, especially in North America [1, 2]. Over the years, concerns around graft quality and long-term patency have been dispelled; ample evidence now exists demonstrating similar survival and major adverse cardiovascular events (MACE) at follow-up when comparing endoscopic harvesting techniques to conventional techniques [3–7]. Additionally, endoscopic harvesting techniques provide many advantages, including a reduction in wound infections, neurological disturbances, pain, and patient satisfaction [8–10]. This was especially evident in patients considered high risk for surgical site infection [11, 12]. Unfortunately, widespread uptake of endoscopic graft harvesting is hindered due to higher surgical costs associated

J. Zacharias (ed.), *Endoscopic Cardiac Surgery*, https://doi.org/10.1007/978-3-031-21104-1_5

with it. However, the initial surgical costs related to the instruments can be mitigated by the significantly lower incidence of perioperative complications, and—as a result—reduced use of resources and personnel for its management (antibiotics, special dressing, advanced wound care and wound care clinic involvement) [13, 14].

To date, endoscopic RA and SVG harvesting can be performed by using sealed or non-sealed systems. The latter avoids the use of a pressurized dissection tunnel, thus mitigating potential detrimental effects described for sealed systems in terms of endothelial damage and graft thrombosis [15, 16]. We aim to provide a thorough and step-by-step description of both RA and SVG endoscopic harvesting approach with a non-sealed system [17, 18].

2 Patient Selection

All patients requiring RA and/or SVG grafts for CABG could potentially benefit from an endoscopic harvesting approach. Allen's test is mandatory in order to confirm effective hand perfusion provided by the ipsilateral ulnar artery and avoid hand ischemia before endoscopic RA harvesting (ERAH). Although both arms may be selected, the non-dominant arm is preferred in most instances. Regarding endoscopic SVG harvesting (ESVH), a careful examination of both legs should be performed in order to detect diffuse signs of chronic venous insufficiency and varicosities that might impact the quality of the graft; furthermore, it is recommended to perform an ultrasound doppler of the saphenous vein on both legs while in the operating room, before patient's prepping.

Tips, tricks and traps: pulse-oximetry can improve sensitivity when Allen's test is performed. Despite not being mandatory, moving to the contralateral arm could be an option in case of recent radial angiography. If both RAs were used for diagnostic tests, ultrasound can rule out signs of dissection or pseudoaneurysm. In most instances, previous orthopaedic surgery (i.e. carpal tunnel syndrome) at the level of the volar surface of the wrist is not an absolute contraindication for ERAH. Furthermore, endoscopic left RA and right internal mammary artery harvesting can be performed without impediment for both operators. Obese patients or patients with particularly muscled forearm, despite not being contraindicated, should be avoided in the initial phase of the learning curve. With respect to doppler assessment of the saphenous vein, it is recommended to place a tourniquet at the level of the thigh in order to improve visualization; furthermore, the entirety of vein course should be marked for improved guidance during the endoscopic phase. Of note, morbidly obese legs are not contraindicated for ESVH.

3 Surgical Instruments

Here is a list of surgical instruments that are required to perform a successful endoscopic RA and/or SVG harvesting by a non-sealed system (Fig. 1):

- Endoscopic re-usable retractor (Bisleri Model, Karl Storz, Tuttlingen, Germany), which is equipped with a 5 mm forward-oblique 45° telescope;
- Impedance-controlled bipolar radiofrequency vessel sealing system (LigaSure Maryland, Medtronic, Minneapolis, MN, USA);
- Left and Right curved pigtail vessel dissector (Hook Ring Dissector, Karl Storz, Tuttlingen, Germany).

4 Endoscopic Radial Artery Harvesting Technique

4.1 Preliminary Details

Selected arm is prepped and draped according to the individual institution's surgical protocols. Hyperextension of the wrist is mandatory by means of a rolled towel placed underneath, thus providing an adequate exposure of the RA.

Tips, tricks and traps: hyperextension at the level of the ipsilateral shoulder must be avoided

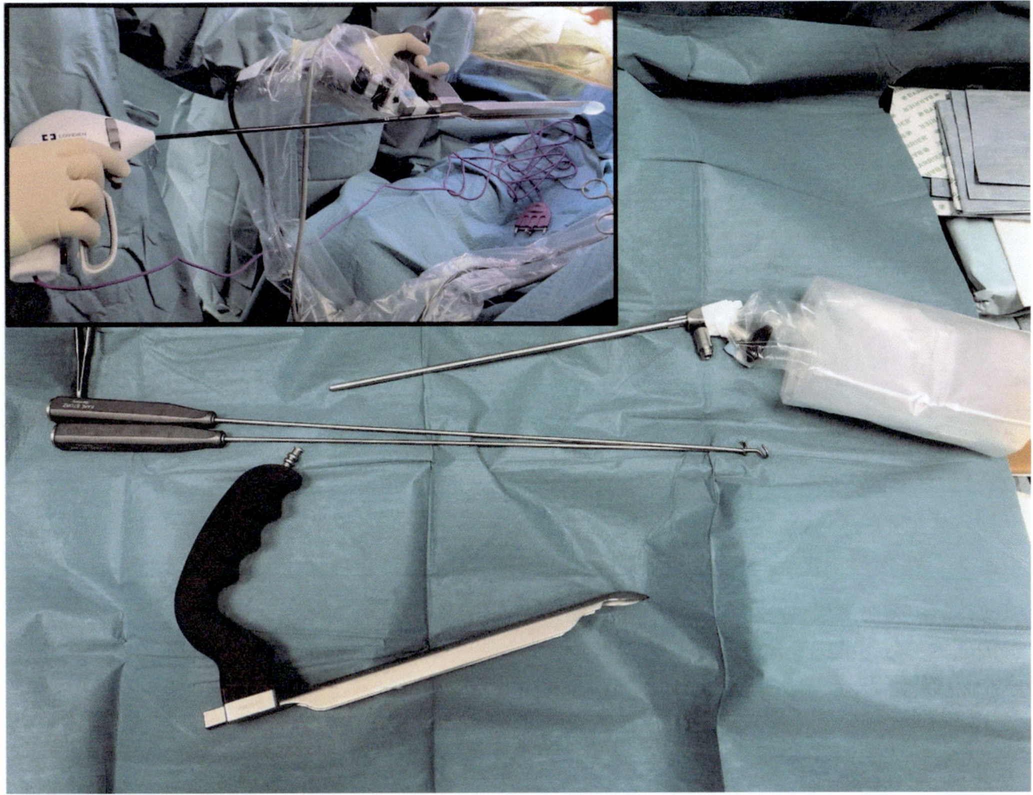

Fig. 1 Surgical instruments required for minimally invasive endoscopic vessel harvesting by means of a non-sealed system. In the box, detail of the vessel sealing system fitting in the dedicated tunnel in the endoscopic retractor

to prevent injuring the brachial plexus. As such, we recommend that the angle between the chest and the abducted arm should be 80° or less. This could be even more important in aged patients with a history of arthritis, or in patients with a history of shoulder interventions/stabilization. Moreover, it is highly recommended to firmly fix the arm to the armboard, in order to avoid unnecessary movement or sliding of the arm during harvesting maneuvers (See Fig. 2 and Video 1).

4.2 Surgical Exposure

Beginning 1 cm above the radial styloid prominence, a longitudinal incision of approximately 2-3 cm is performed along the course of the RA (Fig. 3). A self-retaining retractor is used to spread subcutaneous tissue and expose the fascia between the brachioradialis (BRM) and flexor carpi (FCM) muscles. Dissection of this plane is extended proximally under direct vision, by gently lifting the self-retaining retractor (generally 3-4 cm more from the incision edge). Aim of the surgical exposure is to achieve full mobilization of the RA as a pedicle graft (Fig. 4A, B). Hence, fascia is opened and dissection of surrounding tissues superiorly, laterally, medially and inferiorly to the RA is performed. Impedance-controlled bipolar radiofrequency vessel sealing system (LigaSure Maryland, Medtronic, Minneapolis, MN, USA) is used to divide the pedicle from surrounding tissues until at least 3-4 cm have been harvested under direct visualization (Fig. 4C), then a specifically designed reusable endoscopic retractor (Karl Storz, Tuttlingen, Germany) can be inserted and used to harvest the remaining RA endoscopically.

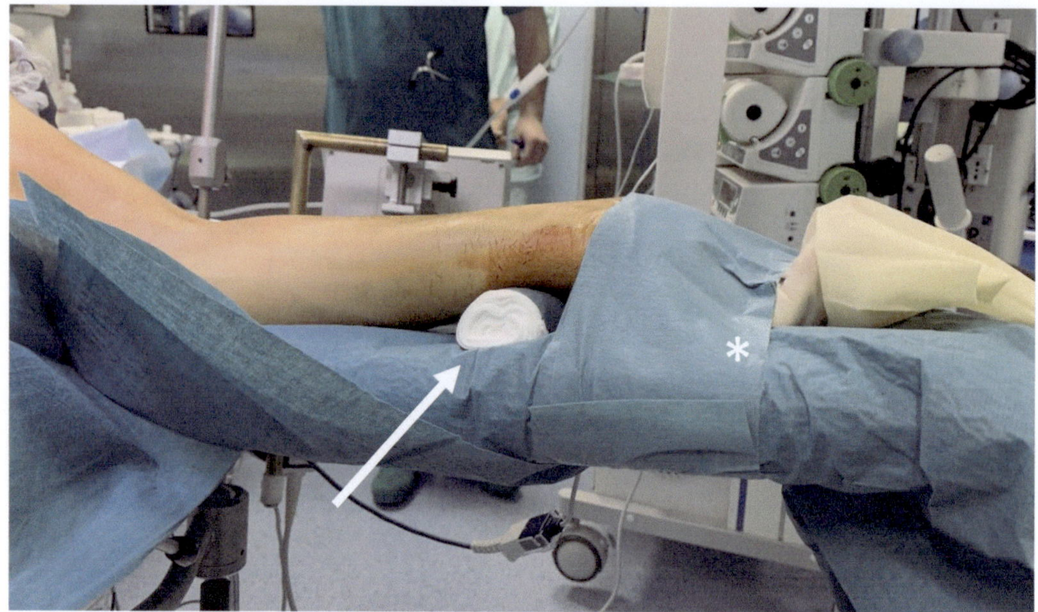

Fig. 2 Left arm positioning: white arrow highlights the use of a rolled pad underneath the wrist in order to adequately hyperextend and expose the RA while the white star shows drapes used to firmly secure the left arm to the surgical armboard

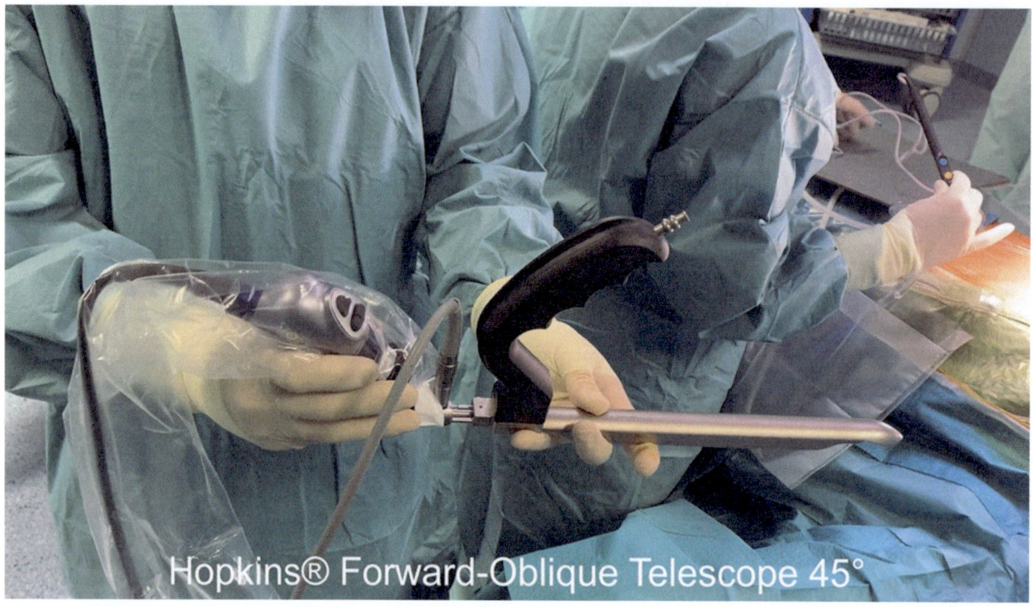

Video 1 Endoscopic Radial Artery Harvesting with a non sealed approach (▶ https://doi.org/10.1007/000-a7a)

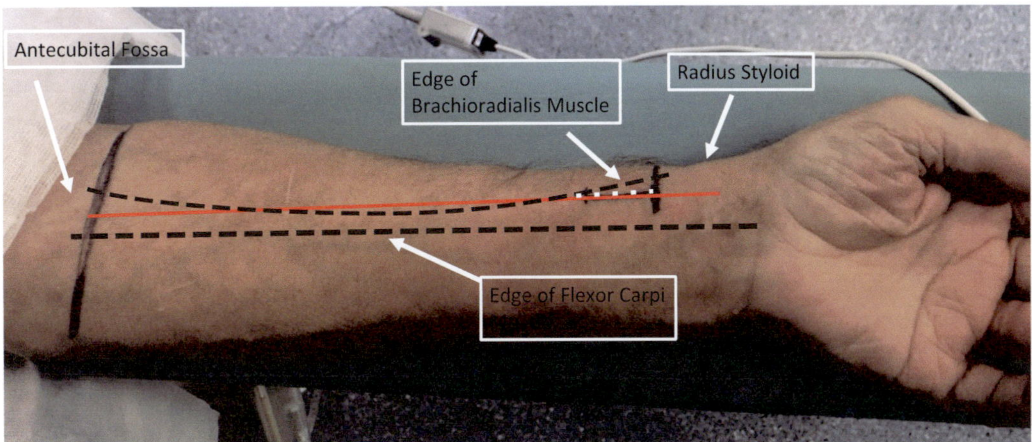

Fig. 3 Schematic left arm anatomy: black dashed lines depict the course of the edge of the brachioradialis muscle (upper line) and the flexor carpi muscle (bottom line). Red dashed line highlights the course of the left RA from the wrist until the antecubital fossa. The short white dotted line shows the initial incision line, 1 cm above the radius styloid and extended proximally for 2–3 cm

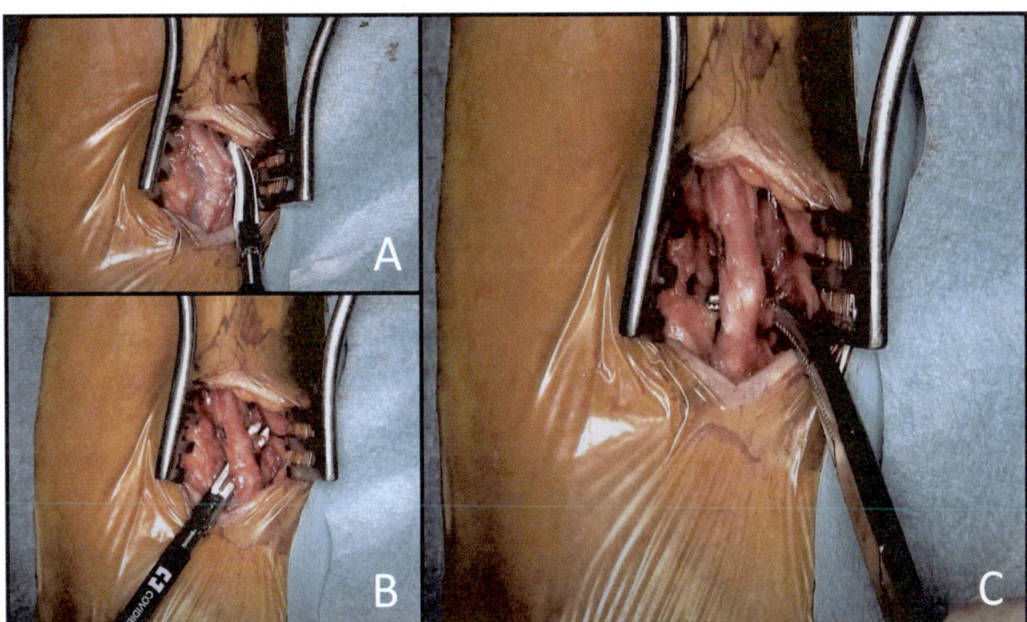

Fig. 4 Left RA is fully isolated as a pedicle before starting endoscopic maneuvers. **A** and **B**: the vessel sealing system during the "open" phase is used to divide side branches and avoid the use of hemoclips; C: Left RA is fully isolated as a pedicle. Note the self-retractor with the handle positioned towards the elbow

Tips, tricks and traps: To manage RA side branches, use of hemoclips must be avoided as they may dislodge or be torn off by the endoscopic retractor, leading to unnecessary bleeding. The ideal position of the self-retaining retractor is as depicted in Fig. 4, with the handle placed towards the antecubital fossa in order to enhance visualization of the dissection tunnel and move the initial dissection as far as possible under direct vision. We strongly recommend following the exact sequence of dissection as described above: first proceed by opening the fascia between the BRM and FCM as far as possible proximally, then, laterally, dividing RA side branches and surrounding tissue from the side of the BRM; next,medially, dividing all side branches and dissect surrounding tissue at the level of the FCM; lastly, divide surrounding tissue inferiorly to the RA. If RA dissection is started medially, traction from the lateral side branches may pull the RA under the BRM, and make the procedure more challenging. Satellite veins at both sides of the RA should be kept as references and surrounding tissue should be divided beyond them (Fig. 4A, B). Pay particular attention when moving the dissection laterally at the level of the wrist: here, the superficial radial nerve might be close, so we strongly recommend avoiding unnecessary traction or digging. Also, the use of a vessel loop around the RA is not helpful, and may, in fact, be dangerous. It is mandatory to correctly prepare and visualize the four dissection planes in order to maintain a "parachute" reference during endoscopic maneuvers.

4.3 Endoscopic Harvesting

As suggested above, we recommend starting by dividing the fascia between BRM and FCM until the antecubital fossa is reached. The endoscopic retractor is slid superior to the muscular fascia in order to divide subcutaneous tissue above the RA course (Fig. 5).

Tips, tricks and traps: the initial dissection plane should be maintained and limited to the fascia. In most instances, the RA, around the mid-portion, tends to dive underneath the BRM:

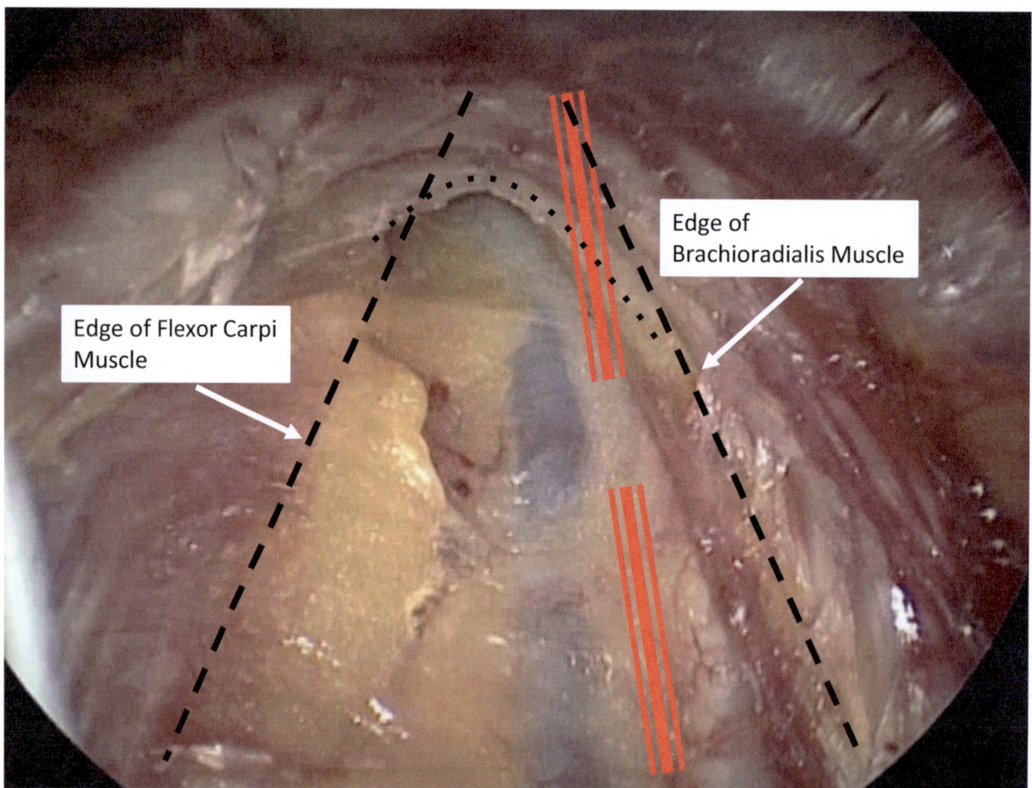

Fig. 5 Endoscopic view: the red-triple line depicts the course of the left RA in its mid-portion tending to run underneath the BRM. The black dotted line highlights the fascia between BR and FC muscles that should be divided as the first step of the endoscopic harvesting

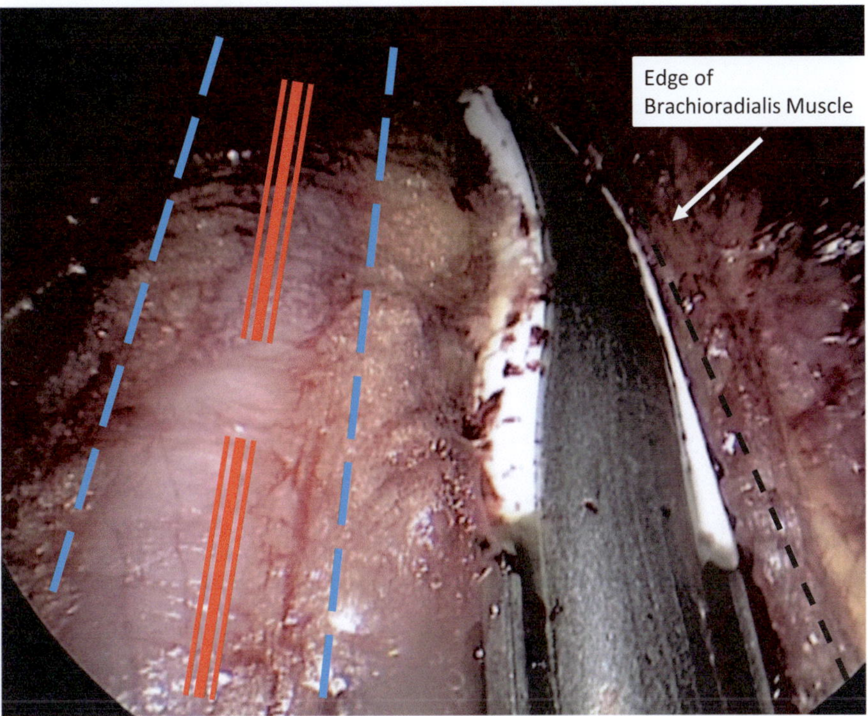

Fig. 6 Endoscopic harvesting at the level of the BRM (lateral) side: red-triple line shows the course of the left RA with the two satellite veins (blue dashed lines). Note the edge of the BRM gently lifted by the endoscopic retractor and the RA running underneath. The vessel sealing system is providing division of lateral side-branches towards the BRM

here, it is important to proceed proximally by dividing the fascia along the BRM edge, as the dissection plane moves slightly medially. While the RA may seem "invisible" at this level, correctly dividing the fascia will lead to the antecubital fossa where the RA tends to superficialize and become clearly visible again. It is very important to avoid division of any muscular structure that may bleed after heparin is given for cardiopulmonary bypass increasing the risk of bleeding and hematoma.

Once the fascia is opened, the retractor is pulled distally, the dissection plane between the RA and the BRM (RA lateral side) is visualized endoscopically, then dissection of the RA itself is started with the goal of reaching the antecubital fossa (Fig. 6).

Tips, tricks and traps: in most instances, the RA runs underneath the BRM, making endoscopic harvesting challenging. This is particularly true for muscular forearms. By using the tip of the endoscopic retractor to gently lift the BRM, a proper visualization of the lateral dissection plane is achieved (Fig. 6). Advancing with small bites of the vessel sealing system can be considered to avoid damaging the RA at this level. Do not move the dissection plane towards the FCM: it should be kept intact since the FCM and RA attachments pull the RA towards the midline, improving exposure, especially in difficult cases.

Similarly, once the previous part is completed, dissection is started at the FCM side from distal to proximal until the antecubital fossa is reached.

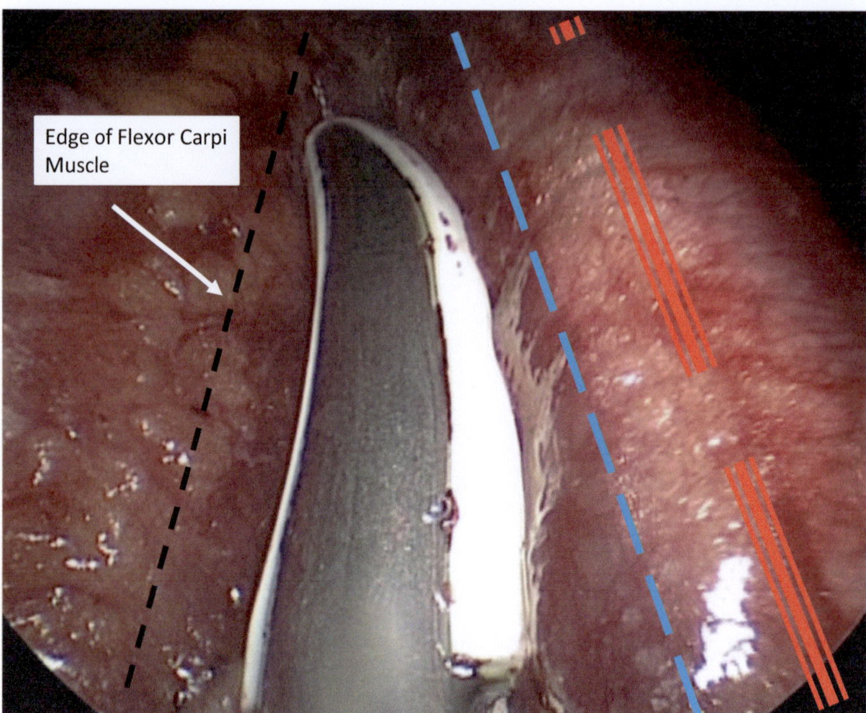

Fig. 7 Endoscopic harvesting at the level of the FCM (medial) side: red-triple line shows the course of the left RA with its medial satellite vein (blue dashed line). Note the edge of the FCM (black dashed line) which is less bulging of the contralateral BRM

During this stage, residual branches at the level of the inferior aspect of the RA are also divided (Fig. 7). It is mandatory to assess the presence of any residual side branches by means of a pigtail vessel dissector (Fig. 8).

Tips, tricks and traps: normally the FCM is smaller compared to the BRM, and does not "bulge" as much. Attention should be paid when approaching the antecubital fossa while performing dissection of the inferior aspect of the RA: in some circumstances, large collateral veins can be visualized close to the division between the RA and ulnar artery. Dissect cautiously and, if extra-length is not required, stop at this level.

Caution should be taken when endoscopically harvesting the right RA. Since we preferentially use the non-dominant arm, operators will become more familiar with the anatomy of the left arm, in which the lateral side of the RA is visualized at the level of the right side of the endoscopic view. Thus, during harvesting maneuvers, especially during the fascia opening phase, the dissection line is moving from right to left proceeding from the wrist towards to the antecubital fossa, in order to avoid the BRM. Conversely, the opposite direction will be taken if the right RA is harvested: an automatic tendency to slightly move from right to left should be avoided keeping in mind that the BRM side (lateral side) of the right RA is positioned to the left side of the screen thus, the ideal direction will be from left to right proceeding from the wrist to the antecubital fossa (Fig. 9).

Otherwise, we recommend following the same steps normally used for the left RA.

4.4 Radial Artery Endoscopic Retrieval

Once heparin is given, operators can proceed to retrieve the full length of the RA. As reported by

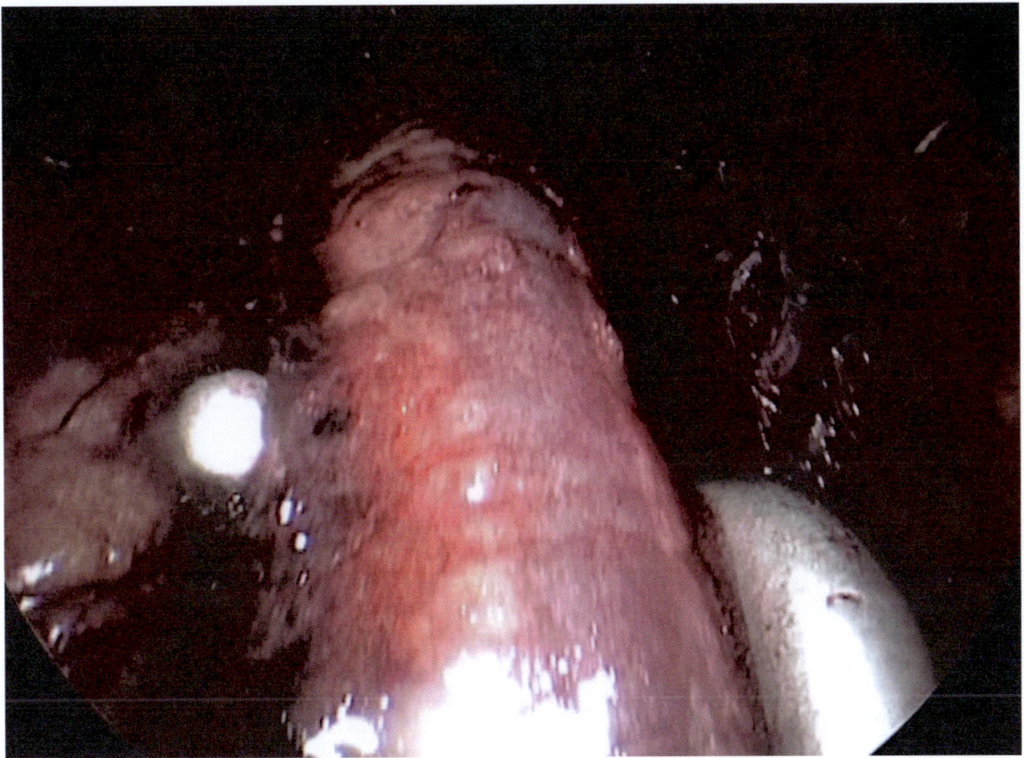

Fig. 8 Pigtail dissector to check the presence of any residual branches

the factory, a proper sealing is guaranteed for up to 7 mm vessel diameter, and, as such, a single incision could be performed safely in each patient: the RA is divided at its proximal end (antecubital fossa) and the graft is then retrieved through the same distal incision at the level of the wrist (single-incision approach) (Fig. 10).

Tips, tricks and traps: if operators are not confident in directly dividing the RA by using the vessel sealing system proximally or if the angle between the RA and the vessel sealing system does not provide a safe direct approach, a counter incision (2 cm max) could be performed at the level of the antecubital fossa above the tip of the endoscopic retractor. Then a blunt dissection is performed under endoscopic control and a tape is passed around the RA. Now, the graft can be divided directly at the level of the wrist and gently pulled from the proximal incision (counter-incision approach). In this context,

it is extremely important to check for any residual side branches before proceeding with the single incision or double incision techniques for graft retrieval.

Incision is sutured in usual fashion after distal ligation of the RA at the level of the wrist. In case sneaky bleeding is present after protamine administration, a small drain can be used and removed following clinical judgement in the first/second postoperative day.

5 Endoscopic Saphenous Vein Harvesting Technique

5.1 Preliminary Details

The course of the great saphenous vein must be marked in every patient by means of ultrasound to identify:

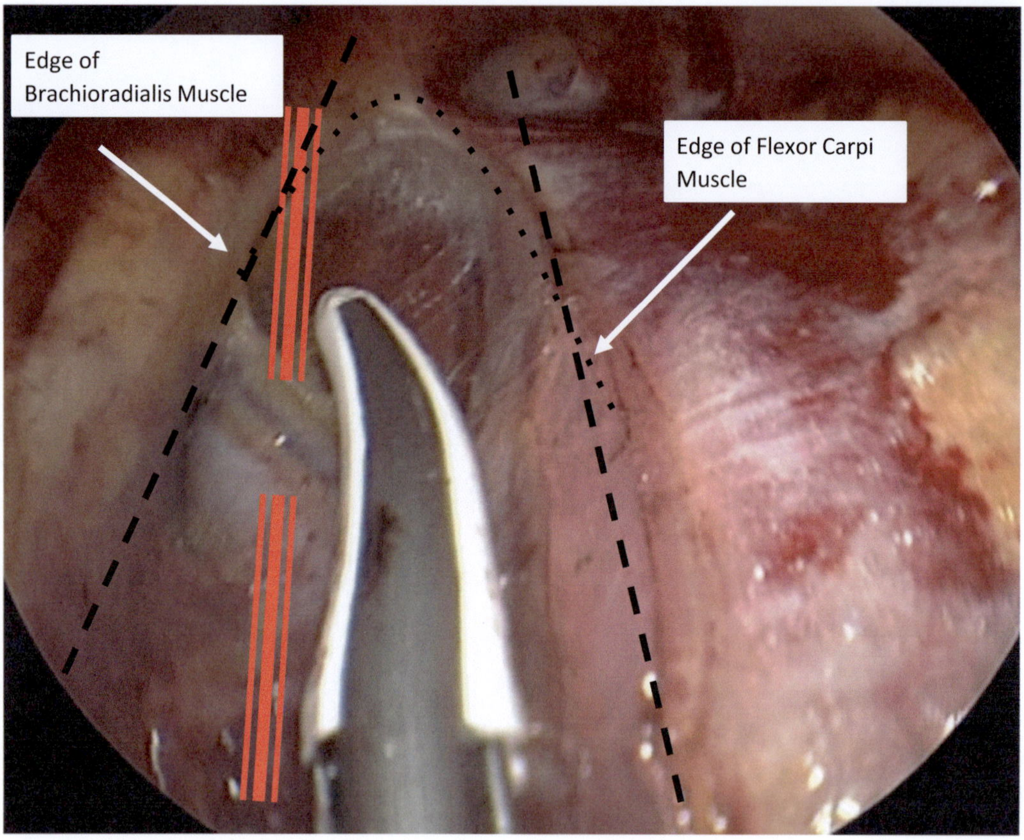

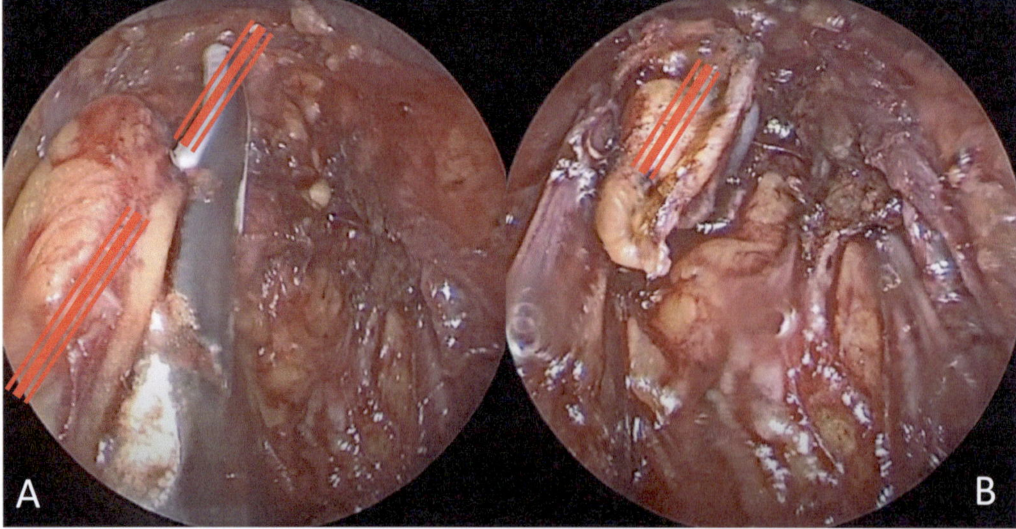

Fig. 9 Endoscopic view of the right RA: the red-triple line depicts the course of the right RA in its mid-portion tending to run underneath the BRM (left side). The black dotted line highlights the fascia between BR and FC muscles

Fig. 10 Radial artery (red-triple line) is directly divided proximally: note the vessel sealing system crossing the radial course (**A**) and the proximal radial artery stump (**B**) left after completing the retrieval procedure

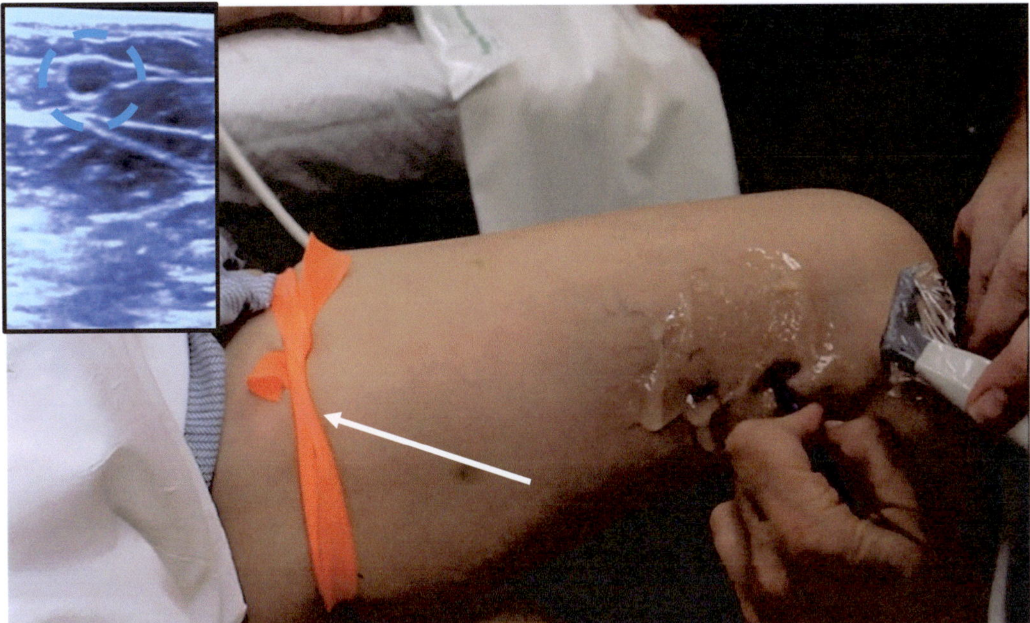

Fig. 11 The course of the saphenous vein is mapped by means of ultrasound. Note the orange tourniquet at the level of the thigh (white arrow) in order to increase saphenous vein diameter for a better visualization (blue dashed circle)

– the site of the initial incision;

– anatomical/pathological variations;

– large side-branches (in experienced hands)

Before mapping, to increase the size of the vein and improve visualization, a tourniquet should be at the level of the thigh (Fig. 11).

Tips, tricks and traps: the best exposure is provided by placing rolled sheets under the knees, with both legs externally rotated, and knees slightly bent in a "frog-like" position. Both knees must be completely supported to avoid position-related neurological complications.

5.2 Surgical Exposure

A 2–3 cm longitudinal incision is made over the course of the SV above the knee. A self-retractor is used to enhance exposure, and the subcutaneous tissue is divided, thereby mobilizing the first 4-5 cm of saphenous vein. Similarly to the RA exposure, impedance-controlled bipolar radiofrequency vessel sealing system (LigaSure Maryland, Medtronic, Minneapolis, MN, USA) may be used at this stage to gently dissect surrounding tissues and side branches.

Tips, tricks and traps: the tissue surrounding SV does not provide stabilization like the muscular structures around the RA. As such, counter traction and stability is crucially provided by a vessel loop passed around the vein. We strongly recommend gently lifting the self-retractor in order to isolate the SV along its course as far as possible under direct visualization. As suggested previously, at this stage, the use of hemoclips should be avoided (Fig. 12).

5.3 Endoscopic Harvesting

A specifically designed reusable endoscopic retractor can be gently inserted through the "open" incision once the SV is isolated. As tissue surrounding SV is mainly composed of subcutaneous fat, dissection is mostly performed by

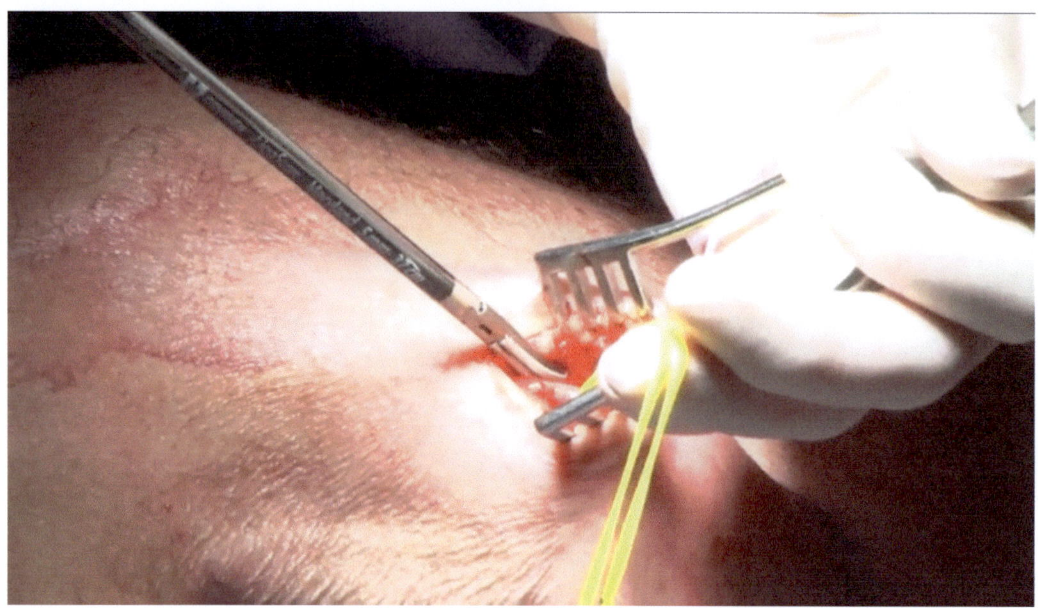

Fig. 12 Saphenous vein is fully isolated as a pedicle through a 3 cm incision above the knee (left side). A vessel loop (yellow string) is passed around the saphenous vein in order to provide stabilization during harvesting maneuvers. Note the operator working position with the handle of the self-retractor used to enhance visualization and isolating the graft as far as possible. The vessel sealing system is used also at this stage to divide side branches thus avoiding the use of hemoclips

gently advancing the endoscopic retractor, while the vessel sealing system can be used to perform smooth dissection and seal side branches.

Tips, tricks and traps: it is strongly recommended beginning the ESVH above the knee, and proceeding with the endoscopic phase towards the groin. This is particularly helpful for beginners since the course of the vein is more linear and side branches usually originate perpendicular to the main axis without vertical side branches that might be damaged while advancing the endoscopic retractor. Moreover, the "frog-like" position allows the operator to work from the patient's feet without conflicts between their maneuvers, patient's knees and the scrub nurse (Fig. 13). This setting can usually provide a 20–25 cm segment (from above the knee to the groin). If extra-length is required, the operator can invert his/her position and proceed towards the knee from the same incision (Fig. 13—right box). Before inverting positions and beginning endoscopic maneuvers, the SV must be isolated at the incision site under direct visualization. At

the level of the knee, the SV receives vertical collaterals from subcutaneous tissue. Hence, advancing the endoscopic retractor might be challenging and should be done carefully.

Alternatively, an incision may be made 3 cm below the knee over the course of the SV: this can either be a starting point for endoscopic harvesting or an additional incision in case extra-length is required. The operator can proceed distally towards the ankle, but they should work from the side of the patient's hips. It is still necessary to keep the legs in a "frog-like" position. In cases where a short segment is required, the operator, according to surgeon's preference, could start endoscopic harvesting from the ankle and proceed proximally towards the knee. We suggest positioning the patient's ankle at the very edge of the surgical table and starting 2-3 cm above the incision you would have normally done for the standard "open" approach. These precautions avoid conflicts between harvesting instruments against medial malleolus and/or the edge of the table.

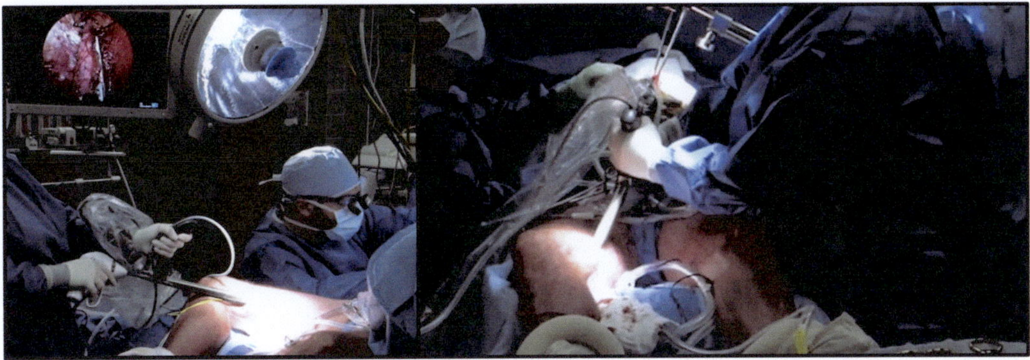

Fig. 13 Left saphenous vein endoscopic harvesting starting above the left knee: the left leg is gently bent in a frog-like position with rolled sheet underneath. Note the operator working position at the patient's feet and the screen positioned to the left. In the right box: operator working position in case extra-length ins required. The frog-like position is maintained, however, operator switched his/her position without affecting surgeon working position during left mammary harvesting

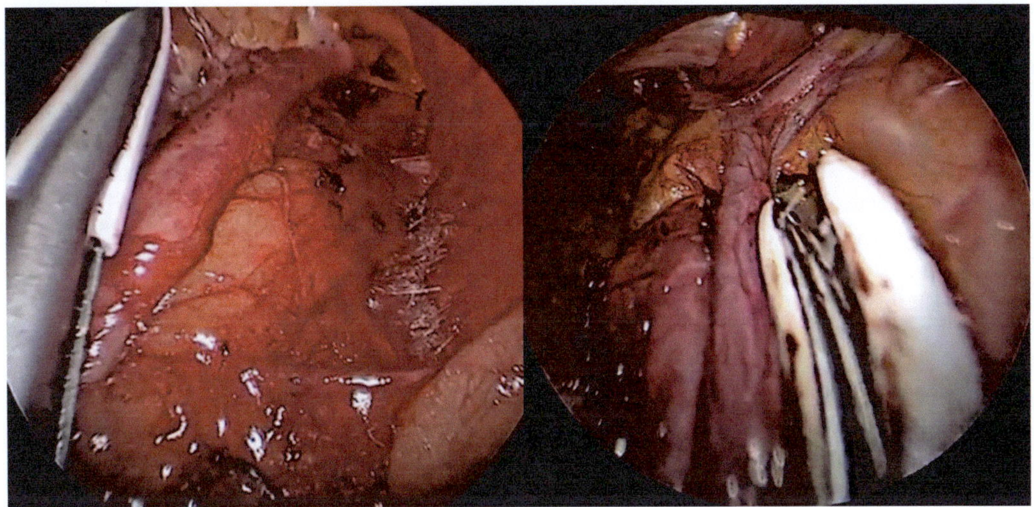

Fig. 14 Endoscopic view of the saphenous vein at the level of the thigh. Side branches can be easily visualized and divided

Generally, as a rule, the ESVH should begin by first dissecting the side where the most traction by side-branches is noted. Thus, harvesting techniques are adapted and altered on a case-by-case basis. This is in stark contrast to endoscopic ERAH technique, which has a predetermined sequence (Fig. 14).

Similarly to the radial artery, a pedicle is feasible and also strongly suggested during endoscopic saphenous vein harvesting: this improves graft quality as it avoids excessive graft manipulation. Moreover, maintaining surrounding tissue around the vein further protects against the minimal thermal spread provided by the vessel sealing system.

5.4 Saphenous Vein Endoscopic Retrieval

Similar to the technique described for radial artery harvest, complete absence of any residual

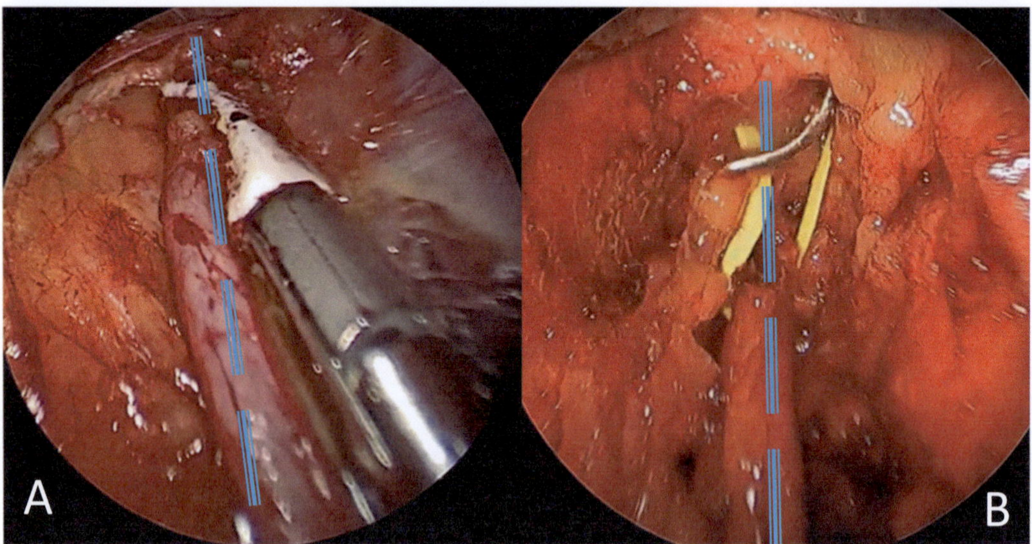

Fig. 15 Saphenous vein retrieval: **A**: single incision technique. The graft (double blue dashed line) is directly divided by means of the vessel sealing system. **B**: double incision technique. The graft is pulled from a small proximal skin incision performed at the tip of the endoscopic retractor, a vessel loop (yellow) is passed around in order to help the retrieval

side branches and surrounding tissue traction is checked by means of specific pigtail vessel dissector (Hook, Karl Storz, Tuttlingen, Germany). The saphenous vein then can be retrieved by a single or double incision technique (Fig. 15).

6 Comments

General considerations applicable to both grafts are described as follows. Endoscopic harvesting approach for radial artery and saphenous vein procurement is a safe and reproducible technique with a feasible learning curve. Particularly, the adoption of a non-sealed system allows operators to avoid potential detrimental effects described with active CO_2 insufflation in a sealed system.

However, with a non-sealed technique as described above, CO_2 could be used as visual flush by connecting an insufflator at the level of a dedicated port of the endoscopic retractor: this allows smoke removal during harvesting maneuvers without increasing pressure in the dissection tunnel or affecting graft quality. Recently, we have reported the feasibility of this approach also without any use of CO_2 in order to minimize the risk of aerosolization during COVID [19].

Additionally, the endoscopic view provides a magnified surgical field. As such, any inadvertent bleeding may appear more severe than it actually is. Nevertheless, if injury to a side branch occurs, we recommend removing the endoscopic retractor and applying external compression. Unless major damage has occurred, such maneuvers are usually effective in achieving hemostasis during both radial artery and saphenous vein harvesting.

During endoscopic harvesting, it is crucial to always visualize both jaws of the vessel sealing system. Pulsatility of the arterial graft is an important landmark that should always be checked before definitively closing the jaws and delivering radiofrequency for sealing. Particular attention should be paid when dividing the inferior aspect of the radial artery: we recommend gently rotating the closed jaws to left/right to ensure the curve-shaped tip of the vessel sealing system is not "biting" the graft. Since saphenous veins are devoid of this landmark, "blind" bites should be forbidden in order to avoid unnecessary risk of graft damage.

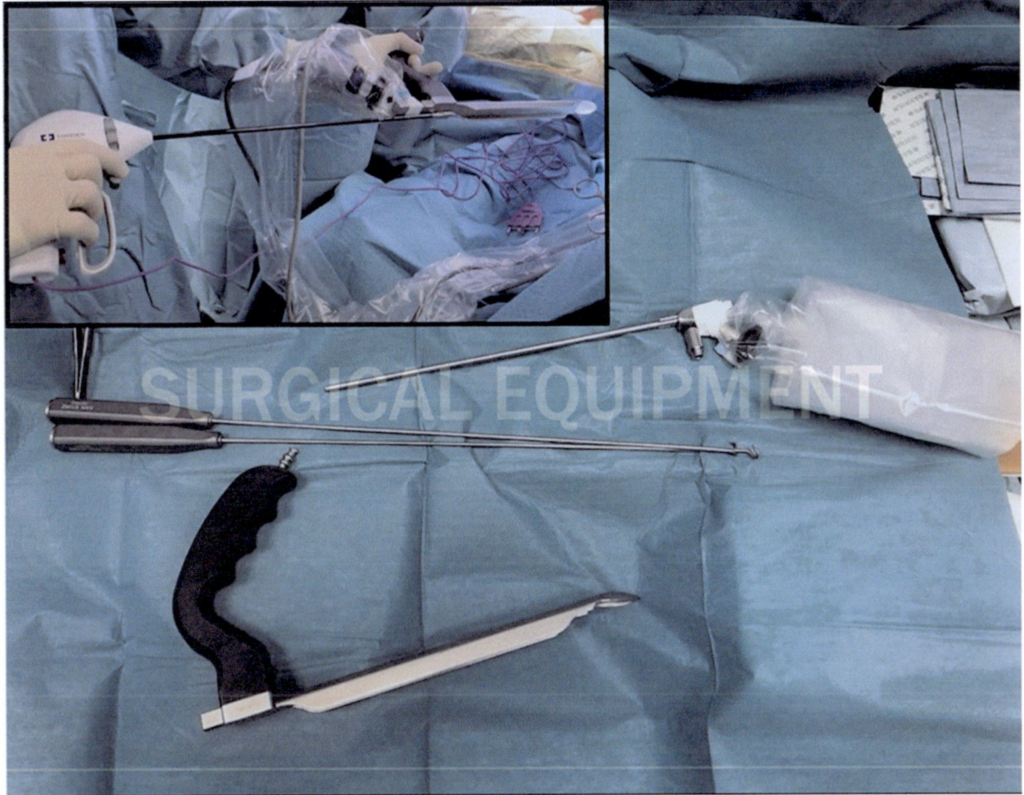

Video 2 Endoscopic Saphenous Vein Harvesting with a non sealed approach (▶ https://doi.org/10.1007/000-a7b)

In conclusion, endoscopic harvesting by means of a non-sealed system can be performed safely after adequate operator training and should be adopted as standard of care.Figure 10Radial artery (red-triple line) is directly divided proximally: note the vessel sealing system crossing the radial course (A) and the proximal radial artery stump (B) left after completing the retrieval procedure (See Video 2).

References

1. Williams J, Peterson E, Brennan J, Sedrakyan A, Tavris D, Alexander J, et al. Association between endoscopic vs open vein-graft harvesting and mortality, wound complications, and cardiovascular events in patients undergoing CABG surgery. JAMA. 2012;308:475–84.
2. Ferdinand FD, MacDonald JK, Balkhy HH, Bisleri G, Hwang HY, Northrup P, Trimlett RHJ, Wei L, Kiaii BB. Endoscopic conduit harvest in coronary artery bypass grafting surgery: an ISMICS systematic review and consensus conference statements. Innovations (Phila). 2017;12:301–19.
3. Burns DJ, Swinamer SA, Fox SA, Romsa J, Vezina W, Akincioglu C, Warrington J, Guo LR, Chu MW, Quantz MA, Novick RJ, Kiaii B. Long-term patency of endoscopically harvested radial arteries: from a randomized controlled trial. Innovations. 2015;10:77–84.
4. Bisleri G, Giroletti L, Hrapkowicz T, Bertuletti M, Zembala M, Arieti M, Muneretto C. Five-year clinical outcome of endoscopic versus open radial artery harvesting: a propensity score analysis. Ann Thorac Surg. 2016;102:1253–9.
5. Lopes RD, Hafley GE, Allen KB, Ferguson TB, Peterson ED, Harrington RA, Mehta RH, Gibson CM, Mack MJ, Kouchoukos NT, Califf RM, Alexander JH. Endoscopic versus open vein-graft harvesting in coronary-artery bypass surgery. N Engl J Med. 2009;361(3):235–44.
6. Sastry P, Rivinius R, Harvey R, Parker RA, Rahm AK, Thomas D, et al. The influence of endoscopic vein harvest on outcomes after coronary artery bypass grafting: a meta-analysis on 276,525 patients. Eur J Cardiothorac Surg. 2013;44:980–9.

7. - Raja SG, Rochon M, Spronson C, Bahrami TT. 4-year outcome analysis of endoscopic vein harvest for coronary artery bypass graft. Vascular Med 2013; https://doi.org/10.1155/2013/517806.

8. Bitondo JM, Daggett WM, Torchiana DF, Akins CW, Hilgenberg AD, Vlahakes GJ, Madsen JC, MacGillivray TE, Agnihotri AK. Endoscopic versus open saphenous vein harvest: a comparison of postoperative wound complications. Ann Thorac Surg. 2002;73:523–8.

9. Bonde P, Graham AN, MacGowan SW. Endoscopic vein harvest: advantages and limitations. Ann Thorac Surg. 2004;77:2076–82.

10. Bisleri G, Giroletti L, Stefini R, Guarneri B, Muneretto C. Neurological study of radial nerve conduction during endoscopic radial artery harvesting: an intra-operative evaluation. J Cardiothorac Med. 2014;2:207–9.

11. Luckraz H, Kaur P, Bhabra M, Mishra PK, Nagarajan K, Kumari N, Saleem K, Nevill AM. Endoscopic vein harvest in patients at high risk for leg wound complications: a cost-benefit analysis of an initial experience. Am J Infect Control. 2016;44(12):1606–10.

12. Goldsborough MA, Miller MH, Gibson J, Creighton-Kelly S, Custer CA, Wallop JM, Greene PS. Prevalence of leg wound complications after coronary artery bypass grafting: determination of risk factors. Am J Crit Care. 1999;8:149–53.

13. - Rao C, Aziz O, Deeba S, Chow A, Jones C, Ni Z, et al. Is minimally invasive harvesting of the great saphenous vein for coronary artery bypass surgery a cost-effective technique? J Thorac Cardiovasc Surg 2008; 135(4):809e15.

14. - Illig KA, Rhodes JM, Sternbach Y, Green RM. Financial impact of endoscopic vein harvest for infrainguinal bypass. J Vasc Surg 2003; 37 (2):323e30.

15. Hussaini BE, Xiu-Gui L, Wolfe JA, Thatte HS. Evaluation of endoscopic vein extraction on structural and functional viability of saphenous vein endothelium. J Cardiothorac Surg. 2011;6:82.

16. Brown EN, Kon ZN, Tran R, Burris NS, Gu J, Laird P, Brazio PS, Kallam S, Schwartz K, Bechtel L, Joshi A, Zhang S, Poston RS. Strategies to reduce intraluminal clot formation in endoscopically harvested saphenous veins. J Thorac Cardiovasc Surg. 2007;134:1259–65.

17. Mahmood D, Rosati F, Petsikas D, Payne D, Torkan L, Bisleri G. Endoscopic radial artery harvesting with a non-sealed approach. Multimed Man Cardiothorac Surg. 2019;9:2019. https://doi.org/10.1510/mmcts.2019.008.

18. Mahmood D, Rosati F, Petsikas D, Payne D, Torkan L, Bisleri G. Endoscopic saphenous vein harvesting with a non-sealed approach. Multimed Man Cardiothorac Surg. 2019;9:2019. https://doi.org/10.1510/mmcts.2019.009.

19. Ali Hassan SM, Palacios CM, Ethier T, Bisleri G. Improved safety of endoscopic vessel harvesting during the COVID-19 pandemic. Ann Thorac Surg. 2020;110(5):e449–50.

Endoscopic Closed Tunnel Conduit Harvesting: Tips, Tricks and Traps

Bhuvaneswari Krishnamoorthy
and Jared Blackmore

Abstract

The introduction of endoscopic conduit harvesting has been a big advance in patient centred care in the surgical revascularisation of patients with coronary artery disease. Like the introduction of all new technology there has been a wide variation in its adoption among teams depending on many factors. The closed tunnel approach was the original technique and has a lot of literature supporting it partly because it has the largest market share of these devices in America. This chapter covers the key steps in using this technique safely and covers both saphenous vein and radial artery harvesting. All new teams and individuals are recommended that they follow the recommended standards from the previous chapter in order to achieve a high quality conduit along with the excellent short term outcomes of this technique.

Supplementary Information The online version contains supplementary material available at https://doi.org/10.1007/978-3-031-21104-1_6. The videos can be accessed individually by clicking the DOI link in the accompanying figure caption or by scanning this link with the SN More Media App.

B. Krishnamoorthy (✉)
Manchester Foundation Trust, Manchester, England, UK
e-mail: b.bibleraaj@salford.ac.uk

J. Blackmore
Miami Valley Hospital, Dayton, OH, US

Keywords

Endoscopic vein harvesting · Endoscopic radial artery harvesting · Closed carbon dioxide tunnel

1 Introduction

This chapter will be aiming to discuss the tips, tricks and traps of closed tunnel conduit harvesting of the greater saphenous vein and radial artery harvesting. Both the authors have a joint experience of carrying out endoscopic conduit harvesting for more than two decades.

The importance of learning endoscopic conduit harvesting is to teach the learners broad based and highly qualified surgical trainees to provide the best care for patients with a wide range of surgical practical strategies [1]. Enhanced practical learning approaches provide an insight of a day-to-day tips, tricks and traps to be considered as part of their learning processes. Each individual practitioner should be taught using these three classifications to avoid any major problems which has not been taught during their training period of conduit harvesting. As we discussed in chapter "Endoscopic Conduit Harvesting: Best Practice Training Guidelines", it is vital for these practitioners to be taught using an e-learning method with theory, structured step by step training, training from simple to complicated cases which will provide an opportunity for the trainee to experience all types of conduits [2]. The trainee and trainers should understand the importance of training points and classification of practical training.

Important Training Points:

- Hands-on training improves the student's self-efficacy [3].
- Using appropriate practical training methods has the potential to raise learning opportunities for the trainees.
- Practical skills learning helps them to improve skills and knowledge around the conduit harvesting and identify the problems earlier rather than later.

Classification of Practical Training Method:

Teaching the surgical trainees with practical tips, tricks and traps is one of the effective methods of teaching and it has been practiced for many years in different surgical fields.

Tips:

Firstly, we should teach the trainee "Important practical tips in surgery". It means 'how it should be carried out' or 'what to know to be able to do the job without struggling'. This way the trainees can learn a step-by-step conduit harvesting procedure by applying their theoretical knowledge about the surgical procedure.

Tricks:

The second step should be about thinking points of a trainee learning the tricks during difficult conduit harvesting. This teaches them recognition of difficult skills learned with some tricks and to find the best solution on how to do it. This provides opportunity for the trainee to learn and act on any difficult situations and have a back up plan of action with a higher level of thinking order.

Traps:

The third step should be about what they have learned and how they can use their knowledge and skills from their experience. At this level, it is important to understand the need of developing the skills and updating their knowledge according to evidence based practice using relevant literature to avoid difficulties and prevent conversions.

2 Greater Saphenous Vein

Introduction:

The most common cardiac surgery performed today worldwide is the Coronary Artery Bypass Grafting (CABG). Several pioneer cardiac surgeons have transformed the CABG procedure for past 100 years. It has evolved from a long scar to small minimally invasive and now percutaneous interventions to treat the coronary artery disease. The use of Great Saphenous Vein (GSV) remains the commonest treatment for multi-vessel coronary artery disease where arterial grafts does not provide length required to graft the posterior wall coronaries such as circumflex and right [4].

Anatomy:

The GSV emerges anterior to the medial malleolus bone as the continuation of the medial marginal vein of the foot and then it ascends along the medial aspect of the tibial bone before emptying into the common femoral vein in the groin. It lies between the compartment delineated by the aponeurotic and the superficial saphenous fascia [5]. The GSV can be identified easily on the transverse scan of the ultrasound as a saphenous eye (Fig. 1a, b), is located within the saphenous compartment within the superficial and aponeurotic deep fasciae [6].

At the level of crease of the groin, saphenofemoral junction is wrapped by the superficial fascia which ends proximal to the inguinal ligament. The GSV has valves which are called as terminal or ostial valves to prevent blood flow back to the lower leg. There are proximal collaterals between these valves from lateral to medial which are the superficial iliac vein, superficial epigastric vein and superficial pudendal vein. They drain venous blood from the abdominal wall and pudendal areas [6].

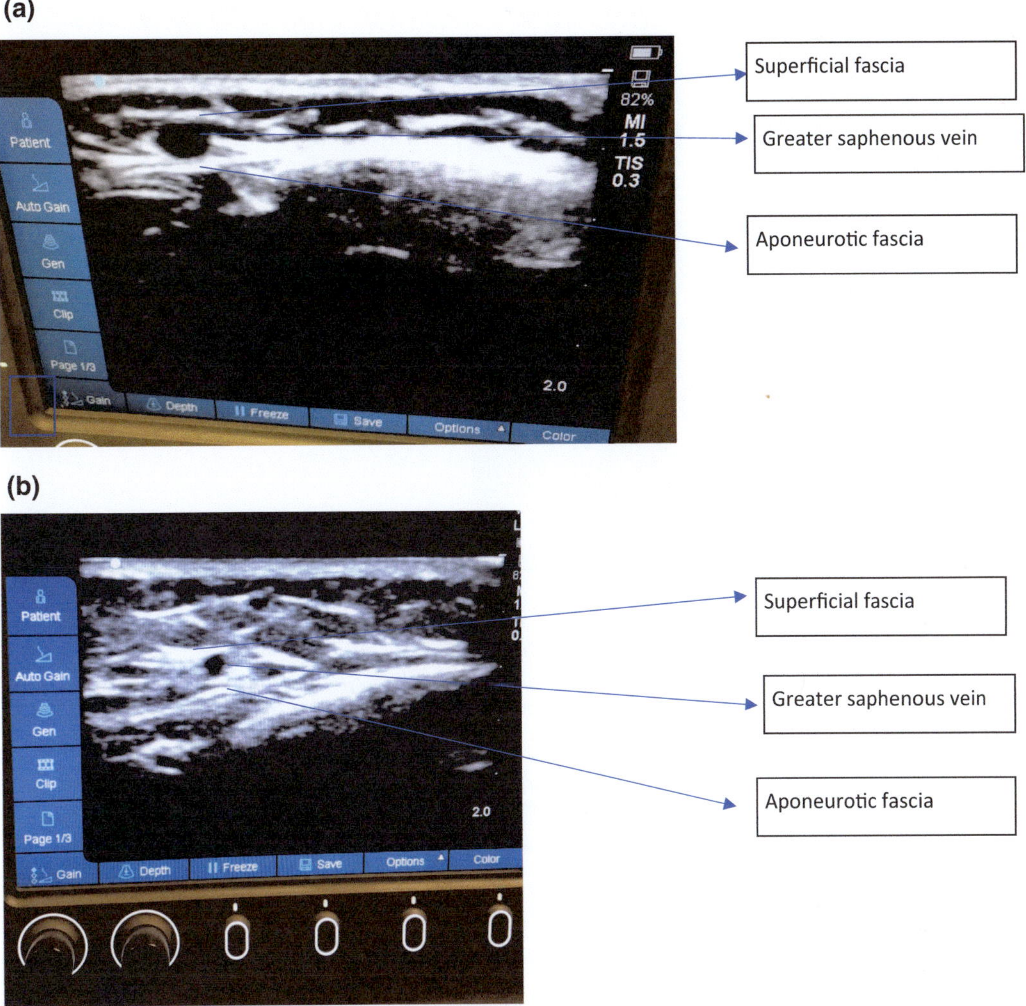

Fig. 1 **a**, **b** Illustrates the placement of greater saphenous vein on the transverse scan of the ultrasound

The anatomical patterns of the GSV in the thigh area can vary from single vein (Fig. 2a, b), divided in two parallel veins within the saphenous compartment (Video 1), GSV running into the saphenous compartment plus a large subcutaneous collateral that joined the GSV by piercing the fascia at the thigh level (Fig. 3) and two veins with two separate eyes in the proximal part of the saphenous compartment (Fig. 4). At the knee level, the anatomy of the vein can be difficult to assess because of the presence of multiple collaterals and perforators packed into a limited space. But, the GSV can be identified by its position in the angle formed by the tibial bone and gastrocnemius muscle which is called the T-G angle [6].

(a)

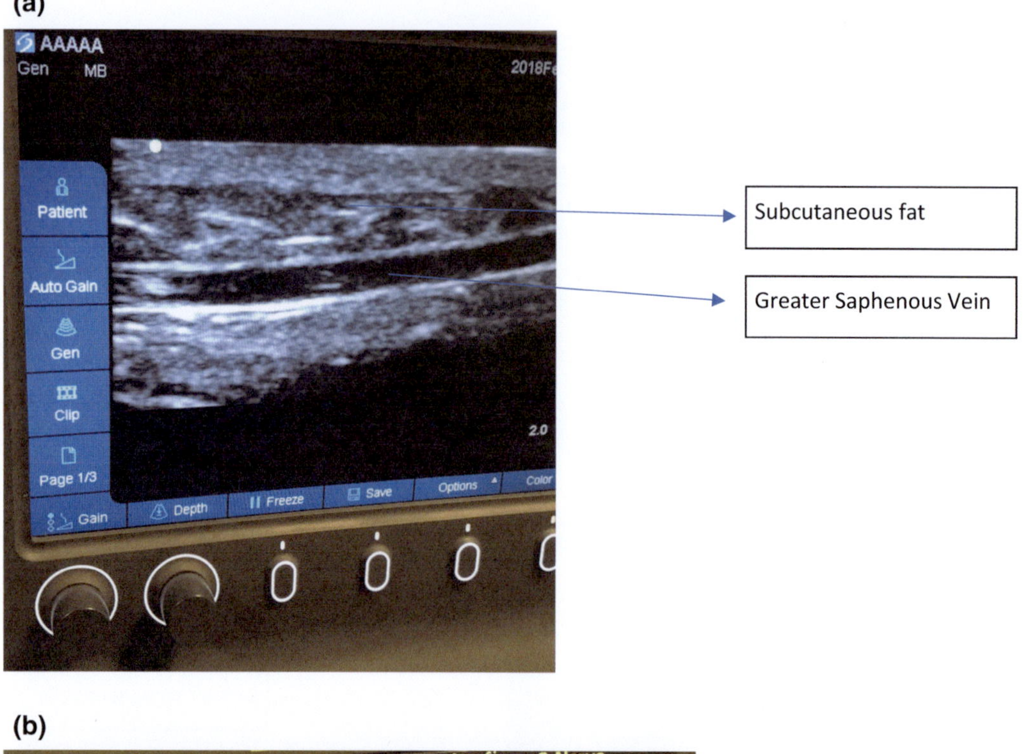

(b)

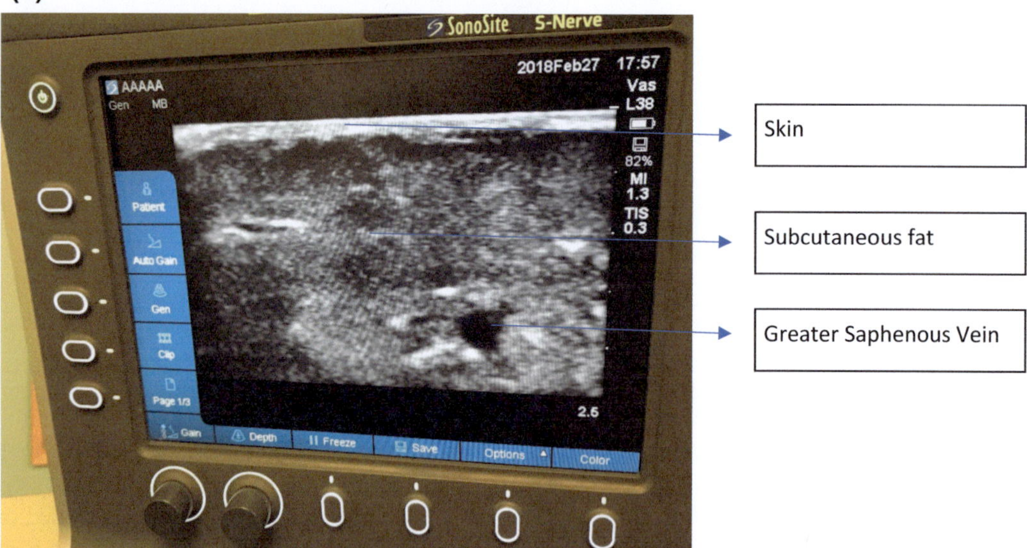

Fig. 2 **a** Single vein on a horizontal scan view on the thigh. **b** Single vein with an cross section view on a transverse scan view on the thigh

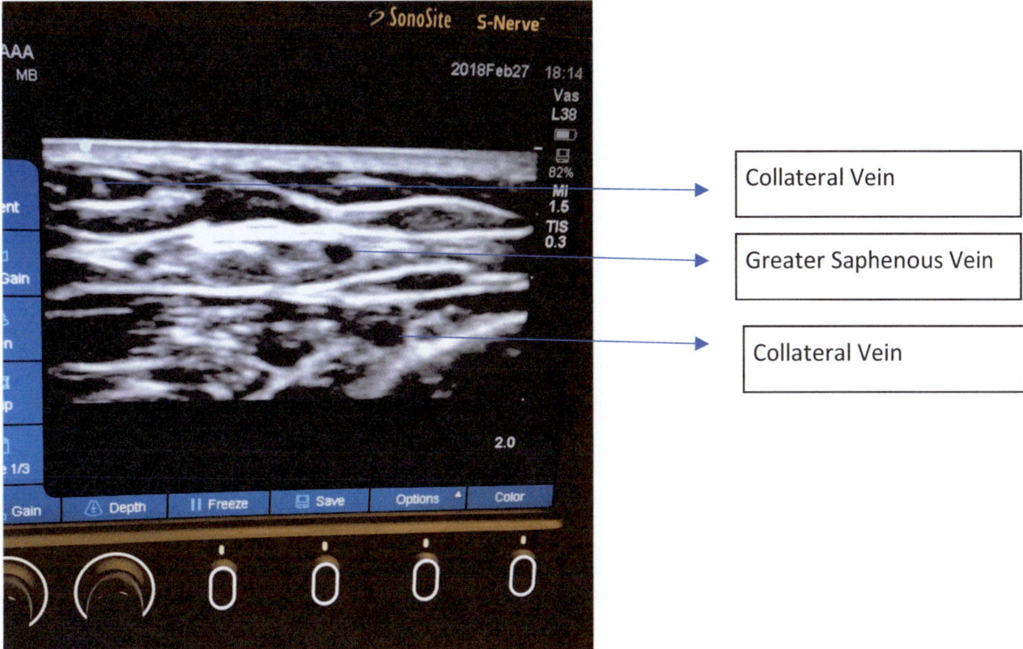

Fig. 3 Illustrates the greater saphenous vein with collateral veins

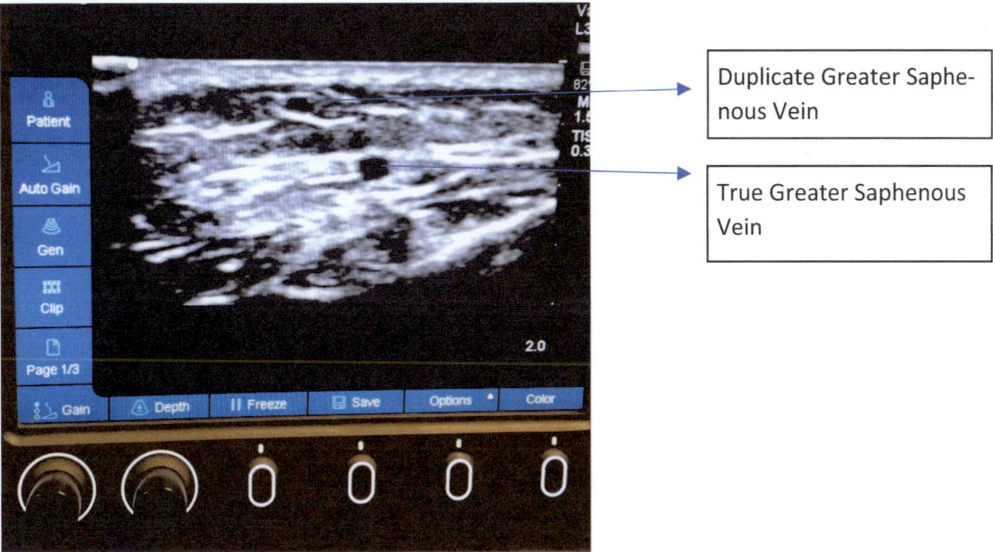

Fig. 4 Two separate vein with ultra sound scanning

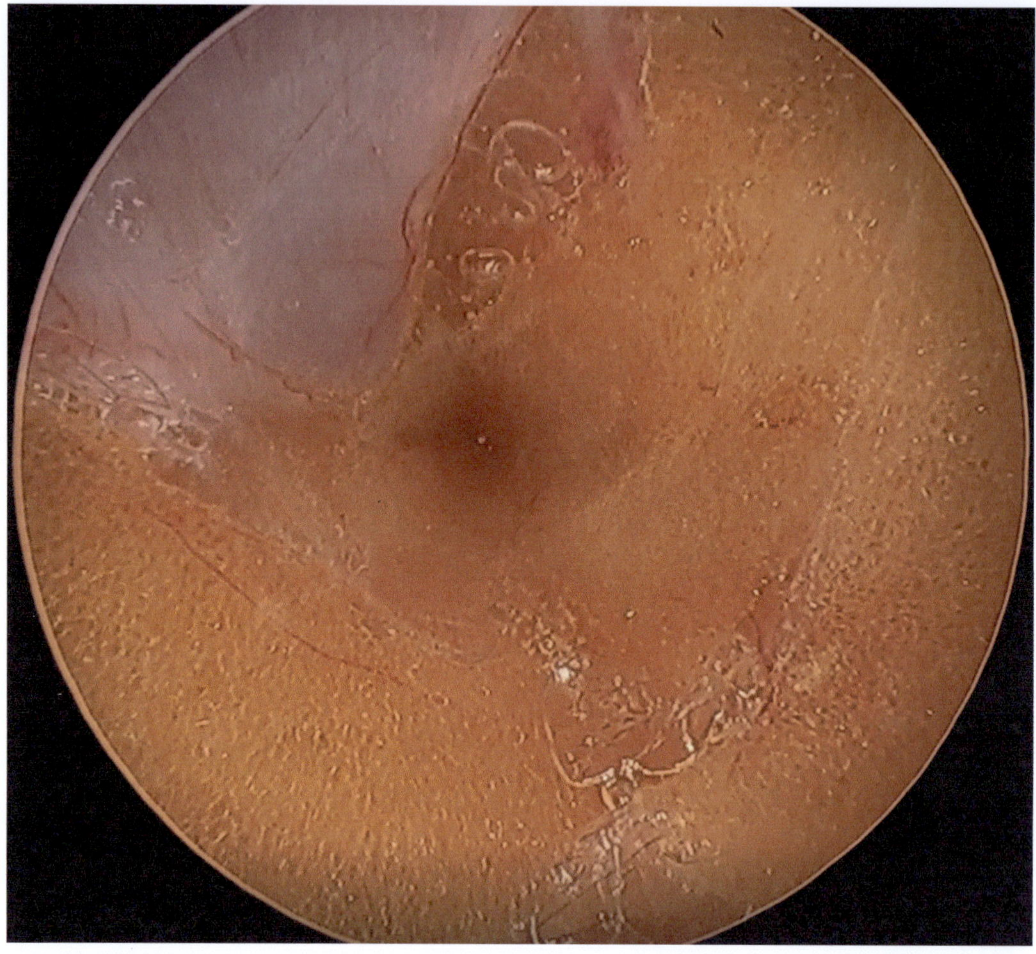

Video 1 Long Saphenous Vein Harvesting (▶ https://doi.org/10.1007/000-a7d)

3 Endoscopic GSV Harvesting

Endoscopic Vein Harvesting (EVH)

A thin endoscope is inserted through a small 2 cm skin incision below the knee and the GSV is harvested under visual guidance. It is well established that the EVH technique is efficacious in reducing leg wound infections with better cosmetic results [7]. This chapter will explore the closed CO_2 tunnel system with tips, tricks and traps to be avoided. It is important to have a good set up, clear protocol, guidelines for performing EVH technique to avoid any common problems during harvesting which will be discussed in the following paragraphs.

Equipments Required for the Closed Tunnel CO_2 EVH:

- Camera stacksystem with camera attachment, digital processor and display monitor.
- CO_2 cylinder with gauge.
- Vein grafting set with skin blade handle, mosquitoes, toothed/non-toothed forceps, needle holder, small langenbeck retractors and west retractors.

- Hemopro 2 delivery unit which can be bought with the company providing the closed tunnel CO_2 EVH disposable.
- 29 cm length 30-degree telescope.
- Fibreoptic light cable.
- Hemopro 2 black lead for the cauterisation. This can be sold as part of a EVH disposable from the EVH company.
- Camera drapes.
- Lens cleaner.
- CO_2 delivery line with filter.
- 20 ml syringe for flushing the vein once harvested.
- Ioban or plain steridrape for the groin.

Patient Consent and Patient Information Leaflet:

Informed consent is the process in which a healthcare professional educates a patient about the risks, benefits and alternatives of a given procedure or intervention. The patient must be competent to make a voluntary decision about whether to undergo the procedure or intervention [8]. There are different types of vein harvesting methods such as open vein harvesting, bridging, open CO_2 and closed CO_2 tunnel endoscopic vein harvesting with their own merits and drawbacks in relation to postoperative complications. We strongly suggest that providing all patients who are undergoing endoscopic vein harvesting with a patient information leaflet will enhance the process of informed consent and shared decision making at the preoperative outpatient clinic appointment. It is important for the reader to obtain local governance and patient directive group approval before implementing any patient related leaflets in clinical practice.

Associated Cost and Business Case for Setting Up Endoscopic Vein Harvesting:

Some hospitals do not adopt endoscopic conduit harvesting technique due to the associated costs of the disposables which can vary from £600 to £800 [9–11] depending on volumes of cases per year. The open vein harvesting has a higher incidence of wound complications compared to endoscopic technique [7, 12]. The endoscopic technique is associated with reduced postoperative pain due to a smaller skin incision compared to a long scar on the open technique [9]. The business case should compose of departmental wound related complications, rationale for introduction of endoscopic technique, benefits of endoscopic techniques with patient/staff satisfaction if available, length of hospital stay and early mobilisation, current literature evidence and business case proposal. Engaging all relevant stakeholders (Consultant cardiac surgeons, theatre manager, clinical director, directorate manager, finance officer and patient directive group member) at an early stage is vital and will support the business case acceptance.

Vein Identification and Incision:

The vein must be identified in three areas for endoscopic techniques depending upon the length of vein required. The first incision can be made 2 cm away and above the medial malleolus bone for patients who a need lower leg vein. The second incision can be made on the lateral border of the tibia and 4 cm below the knee joint for patients who need a full length of GSV. Please note through this incision, the vein can be harvested on the lower leg and upper thigh. The foot end of the table should be lowered during vein harvesting from the thigh which creates space and allows handling of the equipment easier.

Incision One:

Creating a skin incision on the lower leg near the medial malleolus is best for a practitioner who likes to harvest GSV from the bottom of the operating table. However, the practitioners need to take consideration of extending their back, shoulder and neck for a prolonged length of time which can causes damage. The benefit of this technique is that the GSV can be harvested easily because it has less branches on the lower leg. The main drawback is that the feet come in the way of the EVH equipments. That can be managed by positioning all toes and lowering the foot end of the table.

Incision Two:

Creating a skin incision at the lateral border of the tibial bone and 4 cm below the knee joint allows the practitioner to harvest the vein from the thigh and lower leg with one single incision. It is important for the practitioner to stand on the opposite side when harvesting the vein on the leg to avoid too much stress on their neck, back and shoulder. The stalk monitor machine should be placed diagonally to the operating table on the foot end to make sure that practitioner feels comfortable during harvesting. The practitioner should learn the habit of moving from right to left when they harvest the right leg above the thigh (stand on the right side) and lower leg (stand on the left side).

Heparinisation:

Once the vein is identified and dissected, the heparin should be given systemically by the anaesthetic team. The dose of heparin depends on whether the patient had any anticoagulant prior to surgery. If the patient continued their anticoagulant until the day of surgery, 2500 units heparin should be administered and 5000 units for the patient who have stopped their anticoagulants 7 days prior to the surgery [9]. The reason for giving systemic heparin prior to the endoscopic technique is to avoid any intraluminal clot formation inside the GSV which can lead to graft blockage [13]. It is practitioner's responsibility to check the patient notes for anticoagulant administration and confirm this with the patient to avoid any bleeding complications during harvesting and after harvesting.

Important Tips, Tricks for Harvesting:

– Check the stack monitoring, working conditions, level of CO_2 cylinder and electric connections before scrubbing for the surgery. Never assume that someone in the team will check for you.
– White balance the camera, before starting the case.
– Insert the scope on the warm water before starting the case to avoid any fog effect. You can use antifog but better to insert the scope on the warm water will prevent fogging during dissection.
– Do not screw the dissecting glass cone too tightly to avoid any breakage and stress on the tip.
– Place a saline pack with towel under the knee or medium hard knee support to position the leg as half positioned frog's leg which aid in vein harvesting.
– Please note these are small tricks but the practitioner needs to adapt their own style of positioning the patient which is convenient for them to harvest the GSV.
– Lower the foot end of the leg which will allow the practitioner to handle the EVH equipments easily without fighting with the foot.
– Dissect the vein anteriorly with the small west retractor in place and do not dissect the vein posteriorly or laterally to avoid the vein getting trapped or torn during harvesting by the insertion port.
– Insertion port should be left without inflation wherever possible, if needed inject the port bulb with 5 to 10 ml of air which will reduce the pressure on the vein.
– Insert the camera scope with dissecting cone gently:

- Please do anterior dissection for all patients but for patients who are small built and tiny leg circumference, do posterior dissection first (Video 1).
- Once the anterior dissection is completed, do not bring the dissector back to the start. Do lateral dissections on either side of the vein and work backwards to the starting point.
- After successful completion of the anterior and lateral dissections, please do the posterior dissections of the vein until the end of the tunnel.
- Please note that the practitioner should do posterior dissection first, lateral and then anterior dissection for tiny patient with small circumference (<7 cm) of the leg. This creates a space posteriorly, laterally which allows the vein to fall down and

prevents any vein damage caused by the EVH equipment.

- While doing dissection, please isolate the vein branches at least 1 cm around them to have long length vein branches.

In case, the vein branches have split into two or shorter branches. Please go around the branch and divide both branches rather than dissecting/cutting the shorter length which cause damage to the Intimal layer. For shorter and thicker branches which has less than 1 cm length and more than 1 cm width, the vein branches should be cut using intermittent Hemopro technique to avoid any risk of bleeding and thermal heat damages.

Another important trick to dissection is to keep the dissecting cone away from the vein and dissect using the peeling off technique for thin patients and back and forth technique for obese patients will prevent any damage to the patients.

- Cauterisation should be done once the vein is completely dissection to avoid any small branch tear.

Remove the tip of the cone from the scope and add the EVH equipments. Please make sure that you check that the full system working before inserting. You can use wet gauze to check whether the cauterising tip working condition. Insert the tip of the EVH kit in warm water for a few seconds to bring it to body temperature. Insert the unit into the leg and try to avoid any forceful insertion which can tear the vein. This happens due to branches or veins being trapped between the port and the EVH unit. It is important for the harvester to understand that there is a blind spot on the EVH unit. The vein branches should be cut from the lower end to the thigh rather than pushing the EVH unit fully to the end. This technique allows the EVH unit to pass smoothly without tearing any vein branches.

Once the EVH unit is passed to the targeted end whether it is at the thigh or lower end of the leg, the branches can be dissected and cut. Please try not to use the C-ring wherever possible, if needed please do not twist the vein with the C-ring. Twisting the vein with the C-ring can cause histological level damage to the vein. The small branches can get torn very easily from the base of the vein.

- Once the vein is completely mobilised check with C-hook gently, ligate the distal and proximal end of the vein with ligaclips and cut it out or make a small skin incision on the thigh/lower leg area just above the vein and locate the vein and dissect it.
- Insert the vessel cannula on the proximal end of the vein and gently inject heparinised blood, tie all the branches with 4/0 vicryl ties and transfer into the heparinised blood pot.
- Check for any bleeding in the wound site, if satisfactory insert a leg drain and do the normal closure of the incisions with 2/0 vicryl and 3/0 vicryl to the skin.
- Apply small dressing, and pressure bandage from the ankle to the thigh.

Important Traps to Remember While Harvesting:

Technical Errors:

- Switch off everything and start again.
- Ask the theatre staff to check all the electric and non-electric connections, sometimes it gets loosened during connection or transportation.
- Before using the camera, make sure you have done the white balance for image clarity.
- Keep a roll under the knee area to lift the thigh area up and support the knee during harvesting.

- While harvesting thigh, ask the foot end to be lowered down which allows you to handle the EVH equipment smoothly without feet getting in your way.
- While harvesting the lower end of the leg, put the foot end down and stand on the opposite side of the harvesting leg which reduces any stress/injury on your shoulder, back and neck.

Branches:

- Thin patients GSV can be harvested using EVH but good assessment and ultrasound scanning need to be done preoperatively by an experienced practitioner.
- During dissection, the vein needs to be removed from the skin's dermal layer very slowly and gently using the peeling technique and keep the cone away from the vein as much as possible (Video 2).
- During cutting and coagulation, the EVH unit need to be advanced gently by cutting the dermal layer of the skin to create more space inside the leg tunnel.
- The vein should be dissected posteriorly and then anteriorly to give more room for the EVH unit and to avoid damaging the vein adventitial layer.

Bleeding: How to Handle or Avoid?

- Dissect the branches carefully especially a thin hair line branches which can bleed and obstruct the view.

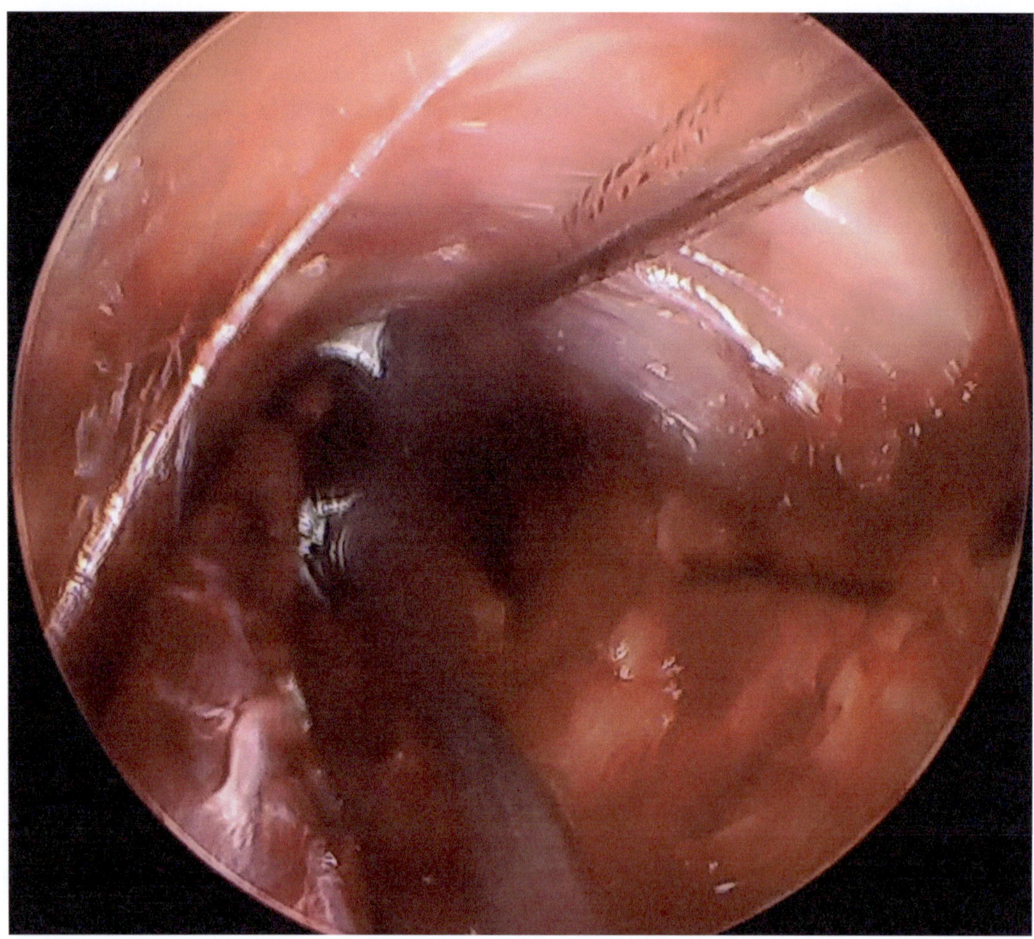

Video 2 Haemopro dissection of vein side branches (▶ https://doi.org/10.1007/000-a7c)

– Do not dissect or hit any adventitial or capillaries network whilst dissecting because it can fill up the leg tunnel quickly.
– Primarily cut and coagulate small branches and cut all the big/thick branches at the end to avoid any bleeding. Use the intermittent coagulation technique rather than continuous which helps to coagulate the vein slowly. For thicker or bifurcating branches which are more than 1 cm thicker, use intermittent coagulation method of 5 s, stop, 5 s, stop and final 5 s and stop technique.
– If there is any minimal amount of bleeding on an isolated area:

  • Please leave that area for few minutes to settle and come back to that area for dissection or branch cutting. Sometimes, you may experience blood clotting or reddish bruising around that area and if you do, please ignore and proceed working.
  • If the amount of bleeding is larger, you can remove the full EVH kit and squeeze the blood out from the tunnel and leave it for a couple of minutes to settle. If it is larger and you are unable to stop it, it is better to convert to bridging technique or put pressure on that area to stop the bleeding.
  • Major bleeding can be avoided by cutting the thicker/larger branches at the end of the vein harvesting procedure. Make sure you check that the full vein is harvested, and all small branches and surrounding tissues are removed and then cut the larger branches before disconnecting the vein.

– Try and avoid injecting any saline to clear the lens if possible because this fills up the leg tunnel. Always try to touch the wall of the leg tunnel to clear your lens.

Vein Damage: How to Avoid It?

– During learning, it is possible to tear the vein or cut the vein into two pieces. It is important to take it slowly as a step by step harvesting method rather than trying to do everything together.
– Vein can get damaged by the tip of the cone which can lead to carbon dioxide embolism. To avoid:

  • Always make sure that your dissecting cone on the middle of the screen during dissection and try to keep the cone away from the vein. Important tip to dissection of the vein is to take vein with surrounding tissues which will avoid any tears or holes on the vein.
  • Set the carbon dioxide level minimum of 10 mmHg with 1-3 L flow to avoid drying the adventitial layer of the vein. 1 L for thin legs and 2-3 L for obese patients.

Obese Patients:

– Scan the leg pre-surgery and mark where your skin incision is and measure the depth of the vein which will help you to find the vein.
– If it is very hard to find the vein if the depth of the vein is above 1 cm. You can use the cone dissector to search for the vein which avoids making pockets or rough dissection.
– Make the skin incision smaller than 2 cm will allow you to keep the insertion port in place with minimal air in the balloon.
– Set the gas flow to 12 mmHg and 3 L rate which will help the fat tissues away. Make sure that you do not create any pockets or distort the fat tissues during dissection.

Vein with surrounding tissues.

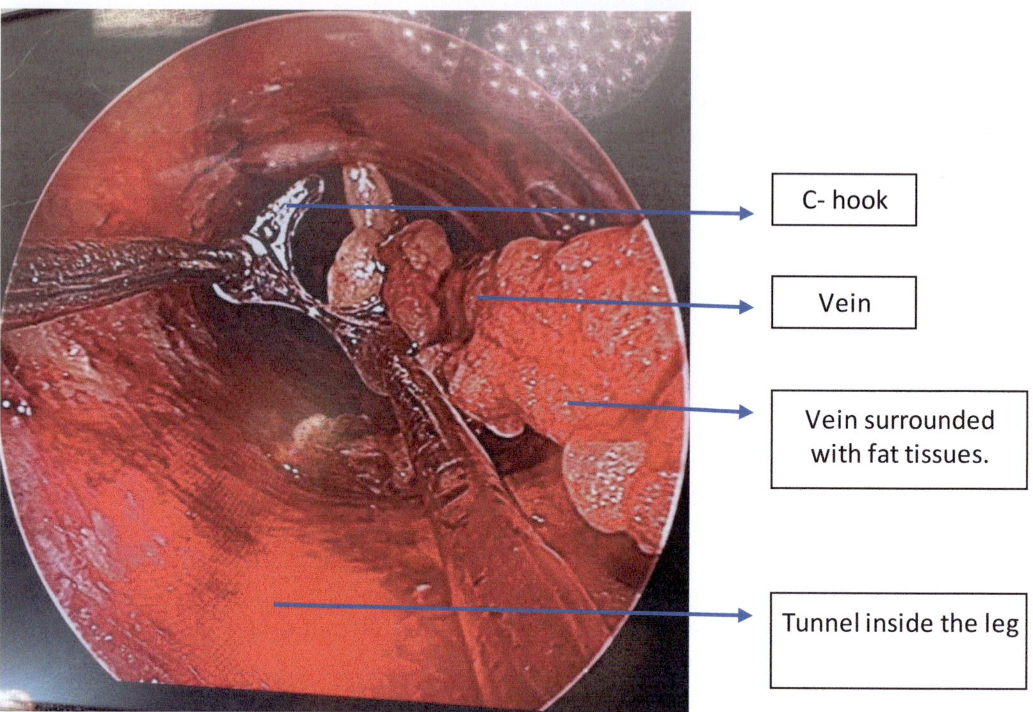

Conclusion:

Endoscopic vein harvesting is an art and the practitioner needs to be trained step by step by the structured training method to obtain the best quality vein for the coronary artery bypass grafting. We strongly believe that nothing is impossible, but we need careful assessment and patient selection which will avoid major problems during vein harvesting. Support mechanisms with clear guidance need to be in place to tackle difficult patients such as obese, thin and patients with segments of varicose veins. The EVH trainees need to be given the chance to learn on patients with no additional co-morbidities for vein harvesting.

4 Endoscopic Radial Artery Harvesting

Historical Context:

The radial artery (RA) was first used as a conduit for coronary artery bypass graft surgery (CABG) in 1971 by Carpentier and colleagues [14]. Use of the RA was abandoned in 1973 due to higher occlusion rates than the saphenous vein. Poor patency rates were attributed to graft spasm, severe intimal hyperplasia due to harvesting technique (skeletonization), and mechanical dilation [15]. A patent RA graft was discovered 15 years after it was previously thought to be occluded, leading to the revitalization of using the RA as a conduit in CABG [16]. Acar et al. [16], published results in 1992 showing 100% early patency rates of radial artery conduits. Three changes were made at that time including harvesting the radial artery as a pedicle, rather than skeletonization, replacing mechanical dilation with pharmaceutical dilation, and adding postprocedural vasodilator therapy with a calcium channel blocker or nitrate. RA use continues to be promoted in recent years with trusted evidence suggesting higher patency rates and survival benefit [17, 18].

Radial Artery Anatomy:

The brachial artery traverses distally through the upper arm until it's bifurcation into the radial and ulnar arteries within the cubital fossa. The RA continues in the lateral aspect of the forearm, while the ulnar continues medially. The RA lies between the flexor carpi radialis and brachioradialis muscles. As the RA continues distally, it becomes more superficial until it can be palpated just laterally to the tendon of the flexor carpi radialis muscle. As the RA approaches the wrist, it bifurcates into deep and superficial branches that proceed to anastomose with the branches of the ulnar artery forming the deep and superficial palmar arches. The first branch of the RA is the radial recurrent artery which has a lateral takeoff just distal to the origin of the RA [19]. The RA is responsible for blood supply to the posterolateral muscles of the forearm, elbow joint, carpal bones, thumb and lateral index finger. The superficial radial nerve traverses along the RA, deep to the brachioradialis muscle, then over the distal radius and radial fossa. The superficial radial nerve provides sensory innervation to the thumb, index, middle, and lateral half of the ring fingers in addition to the dorsal hand area of those fingers [20].

Endoscopic Radial Artery Harvest (ERAH)

Indications:

The RA should be considered for use in CABG when the coronary angiogram displays stenoses of >70% within the left anterior descending and left circumflex systems and >90% within the right coronary artery system (Fig. 5) for coronaries perfusing the LV myocardium [21]. The RA has been shown to have superior surgical outcomes to the saphenous vein (SV) and comparable surgical outcomes to the right internal thoracic artery (RITA) (while having a lower incidence of deep sternal wound infection), therefore it should be the second conduit of choice behind the left internal thoracic artery (LITA) [22–24]. The patient should be less than 75 years old as this has been shown to be the cutoff for loss of benefit for RA use [18].

Contraindications:

Contraindications for RA harvest include recent catheterization, Raynaud's disease, rheumatoid arthritis, scleroderma, subclavian stenosis, renal failure requiring hemodialysis (need for AV fistula), and poor forearm or hand collateral circulation [25]. Dupuytren's contracture was listed in this cited publication as a contraindication, however it is this author's opinion that Dupuytren's is not of vascular origin and neither its existing condition nor eventual repair would be affected by harvesting the RA. Additionally, carpal tunnel syndrome (CPS) was also listed in this reference as a contraindication, but in our experience, we have found that patients with surgically treated CPS can safely undergo RA harvest without complication.

Preoperative Planning

Collateral Circulation of the Hand:

The RA is predominantly responsible for blood supply to the thumb and radial side of the index finger [26]. The radial and ulnar arteries feed into the hand, forming superficial and deep palmar arches. A complete superficial palmar arch in which the ulnar artery is dominant and can adequately perfuse the entire hand is found in 84.4% of the population [27]. A combination of non-invasive techniques form the modified Allen's Test which can accurately determine the completeness of the palmar arch. This is performed

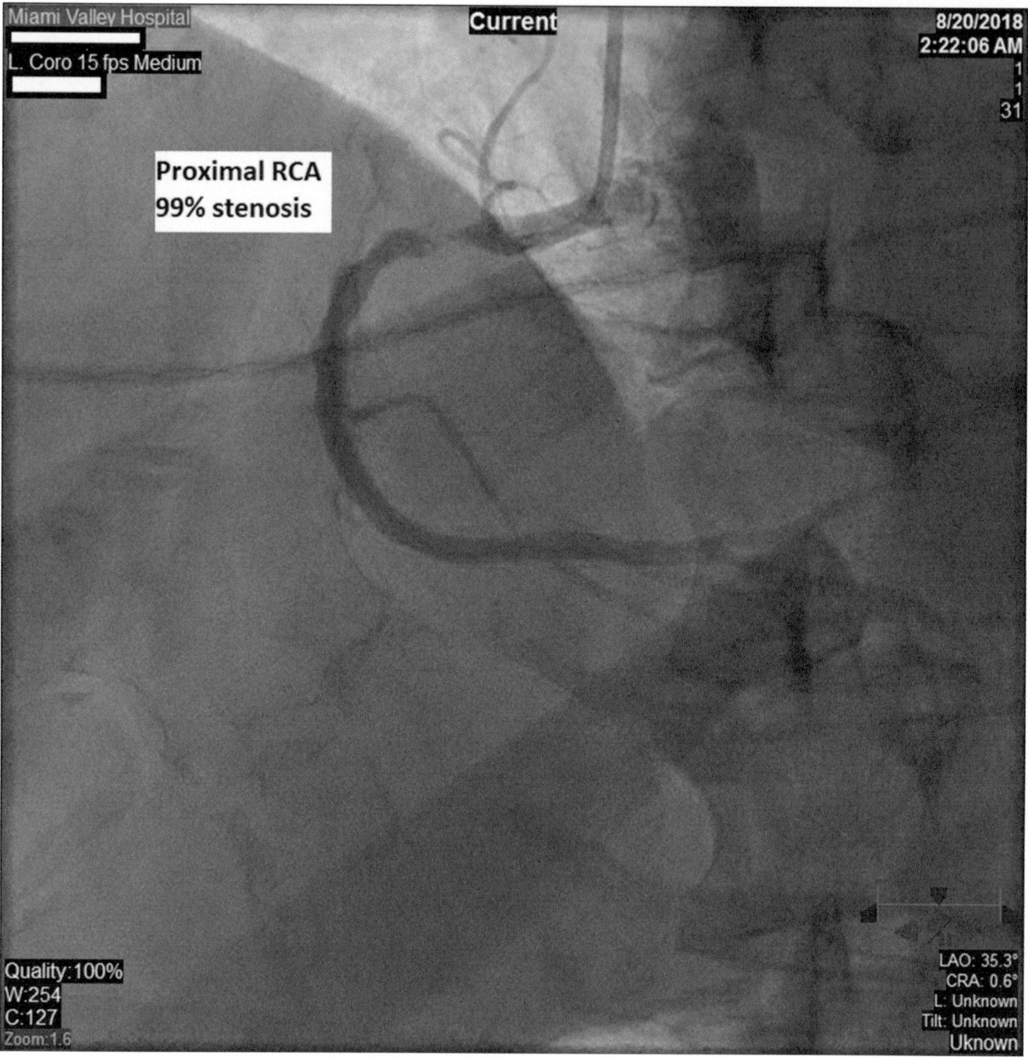

Fig. 5 Coronary artery angiogram displays stenoses >90% in the right coronary artery system

by applying a continuous pulse oximeter/ plethysmometer on the thumb. Once a baseline waveform amplitude and oxygen saturation are established, the radial and ulnar arteries are compressed while the patient is asked to clinch their fist. When the waveform amplitude has flattened and the oxygen saturation has diminished, the patient opens and relaxes their hand while the ulnar artery compression is lifted. The RA remains occluded by compression currently. Return of the pulse waveform to 50% amplitude or greater and baseline oxygen saturation is considered a negative test indicating the RA can be safely harvested without concern for hand ischemia.

Ultrasound:

Ultrasound (US) should be utilized preoperatively on every RA harvest case. The RA can be easily identified with the venae comitantes and visible pulsations. Measurements can be made quickly and accurately via US with the target diameter greater than 2 mm. The US can also be used to follow the length of the artery to evaluate

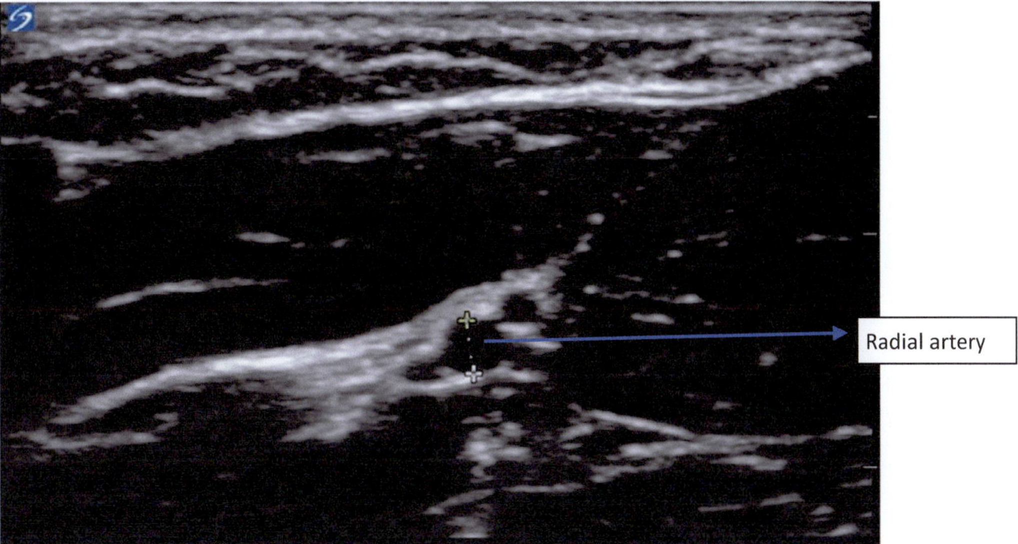

Fig. 6 Illustrates the ultrasound image of the radial artery

for any anatomical anomalies or intraluminal plaques (Fig. 6).

Surgical Steps:

Routine Setup:

Two arm boards are attached to the bed, and the arm is laid out to an angle slightly less 90°. If using a tourniquet; a non-sterile webril and tourniquet are placed on the upper arm. With a permanent marker, draw a line two finger widths below the antecubital fossa to demarcate the proximal limit of dissection. Draw a line on the wrist crease to demarcate the distal limit of dissection. Circumferentially prep from fingertips to the tourniquet per hospital protocol. After prep, exclude the non-sterile tourniquet with two 1010 drapes. The arm boards are then draped with a sterile Mayo stand cover. The arm is placed down with a rolled towel under the wrist (Fig. 7) to extend the incision sit.

Heparinization: Preoperative heparinization is initiated depending on surgeon preference.

Tourniquet Use:

A common debate within the RA harvesting community is whether or not to use a tourniquet for the procedure. The RA and its branches are significantly more delicate than that of the SV and the harvesting tunnel is often smaller than what is found in the leg. The use of a tourniquet ensures a bloodless field providing the best environment for precise dissection and cauterization of the branches and connective tissue. Often the argument is made to have the tourniquet in place and deflated, only to be inflated if significant bleeding is encountered. This scenario place's reliability on OR staff to quickly inflate the tourniquet and leaves a bloody environment in which additional harvesting would be more challenging due to compromised visualization. Use of the tourniquet is not without risk. Potential complications include nerve injury (1:6200 for upper limb), muscle injury, vascular injury, skin injury. The most common side effect seen with upper extremity tourniquet use is sudden decrease in CVP and MAP due a combination of the release of anaerobic metabolites into the systemic circulation and shift in blood volume back into the extremity. For this reason, it is important to communicate with your anesthesia provider about the tourniquet deflation. One to three hours has been described as a safe time

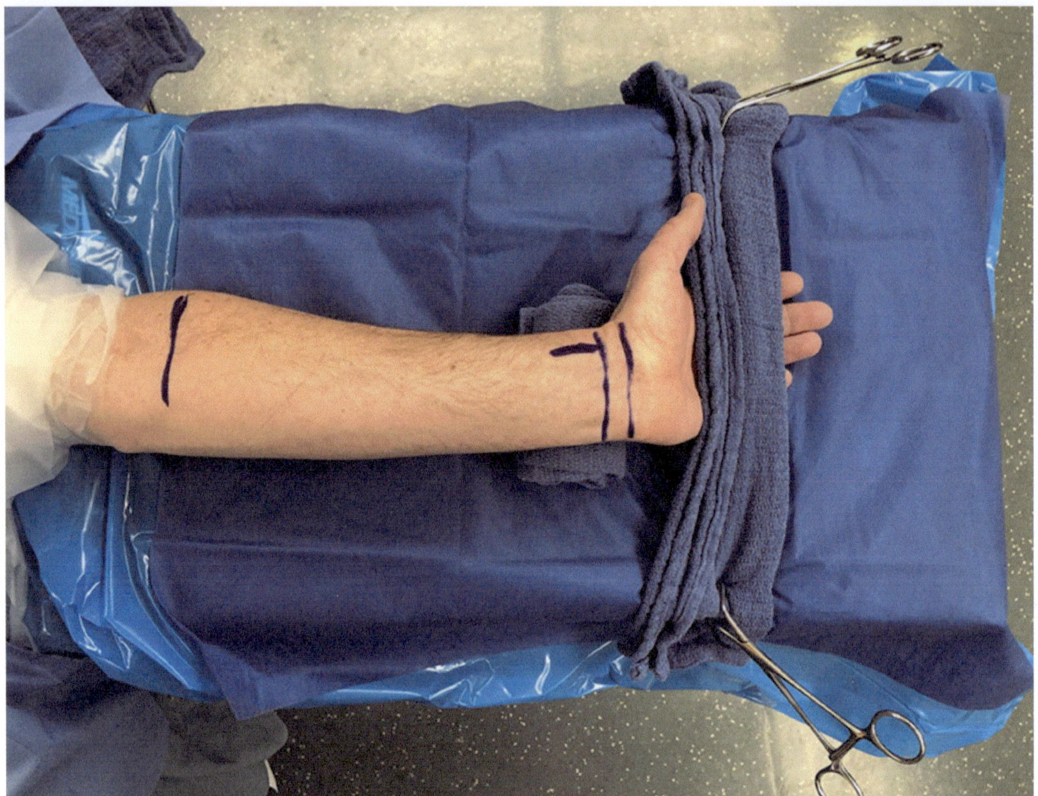

Fig. 7 Illustrates the hand position and setup before harvesting radial artery

limit for tourniquet use, however, with this procedure, no more than one hour should be needed nor exceeded [28].

Vasodilators:

Preoperative initiation of a vasodilator can aid in avoiding spasm of the RA. A nicardipine or diltiazem drip is started prior to incision at a modest rate of 2.5 mg/hr as tolerated by the patient's hemodynamics. The vasodilator drip is continued postoperatively until a PO calcium channel blocker can be started. Our practice prefers starting Amlodipine at 2.5 mg PO on postop day 1 with a 2 h overlap of the IV infusion prior to cessation. The calcium channel blocker is continued postoperatively for three months to one year, depending on institutional preference and patient tolerance [29].

Closed Tunnel Harvesting Technique:

Dissection:

An approximately 3 cm longitudinal incision is made over the RA just lateral to the tendon of the flexor carpi radialis muscle. A thin layer of adipose tissue will be dissected away to reveal the fascia (Fig. 8) covering the RA. The fascia can be cut away with Jameson scissors revealing the RA and satellite veins. There are numerous vascular branches in this area requiring delicate and precise ligation to avoid bleeding. Small clips are adequate to aid in the ligation of the branches; however, an ultrasonic scalpel is preferred for increased efficiency. Once the RA and accompanying veins are isolated, a vessel loop is passed (Fig. 9) under the pedicle. A soft bulldog clamp is applied to the RA and the modified

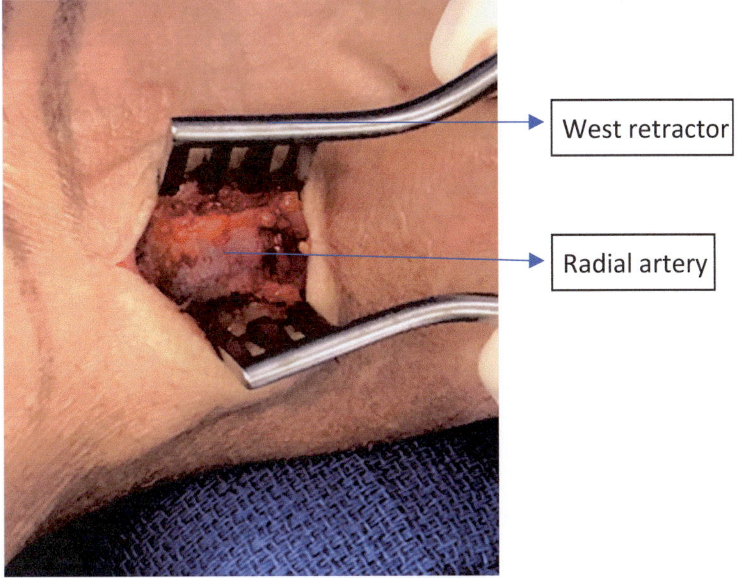

Fig. 8 Illustrates the initial exposure of the radial artery in the wrist

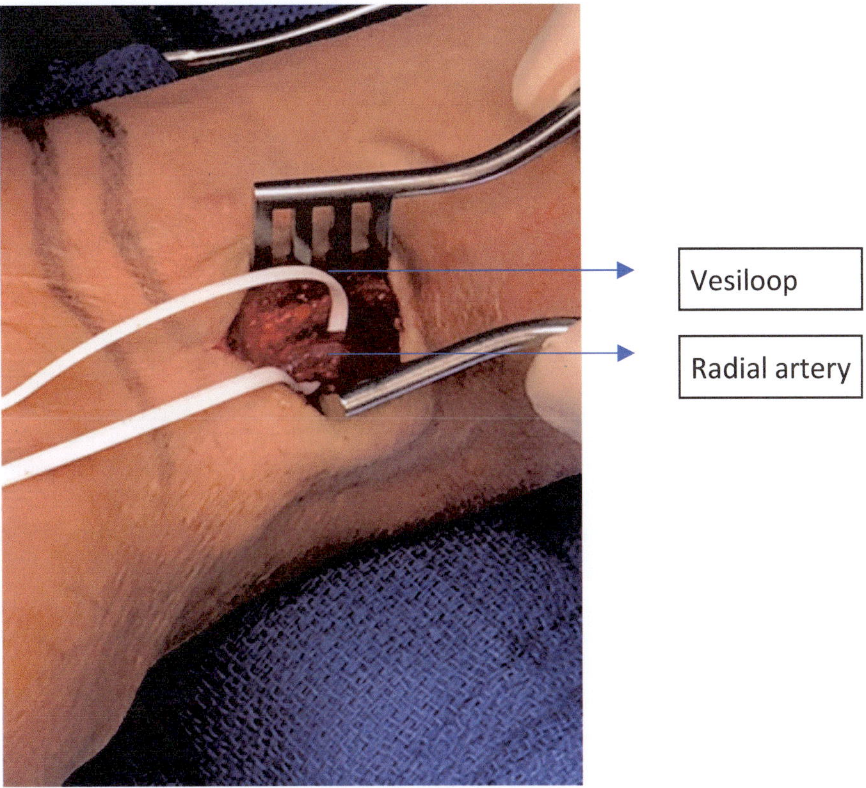

Fig. 9 Illustrates the isolated radial artery before harvesting

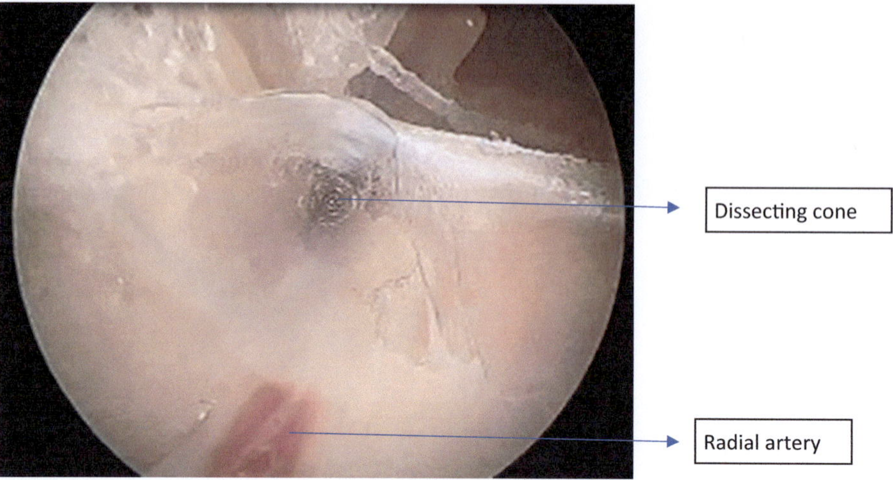

Fig. 10 Illustrates the tunnel in the hand and the endoscopic dissection tip

Allen's Test is again performed to ensure adequate hand perfusion by the ulnar artery. The bulldog clamp is then removed, and additional dissection of the RA pedicle and anterior fascia is performed as far proximal as possible to allow for safe entry of the endoscopic harvesting device. Exsanguinate the arm with an Esmark bandage and inflate the tourniquet.

The endoscopic harvesting device is then introduced into the incision (Fig. 10) in between the RA pedicle and the anterior fascia. Dissection is performed initially by an anterior pass following along the vena comitantes on either side. An additional posterior pass is then performed to identify any branches and connective tissue on the posterior aspect of the pedicle. During these dissection passes, it is important to glance away from the monitor down to the surgical field on occasion to assess the progress up the arm. The length of the RA is shorter than what a harvester will be accustomed to with the SV, therefore the proximal limit of dissection may be reached sooner than anticipated. The RA harvest differs from that of the SV in that the entirety of the harvesting device will not be needed to reach the endpoint. As the proximal limit of dissection is approached, there will be an increase in adipose tissue (Fig. 11) on and around the radial pedicle. Take caution when approaching branches for dissection as they are much more fragile than those of the SV (Fig. 12).

Cauterization:

Blunt tissue dissection is followed by the cauterization step. Introduce the device into the trocar, but do not proceed all the way into the tunnel. This pause allows you to evaluate the tunnel directly in front of the trocar. At this point, you can advance the cautery sheers to ligate any branches that would impede progression of the device and to also begin the anterior fasciotomy (Fig. 13). Continue the anterior fasciotomy approximately 1/3 the distance up the forearm, following the tendon of the brachioradialis muscle. Conclude the fasciotomy as the tendon crosses to the opposite side of the tunnel. Cauterize each branch as they are encountered to avoid avulsion injury. Branches of the RA are extremely small and fragile making them susceptible to avulsion. When the proximal limit of dissection has been reached, retrace the length of the pedicle to ensure that all branches and connective tissue have been ligated.

The harvesting device is then inserted the length of the tunnel to the proximal limit of dissection. Palpate the distal end of the device while watching the monitor to determine the desired ligation point. Using an #11 scalpel,

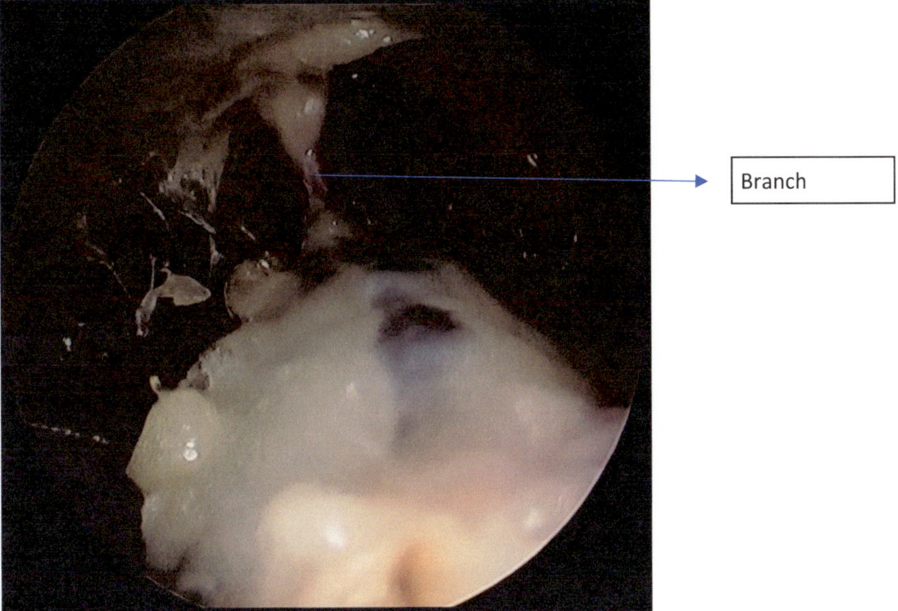

Fig. 11 Illustrates the clear hand tunnel and branches of the radial artery

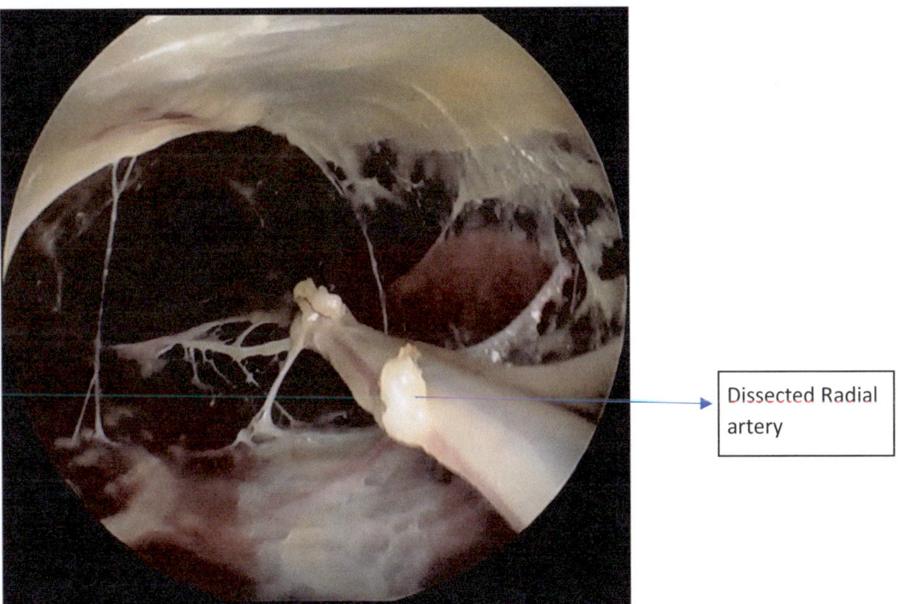

Fig. 12 Illustrates the dissected radial artery within the tunnel in the hand

puncture the skin down to the distal tunnel, carefully observing the tip of the blade to avoid injury to the pedicle. Insert a tonsil hemostat through the incision site and open the tips to stretch open the anterior fascia. When clamping the pedicle, consider the depth of the tunnel that it will need to be pulled through. This depth should coincide with an equal length on the

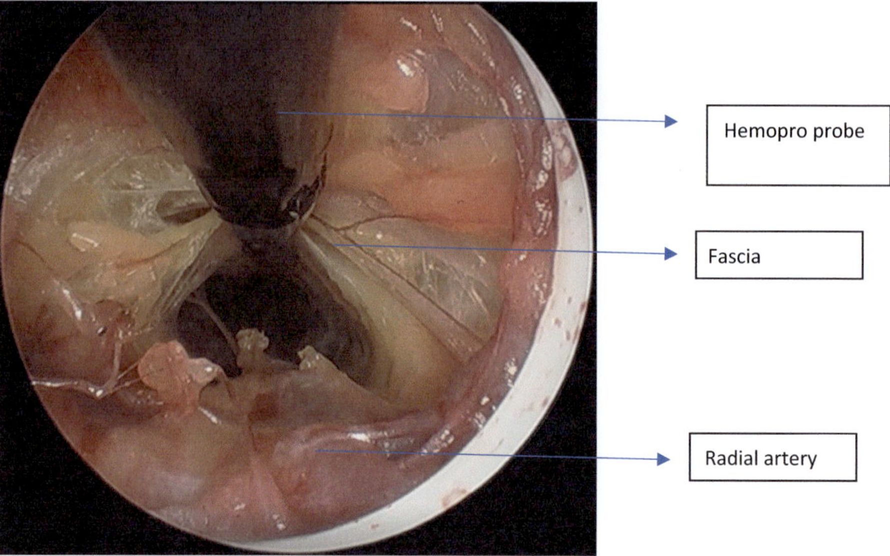

Fig. 13 Illustrates the anterior fasciotomy

proximal side of the clamp to avoid tension. With the pedicle clamped, remove the hemostat from the tunnel. Divide the pedicle under direct vision and ligate the proximal stump with a stick-tie using a 2–0 silk suture.

Conduit Preparation:

When the pedicle has been completely removed from the tunnel, deflate the tourniquet, if using. At this point, the distal end remains intact and blood flow should be observed from the proximal, ligated end. Place a soft bulldog on the ligated end and irrigate the pedicle with Papaverine (Fig. 14). Using a small clip applier, inspect the pedicle for branches and clip as they are encountered. A large clip can be applied to the connective tissue to denote the proximal end of the conduit to aid in maintaining orientation. Clamp the distal end of the radial pedicle with a right-angle hemostat and ligate with a scalpel. The distal RA stump is then tied off with a silk tie. Engage the proximal end of the RA and flush with vessel solution. The pedicle is then placed in a specimen cup with vessel solution and stored in a warmer at 37 °C (98°F). The wrist incision is closed in usual fashion. The stab-and-grab incision is closed with a single figure-of-eight subcutaneous stitch using a 3–0 Vicryl (Fig. 15). Cover each incision with appropriate bandages. The arm is wrapped with a Kerlex dressing followed by an ACE wrap. A continuous pulse oximeter is placed on the thumb to verify adequate perfusion. The wraps are removed on POD 1 to inspect for hematoma formation and baseline strength and sensation of the hand and arm.

Body Habitus Considerations:

The body habitus of the patient can provide additional variables that further complicate the procedure. Thin patients generally provide harvesting advantages as the initial dissection to the RA is simplified, the tunnel is easily maintained, and the depth of which the RA pedicle needs to traverse for ligation is minimal. Obese and muscular patients, however, provide certain procedural difficulties. A wrist with excess adipose tissue causes the initial dissection down to the RA to become challenging. If using a closed-

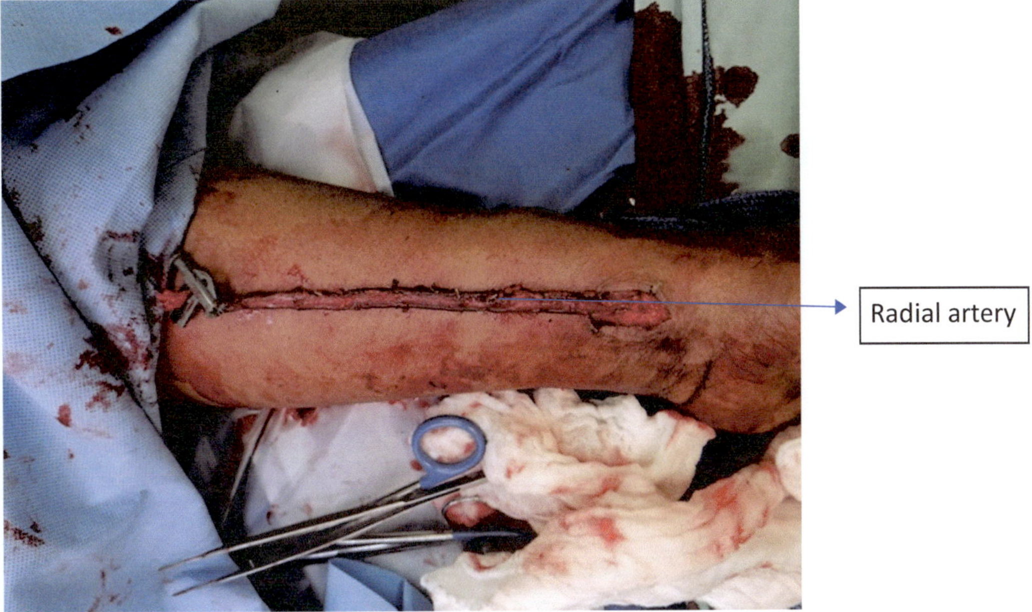

Fig. 14 Illustrates the harvested radial artery with bulldog clip

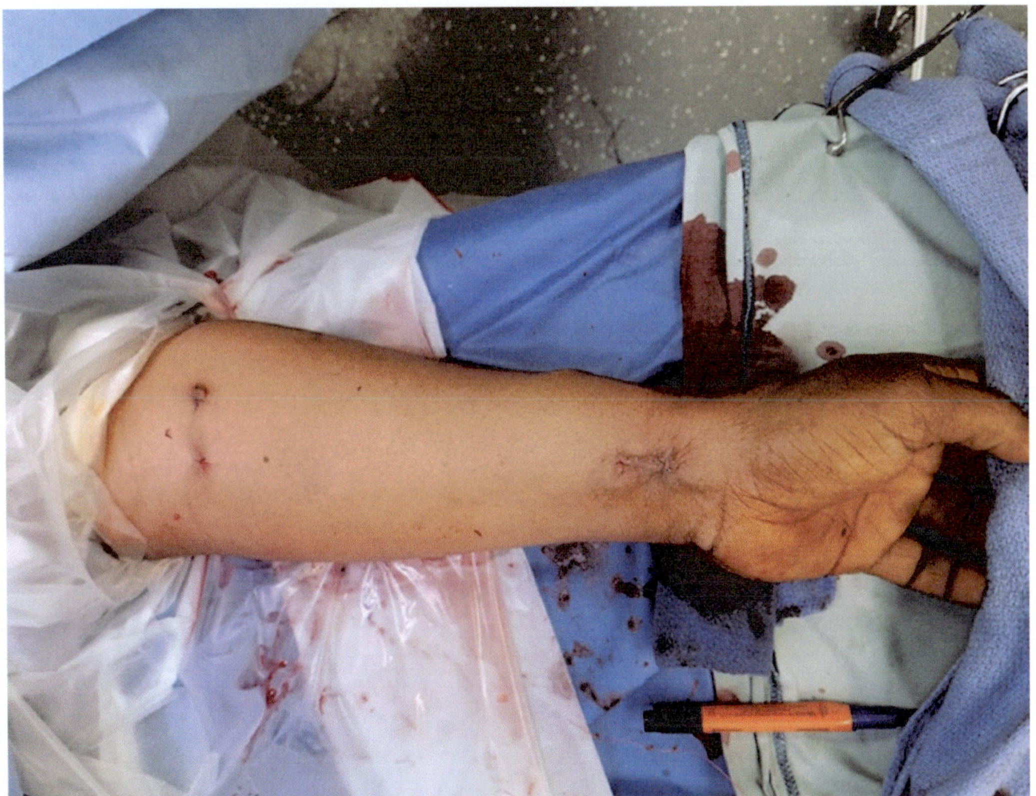

Fig. 15 Illustrates the closed arm after radial artery harvesting

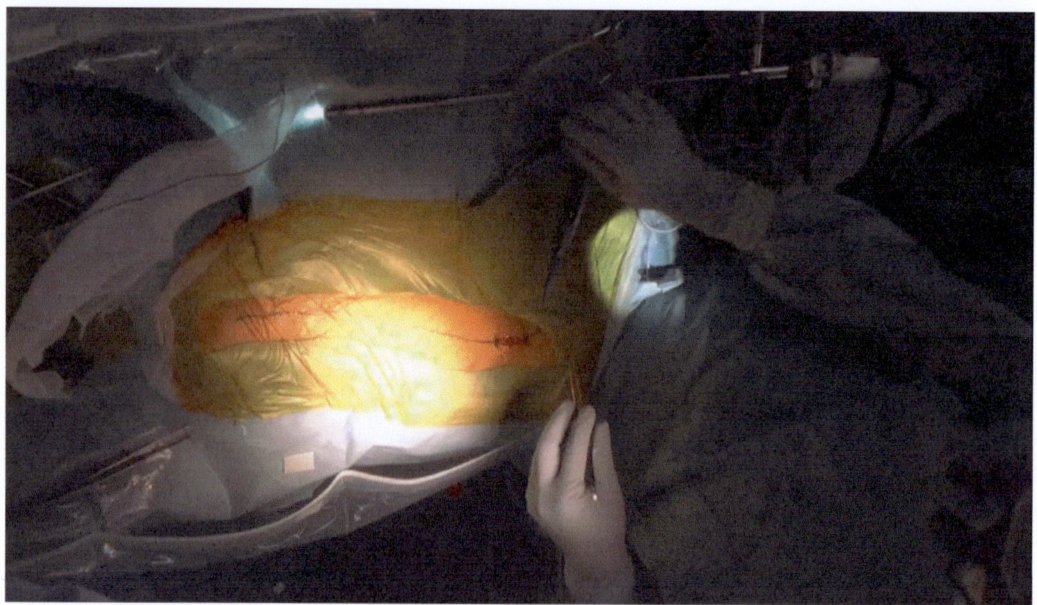

Video 3 Endoscopic radial artery harvest (▶ https://doi.org/10.1007/000-a7e)

CO_2 tunnel, an obese arm can cause the tunnel to collapse. In addition to collapsing the tunnel, the main disadvantage that a muscular arm produces is that of the depth which the radial pedicle must be retrieved for the stab-and-grab ligation (Video 3).

General Concepts:

A harvester should be experienced and proficient with endoscopic saphenous vein harvesting before attempting an endoscopic radial artery harvest. The branches of the RA are prone to avulsion and the risk of vasospasm is high due to vessel manipulation. Harvesters should have completed 50–75 endoscopic SV harvests independently prior to pursuing ERAH. If possible, formal training in a cadaver lab should be obtained prior to attempting in the operating room. In our experience, the non-dominant hand should be the first choice, but the dominant hand does not need to be avoided if that

RA proves to be the best conduit for harvesting. Internal evaluation of the patient's grip strength 3 months after surgery has shown no loss of strength from the donor arm.

5 Conclusion

Evidence continues to suggest the RA provides superior patency rates compared to the SV and comparable patency rates to the RITA. There is less risk associated with using the RA compared to the RITA. For these reasons, the RA should be the second choice for coronary revascularization conduit, following the LITA. ERAH has been proven to be a safe surgical technique with no effects on graft patency or mortality [30]. Compared to open harvesting, ERAH results in improved cosmesis, less pain, and fewer neurologic complications [31, 32].

References

1. Collins JP. New standards and criteria for accreditation of hospitals and posts for surgical training. ANZ J Surg. 2008;78(4):277–81.
2. Krishnamoorthy B, Critchley WR, Bhinda P, Crockett J, John A, Bridgewater BJ, et al. Does the introduction of a comprehensive structured training programme for endoscopic vein harvesting improve conduit quality? A multicentre pilot study. Interact Cardiovasc Thorac Surg. 2015;20(2):186–93.
3. Klassen RM, Klassen JRL. Self-efficacy beliefs of medical students: a critical review. Perspect Med Educ. 2018;7(2):76–82.
4. Goldman S, Zadina K, Moritz T, Ovitt T, Sethi G, Copeland JG, et al. Long-term patency of saphenous vein and left internal mammary artery grafts after coronary artery bypass surgery: results from a Department of Veterans Affairs Cooperative Study. J Am Coll Cardiol. 2004;44(11):2149–56.
5. Mitchel P. Goldman RAW. Chapter 12: Clinical Methods for Sclerotherapy of Telangiectasias,: Elsevier; 2017.
6. Chen SS, Prasad SK. Long saphenous vein and its anatomical variations. Australas J Ultrasound Med. 2009;12(1):28–31.
7. Krishnamoorthy B, Critchley WR, Glover AT, Nair J, Jones MT, Waterworth PD, et al. A randomized study comparing three groups of vein harvesting methods for coronary artery bypass grafting: endoscopic harvest versus standard bridging and open techniques. Interact Cardiovasc Thorac Surg. 2012;15(2):224–8.
8. Slim K, Bazin JE. From informed consent to shared decision-making in surgery. J Visc Surg. 2019;156 (3):181–4.
9. Krishnamoorthy B, Critchley WR, Thompson AJ, Payne K, Morris J, Venkateswaran RV, et al. Study Comparing Vein Integrity and Clinical Outcomes in Open Vein Harvesting and 2 Types of Endoscopic Vein Harvesting for Coronary Artery Bypass Grafting: The VICO Randomized Clinical Trial (Vein Integrity and Clinical Outcomes). Circulation. 2017;136(18):1688–702.
10. Illig KA, Rhodes JM, Sternbach Y, Green RM. Financial impact of endoscopic vein harvest for infrainguinal bypass. J Vasc Surg. 2003;37(2): 323–30.
11. Garcia-Altes A, Peiro S. A systematic review of cost-effectiveness evidence of endoscopic saphenous vein harvesting: is it efficient? Eur J Vasc Endovasc Surg. 2011;41(6):831–6.
12. Luckraz H, Cartwright C, Nagarajan K, Kaur P, Nevill A. Major adverse cardiac and cerebrovascular event and patients' quality of life after endoscopic vein harvesting as compared with open vein harvest (MAQEH): a pilot study. Open Heart. 2018;5(1): e000694.
13. Brown EN, Kon ZN, Tran R, Burris NS, Gu J, Laird P, et al. Strategies to reduce intraluminal clot formation in endoscopically harvested saphenous veins. J Thorac Cardiovasc Surg. 2007;134 (5):1259–65.
14. Carpentier A, Guermonprez JL, Deloche A, Frechette C, DuBost C. The aorta-to-coronary radial artery bypass graft. A technique avoiding pathological changes in grafts. Ann Thorac Surg. 1973;16 (2):111–21.
15. Verma S, Szmitko PE, Weisel RD, Bonneau D, Latter D, Errett L, et al. Should radial arteries be used routinely for coronary artery bypass grafting? Circulation. 2004;110(5):e40–6.
16. Acar C, Jebara VA, Portoghese M, Beyssen B, Pagny JY, Grare P, et al. Revival of the radial artery for coronary artery bypass grafting. Ann Thorac Surg. 1992;54(4):652–9; discussion 9–60.
17. Collins P, Webb CM, Chong CF, Moat NE, Radial Artery Versus Saphenous Vein Patency Trial I. Radial artery versus saphenous vein patency randomized trial: five-year angiographic follow-up. Circulation. 2008;117(22):2859–64.
18. Gaudino M, Benedetto U, Fremes S, Biondi-Zoccai G, Sedrakyan A, Puskas JD, et al. Radial-Artery or Saphenous-Vein Grafts in Coronary-Artery Bypass Surgery. N Engl J Med. 2018;378(22):2069–77.
19. Marchese RM, Geiger Z. Anatomy, Shoulder and Upper Limb, Forearm Radial Artery. StatPearls. Treasure Island (FL); 2021.
20. Glover NM, Murphy PB. Anatomy, Shoulder and Upper Limb, Radial Nerve. StatPearls. Treasure Island (FL); 2021.
21. Hillis LD, Smith PK, Anderson JL, Bittl JA, Bridges CR, Byrne JG, et al. 2011 ACCF/AHA guideline for coronary artery bypass graft surgery: executive summary: a report of the American College of Cardiology Foundation/American Heart Association Task Force on Practice Guidelines. J Thorac Cardiovasc Surg. 2012;143(1):4–34.
22. Baudo M, Gaudino M. Radial artery and right internal thoracic artery: jousting for the throne of coronary artery bypass grafting. Ann Transl Med. 2017;5(17):354.
23. Gaudino M, Lorusso R, Rahouma M, Abouarab A, Tam DY, Spadaccio C, et al. Radial artery versus right internal thoracic artery versus saphenous vein as the second conduit for coronary artery bypass surgery: a network meta-analysis of clinical outcomes. J Am Heart Assoc. 2019;8(2): e010839.
24. Tranbaugh RF, Schwann TA, Swistel DG, Dimitrova KR, Al-Shaar L, Hoffman DM, et al. Coronary artery bypass graft surgery using the radial artery, right internal thoracic artery, or saphenous vein as the second conduit. Ann Thorac Surg. 2017;104(2):553–9.
25. Navia JL, Olivares G, Ehasz P, Gillinov AM, Svensson LG, Brozzi N, et al. Endoscopic radial artery harvesting procedure for coronary artery

bypass grafting. Ann Cardiothorac Surg. 2013;2 (4):557–64.

26. Nguyen JD, Duong H. Anatomy, Shoulder and Upper Limb, Hand Arteries. StatPearls. Treasure Island (FL); 2021.

27. Gellman H, Botte MJ, Shankwiler J, Gelberman RH. Arterial patterns of the deep and superficial palmar arches. Clin Orthop Relat Res. 2001;383:41–6.

28. Kumar K, Railton C, Tawfic Q. Tourniquet application during anesthesia: "What we need to know?" J Anaesthesiol Clin Pharmacol. 2016;32(4):424–30.

29. Gaudino M, Benedetto U, Fremes SE, Hare DL, Hayward P, Moat N, et al. Effect of Calcium-Channel Blocker Therapy on Radial Artery Grafts After Coronary Bypass Surgery. J Am Coll Cardiol. 2019;73(18):2299–306.

30. Rahouma M, Kamel M, Benedetto U, Ohmes LB, Di Franco A, Lau C, et al. Endoscopic versus open radial artery harvesting: A meta-analysis of randomized controlled and propensity matched studies. J Card Surg. 2017;32(6):334–41.

31. Bisleri G, Giroletti L, Hrapkowicz T, Bertuletti M, Zembala M, Arieti M, et al. Five-Year Clinical Outcome of Endoscopic Versus Open Radial Artery Harvesting: A Propensity Score Analysis. Ann Thorac Surg. 2016;102(4):1253–9.

32. Patel AN, Henry AC, Hunnicutt C, Cockerham CA, Willey B, Urschel HC, Jr. Endoscopic radial artery harvesting is better than the open technique. Ann Thorac Surg. 2004;78(1):149–53; discussion-53.

Endoscopic Vein Harvest Using an Open System (Terumo®)

Donna Croft, Steven Power, and Louise Parry

Abstract

The advent of endoscopic vein harvesting (EVH) has allowed operators to harvest the long saphenous vein (LSV) through small incisions. This has translated into a reduction in leg wound infections, pain, hospital length of stay and recent studies demonstrate it to be equal to open vein harvesting (OVH) with regards to long term vein graft patency. Within our institution, EVH is routinely performed by a Surgical Care Practitioner (SCP) for most patients undergoing coronary artery bypass grafts (CABG). The EVH system routinely used at our institution is the Terumo® Virtuosaph® Plus Endoscopic Vessel Harvesting System. The learning curve for EVH is steep and although we have encountered many traps along the way, we have developed some tips and tricks that we would like to share with you within this chapter. Drawing on our experiences at Blackpool this chapter will walk the operator through the steps required to ensure successful EVH for patients undergoing CABG. It will begin with the preoperative assessment of patients for EVH, followed by the procedure. This is broken down into two parts; the dissection and the harvest, followed by postoperative complications.

Keywords

Endoscopic vein harvesting · EVH · Terumo · Long saphenous vein · Coronary artery bypass surgery · CABG

Supplementary Information The online version contains supplementary material available at https://doi.org/10.1007/978-3-031-21104-1_7. The videos can be accessed individually by clicking the DOI link in the accompanying figure caption or by scanning this link with the SN More Media App.

D. Croft (✉) · S. Power · L. Parry
Lancashire Cardiac Centre, Blackpool Teaching Hospitals NHS Foundation Trust, Blackpool, UK
e-mail: donna.croft2@nhs.net

1 Introduction

Use of an Endoscopic Vein Harvest (EVH) technique, when harvesting the Long Saphenous Vein (LSV) for Coronary Artery Bypass Graft Surgery (CABG), has been shown to reduce leg wound complications when compared to open vein harvesting, with no significant difference in the rate of major adverse cardiac events [1].

The EVH programme was initiated at Blackpool Teaching Hospitals NHS Foundation Trust in 2007 and has become the standard practice for all patients undergoing CABG. Currently, approximately 75% of patients undergoing CABG surgery at the trust receive EVH using the Terumo™ EVH system.

2 Pre-operative Considerations

2.1 Equipment Preparation

Prior to undertaking your first EVH procedure, it is important to ensure you have all the equipment available, that it is working and that all the equipment is compatible with each other.

The following equipment is essential (Fig. 1):

Non-disposable

- Video stack system and camera.
- CO_2 insufflation system.
- A compatible light lead.
- A compatible generator (See Table 1).
- Terumo™ Endoscope (MCENDO550).

Disposable

- Virtuosaph® Plus Endoscopic Vein Harvesting System.
- Camera cover.
- CO_2 insufflation tubing.

2.2 Orientation to the Terumo System (See Video 1)

See Fig. 2

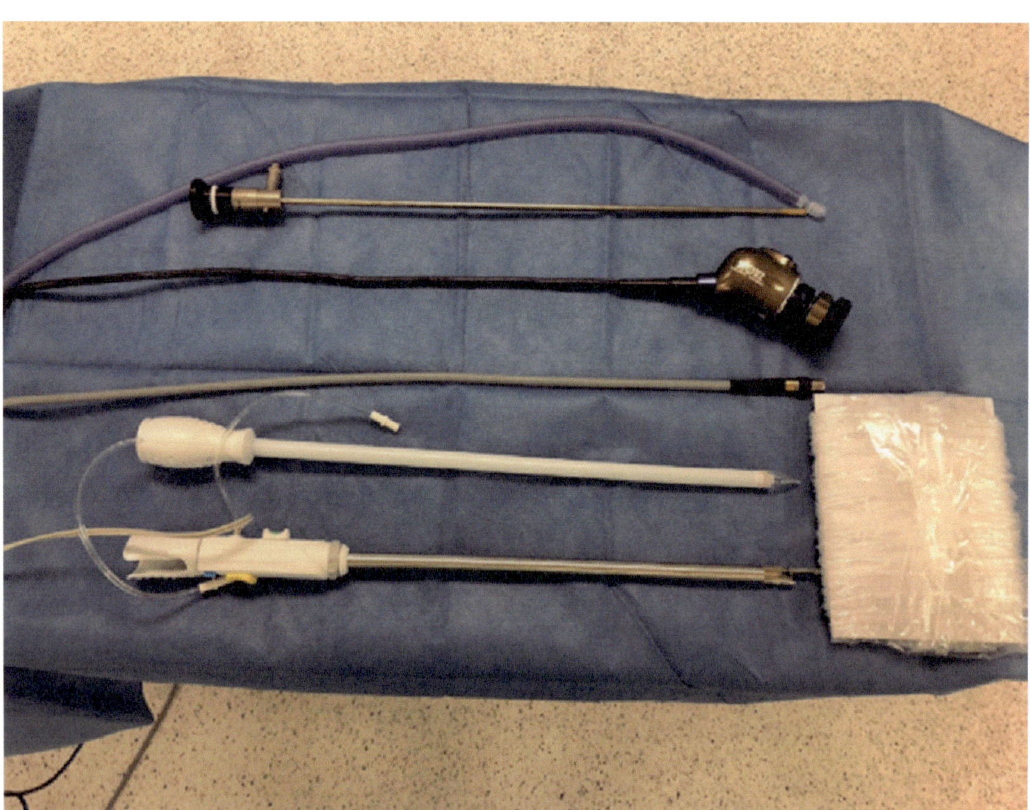

Fig. 1 EVH equipment

Table 1 Compatible generators

Generator	Model	Foot Pedal Type	Mode	Settings range (W)
Olympus®	UES-40	Dual (Cut/Coag)	Bipolar cut	8–12
ValleyLap™	Force FX	Single	Bipolar Macro	14–18
ValleyLap™	Force FX-C	Single	Bipolar Macro	14–18
Bovie®	Aaron® ORIPRO 300	Single	Bipolar Macro	8–10
ConMed®	System 5000™	Single	Bipolar Macro	6–8
Olympus®	ESG-400	Dual (cut/coag)	Bipolar BiSoft Coag effect	8
Covidien®	Force triad™	Single	Bipolar Macro	6–7

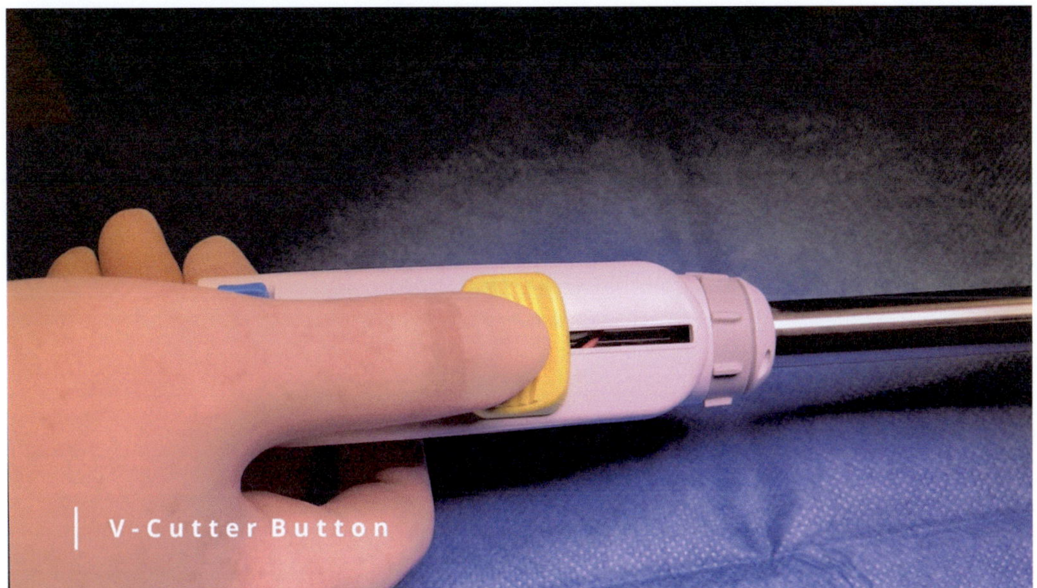

Video 1 Orientation to Terumo scope (▶ https://doi.org/10.1007/000-a7h)

2.3 Theatre Set-Up

Prior to commencing each EVH procedure, get into a routine of ensuring that the equipment is set up and ready for use in a timely manner (Fig. 3). This allows for any issues to be fixed prior to commencing the procedure and reduces the chances of issues occurring during the EVH. Issues occurring mid procedure can make the EVH more difficult, increase the length of harvest time and create added and unnecessary stress.

- Plug in the stack system and diathermy and test the equipment where possible to ensure that it is working.
- Set the screen of the stack system up so the height is level with your head and is opposite where you are standing. This ensures minimal strain is placed on your neck and back.
- Ensure all the equipment is set on the appropriate settings, ready for use.
- Ensure there is enough CO_2 gas in the canister for the EVH.

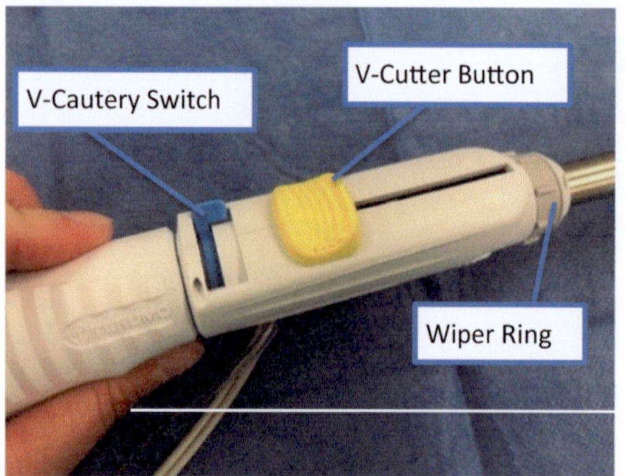

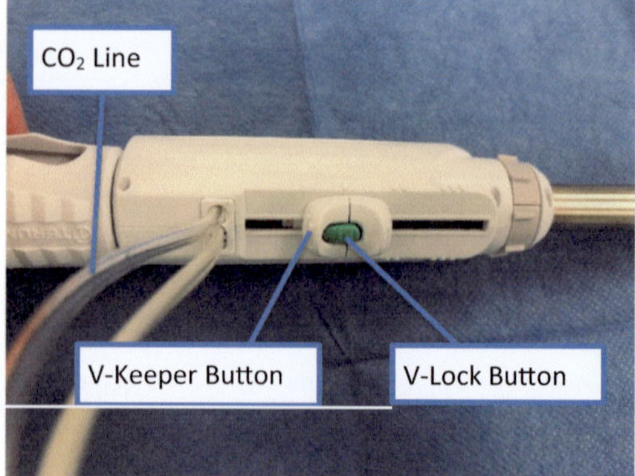

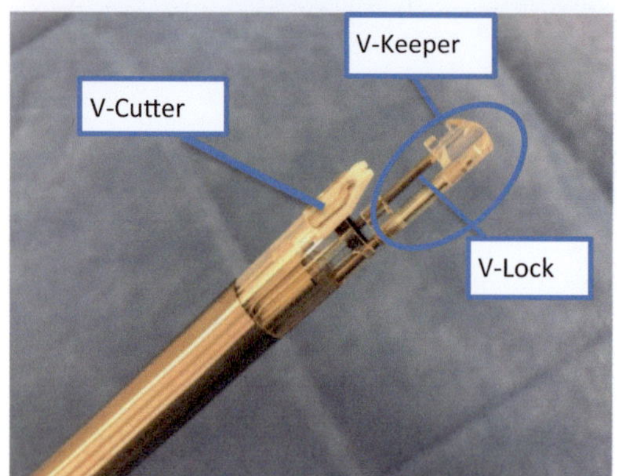

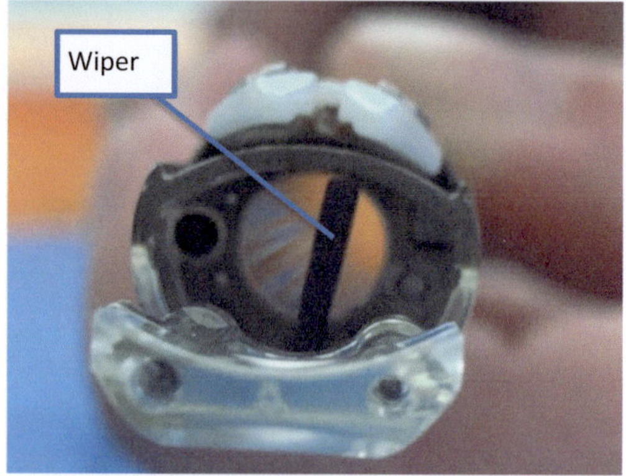

Fig. 2 Equipment orientation

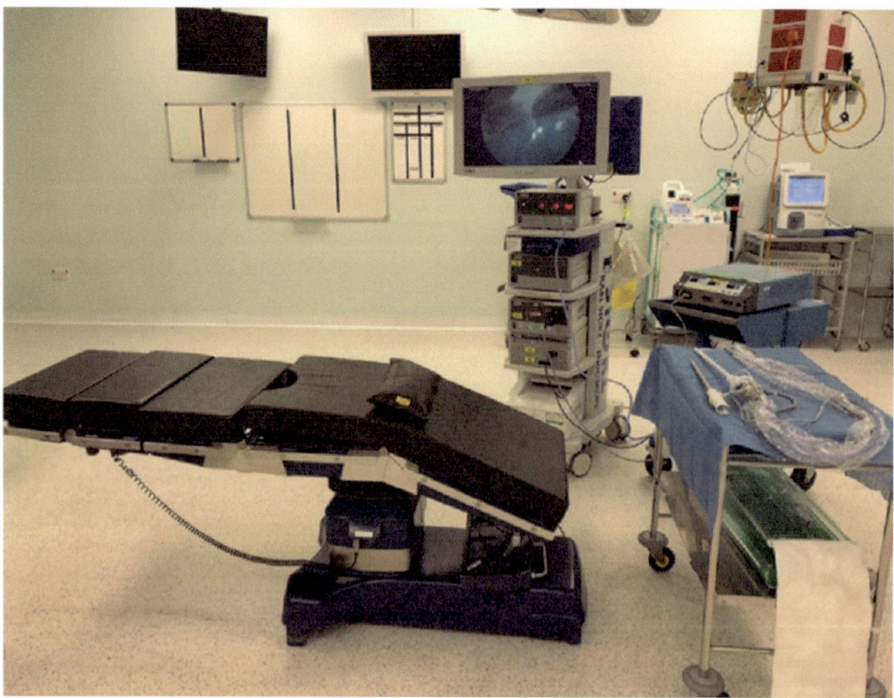

Fig. 3 Theatre set up

- Ensure the necessary surgical instruments are available for use.
  - Basic instruments including a Scalpel, Scissors and Forceps
  - A Small Langenbeck
  - Artery forceps, such as Mosquitos
  - A long-handled artery forcep, such as a Sawtell

Note: Ideally, learn to harvest the vein by standing on the same side as the leg from which you are harvesting. Although, only a minor movement, harvesting from the opposite leg can cause pain in the lower back from reaching over. When all the equipment is placed ergonomically, EVH allows the operator to maintain a better posture and sustain the body's three natural curves [2].

2.4 Pre-operative Patient Assessment

When beginning an EVH programme, initial patient selection is vital. The first 20–30 cases will be focused on becoming familiar with the equipment and its application, alongside consolidating the muscle memory and hand–eye coordination required for EVH. Choosing the initial patients carefully means there will be an increased chance of a successful harvest and minimal damage to the conduit. Once the use of the equipment has been mastered, it will be easier to utilise the techniques discussed later in the chapter to adapt to more difficult harvests.

Prior to commencing each EVH ensure you are aware of the patients past medical history and carry out a clinical examination of the lower limbs, including ultrasound assessment if appropriately trained. If any of these indicate that a harvest may be more difficult when done endoscopically, then consider using an alternative method. The quality of the conduit is the optimum priority and if there is a risk that this may be compromised by using an endoscopic approach, then an alternative method should be utilised until the operator is more experienced.

2.5 Patients Past Medical History

Although the past medical history of the patient should be reviewed prior to any conduit harvest, some patient history can indicate whether harvesting the vein using an EVH method may be more difficult.

- **Patients on anticoagulant treatment** immediately prior to surgery can mean a greater chance of bleeding within the tunnel.
- **Patients who have had previous trauma to the lower extremities** may develop tissue fibrosis, which can make manipulation of the scope difficult or may prevent a tunnel forming. This can be dependent on the type and location of the trauma.

2.6 Clinical Examination

Clinical examination of a patient's lower limbs can also indicate when an EVH may be more challenging.

- **Large legs** can mean the vein is located deeper in the leg and means an increased chance of fatty tissue falling into the tunnel, which can reduce your vision. You could consider harvesting the vein in the calves of these patients, if the LSV is suitable.
- **Small legs** can mean the vein is located more superficially within the leg. This makes manipulation of the scope within the tunnel difficult when dissecting the fat from the vein and can lead to significant bruising on the surface of the skin.
- **Fragile patients** can mean fragile tissues and fragile veins, which are more prone to damage. These veins commonly may also have tiny, hair-like tributaries, which can easily become avulsed by the endoscope.

2.7 Ultrasound

Using ultrasound prior to harvesting the LSV has been shown to reduce both the length and quantity of incisions and reduce the harvesting of unsuitable conduit, in multiple studies [3] (Fig. 4). Ultrasound is also non-invasive and relatively easy to use once trained. In EVH, pre-operative ultrasound also has the added benefit of providing an accurate location of the LSV, at the medial aspect of the upper calf, where the initial EVH incision is made. Identifying the LSV for EVH can sometimes be difficult in the absence of ultrasound when compared to the use of land-mark techniques commonly used for open vein harvest. Ultrasound can also identify a superficial or deep LSV, which can make EVH more challenging. The use of ultrasound in EVH therefore has two advantages.

Pre-operative ultrasound aids in identifying the location of optimum LSV by:

- **Confirming the presence of the LSV** and that it has not been removed during a previous surgery.
- **The diameter of the LSV**—Studies have reported that the most optimum LSV size for CABG surgery as measured by ultrasound is (2–5 mm) [3].
- **Highlighting any calibre changes or bifurcations.**
- **Identifying any varicosed of unusable segments,** due to dilation or tortuosity or whether there is just one small area effected.
- **Identifying any thrombosed segments,** which should be avoided.

Pre-operative ultrasound can be used to assess EVH difficulty by:

- **Providing a means of locating the LSV for the initial incision** at medial aspect of upper calf. This can be marked using an indelible skin marker (Fig. 5).
- **Identifying whether the LSV is superficial or deep,** which can make the harvest more difficult.

- **Identifying whether the vein is located posteriorly.**
- **Identifying locations where the vein takes a sudden change in direction,** or a large tributary which may distort the location of the true LSV once carrying out EVH. These locations can be marked using an indelible skin marker. Large tributaries can also be more difficult to seal effectively using the diathermy. Tips to overcome this are discussed later in the chapter.
- **Identification of 'red-herring' veins.** In some patients, superficial veins may run near the true LSV. Early identification reduces the chances of following a vein other than the LSV. Again, indelible skin markers can be used to identify the course of the true vein, so the practitioner ensures they stay on course.
- **Identifying any varicose veins,** which are fragile and thin walled areas of vein and are more likely to perforate and cause bleeding within the tunnel.

2.8 Other Points to Note

- **Calf vein can be more difficult to harvest,** especially in patients with smaller legs. This is because in the calf the LSV runs along the medial aspect of the tibia and manipulation of the scope against the bone can be difficult. In the calf, the Saphenous nerve is also more likely to be present in very close proximity to the LSV and extra care and dexterity is needed to preserve its integrity and prevent nerve damage.
- **Consider choosing cases that require less segments of vein.** Beginning to learn EVH by harvesting just one segment of vein would be ideal, however, two segments is reasonable. More than two segments can take a significantly longer time until the user builds up the dexterity required to confidently harvest.
- **If there is a risk of conduit damage** and there being no further conduit available, then consider using an alternative method to EVH until more experienced.

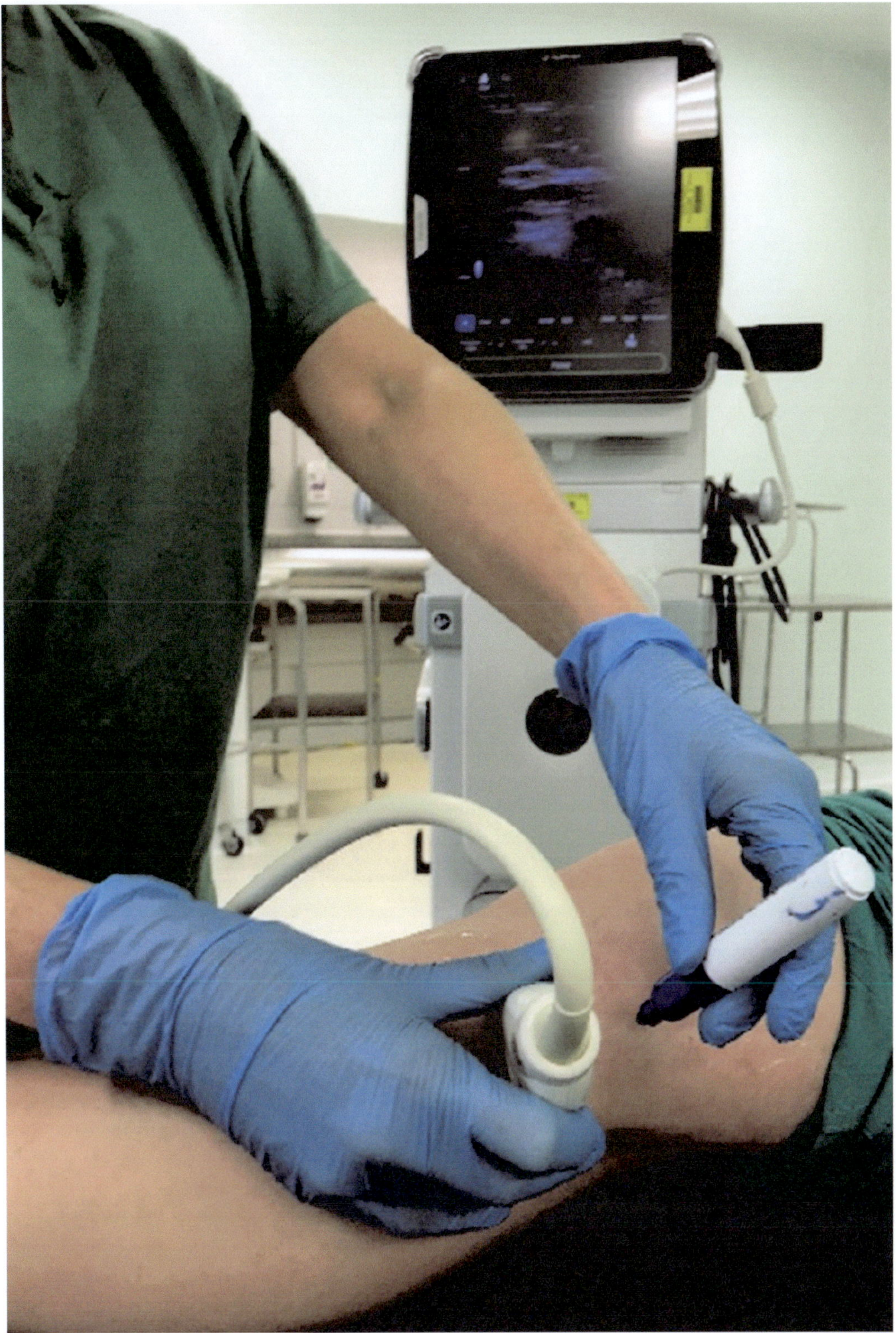

Fig. 4 Identifying the LSV using ultrasound scanning

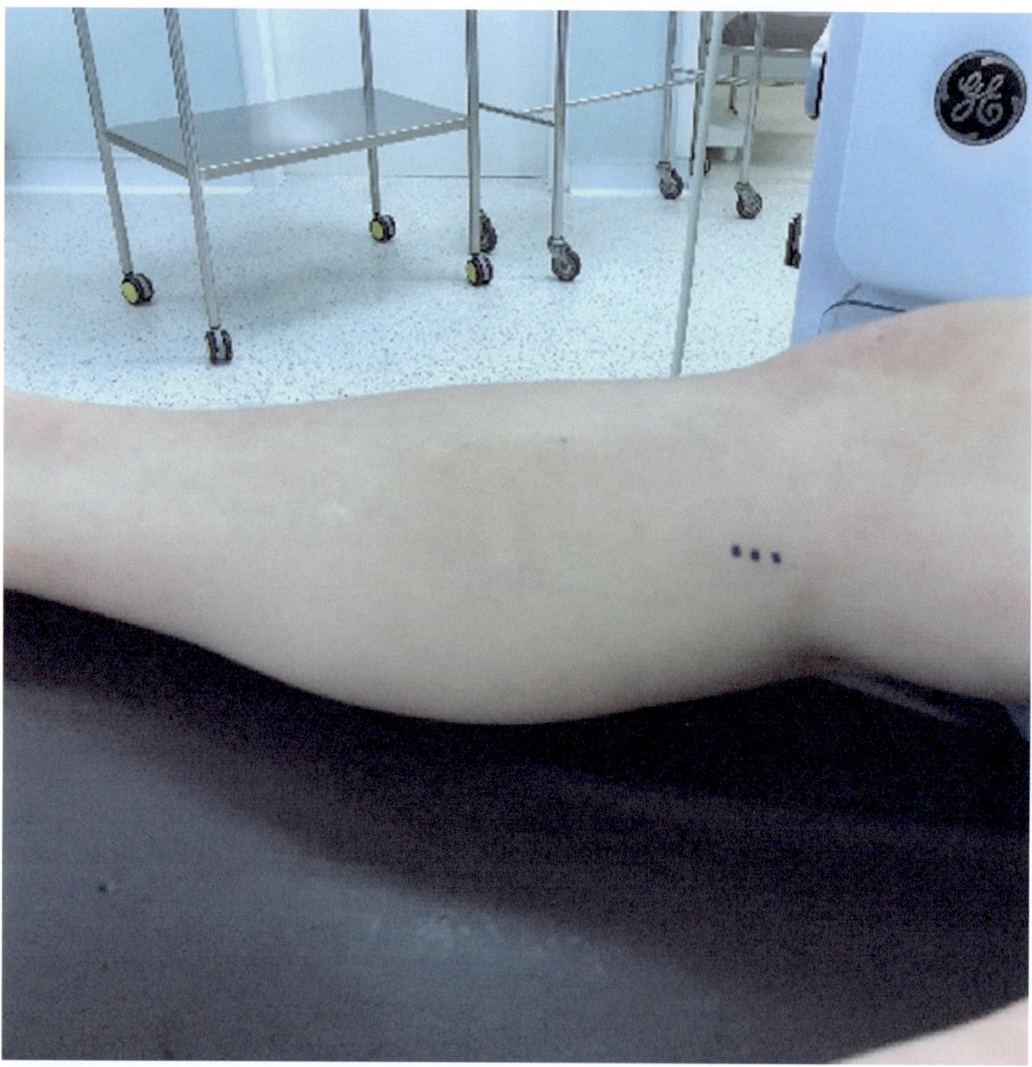

Fig. 5 Marking the vein after identification

3 Intra Operative Procedure

3.1 Patient Positioning

Position the patient supine with legs slightly bent and externally rotated using appropriate pressure relieving devices under the knees and heels, allowing access to the long saphenous vein (LSV) medially.

Assemble equipment

1. Attach the light source to the endoscope.
2. Apply sterile camera cover to camera.
3. Attach the camera head to the endoscope and adjust the focus to ensure clear vision.
4. Set light source at 30%.
5. Attach insufflation tubing ensuring it is not occluded (set to 2.0 L per minute and a pressure of 10 mmHg).

Procedure

The LSV is usually harvested endoscopically just below the medial aspect of the knee ascending in the direction of the thigh particularly if two segments of vein are required (Fig. 6). If a third segment is required or vein above the knee is unsuitable for harvesting the direction of the dissection and harvest descends downwards from the knee to the ankle (Fig. 7).

In our experience at Blackpool, we give a single 5000 IU bolus of intravenous heparin prior to the initial incision at the leg, as we have occasionally observed macroscopic intraluminal clot within the LSV during harvesting.

Make a transverse or oblique incision approximately 2 cm at the appropriately identified point along the leg.

Locate the LSV using direct vision and dissection, once exposed isolate with a sling, tie or tape.

Now open the Terumo VirtuoSaph® Plus Endoscopic Vessel Harvesting System. Insert the endoscope into the dissector, attach the insufflation tubing and switch on the CO_2 using the camera head controls. Perform a white balance. You are now ready to commence the dissection process.

Dissection

- Using the tip of the dissector locate the LSV at the incision site (isolated by the sling/tie or tape) and advance the tip through the fat anteriorly to the vein (Fig. 8).
- NB If using trocar, slide this over the dissector before inserting into the incision.
- Continue the same process posteriorly then dissect all the tributaries along the way. Ensure a sufficient tributary length is dissected to allow safe cut and cautery (Fig. 9).
- Disconnect the insufflation tubing and remove the dissector from the endoscope as the dissection process is now complete.
- Insert the endoscope into the harvester and connect the bipolar diathermy cable to the appropriate machine and setting, ensuring you have the bipolar foot pedal nearby ready for use. Connect the insufflation tubing to the handle of the harvester and switch on the CO_2.

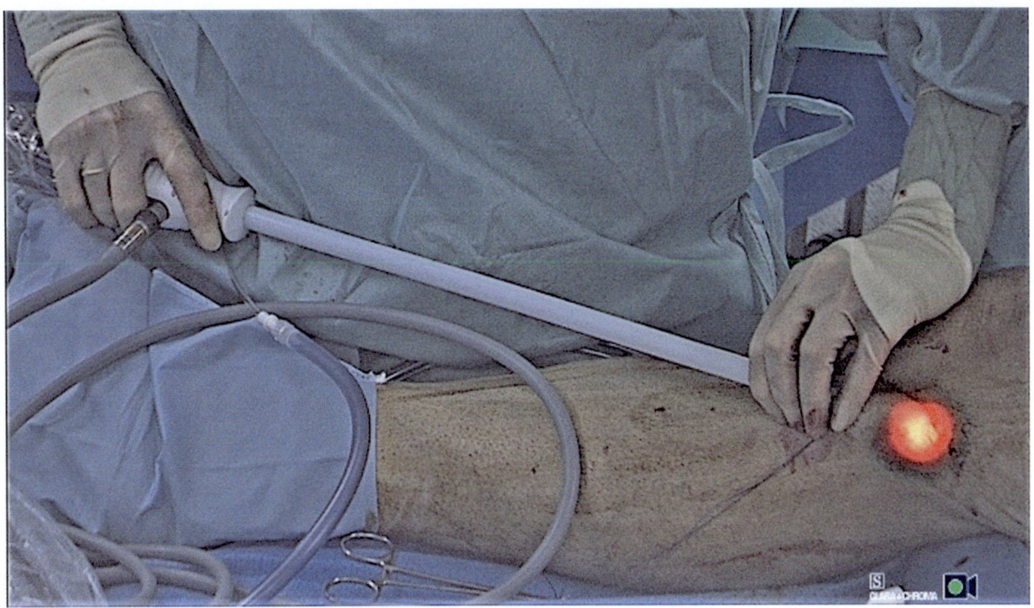

Fig. 6 Initial dissection up the thigh

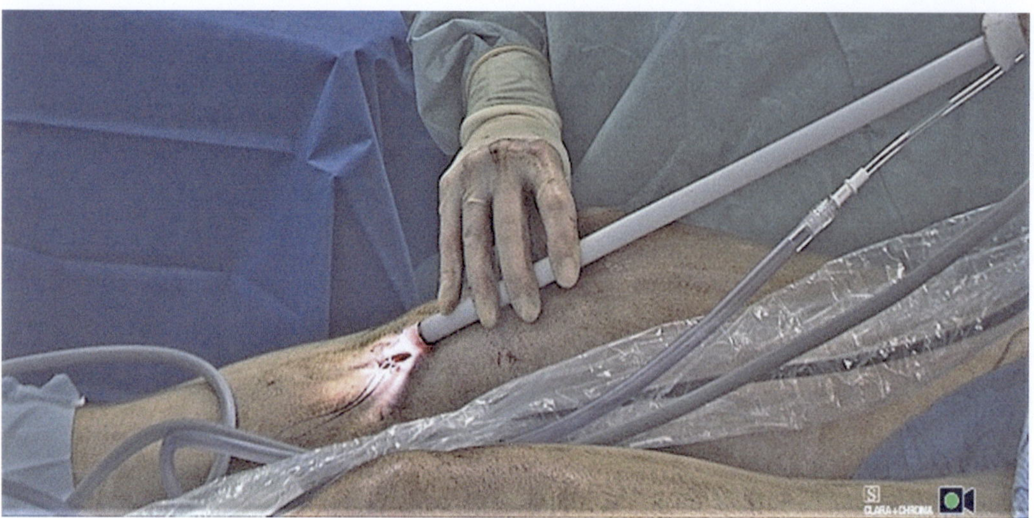

Fig. 7 Dissection down the calf

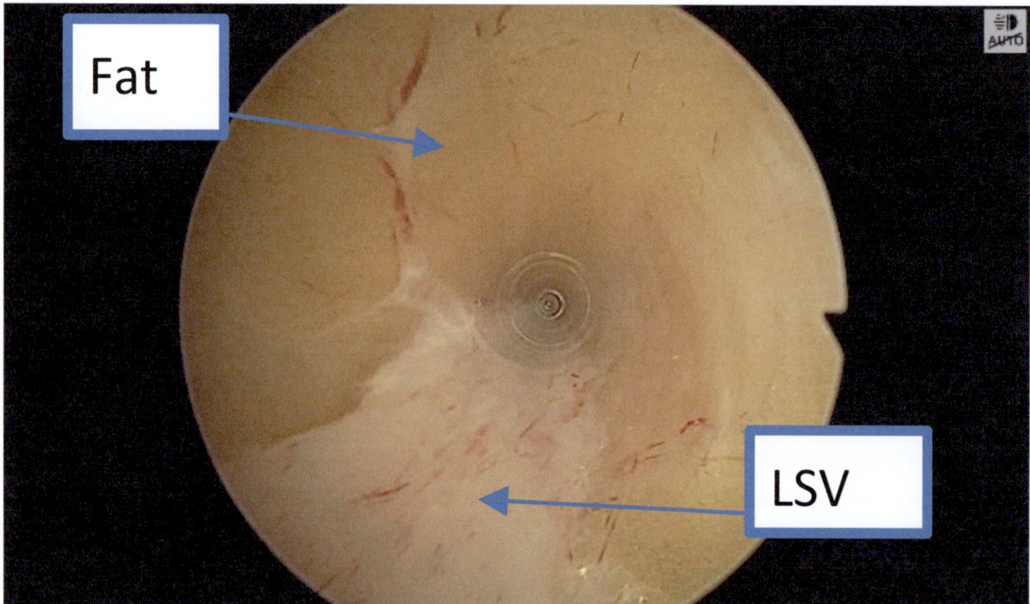

Fig. 8 Anterior dissection of the fat plane

- You are now ready to commence the harvest process. (see Video 2).

Note: Be aware of the proximity of the saphenous nerve in relation to the vein especially when dissecting, and ensure it is not caught in the V Keeper when harvesting.

Harvest

- Ensure the V keeper is closed, the V cutter retracted and insert the harvester through the incision into the tunnel (Use a Langenbeck to lift open the incision OR rotate the harvester 180° to prevent the V cutter from catching the

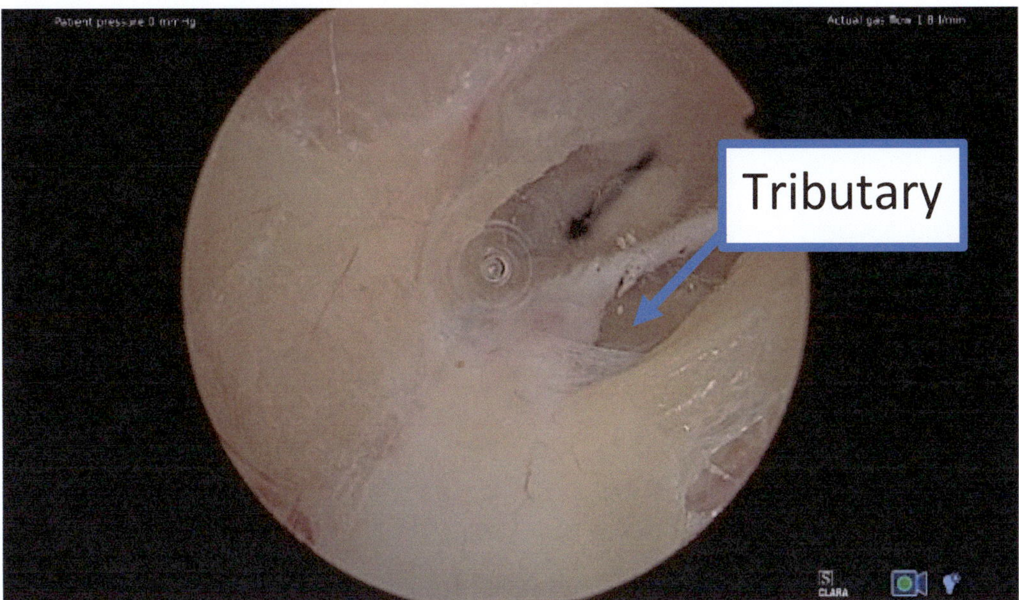

Fig. 9 Dissection of the tributaries

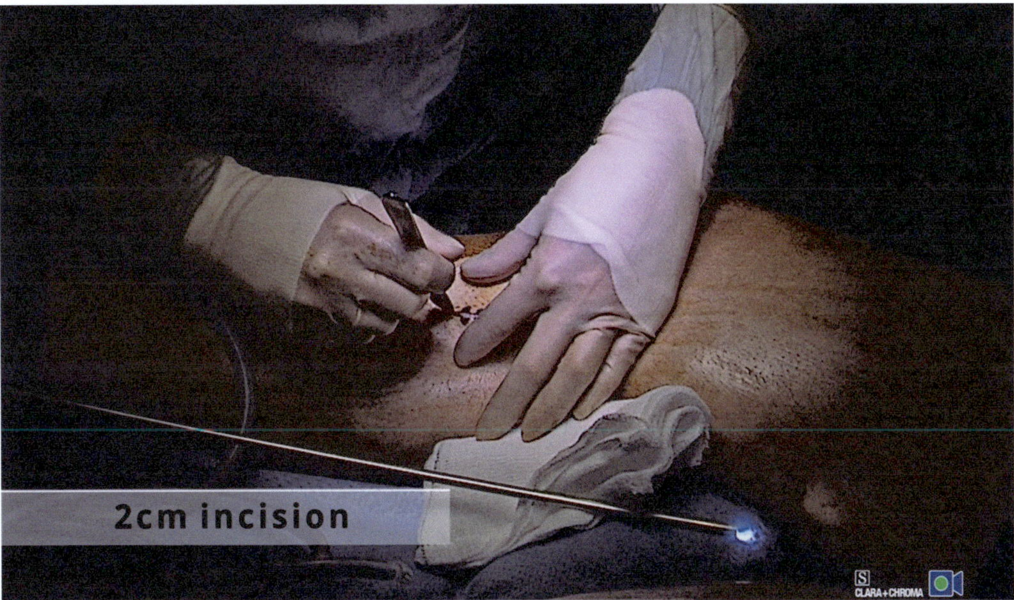

Video 2 Dissection of LSV (▶ https://doi.org/10.1007/000-a7g)

skin during insertion. If there is a tributary near the entrance of the tunnel obstructing the insertion of the harvester, it may be necessary to cauterise and cut the tributary to allow initial insertion.

- Rotate the harvester, whilst advancing through the tunnel, to avoid tributaries and tissue until the end of the dissected vein is reached. Ensure the harvester is positioned over the vein throughout. Advance the V keeper, open the V

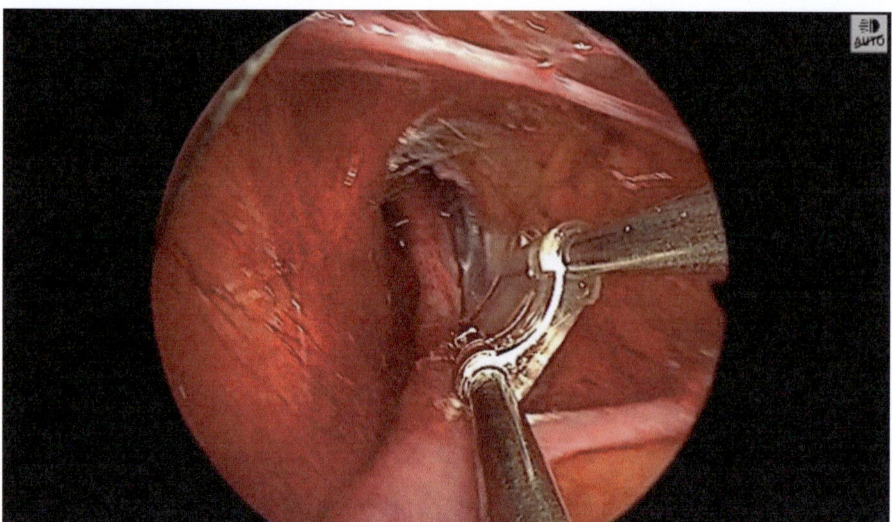

Fig. 10 Open V lock

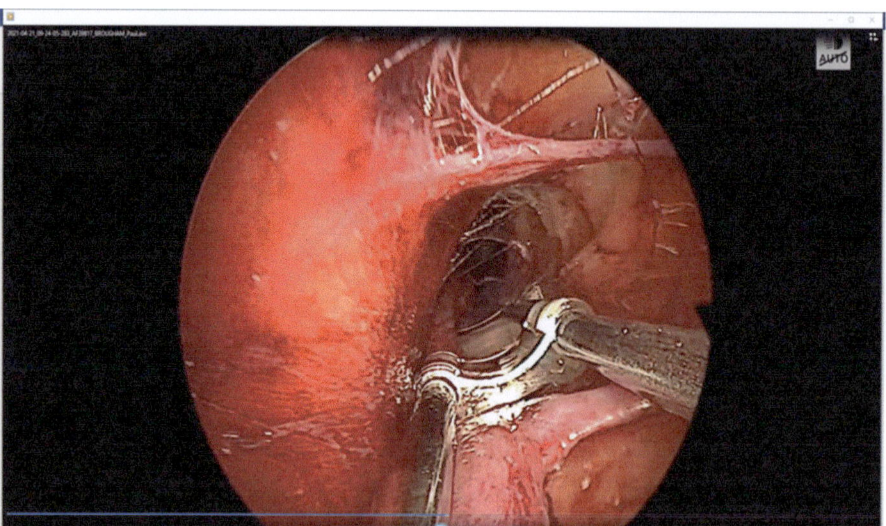

Fig. 11 Position vein in V keeper

lock and position the vein into the V keeper (please note the direction of insertion into the V keeper then close the V lock and retract the V keeper ensuring the vein is free of the saphenous nerve (Figs. 10 and 11).

- At this point perform a stab incision in the thigh using endoscopic guidance, insert an artery clip and grab the vein (Fig. 12).

- Leave the clip in situ and begin moving the harvester towards the knee until a tributary is encountered. Be aware of the vein buckling as there may be a tributary present which is buried amongst the fat and not visible on the monitor.

- If there is a tributary located on the right of the LSV seen on the monitor, rotate the harvester clockwise to allow the tributary to become taut and advance the V cutter using the V cutter

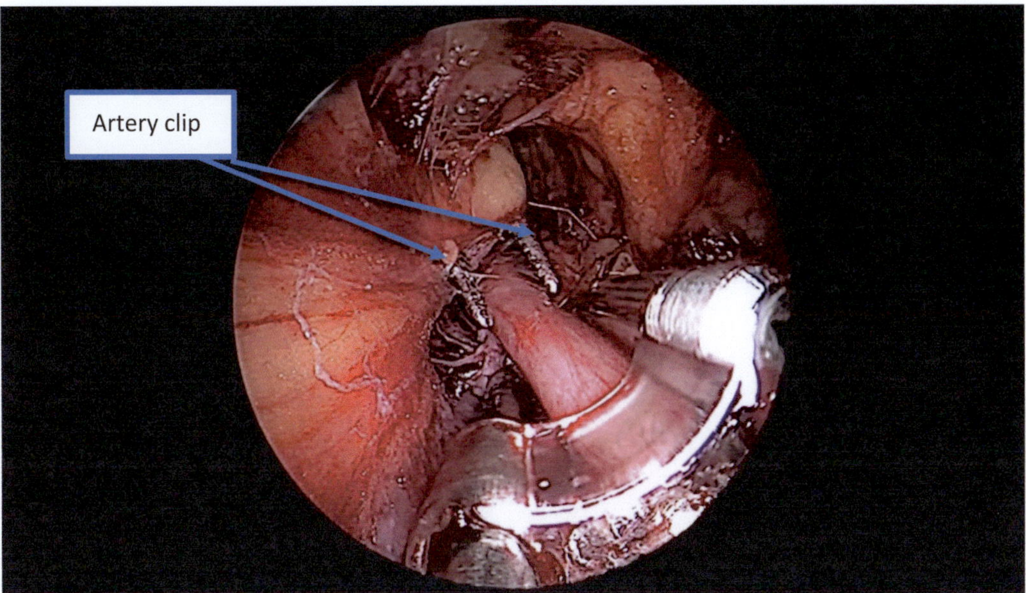

Fig. 12 Grabbing the LSV

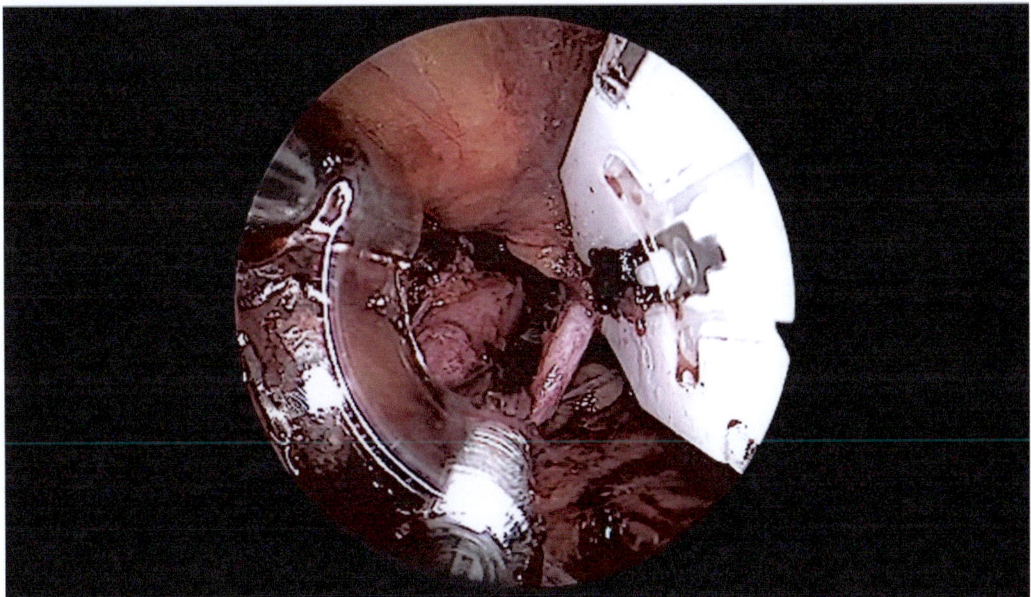

Fig. 13 Tributary on right

button (this will advance from the right-hand side) so the tributary sits in the slit between the bipolar tips of the V cutter (Fig. 13).

Ensure the ground electrode on the V cutter is placed against the tunnel wall. Slowly advance the V cutter button forwards whilst pressing the diathermy foot pedal until the tributary is cauterised and cut. Similarly, if there is a left sided tributary, rotate the harvester anticlockwise and the V cutter will advance from the left (Fig. 14).

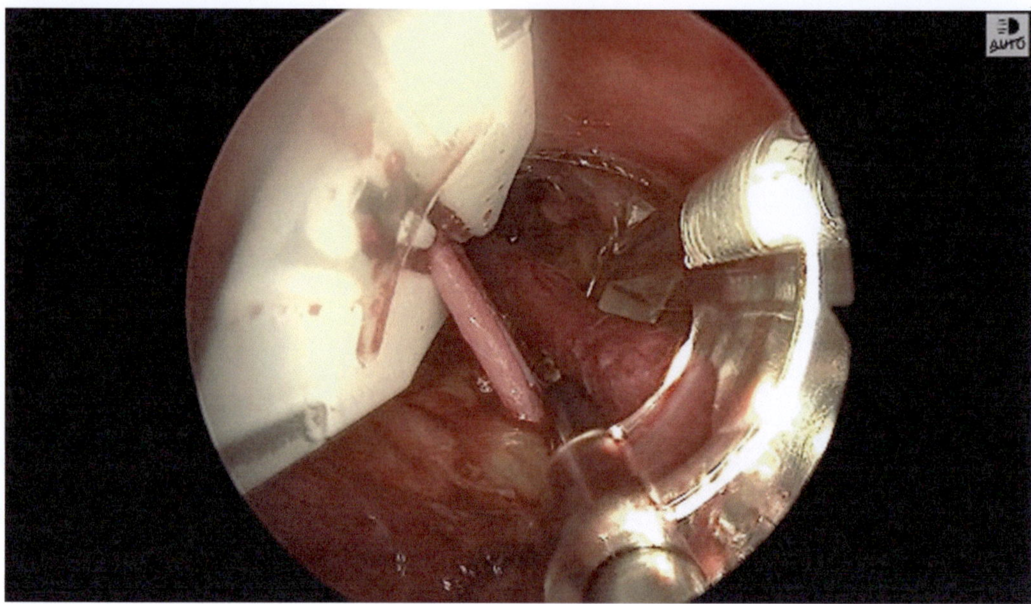

Fig. 14 Tributary on left

- If haemostasis is not achieved at this point, then spot cautery can be used. This is done by releasing the vein from the V keeper and positioning the ground electrodes of the V cutter into the area of the tunnel wall that is bleeding. Move the blue cautery switch across laterally and hold whilst pressing the foot pedal to cauterise the area, releasing after 2 s.
- The grey wiper ring on the handle of the harvester operates a wiper blade which cleans the endoscope lens if required.
- There is the option to cauterise and cut by performing tributary isolation. This is achieved by releasing the LSV from the V keeper and capturing the specific tributary. If the tributary is on the right, insert into the V keeper with the V lock at the bottom. For a left sided tributary insert the vein with the V lock at the top. Follow the previous steps for rotating the harvester and advancing the V cutter.
- Continue the harvesting process until all the tributaries have been cauterised and cut. Release the vein from the V keeper and turn off the CO_2 and light source. The vein can now be divided proximally in the thigh or distally (if the lower leg vein is harvested) and then pulled out through the incision.
- After ligating or clipping the tributaries, flush the vein as per institutional protocol to remove any potential clots. Evacuate any blood from the tunnel before closing the skin incision with a subcuticular suture and the stab incision with an interrupted suture (See Video 3).

Note: There may be occasions when extending the incision is necessary to access tethered tributaries at the entrance of the tunnel. Similarly have a low threshold to open certain points along the harvest site if difficulties arise.

4   Traps, Tips and Tricks

4.1   Bleeding

If haemostasis is not achieved internally by spot cautery, bleeding within the tunnel may obstruct the view of the operator. In this case remove the harvester from the tunnel and apply pressure to the area externally for approximately 3 to

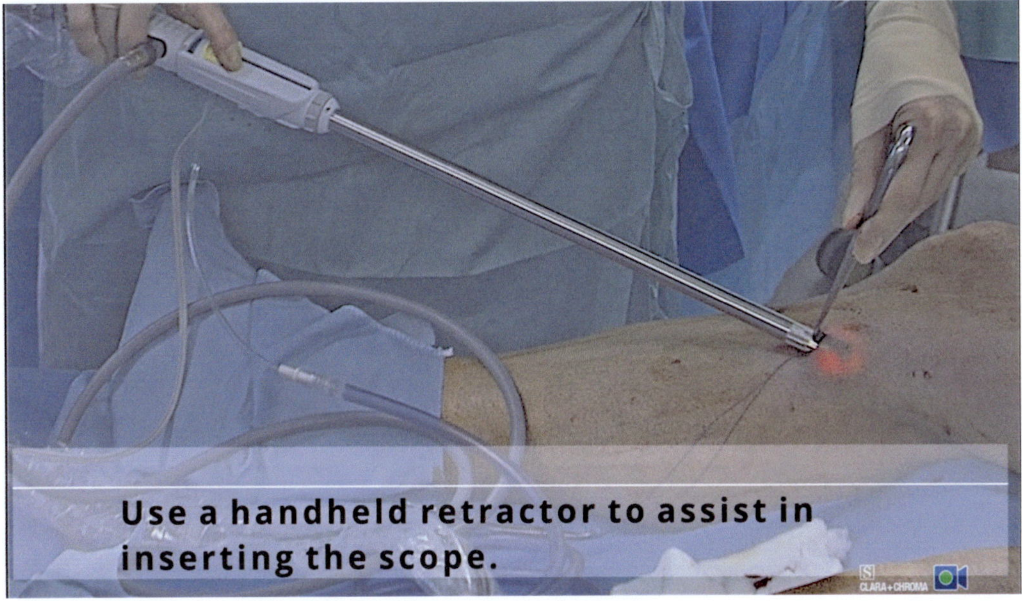

Video 3 Harvest of LSV (▶ https://doi.org/10.1007/000-a7f)

5 minutes then continue (Fig. 15). A suction catheter attached to a cell salvage system can be used to evacuate blood from the tunnel (Fig. 16). If bleeding persists then it may be necessary to insert a drain (as per surgeons' guidance or local protocol).

Tips to avoid bleeding

During the dissection, advance the dissector forwards then backwards, this allows the tunnel to inflate with CO_2 thus enabling a better visual field and will reduce the risk of damage to the vein, bleeding or fat disruption.

During harvesting keep the vein in the middle of the tunnel and avoid dragging the harvester on the bottom, this will avoid bleeding and fat disturbance.

4.2 Large or Bifurcating Tributaries

These can sometime tether the vein and it can be difficult to dissect. Manipulation of the dissector within the tunnel manually can enable the operator to accurately direct the tip of the dissector around such tethered tributaries. Large tributaries may sometimes bleed after cauterising and cutting which can obstruct the view of the operator, therefore leaving them till the end when all other tributaries have been divided, may prevent this. Note: It may be helpful to perform tributary isolation to have better exposure of the large tributary. Alternatively, the operator can divide the tributary by performing a stab incision and grab the large tributary with an artery clip.

4.3 Fat in Tunnel

Fat disruption, particularly at the beginning of the harvest when inserting the harvester or producing a false tunnel, can obstruct the view and cause endless problems with the harvesting process. If this occurs the harvester will need to be removed, cleaned of fat debris and reinserted. It is important to disrupt as little fat as possible ensuring a clean dissection and thus a fat free tunnel.

Tip

To ensure minimal fat disruption keep the cone tip in the plane between the vein and fat during the posterior and anterior dissection.

Fat stuck to the tip of the harvester can sometimes be removed by extending the V

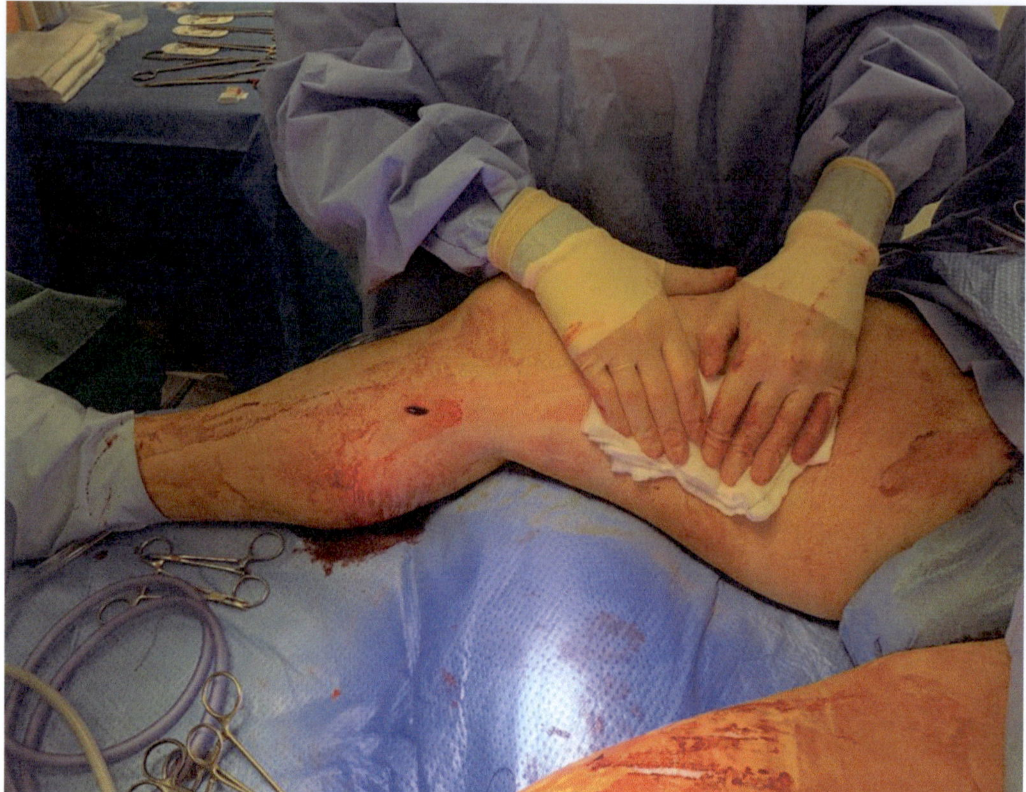

Fig. 15 Dealing with branch bleeding

keeper in the hope it will become dislodged from the end of the harvester to allow the harvesting process to progress (See Video 4).

4.4 Superficial Saphenous Vein

In our experience, these veins tend to be difficult to dissect due to their adherence to the anterior tunnel wall. Performing a posterior dissection first can make the anterior dissection easier. Thin legs and vein adherence can be challenging to dissect as too much pushing may cause damage to the vein and there is a danger of perforating the skin with the tip of the dissector.

Tip

When it is difficult to advance the dissector through the fat it may be necessary to adopt a twisting action side to side to aid advancement whilst applying external counter-pressure at the tip of the dissector. In these situations, have a low threshold to perform an open vein harvest.

4.5 Orientation

The camera can inadvertently twist which will produce an incorrect position of the vein on the monitor. To avoid this the operator must maintain correct positioning of equipment during the harvesting process to ensure optimum orientation of the image (Fig. 17).

4.6 CO_2 Blockage

Fat and debris may occlude or impair CO_2 insufflation, if this occurs remove the harvester

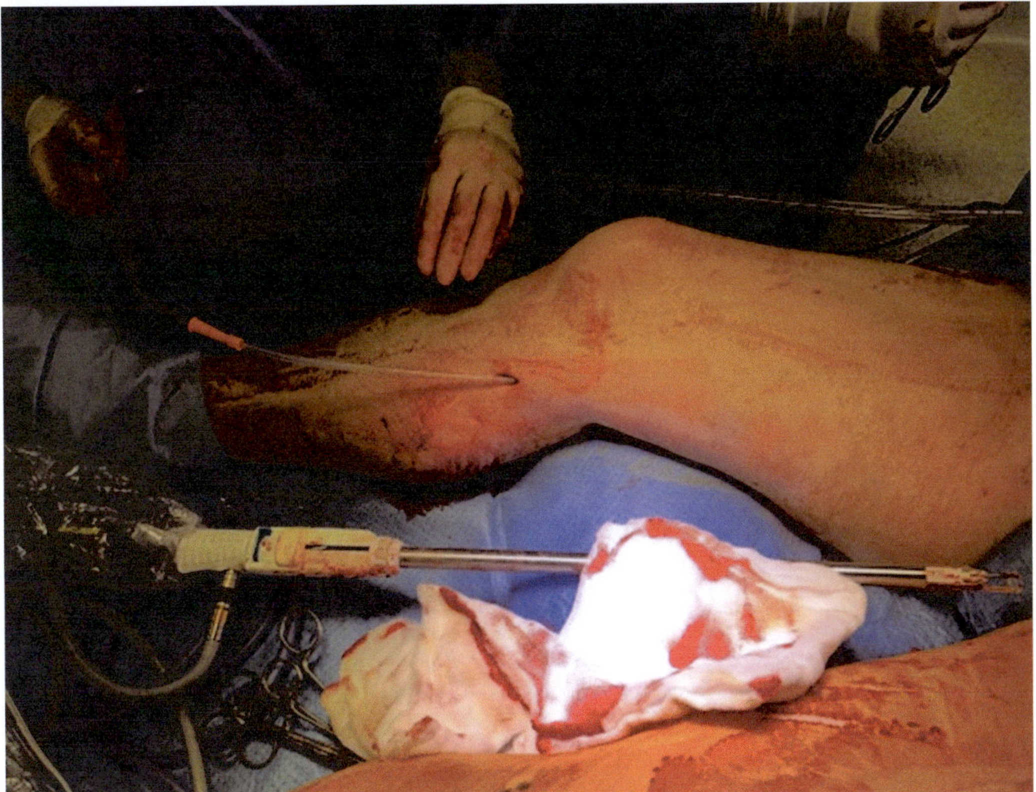

Fig. 16 Use of suction

and clean the end with a damp swab. The CO_2 tube on the harvester may also be evacuated by using a 20 ml syringe of air.

4.7 Thermal Spread

Dissect enough tributary length to avoid the spread of thermal damage when cauterising and cutting tributaries.

4.8 Twisted/Tangled Vein

If the vein becomes twisted around or tangled within the V Keeper, then release the V Lock and carefully free the vein. Once freed, recapture the vein in the V Keeper and continue with the harvest. In the event of a tangled or twisted vein

around the V Keeper, where the view is obstructed by blood or debris, open the leg to safely free the vein under direct vision.

5 Post-operative Complications

5.1 CO_2 Embolus

Although rare, carbon dioxide insufflation during EVH can enter a tributary or damaged saphenous vein. This is potentially fatal and can cause CO_2 bubbles to collect in the right atrium (which may be visible on trans-oesophageal echocardiogram (TOE)) and may result in changes to the haemodynamic status of the patient. In such circumstances discontinue CO_2 insufflation immediately and treat the haemodynamic status of the patient accordingly [4].

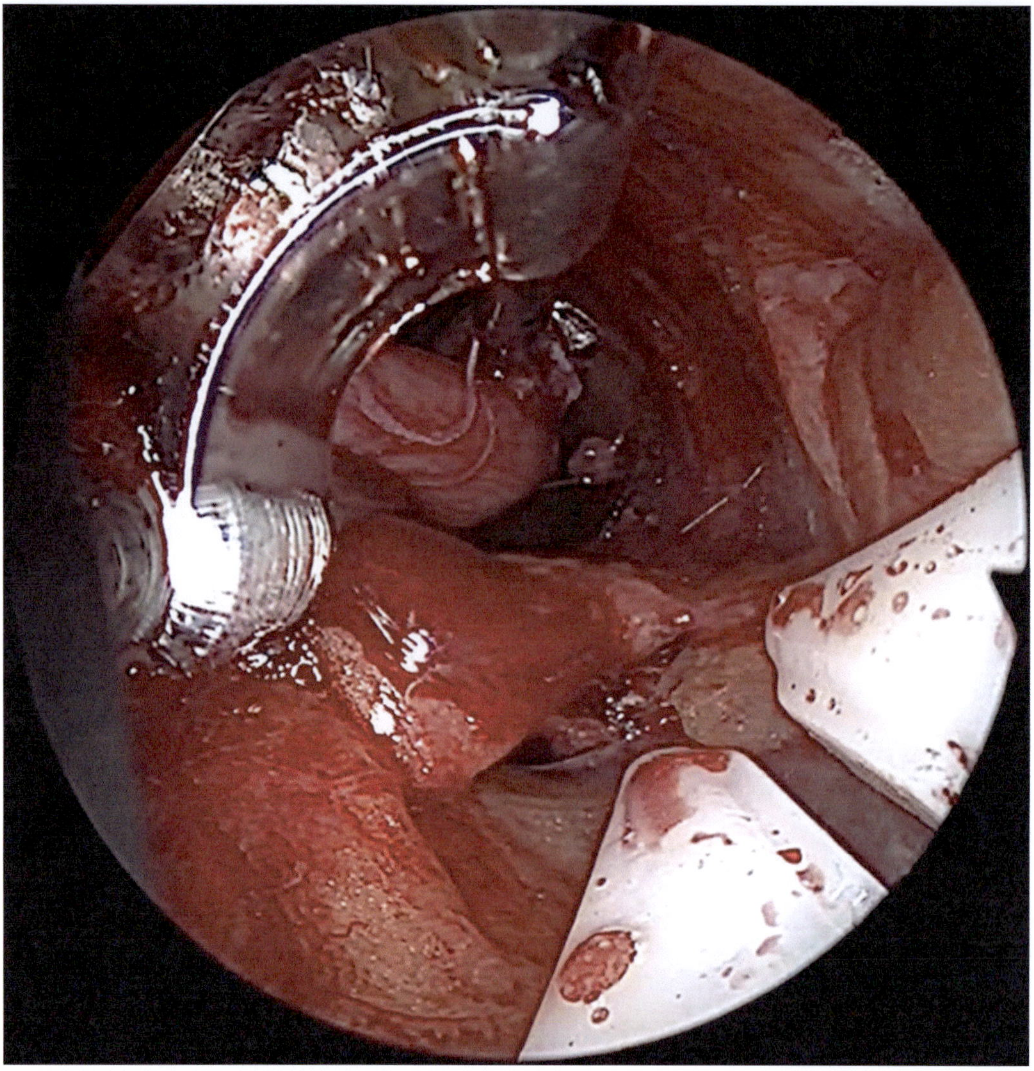

Video 4 Traps, tips and tricks (▶ https://doi.org/10.1007/000-a7j)

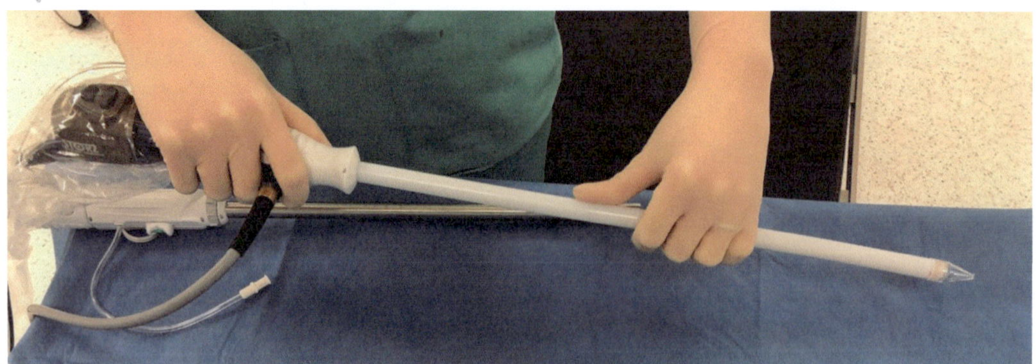

Fig. 17 Correct orientation

5.2 Saphenous Nerve Injury

In the thigh there can be altered sensation and increased pain from injury to the medial femoral cutaneous nerve. Similarly, the medial surface of the lower leg can be affected when harvesting LSV from below the knee. These symptoms are temporary and should resolve in approximately 6 months [5].

As with open vein harvesting haematoma and infection are post-operative complications and treatment will follow institutional guidelines.

References

1. Zenati MA, Bhatt DL, Bakaeen FG, Stock EM, Biswas K, Gaziano M, Kelly RF, Tseng EE, Bitondo J, Quin JA, Hossein Almassi G, Haime M, Hattler B, DeMatt, E, Scrymgeour A. GD Huang 2019 Randomized trail of endoscopic or open vein-graft harvesting for coronary-artery bypass. 2019;380:132–41.
2. Health and Safety Executive.:Back Pain. https://www.hse.gov.uk/msd/backpain/index.htm. Accessed 21 May 2021.
3. Cohn JD, Korver KF. Optimizing Saphenous vein site selection using intraoperative venous duplex ultrasound scanning. Ann Thorac Surg. 2005;79:2013–7.
4. Lin TY, Chiu MK, Wang MJ, Chu SH. Carbon dioxide embolism during endoscopic saphenous vein harvesting in coronary artery bypass surgery. J Thorac and Cardio Surg. 2013;126(6):2011–105.
5. Raja SG, Sarang Z. Endoscopic vein harvesting: technique, outcomes, concerns and controversies. J Thorac Dis. 2013;5 Suppl 6:630–7.

Further Reading

6. 888627_VS-PLUS-Brochure_USletter_MAR2018_FINAL-LR.pdf (terumo-cvs.com)

Endoscopic Mitral Valve Surgery Using the External Clamp

Patrick Perier

Abstract

Fear change and it will destroy you, embrace change and it will enlarge you.
Elizabeth Moon in the Speed of Dark

Minimally "invasive" mitral valve surgery has become along the years more and more accepted by the surgical community, and more and more demanded by the patients. In Germany, isolated mitral valve repair is performed minimally invasively in more than 50% of the cases. Many different approaches are existing: direct Vision, totally endoscopic operation, peripheral cannulation, central cannulation, depending on the surgeon's preferences. One differentiation is the use of external clamp or endo aortic occlusion. We will concentrate in this article on the description of our use of the external clamp. Emphasis has to be placed on the advantages of the totally endoscopic approach: limited incision, no rib spreading to ensure limited postoperative pain and a quick recovery. Moreover; everyone in the operating room can follow the operation, which strengthens the links between the members of the team, but also this allows to train in a very effective way.

Keywords

Heart valve · Mitral valve repair · Mitral valve · Valve disease · Surgery · Minimally invasive approach · External clamp

Minimally invasive mitral valve surgery started in 1996 when Alain Carpentier performed the first successful video assisted mitral valve repair [1]. Pioneers like Fred Mohr [2] and Hugo Vanermen [3] have further developed the technique which progressively has become a routine approach for mitral valve surgery in many centers. In Germany, more than half of the operation on isolated mitral valve regurgitation are performed minimally invasively. The presumed benefits of this approach for both mitral valve repair and mitral valve replacement include improved cosmetic, but also a reduction in postoperative pain, blood loss, blood transfusion, hospital stay, and time to return to normal activity; of course, there is no risk of sternal infection. Numerous studies have confirmed the safety of this approach, and the excellent midterm outcomes [4]. It has been shown that mitral

Supplementary Information The online version contains supplementary material available at https://doi.org/10.1007/978-3-031-21104-1_8. The videos can be accessed individually by clicking the DOI link in the accompanying figure caption or by scanning this link with the SN More Media App.

P. Perier (✉)
Herz und Gefäß Klinik, Salzburger Leite 1, 97616 Bad Neustadt/Saale, Germany
e-mail: pperier@club-internet.fr

valve repair can be performed with the same efficiency as a standard sternotomy, and with the same rate of repair [5].

Minimally invasive mitral valve surgery is a spectrum, with different varieties of incisions, means of cannulation and means of visualization. Schematically it can be divided in two groups. In the first group, direct vision is used. It is the most popular, but it is associated with a longer incision and most often a rib-spreading retractor is needed. This minimizes the full advantage of minimally invasive approach. In the second group, endoscopic guidance (whether traditional or robotic) with improved visualization allows to further reduce invasiveness and trauma, thus enhancing the advantages of minimally invasive surgery [6, 7]. The recent development of 3-D visualization has greatly improved the comfort, the precision and has led to a decrease in the operating and ischemic time.

To achieve good results and master this approach, a learning curve is necessary which may create a reluctancy to adopt this technique [8–10].

Two different methods of cross clamping the aorta is available: the endo-aortic balloon occlusion or the external trans thoracic cross clamping which is the subject of this chapter. There is little evidence to choose one option or the other, and in end effect it is more a question of personal inclination [11].

1 Arguments for the External Clamp

Surgeons performing minimally invasive mitral valve repair usually adopt one way of clamping the aorta external or internal and stick to this method. Since the beginning of our experience, we have chosen to use the external clamp for its ease of use. Other elements are to be taken into consideration, among which the economic aspect plays is key. It is a fact that the price of the endo-aortic balloon system is significant, whereas for the external clamp, apart from the clamp bought once for all, the only expenses are a 4-0 suture and a cannula for the injection of the cardioplegia.

Another point that will become increasingly important is the environmental impact. The amount of waste in the operating room after using an endo clamp is considerably greater (Fig. 1) than after using an external clamp (Fig. 2) as shown in the attached pictures, and that is not considering the negative impact on the environment of the manufacture of this material. In comparison, the carbon footprint of the external clamp is negligible.

The external clamp is always ready for use. In contrast over the years, due to technical failures, the production of the endo-balloon has been stopped several times, sometime for a long period, obliging its users to switch to another method. The reliability of the device is questionable.

2 Preoperative Decision Making Process

Once the indication for mitral surgery has been retained, it is necessary to decide if the patient can be operated minimally invasively, and this depends on the level of expertise.

In advanced centers where minimally invasive mitral valve surgery is routinely performed, all patients referred for mitral surgery are operated minimally invasively with or without concomitant tricuspid repair, atrial fibrillation ablation or ASD. The contraindications are patients with previous right thoracotomy, severe peripheral vascular disease, or particularly important bar of calcium of the posterior annulus, which may be a relative contraindication. A previous sternotomy is not a contraindication.

For surgeons with less experience, the selection of patients is crucial, and a step-by-step strategy is mandatory to ensure a safe outcome with a good result. Easy patients should be tackled first, isolated mitral valve dysfunction like annular dilatation, mitral valve replacement, easy prolapse of the posterior leaflet. The

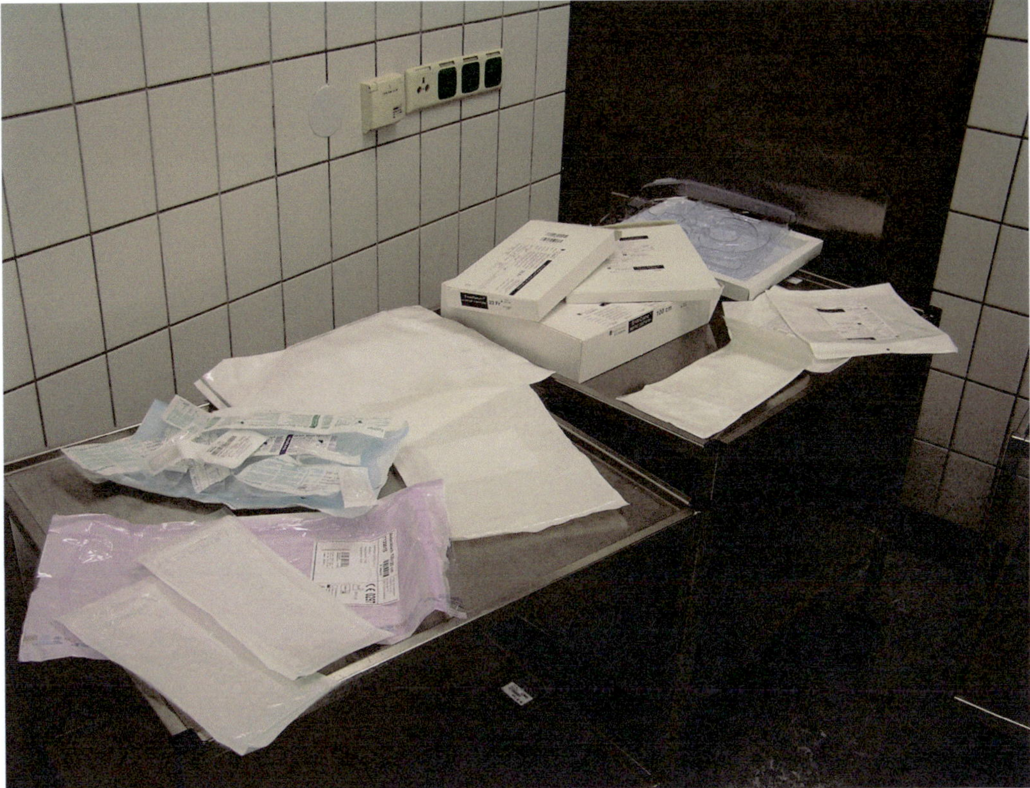

Fig. 1 Waste in the OR after the use of an endo-clamp

difficulty of the cases may be progressively increased, and then it is possible to add ablation, then tricuspid repair and then a combination of the three.

3 Preoperative Radiological Examinations

A computed tomographic angiography from the neck to the thighs may be performed. It will assess:

– The ascending aorta (dimensions and quality)
– The presence of significant mitral calcifications
– The most appropriate intercostal space to access the mitral valve.
– The descending and abdominal aorta

– The iliac and femoral vessels ruling out aneurysm, severe arteriosclerotic disease, or dissection.

In our center, we do not perform this examination routinely, except for patients above 75 years of age, or patients with history of peripheral vascular disease.

4 Anesthesia and Positioning of the Patient

A routine anesthesia is performed. The only particular point for minimally invasive surgery is the question of intubation: single lumen or double lumen tube. There are advantages to both approaches. With the single lumen tube, one has

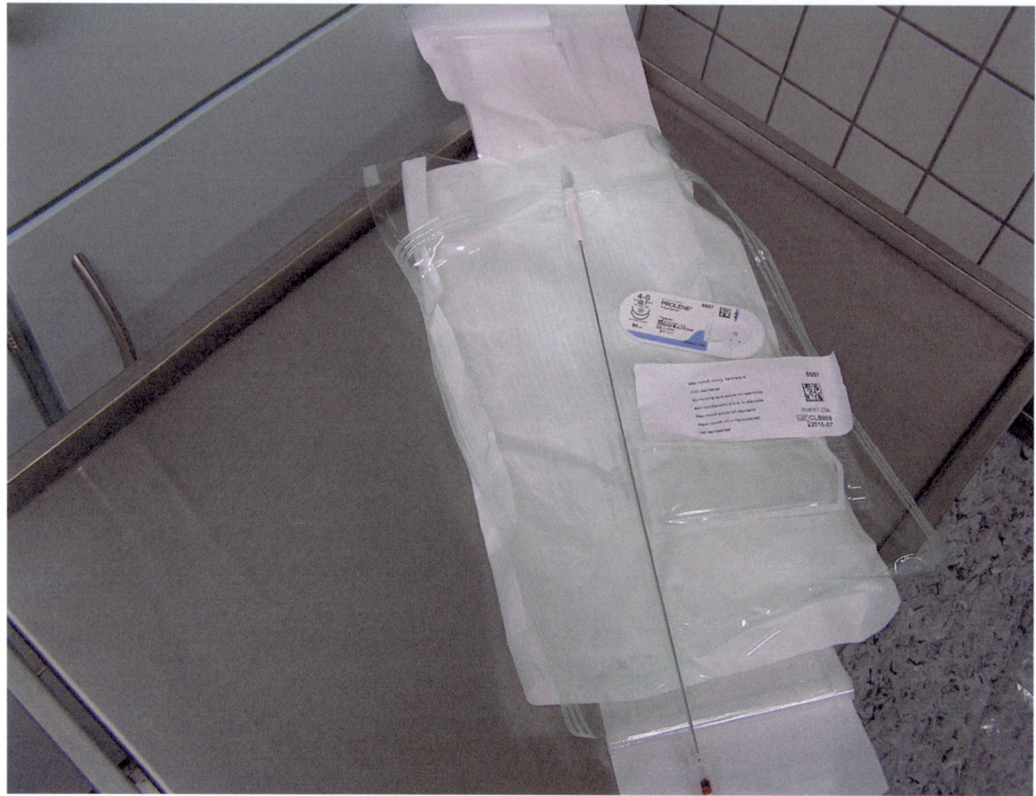

Fig. 2 Waste in the OR after the use of an external clamp

to start the heart lung machine after having opened the thorax and wean the patient off bypass when the thorax is ready to be closed. On the contrary, the use of a double lumen tube allows to shorten the hear lung machine time, but the operation altogether is longer, because of the placement of the tube, the necessity to change it at the end of the operation. Many centers use one lumen tube.

The patient is in supine position, with a small elevation of the right hemithorax with the right arm minimally hyper-extended so that the forearm is just below level of the table (Fig. 3). Special care is taken to protect the bony prominences of the right arm.

Drape ensuring exposure of the right neck, sternum, right chest superiorly to axilla and posteriorly to the posterior axillary line, both groins and both legs. It is necessary to be able to control the colour and the aspect of the leg after cannulation to make sure that the cannula is not obstructing distal blood flow. Mark the groin creases and femoral pulses bilaterally. Mark the sub-mammary fold, including the 4 cm limits of the planned skin incision.

The Iron-Assist™ instrument holder (Geister Medizintechnik GmbH, Tuttlingen, Germany) and camera holder are positioned at the left and right head of the table respectively.

5 Cannulation and Cardiopulmonary Bypass (Video 1)

Routinely a single femoral venous cannula is used except when the patient is above 1, 9 m or weighs more than 100 kg. In those instances, an Edwards Fem-Flex II 16 FR cannula (Edwards Lifesciences, Irvine, CA) is placed by the

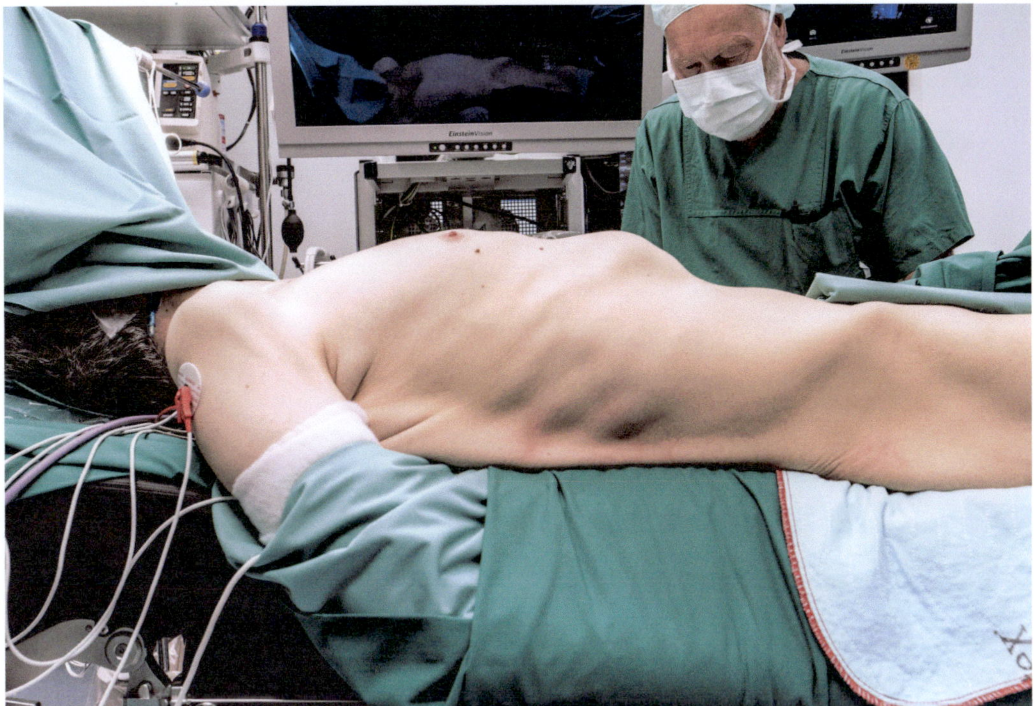

Fig. 3 Position of the patient

anesthesiologist in the jugular vein under transoesophageal echocardiographic (TEE) guidance. In case of tricuspid repair, a dual stage venous canula is used, and the IVC and SVC are snared on the canula, controlling that the portion without side holes is in the right atrium.

A longitudinal 3 cm skin incision, 2-fingers lateral to the femoral pulse, has been observed to reduce seroma formation. Dissection proceeds medially to expose the anterior aspect of the femoral vessels only, without encircling. After palpation of these vessels confirms them to be suitable a full dose of heparin is given. 2 adventitial arterial and 1 partial thickness venous 5-0 Prolene® (Ethicon, Somerville, United States)

purse strings are placed and the bypass lines are handed out.

Using the TOE bicaval view for Seldinger guided venous cannulation the wire is crossed to the SVC ensuring no kinks or confusion with other lines occur. The dilator is used and a 1–2 mm cut anteriorly placed on the vein onto the dilator. A 22, 24 or 28French QuickDraw™ single stage venous cannula (Edwards, Irvine, Unites States) is inserted with TOE. The arterial cannula with Seldinger wire and a 1 mm anterior cut onto the dilator is placed. (16, 18 (up to 5 l/min), 20, 22French EOPA® arterial cannula, collar at 5 cm (see Video 1).

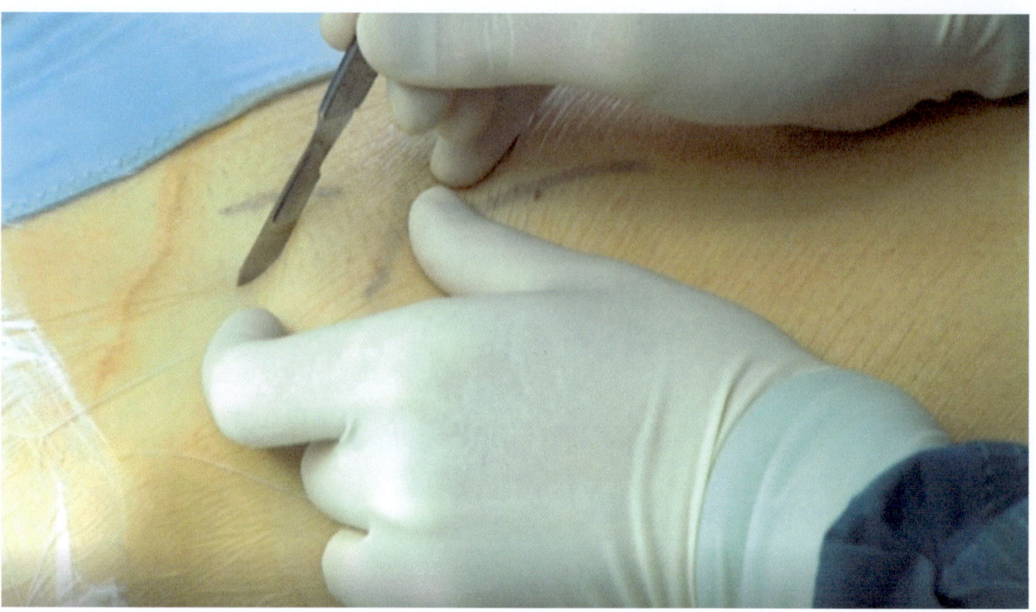

Video 1 Safe peripheral cannulation (▶ https://doi.org/10.1007/000-a7n)

It is also possible to cannulate the femoral vessels percutaneously.

Bypass is commenced before entry into the pleural space to allow the ventilator to be disconnected, and the patient is cooled to 32 °C. All peripheral venous lines must be closed before the vacuum-assist bypass is initiated. If adequate bypass flow is not achieved have a low threshold for bilateral femoral arterial cannulation.

Visually inspect the leg for adequate perfusion periodically during bypass. Poor leg perfusion will necessitate distal femoral artery cannulation, via the main femoral cannula's side arm, using an 8French cannula and purse string.

6   Surgical Access

Most often it is possible at palpation to feel the 4th intercostal space and therefore to guide where the incision should be located. Most of the time it is in the immediate vicinity of the nipple. In men, a 2 to 3 incision is made at the border of the areolar depending on the location of the intercostal space between 11 and 5 or 9 and 3 (Fig. 4 and Video 2). In women, if possible, a peri areolar incision is performed in the same way, but sometimes it would be too anterior, which will lead to an approach of the mitral valve with a too marked angle, making the operation difficult. In this case a more lateral incision trough the breast is indicated. A posterior incision in the mammary groove is too posterior and will increase the distance between the incision and the mitral valve, furthermore, there will be no angle with the mitral valve, making the visualization of some aspect of the mitral apparatus difficult. After opening the intercostal space, a soft tissue retractor is placed to spread the tissues and to avoid that debris are brought in the cardiac cavity with the motions of the instruments. No rib retractor should be used! The port for the endoscope is placed in the same intercostal space as the incision (Video 2).

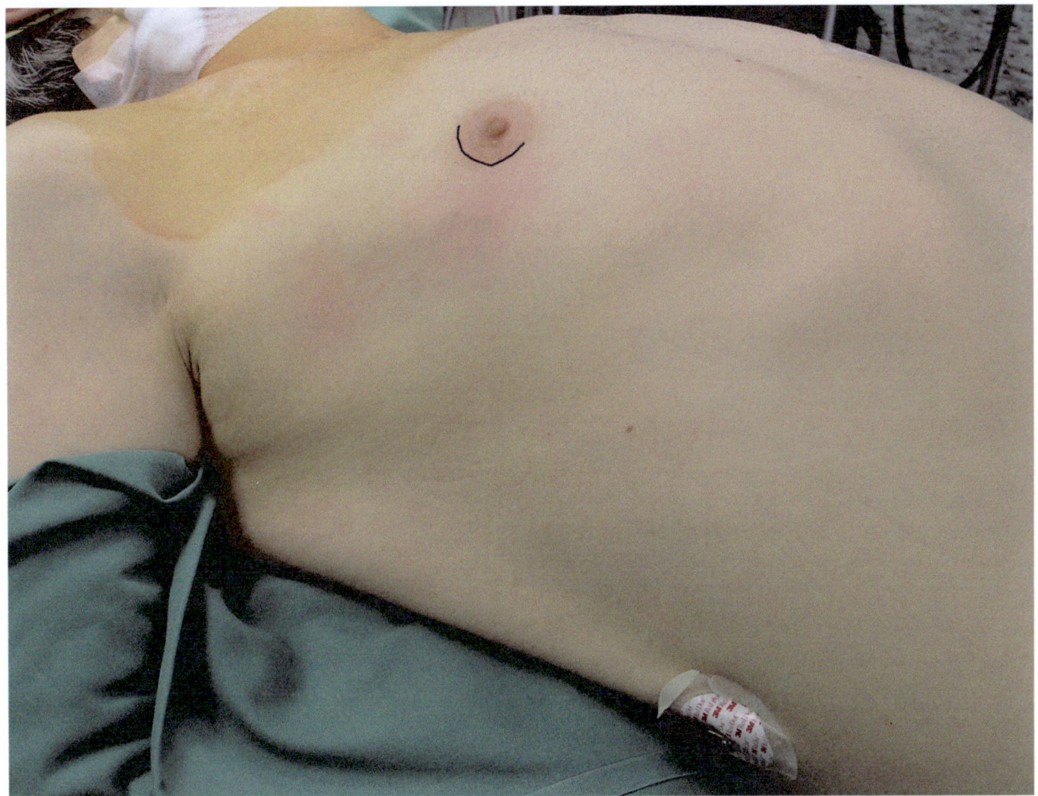

Fig. 4 Peri-areolar Incision 9-3

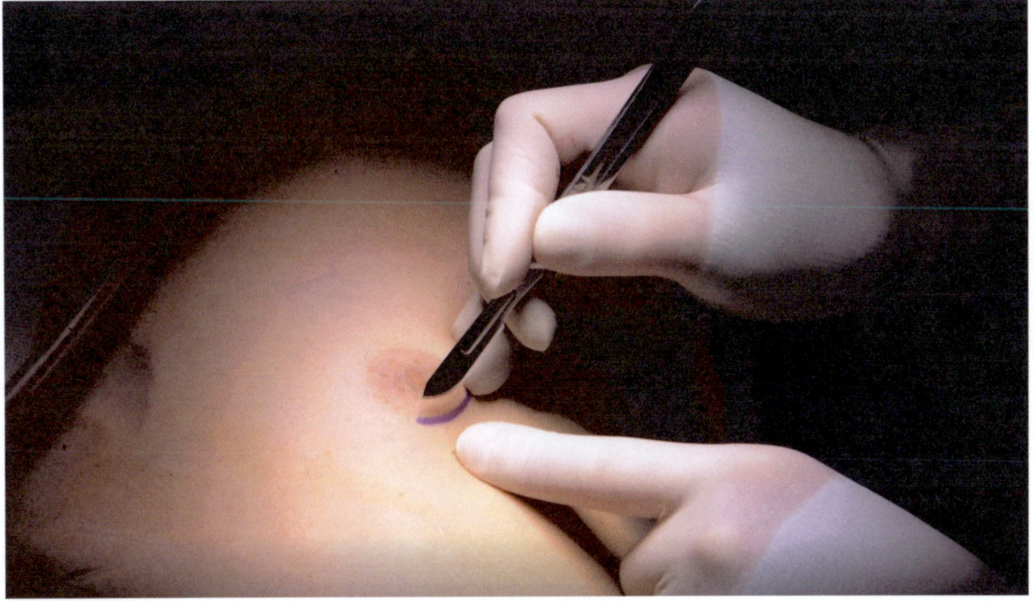

Video 2 Creating the Peri-areolar incision (▶ https://doi.org/10.1007/000-a7m)

7   The Set Up (Figs. 3, 4, 5 and 6)

Everything should be made as simple as possible, but not simpler.

Albert Einstein

The set up should always be the same and kept simple. A 10 mm 30° angle high-definition 3D endoscope is inserted through a port made in the 4th intercostal space, posterior to the internal part of the soft tissue retractor. Significant pericardial fat at the sterno-diaphragmatic area is removed. An L-shaped incision is cut in the pericardium far away from the phrenic nerve using the diathermy, from the diaphragm to the aortic reflection superiorly, then adjacent to the diaphragm surface, posteriorly, to a level just anterior to the inferior vena cava (IVC) avoiding the phrenic nerve (Video 3).

Three 2-0 Vicryl® (Ethicon) pericardial stay sutures are placed with the Endo Close™ (Medtronic) using a finger to protect the lung, posterior to the camera port, 2 intercostal spaces below (posterior axillary), and 1 space above (axillary) where they are clipped in place or tied around rubber tubing. The inferior pericardial stay suture should be placed close to the diaphragm, pulling on the suture will take the diaphragm out of the way, avoiding placing stay sutures directly on the diaphragm.

The pericardial reflection posterior to the IVC is opened with long Metzenbaum scissors then rough sucker. This facilitates the left atriotomy; the inferior vena cava is encircled twice with a 0 black silk to snare the IVC, if required, in case of concomitant tricuspid surgery. A small stab and blunt dissection are made-1-2 rib spaces inferior to camera port, midaxillary, for the sump sucker. This is temporarily positioned posterior to the IVC.

Ensure the heart is empty and properly decompressed when entering the pericardium. The operation should not be started if the venous return is not satisfactory. A simple measure is to make sure that the venous canula is at the top of the thorax, at the level of the innominate vein, at the limit of the camera view.

If a SVC snare is necessary, the pericardial incision is extended superiorly for full exposure. The pericardial reflection over the SVC is cut and a right-angle clamp is used to blunt dissect.

The operative field should be flooded with CO_2 to avoid air in the heart cavities and to

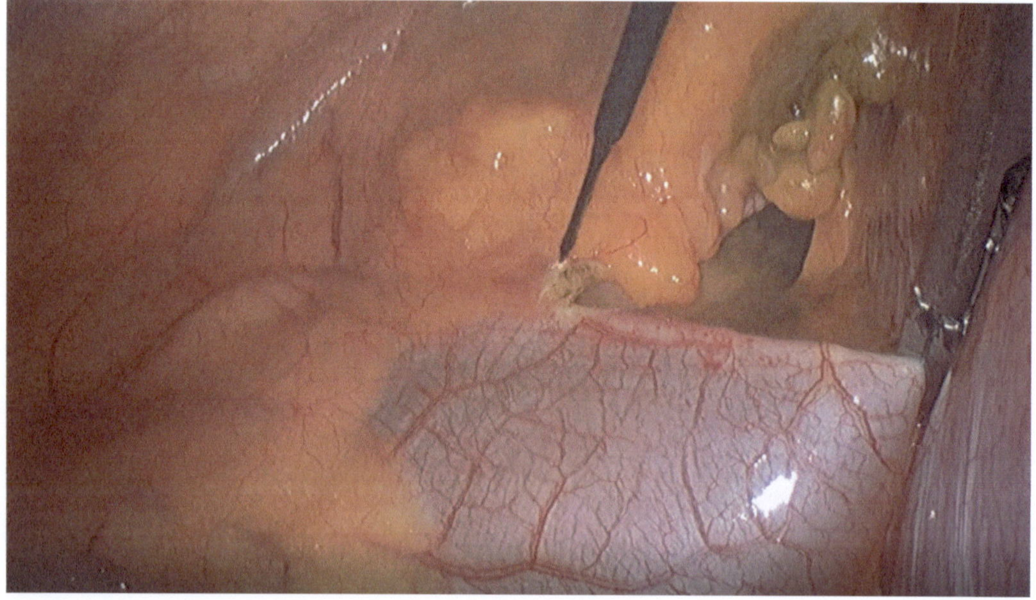

Video 3 Opening the pericardium (▶ https://doi.org/10.1007/000-a7k)

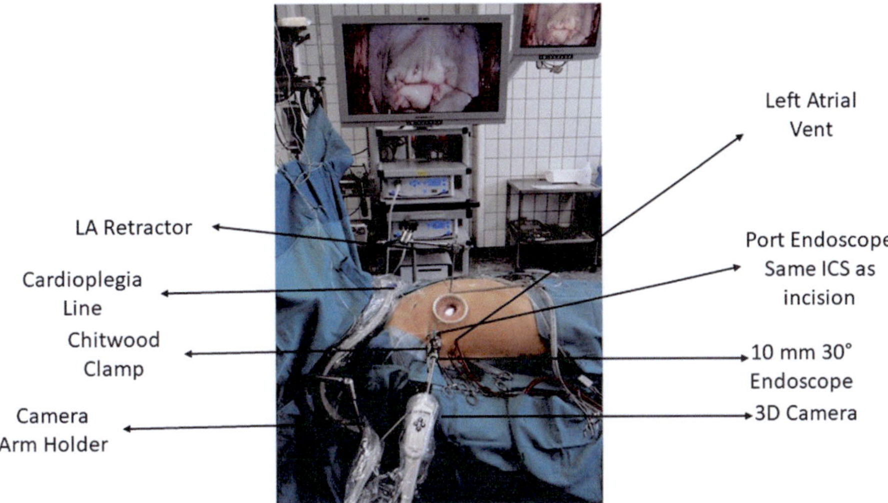

Fig. 5 The setup

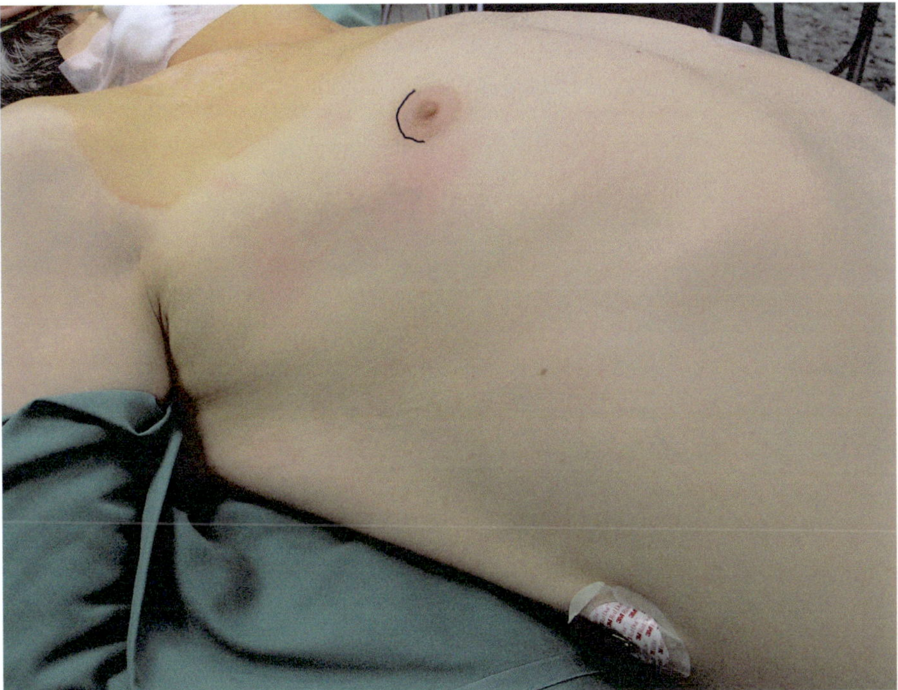

Fig. 6 Peri-areolar incision

facilitate the deairing. At the beginning of our experience, we started CO_2 insufflation as soon as the thorax was open at a rate of 3 L/Mn. The perfusionists and the anesthetists complained because of blood acidosis and hypercapnia. We progressively reduced the flow to 1 L/Mn, which was not enough. At the present time, we start CO_2 insufflation when we place the sutures for the ring, at the end of the repair, with the same efficiency.

8 Placement of the External Clamp (Video 4)

It is certainly possible to place the external clamp in the transverse sinus, but there are drawbacks: the left appendage is in the vicinity vulnerable to injury as well as the pulmonary artery. Moreover, there is not much space left on the ascending aorta below the clamp for the cardioplegia needle. After having had all the complications mentioned, we looked for another method.

We lift the aorta away from the pulmonary artery with long-shafted forceps, divide the adventitia with long-shafted scissors. Proceed between the aorta and the pulmonary artery towards the left shoulder with blunt dissection, using the rough sucker and long-shafted forceps until the contralateral pericardial space is entered, and the pericardium seen. Using a small stab with blunt dissection 1 or 2 intercostal space superior to camera and working port, mid-axillary at the level of the video port, insert the aortic clamp curved caudally, and once in the thorax turn it cranially. Place the clamp across the aorta at its upper visible limit, taking care to avoid the pulmonary artery and left atrial appendage, and leave open.

Clear any significant fat on the ascending aorta to make a suitable landing zone for the cardioplegia canula. A double purse string with 4-0 nonabsorbable polypropylene is placed. This is proximal to the aortic clamp and lateral to the uppermost aortic aspect, using forceps to stabilize and ease the placement of the sutures. A long, single lumen cardioplegia cannula (2 notches for stays) is placed, snared and spigoted. Tuck the snare away in the left pericardial cavity. A mid-clavicular stab in the 2nd intercostal space is used to externalize and connect the clamped cardioplegia line.

A 5 cm jaw transthoracic aortic clamp is usually used although a 7.5 cm transthoracic aortic clamp is preferable with larger aortae or obstructive shoulders or patient with a large thorax.

The end of the cardioplegia cannula is cut off to remove fat debris before connecting it to the cardioplegia line via a 3-way tap.

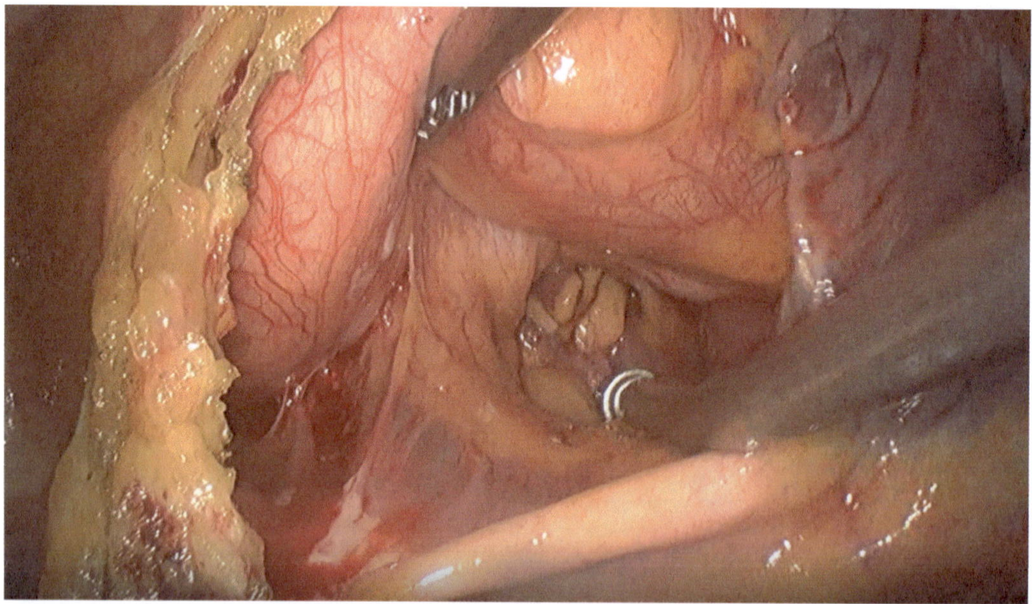

Video 4 Placement of the external clamp (▶ https://doi.org/10.1007/000-a7p)

Cardioplegia is then given. We use Bretschneider solution. Typically, the heart arrest occurs after 200–300 ml. If cardioplegic arrest is delayed it may be due to an aortic insufficiency, a displacement of the cardioplegia canula or a lack of efficiency of the aortic clamp. It is necessary to find the cause of this delay. We routinely infuse 1500 ml for patients above 80 kg; for those with a lower weight to decrease the evolution we infuse only 1000 ml. After 90 mn of aortic cross clamping, if obviously the operation will last longer than 2 h, we inject another 500 ml cardioplegia.

9   Atriotomy

A 2-0 Vicryl® stay suture is placed in the fat anterior to the interatrial groove, exerting traction will improve the exposure of the left atrium, for the opening, the closure and later to control the lack of bleeding. A long needle is used as a guide by placing through the chest wall lateral after having palpated the intercostal space (4th) the needle has to be delicately handled; its role is to avoid hitting the internal mammary vessel. Internally this is located just medial to the Alexis® inner ring using fingertip proprioception. A 5 mm stab is done at the level of the exploring needle and pass the interatrial stay suture and the shaft for the left atrial retractor.

Incise the left atrium midway between the right inferior and towards the right superior pulmonary vein. A hand held sump sucker in left atrium retracting inferiorly provides a good view. A 2-0 Ethibond® atriotomy stay suture is placed in the fat anterior to the interatrial groove. A long needle is used as a guide by placing through the chest wall lateral to the internal mammary artery, level with working ports, and left atrium. Internally this is located just medial to the Alexis® inner ring using fingertip proprioception. A 5 mm stab lateral to the needle is made and a Pean artery clip is used to develop the tract. Use the above stab hole to pass through the atriotomy stay suture and site the shaft of atrial retractor.

Incise the left atrium midway between the right inferior and towards the right superior pulmonary vein. A handheld sump sucker in left atrium retracting inferiorly provides a good view. The left atrial incision is carried out with long shafted scissors towards the roof of the left atrium and under the IVC. The atrial wall is retracted anteriorly by inserting the blade of the atrial retractor and fixing the shaft with the Iron-Assistant™ and clamp at the base of the atrial retractor shaft. Most of the time the inferior wall of the left atrium is blocking the view of the mitral valve.

A 4-0 Prolene is passed through the atrial wall at around 5 o'clock, 2 cm behind the inferior wall and will nicely expose the mitral valve. The endoscope is then placed to have the mitral valve in full view, in the middle of the screen. Instead of bringing the endoscope close to the mitral valve, it is preferable to use the zoom properties of the equipment. The endoscope should remain as close to the thorax wall as possible to avoid conflicts with the instruments.

10   Mitral Valve Repair

Mitral valve repair is performed according to the standard techniques. After careful analysis, the proper technique can be selected and implanted according to the lesions. Surgery must be driven by the strategy, which is to restore a good surface of coaptation, smooth and regular, as long as possible and located in the inflow of the left ventricle.

A ring annuloplasty is routinely used, special care has to be taken to avoid an injury of the aortic valve or the circumflex artery.

11   Mitral Valve Replacement

Any type of mitral valve replacement can be carried out, mechanical or biological. The only particularity is that the incision of the working port is planned long enough to accommodate to the bulky prosthesis. Using the Cor-knot® device (LSI Solutions) may help to have a standard tension on the knots.

12 Concomitant Tricuspid Repair

In case of indication of a tricuspid repair, it is necessary to carefully take this into account in the planning of the operation. In contrast to an operation performed through sternotomy, a minimally invasive tricuspid repair is time consuming, around 45 mn. The exposure is not always easy, and the closure of the right atrium has to be perfect with no bleeding, and this takes time.

In our daily practice we start with the tricuspid repair before the mitral valve. It avoids having the stay suture in the way.

13 End of the Operation and Deairing

It is crucial that, after the closure of the left atrium and before deairing, when the heart is still totally decompressed, a pacemaker wire is placed on the diaphragmatic face of the right ventricle.

A left vent is placed in the left ventricle, suction is applied on the cardioplegic needle, the heart is filled. Deairing should be controlled with echocardiography. CO_2 is very potent and most of the time, there are just isolated bubbles, at the most.

After unclamping the aorta, and some reperfusion, ventilation may be resumed, and the HLM flow may be reduced to ½ liter, while controlling the oxygen saturation. A "preview" echocardiographic control is performed. It saves a lot of time if at that stage the result is not satisfactory, and if it is necessary to improve the result of the repair. Everything is still in place.

In case of a good result, the HLM can proceed again full flow, the ventilation has to be stopped. The cardioplegia line is removed and the hole is secured with a 4-0 Prolene.

Closure, hemostasis, discontinuation of CPB, decannulation and echocardiographic control are performed in a normal way.

This minimally invasive mitral surgery is increasingly being shown to yield comparable or better results to open mitral surgery with all the added benefits associated with endoscopic procedures, and foremost is associated with an extremely high patient satisfaction. One motto is never losing sight of patient safety and quality of the results. This non compromise attitude is best achieved with a dedicated team approach. A team is made of surgeons, anesthetists, perfusionists, and nurses. As Simon Sinek as taught us, "a team is not only a group of people working together, but a team is also a group of people trusting each other". Another point is the necessity of building a routine, which will allow the team to develop the required skills and to build an experience on which everyone can rely. It means that a minimal number of cases per year is necessary to start a program of minimally invasive mitral surgery. It is even more important in the beginning to be able to select patients according to one's level of expertise.

Endoscopic minimally invasive mitral surgery is a fantastic training tool. The trainees can perfectly see what the senior surgeon is doing, contrary to what happens in the conventional surgery. When assisting a younger surgeon, it is possible to totally control each manoeuvre of the operation.

Tips

1. Maintaining a regular theatre team allows for a smooth procedure.
2. Having good TOE images are crucial for safe peripheral cannulation.
3. The external clamp is best placed by making the incision on the upper border of the rib to avoid the neuromuscular bundle running at the lower aspect of each rib.

Tricks

1. Incising the tissue over the pulmonary artery and creating the bloodless field below the aorta gives extra space to apply the clamp and avoids injury to the left atrial appendage.

2. A circular suture in the adventitia of the aorta placed above the sino-tubular junction acts as a safe way to anchor the cardioplegia cannula.
3. If an extra suture is required at the cardioplegia site a pledged braided suture can be tied with a CorKnot to control the bleeding. This is best done with a reduced pump flow.

Traps

1. In large patients with a lot of adipose tissue over the pericardium an energy source is useful to dissect the fat off the pericardium prior to opening it.
2. In patients with short aortas avoid the temptation to place the cardioplegia cannula in the non coronary sinus area as this can be difficult to control in some patients.
3. In case of bleeding from the stab incisions a period of pressure applied by a peanut swab until heparin is reversed helps to localise the cause and often this can then be dealt with diathermy to the site.

References

1. Carpentier A, Loulmet D, Carpentier A, Le Bret E, Haugades B, Dassier P, et al. Open heart operation under videosurgery and minithoracotomy. First case (mitral valvuloplasty) operated with success. C R Acad Sci III. 1996;319(3):219–23.
2. Mohr FW, Falk V, Diegeler A, Walther T, van Son JA, Autschbach R. Minimally invasive port-access mitral valve surgery. J Thorac Cardiovasc Surg. 1998;115(3):567–74;discussion 74–6.
3. Vanermen H, Wellens F, De Geest R, Degrieck I, Van Praet F. Video-assisted Port-Access mitral valve surgery: from debut to routine surgery. Will Trocar-Port-Access cardiac surgery ultimately lead to robotic cardiac surgery? Semin Thorac Cardiovasc Surg. 1999;11(3):223–34.
4. Cheng DCH, Martin J, Lal A, Diegeler A, Folliguet TA, Nifong LW, et al. Minimally invasive versus conventional open mitral valve surgery: a meta-analysis and systematic review. Innov Technol Tech Cardiothorac Vasc Surg. 2011;6(2):84–103 https://doi.org/10.1097/IMI.0b013e3182167feb.
5. Perier P, Hohenberger W, Lakew F, Batz G, Diegeler A. Rate of repair in minimally invasive mitral valve surgery. Ann Cardiothorac Surg. 2013;2 (6):751–7.
6. Casselman FP, Van Slycke S, Wellens F, De Geest R, Degrieck I, Van Praet F, et al. Mitral valve surgery can now routinely be performed endoscopically. Circulation. 2003;108 Suppl 1:II48–54.
7. Suri RM, Antiel RM, Burkhart HM, Huebner M, Li Z, Eton DT, et al. Quality of life after early mitral valve repair using conventional and robotic approaches. Ann Thorac Surg. 2012;93(3):761–9.
8. Murzi M, Cerillo AG, Bevilacqua S, Gasbarri T, Kallushi E, Farneti P, et al. Enhancing departmental quality control in minimally invasive mitral valve surgery: a single-institution experience. Eur J Cardiothorac Surg. 2012;42(3):500–6.
9. Holzhey DM, Seeburger J, Misfeld M, Borger MA, Mohr FW. Learning minimally invasive mitral valve surgery: a cumulative sum sequential probability analysis of 3895 operations from a single high-volume center. Circulation. 2013;128(5):483–91.
10. Vo AT, Nguyen DH, Van Hoang S, Le KM, Nguyen TT, Nguyen VL, et al. Learning curve in minimally invasive mitral valve surgery: a single-center experience. J Cardiothorac Surg. 2019;14 (1):213.
11. Rival PM, Moore THM, McAleenan A, Hamilton H, Du Toit Z, Akowuah E, et al. Transthoracic clamp versus endoaortic balloon occlusion in minimally invasive mitral valve surgery: a systematic review and meta-analysis. Eur J Cardiothorac Surg. 2019;56 (4):643–53.

The Endo-Aortic Balloon Technique in Totally Endoscopic Atrioventricular Valve Surgery

Karel M. Van Praet, Markus Kofler,
Axel Unbehaun, Volkmar Falk,
and Jörg Kempfert

Abstract

Minimally invasive cardiac surgery through a right (antero) lateral mini-thoracotomy approach evolved as standard of care for the treatment of pathologies affecting the atrio-ventricular valves. To perform this procedure, surgeons across the world either use the external trans-thoracic aortic cross-clamp (TTC), which can be applied directly across the ascending aorta from the right chest or perform endo-aortic balloon occlusion with a balloon clamp introduced from the groin into the ascending aorta just above the sinotubular junction. The endo-aortic balloon occlusion catheter carries the balloon at its tip and consists of three lumina (one for delivery of cardioplegia and aortic root venting; one for balloon inflation and deflation; one for aortic root pressure monitoring). Balloon placement is facilitated by transesophageal echocardiography and is contraindicated in cases of ascending aorta diameter >42 mm.

Supplementary Information The online version contains supplementary material available at https://doi.org/10.1007/978-3-031-21104-1_9. The videos can be accessed individually by clicking the DOI link in the accompanying figure caption or by scanning this link with the SN More Media App.

K. M. Van Praet (✉) · M. Kofler · A. Unbehaun ·
V. Falk · J. Kempfert
Deutsches Herzzentrum der Charite (DHZC),
Department of Cardiothoracic and Vascular Surgery,
Augustenburger Platz 1, 13353 Berlin, Germany
e-mail: vanpraet@dhzb.de;
karel.van-praet@dhzc-charite.de;
karel.vanpraet@gmail.com

Charité—Universitätsmedizin Berlin, corporate
member of Freie Universität Berlin,
Humboldt-Universität zu Berlin, Charitéplatz 1,
10117 Berlin, Germany

DZHK (German Center of Cardiovascular Research),
Partner Site Berlin, Berlin, Germany

V. Falk
Translational Cardiovascular Technologies, Institute
of Translational Medicine, Department of Health
Sciences and Technology, Swiss Federal Institute of
Technology (ETH) Zurich, Zurich, Switzerland

Keywords

Cardiac surgery · Endo-Aortic Balloon Occlusion (EABO) · EAB technique · IntraClude · Aortic cross-clamp · Mitral valve · Tricuspid valve · Minimally Invasive Mitral Valve Surgery · Endoscopic surgery

1 Operative Theatre Design for Totally Endoscopic Cardiac Surgery and Patient Selection

Setting up state-of-the-art minimally invasive valve surgery (MIVS) operating rooms requires consideration of both basic and complex factors [1]. Such elements as a safe and yet efficient workflow, theatre hygiene, access and lights are to be integrated into the layout alongside instruments such as a cardiac anaesthetic and transesophageal echocardiography (TEE) machine, an endoscopic camera and CO_2 delivery stack, a cardiopulmonary bypass (CPB) machine, various synchronized screens for neuro-cardio-respiratory, TEE and 2D and 3D endoscopic image projection. Furthermore, these MIVS and totally endoscopic cardiovascular operating rooms must suit the appropriate requirements of two surgeons, a theatre nurse and a support nurse, the anesthesiologist and a perfusionist needing ready access to all standard cardiovascular apparatus, grafts, guidewires, stents and sutures. While the first surgeon looks at the main video screen, the assisting surgeon should be able to follow the operation on a second screen (slave monitor—in some cases even wireless). Streamlined videotaping of the case is useful for didactic and teaching purposes.

Patient selection plays a crucial role especially as the volume of surgical programs is steadily decreasing [1]. Discretion should be employed during the primary selection of patients and valve pathology alongside the routine preoperative investigations. Contrasted computed tomography (CT) should be utilized in the evaluation of the aorta-iliac-femoral arterial axis.

2 Preoperative Planning of the Procedure

The optimal preoperative ECG-synchronized computed tomographic angiography (CTA) reaches from the upper thoracic aperture to the lesser trochanter [2]. This is to include the thoracic cage as well as the thoracic and abdominal aorta, the iliac arteries and common femoral arteries, the latter constituting the most common vascular access site in MIVS [3]. The following needs to be considered when evaluating the CTA-scan: any aortic diseases (calcification, aneurysms, dissections, thrombus), significant MV annular calcification and other anatomic abnormalities [4]. In aortas with a

diameter of more than 4 cm, complete occlusion with the endo-aortic balloon occlusion technique becomes less consistent. There are central cannulation techniques available for performing MIS although most surgeons prefer peripheral cannulation [5]. This involves minimizing the thoracotomy and rib spreading and provides clear access to the MV but demands thorough knowledge of the peripheral vascular anatomy [6].

Thorough knowledge of peripheral vascular anatomy is needed for this approach and a CTA of the chest, abdomen and pelvis, preferably with contrast, supplies the most useful information. Without contrast, the CT-scan is still useful but may not expose subtleties in soft plaque which are important for peripheral cannulation and retrograde arterial perfusion (RAP).

Femoral and iliac arteries and the aorta which have minimal aneurysmal disease, thrombus or calcium and any indication of an iliac or femoral artery dissection is a contraindication for peripheral arterial cannulation [7]. Patients with a history of peripheral vascular disease should undergo evaluation with lower extremity non-invasive studies and/or lower extremity CTA, as cannulation can result in lower-extremity ischemia while on CPB. Regarding borderline arterial femoral diameter cases, additional distal leg perfusion through an extra smaller cannula may be preferable. Besides, three-dimensional (3D) reconstructions of preoperative CT-scans greatly support the better understanding of complex cardiac anatomy, preoperative surgical planning and improve communication within the multidisciplinary team [8]. Once a procedure employing a percutaneous access via the common femoral artery (CFA) is complete, it is common to use vascular closure devices (VCDs) to attain hemostasis [9]. Complications such as infection, lymphoma or hematoma may be evaded by the use of percutaneous femoral vessel cannulation for MIVS, yet these are apt to typical drawbacks (i.e. bleeding and vascular complications) associated with transcatheter devices.

3 Anesthesia

The role of anesthesia in MIVS is to reduce postoperative recovery time by facilitating speedy treatment including early extubation and ambulation. Prior to the administration of general anesthesia (and the initial short-acting drugs such as propofol, remifentanil and rocuronium) the monitors are put into place. These comprise a sedation monitor and a cranial near-infrared spectroscopy (NIRS) to monitor any possible upper-body venous drainage difficulties [2].

One unilateral radial arterial catheter is enough when planning TTC which is in contrast to the bilateral radial pressure monitoring needed in the endo-aortic balloon occlusion cross-clamping technique. Should the endo-aortic balloon become displaced into the innominate artery, bilateral radial arterial catheters will provide immediate warning. Alerts will also be made for the following innominate arterial obstruction leading to an eventual decrease of NIRS.

4 Peripheral Vascular Cannulation and IntraClude™ Positioning

During the initial learning period, it is worth using supplementary venous drainage as in a right internal jugular venous cannula (16–18 Fr, FemFlex, Edwards Lifesciences, Irvine, California, USA) [1]. More experienced centers, however, may only depend on one single femoral venous cannulation reinforced by vacuum assisted drainage.

To afford entry to the right common femoral artery and vein, a 3–4 cm incision is made across the right groin (if opted for open surgical cannulation). Great care should be taken here in order to avoid the medial lymphatic areas. The femoral vein is initially punctured using the Seldinger technique after systemic heparinization and confirmation of an activated clotting time more than 400 s. Using TEE or fluoroscopy, a radio opaque guidewire is navigated into the right atrium (and even further into the SVC if only one venous cannula is used) and then the (mostly 25 FR)

Quickdraw™ venous cannula is lead over the guidewire and anchored with the cannula tip into the SVC. Likewise, the common femoral artery is punctured above the deep branch bifurcation and the guidewire is navigated by TEE into the descending aorta. The guidewire should be freely moving on TEE to ascertain correct placement intraluminally into the descending aorta. The artery is then dilated and an appropriately sized (rule of thumb: 21 FR for female patients; 23 FR for male patients) EndoReturn™ cannula inserted, de-aired, secured and observed for pulsatile waveforms. To monitor for leg ischemia throughout peripheral CBP, some centers employ peripheral limb saturation monitoring. However, the controversial use of distal perfusion strategies including extra cannulation as a standard is not supported. The Intraclude™ catheter device is inserted through the Endoreturn™ side-arm, de-aired and navigated using TEE across the descending aorta, the aortic arch and into the ascending aorta and is then locked into position. Experience is the key and although executing total percutaneous cannulation using vascular closure devices is beneficial, without the significant experience it is not encouraged. There are acknowledged reports of CPB pressures of more than 300 mmHg needing contralateral cannulation and an interruption to temporary flow yet arterial line pressures (behind the oxygenator) of maximum 450 mmHg, accepted at our institution, are rarely observed. Nevertheless, this is still a topic of discussion. If the CPB arterial line pressure exceeds 450 mmHg, a bail-out option of an extra contralateral arterial outflow cannula should be in place. CPB and systemic hypothermia to 34 degrees Celsius are meticulously introduced. The importance of detailed preoperative aorta-iliac-femoral axis evaluation, access planning and the exact use of guidewire navigation cannot be stressed enough. A lack thereof can lead to insufficient CPB flow, guidewire resistance and cannulation related aortic dissection. A further option for cannulation access, although not proposed for the primary MIMVS learning experience, is direct central aortic cannulation or through the right axillary artery.

5   Aortic Cross-Clamping: Balloon Inflation, Antegrade Cardioplegia Delivery and Venting

The insertion of an EAB clamp temporary attains obstruction of the aorta during cardiac surgery including mitral valve repair or replacement and minimally invasive coronary artery bypass grafting (CABG). It is commonly used as part of the technology for minimally invasive cardiac surgery comprising endovascular aortic occlusion, cardioplegia and left ventricular decompression. After the balloon catheter is navigated towards the aortic root (through the skin and usually into the femoral artery in the groin), aortic occlusion is attained by filling the balloon at the tip of the catheter with saline. In this way the blood flow is blocked, although to pick up any balloon migration, constant echocardiographic monitoring is required. Most MIMVS surgeons start by performing TTC. This technique is familiar and enables the direct clamping of the aorta in the same way as one would do in a sternotomy. It works like a 'lobster pincer' since only one of the two branches is actuated by the handle while the other is straight.

The EABO technique provides both aortic occlusion and cardioplegia, based on the use of an endo-luminal balloon catheter inserted through the femoral artery. Another use of EABO are re-do procedures where external cross-clamping can be complicated by the presence of adhesions. Although the endo-aortic balloon occlusion technique has been associated with higher risk of periprocedural aortic dissection in the past, currently both techniques are considered safe and have similar rates of stroke and survival.

Antegrade cardioplegia delivery, aortic root venting and pressure monitoring for ascending aorta sizes ranging 20–42 mm is performed by IntraClude™ (Edwards Lifesciences, Irvine, California, USA). This is a composite endo-aortic balloon occlusion device (10.5 Fr, 100 cm length) which is guided by TEE or fluoroscopy into the sinotubular junction via a 200 cm 0.0038 J-tip guidewire and is fed through the side arm of the EndoReturn™ femoral arterial cannula (21–23 Fr, Edwards Lifesciences, Irvine, California, USA).

The preparedness of the team and the parameters are initially confirmed before the assisting surgeon stabilises the EndoReturn™ cannula with his/her right hand and the TEE then reconfirms position of the IntraClude™ device.

To attain rapid diastolic cardiac arrest, this device is then partially inflated to approximately 75% of the volume of the ascending aorta by manually flushing adenosine (0.25 mg/kg) via a syringe through the device port. As antegrade cardioplegia is delivered and monitored by aortic root and cardioplegic line pressures, the balloon is fully inflated and, guided by TEE, placed between the sinotubular ridge and innominate artery. The surge of the retrograde CPB inflow will push the balloon towards the aortic valve. To safeguard the position of the device at the sinotubular junction, it is vital to retract the device under the guidance of TEE. The right arterial line pressures are secured as the balloon is locked into position and TEE positioning is confirmed using endoscopic visualisation and palpation of the aorta with a rigid sucker. Repositioning of the device could be contemplated when there is no trace of the radial artery which suggests innominate artery obstruction due to dislodgement.

Tips, Tricks & Traps.

- **Actual endo-aortic balloon cross-clamping sequence in a normal MIMVS case:**

  - The ideal mean arterial start-off pressure is 70 mmHg.
  - Firstly, inflate the balloon with only half of the calculated volume with normal saline. The half-inflated balloon will then hover above the aortic root suspended by the CPB flow. The new formula for *calculated volume* is the diameter of the ascending aorta minus 7. For example, if the ascending aorta measures 32 mm in cross-sectional diameter, a total of 25 mL (32 − 7 = 25) should be administered into the balloon upon full completion of endo-aortic balloon occlusion.

- Prompt and efficient administration of adenosine (simplified dosing is 4 ampules; official recommendation 0.25 mg/kg body weight) will induce a temporary atrioventricular block, usually causing proximal movement of the balloon. This is the moment when the slack in the system (the balloon catheter) is retracted.
- Then the balloon is inflated with the remaining calculated volume, thereby sealing off the ascending aorta intraluminally.
- Upon full inflation, balloon pressures of around 400 mmHg are safe and to be expected.
- Cardioplegia should commence immediately at a line pressure of at least 350 mmHg, inducing a cardioplegia flow of approximately 250-300 mL/min. Consider a single dose cardioplegia type and apply *fire and forget strategy* (i.e. Custodiol or DelNido). Cardioplegia should begin immediately to avoid cardiac contractions which could cause distal displacement of the balloon.
- Due to administration of cardioplegia, a loss of systemic vascular resistance will be seen (less pronounced with DelNido; more pronounced with Custodiol). In order to avoid distal displacement of the balloon, noradrenalin should be given to maintain systemic arterial pressures and counterbalance distal balloon migration.
- During administration of cardioplegia, the balloon should be in the proximity of the innominate artery yet not occlusive. This is on account of the disappearance of the balancing force (cardioplegia-force) after cardioplegia is completed and the balloon will only be able to relocate proximally (due to CPB flow).
- Balancing forces on the balloon during cardioplegia are:
  The yellow pressure line on the monitor (pressure measured at the tip of the balloon) will move the balloon distally.
  The white pressure line (CPB flow) will push the balloon proximally.

- After cardioplegia is fully administered, venting via the tip of the balloon should be started (firstly negative pressures will arise and secondly, depending on the anesthesia monitoring system, an "X" or dashed lines will appear).

- **Troubleshooting**:

  - Difficulties in navigating the balloon into the ascending aorta.
    Position the balloon in the proximal descending aorta (distally from the aortic arch) and then, after fully retracting the guidewire, re-advance the guidewire. The composite endo-aortic balloon occlusion device (10.5 Fr, 100 cm length) will act as a type of catheter helping to navigate the wire around the aortic arch.
  - Should a permanent pacemaker be implanted, the administration of adenosine will not be effective.
    Electrical induction of ventricular fibrillation can be used in this case.
  - In general, short and slightly dilated (ascending) aortic anatomy and/or tortuous vascular anatomy might lead to less stable balloon positioning.
    These anatomical findings might not be the ideal starter case.
  - Instead of left and right radial arteries, right brachial and femoral arteries can also be used for arterial pressure line monitoring.
    Some centers even use isolated right radial pressure monitoring (yet this is not advised). Consider routine bilateral cerebral NIRS monitoring.
  - In the case of distal balloon migration during administration of antegrade cardioplegia via the tip of the balloon, it is critical to understand that the balloon can not be actively positioned more proximally since the catheter can only be pulled, not pushed.
    As a solution, increase systemic arterial pressure (> root pressure) or reduce the root pressure by lowering or stopping the cardioplegia flow.

– Open the left atrium only after full administration of cardioplegia. Once the left atrium is opened and filled with air, TEE visualization of the precise position of the balloon is significantly impaired.

– Be aware of the fact that in case of significant balloon migration (distal from the innominate artery!), cardioplegia is going to be washed out due to collateral flow coming from the innominate artery.

– Unrealistically high aortic root pressure values during administration of cardioplegia (>100 mmHg) are a typical sign of balloon over-inflation.
In this case reduce the filling pressure (remove some volume) of the balloon.

– During the stable phase of endo-aortic balloon occlusion, the balloon will not cause any difficulty as long as the "X" or dashed lines are seen, indicating complete sealing of the ascending aorta, and left/right arterial blood pressure lines are matching, indicating no obstruction of the innominate artery. Actual balloon pressure readings are less of a concern.

– In the case of changes in "X" or dashed lines into positive root pressure readings, consider the following:
Increase vent suction via the tip of the balloon
Slightly pull on the balloon catheter to make the balloon occlusive
Add 1-2 mL of balloon volume

– In the case of balloon perforations (e.g. needle perforation during mitral valve replacement, heavy calcifications, TAVI prosthesis in aortic valve position) or any other significant problems associated with endo-aortic balloon technique:
Consider balloon deflation (this will induce cardiac reperfusion) and consider finishing the procedure on a fibrillating or beating heart.

– Be aware of possibly locating and visualizing the balloon directly in the ascending aortic position using a sucker, especially in case of poor TEE visualization.

– Systemic vascular tortuosity might result in vascular stretching during the course of the ischemic phase of the MIMVS procedure leading to balloon dislocation. Repositioning of the balloon might be needed over time.

6 Discussion

There is a strong case for endo-aortic balloon occlusion as the alternative to trans-thoracic external aortic cross-clamping. A clear advantage is the omission of a cardioplegia puncture hole in the ascending aorta, eliminating the need to suture the aorta as well as the risk of bleeding from the puncture site. Moreover, it comes into play for re-do procedures where the adhesions can prove awkward for cross-clamping. The need to place the endo-aortic balloon device through the arterial cannula is a disadvantage, however, because the operative size of the arterial cannula is then reduced. A second arterial cannula can be placed if the result is high line pressures or inadequate flow. Regarding distal balloon migration, it has been noted that it can occur and results in innominate artery occlusion. Yet this migration tendency can be curbed by retracting the slack of the catheter during inflation and detected without difficulty by observing the bilateral radial artery pressures. Past concerns about the endo-aortic balloon's association with aortic dissection have been quashed since the routine use of CT angiography to assess the general risk of retrograde perfusion in certain anatomies and the acceptance of essential training in basic wire skills. The operational field, especially the left fibrous trigone, can also be potentially obscured due to proximal migration. A further disadvantage is that it could become non-occlusive to the sinus of Valsalva culminating in perfusion of the coronary ostia. The potential for puncturing or rupturing of the balloon during the procedure, the required bilateral arterial lines for monitoring the installation and the cost of the catheter itself are all further disadvantages.

The little existing data comparing TTC with the endo-aortic balloon technique is retrospective in nature, drawing attention to the fact that there is not much difference in the safety profiles of either technique. Both have a markedly lower stroke rate than fibrillatory arrest and there is no difference in retrograde aortic dissection, bleeding, or adequacy of myocardial protection. Kowalesky et al. [10] suggested that (1) in a preoperative patient the key is to predict and prevent complications with femoral cannulation and to evaluate optimal perfusion; (2) there are no noted differences in both techniques regarding aortic cross-clamping and CPB timing; (3) there is associated risk found in the endo-aortic balloon technique with an increase in relative risk of limp ischemia and vascular complications; (4) a mandatory yet inadequate learning curve can lead to more frequent complications for surgeons with initial experience of the endo-aortic balloon technique; (5) between TTC and the endo-aortic balloon technique there are no major differences in the number of acute kidney injury or mortality incidents or cerebrovascular accidents.

The initial learning curve preferably involves simple atrial septal defect, intraatrial myxoma and uncomplicated valve procedures. Regarding a steeper learning curve, seven key aspects have been identified by Hunter et al. [11]: atrioventricular valve repair techniques, TEE navigated cannulation, incision placement and setup, transition to single shaft instrument use, atrioventricular valve visualization and CPB strategies. To overcome the learning curve it has been suggested that a typical number of operations should lie between 75 and 125 procedures. Furthermore, to uphold the resulting standards, it is recommended that more than 1 procedure per week should be performed. De Praetere et al. [12] preferred 30 procedures for a successful learning curve with the aortic cross clamp time to be considerably reduced before and after the end of the learning curve. It is crucial to perform simulation team training due to the stark decrease in surgical volume (Videos 1 and 2).

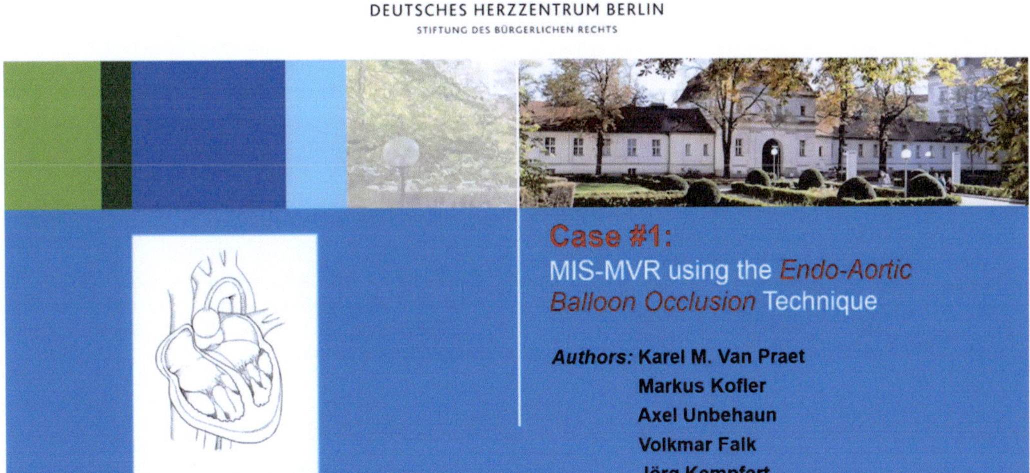

Video 1 Case 01—MIS-MVR using the endo-aortic balloon occlusion technique (▶ https://doi.org/10.1007/000-a7q)

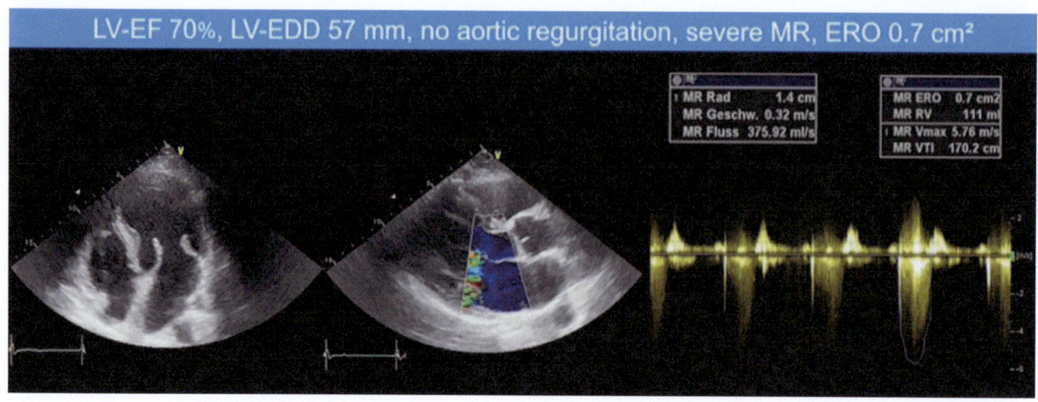

Video 2 Case 02—MIS-MVR using the endo-aortic balloon occlusion technique (▶ https://doi.org/10.1007/000-a7r)

References

1. Van der Merwe J, Casselman F, Van Praet F. The principles of minimally invasive atrioventricular valve repair surgery utilizing endoaortic balloon occlusion technology: how to start and sustain a safe and effective program. J Vis Surg. 2019;5:72–72. https://doi.org/10.21037/jovs.2019.08.01.

2. Van Praet KM, Kofler M, Montagner M, et al. Minimally invasive mitral valve repair using external clamping — pearls and pitfalls. J Vis Surg. 2020;6 (45). doi:https://doi.org/10.21037/jovs-2019-amvis-07

3. Van Praet KM, Kempfert J, Jacobs S, et al. Mitral valve surgery: current status and future prospects of the minimally invasive approach. Expert Rev Med Devices. 2021. https://doi.org/10.1080/17434440.2021.1894925.

4. Van Praet KM, Kofler M, Unbehaun A, et al. Reply to Del Giglio, Tamagnini, Biondi, and Di Mauro. J Card Surg. 2020:4–7. doi:https://doi.org/10.1111/jocs.14998

5. Karel M Van Praet, Markus Kofler, Stephan Jacobs, Volkmar Falk, Axel Unbehaun JK. The MANTA Vascular Closure Device for Percutaneous Femoral Vessel Cannulation in Minimally Invasive Surgical Mitral Valve Repair. Innov . 2020:1–4. doi:doi:https://doi.org/10.1177/1556984520956300.

6. Van Praet KM, Stamm C, Sündermann SH, et al. Minimally invasive surgical mitral valve repair: State of the art review. Interv Cardiol Rev. 2018;13(1):14–9. https://doi.org/10.15420/icr.2017:30:1.

7. Van Praet KM, Kofler M, Sündermann SH, et al. Minimally invasive approach for infective mitral valve endocarditis. Ann Cardiothorac Surg. 2019;8 (6):702–4. https://doi.org/10.21037/acs.2019.07.01.

8. Van Praet KM, van Kampen A, Kofler M, et al. Minimally invasive surgical aortic valve replacement: the RALT approach. J Card Surg. 2020:1–6. https://doi.org/10.1111/jocs.14756

9. Van Praet KM, Van Kampen A, Kofler M, Unbehaun A, Hommel M, Jacobs S, Falk V, Kempfert J. Minimally invasive surgical aortic valve replacement through a right anterolateral thoracotomy. Multimed Man Cardiothorac Surg.

10. Kowalewski M, Malvindi PG, Suwalski P, et al. Clinical safety and effectiveness of endoaortic as compared to transthoracic clamp for small thoracotomy mitral valve surgery: meta-analysis of observational studies. Ann Thorac Surg. 2017;103(2):676–86. https://doi.org/10.1016/j.athoracsur.2016.08.072.

11. Hunter S. How to start a minimal access mitral valve program. Ann Cardiothorac Surg. 2013;2:774–778.

12. De Praetere H, Verbrugghe P, Rega F, Meuris B, Herijgers P. Starting minimally invasive valve surgery using endoclamp technology : safety and results of a starting surgeon. Interact Cardiovasc Thorac Surg. 2015;20(30):351–8. https://doi.org/10.1093/icvts/ivu394.

Endoscopic Tricuspid Valve Surgery: Planning and Deployment

Marco Solinas and Giacomo Bianchi

Abstract

Tricuspid valve surgery, either in isolation or in combination with mitral valve surgery, can be easily implemented and performed through fully endoscopic access. Targeted measures are required for rapid, correct, and effective execution. As in the more general strategy of minimally invasive valve surgery, proper patient selection and planning based on imaging techniques are the secure foundation on which to base the surgical framework. Proper surgical access, ergonomics of instruments and movement, adequate venous drainage via cardiopulmonary bypass, and a bloodless field with minimal risk of gas embolization along with proper interaction between endoscopic optics and stitch placement to avoid minimal interference are the key points for performing the surgery. In this chapter, we describe our experience and workflow together with "tips and tricks" for successful intervention with a fully endoscopic approach, with attention to "traps" that may emerge.

Keywords

Tricuspid valve · Minimally invasive · Full endoscopic · Repair · learning curve

1 General Consideration

Minimally invasive mitral valve surgery through a mini-thoracotomy approach has gained increasing popularity in recent years; although with alternating phases since it was first proposed [1, 2], after 30 years it has demonstrated its superiority over the conventional approach [3–6]. This is due to the diffusion of " "Valve Centers" able to ensure a high reparative standard and results independently from the surgical approach.

The adoption of the mini-thoracotomy approach in cardiac surgery led to an initial resistance in implementing multi-valvular surgery; this resistance was essentially due to the adaptation of the surgeon to the new setup, in focusing the technical gesture to the minimally invasive approach providing the same qualitative results as a median sternotomy, and to the fear of increased clamping time.

Supplementary Information The online version contains supplementary material available at https://doi.org/10.1007/978-3-031-21104-1_10. The videos can be accessed individually by clicking the DOI link in the accompanying figure caption or by scanning this link with the SN More Media App.

M. Solinas · G. Bianchi (✉)
Department of Adult Cardiac Surgery, Ospedale del Cuore "G. Pasquinucci"—Fondazione Toscana "G. Monasterio", Massa, Italy
e-mail: gbianchi@ftgm.it

M. Solinas
e-mail: marco.solinas@ftgm.it

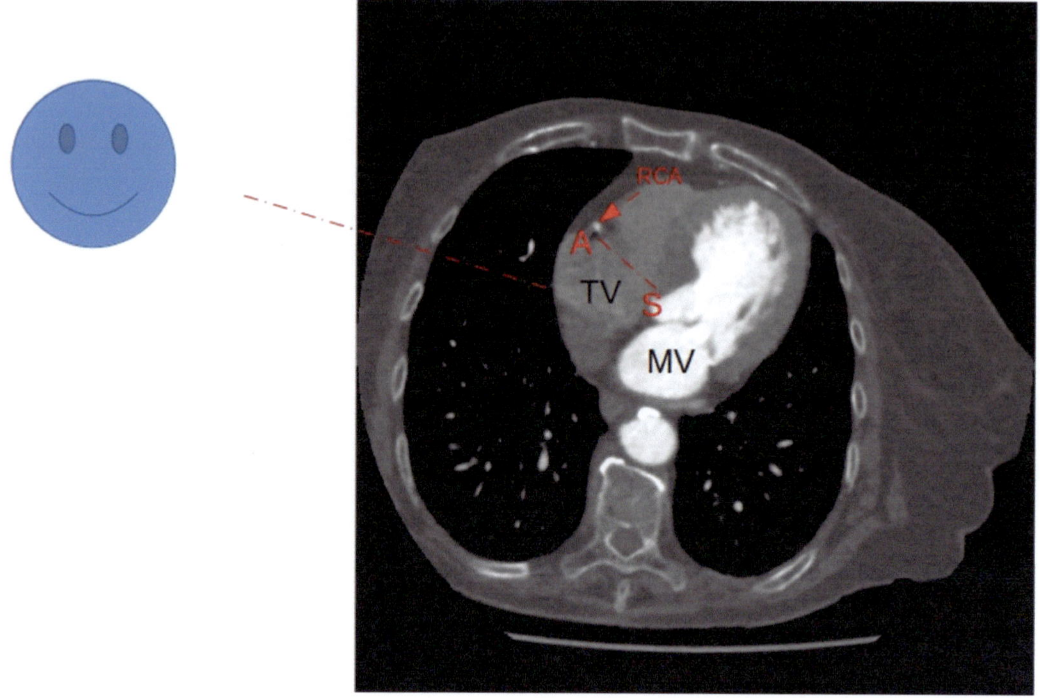

Fig. 1 Spatial ergonomics of endoscopic tricuspid valve surgery; the dashed line is the path of surgeon's instruments. TV: tricuspid valve; A: anterior leaflet; S: septal leaflet; RCA: right coronary artery; MV: mitral valve

In particular, the tricuspid valve has suffered a fate of further " "abandonment": first, because of the erroneous hypothesis of a regression of the pathology after surgical correction of the left valve pathology; second, in the context of minimally invasive surgery, because of the fears expressed above, associating the correction of concomitant tricuspid pathology with mitral pathology has been an infrequent eventuality.

In more recent times, with the increased spread of minimally invasive surgery, development of shared frameworks tailored to each Center, and progressive accommodation of surgeons to the approach, associated procedures have increased, such as ablation of atrial fibrillation, closure of septal defects, and tricuspid valve surgery.

In minimally invasive tricuspid surgery, both video-assisted and endoscopic, the fundamental difference from the sternotomy approach is that the valve structure remains in its anatomical position: the tricuspid valve is normally oriented at an obtuse angle with respect to the sagittal plane, i.e., it looks toward the lower right side, hence the need to perform some maneuvers for surgical exposure. In fact, while in median sternotomy after the opening of the right atrium the exposure involves rotation toward the observer until the valve plane is orthogonal to the operator, and in the minimally invasive approach the surgeon is parallel to the valve plane and limited in exposure by the sternum and intact rib cage, thus having fewer degrees of freedom and greater physical impediments (Fig. 1).

The key to success for rapid and reproducible tricuspid valve surgery essentially lies in optimal exposure, whether annuloplasty or prosthetic replacement is planned. This is even more important in the case of a fully endoscopic approach.

Below we illustrate the preoperative workup to plan and then implement endoscopic tricuspid valve surgery; it goes through the analysis of chest radiography, possibly CT scan of the chest, corroborated by some tips and tricks in the surgical setup.

2 Preoperative Planning

2.1 Chest X-Ray and CT Scan

The first, easiest, and most widely accessible imaging of the patient's anatomy is the two-projection chest radiography. This diagnostic test is particularly informative as it can delineate factors that absolutely or relatively contraindicate minimally invasive or endoscopic surgery from a mini-thoracotomy approach. In Table 1, we report what we believe represent absolute and relative contraindications to these approaches.

The presence of chronic lung disease, fibrothorax, previous lung surgery, or other pathological conditions that advise against manipulation of the lung should be considered as exclusion criteria for this type of surgery. Relative contraindications should be adapted on the basis of the experience of the Center; in our Institute, right thoracic wall surgery combined with radiotherapy is not usually considered a relative contraindication, but a "red flag" regarding the possibility of tenacious adhesions and therefore possible conversion to sternotomy.

The analysis of the radiogram of the chest in latero-lateral projection deserves a specific evaluation. As we have previously described, tricuspid valve exposure in video-assisted and endoscopic mini-thoracotomy enjoys fewer degrees of freedom in projecting the valve plane toward the observer (surgeon's eyes and/or endoscope) by conventional tools (dedicated traction/exposure stitches) and atrial retractors. One of the limiting factors is the rib cage and the sternum: the shallower the chest, the less the possibility to expose the valve, as the sternum limits the retractor stroke. From our experience of about 500 cases of endoscopic mitro-tricuspid surgery, we have deduced that a distance between the sternum and the vertebrae, calculated at the level of the pulmonary hilum, less than or equal to 14 cm is associated with a difficult exposure of the mitral and tricuspid valve (personal data).

Therefore, we believe that the presence of Pectus excavatum or other rib cage deformities represents an additional limitation to exposure, which at least initially should be avoided by a Center starting a minimally invasive program or becoming familiar with a fully endoscopic approach.

Elevation of the right hemi-diaphragm can make exposure of cardiac structures particularly difficult, although, as we will see in the dedicated section of this chapter, a few tricks allow the diaphragm to be safely retracted with a step-by-step approach.

Reinterventions, especially in the case of previous sternotomies, are not considered by our Center to be even a relative contraindication, but a true indication for endoscopic minimally invasive surgery [7–11].

The CT scan of the chest, with and without contrast medium, performs a dual task: first, it deepens the findings of the chest X-ray (Table 2), and secondly it gives the possibility through the software in clinical use (most of them are open source and free to use) to perform three-dimensional reconstructions for preoperative planning and effective surgery deployment [10].

Table 1 Absolute and relative contraindication to endoscopic right mini-thoracotomy

Absolute contraindications	Relative contraindications
Severe chronic obstructive pulmonary disease	Right Chest Surgery and radiotherapy
Fibro-thorax	Lung adhesion
Previous lung surgery	Dilated Ascending Aorta (>40 mm)
Bullous emphysema	Severe peripheral disease
	Aortic regurgitation more than mild
	Pectus Excavatum
	High right hemi-diaphragm

Table 2 Anatomical findings at CT scan and considerations for minimally invasive surgery

Findings	Considerations
Aorta	Evaluate degree, location, and type of atheroma, including hard versus soft plaque; measure diameter of ascending aorta (must be < 4 cm for endoaortic balloon)
Great vessels	Rule out aberrant anatomy, including patent ductus arteriosus, persistent left SVC, and aberrant right subclavian artery, which may make monitoring of an endoaortic balloon difficult
Mitral valve	Evaluate degree of mitral annular calcification
Iliac artery	Rule out aneurysm, tortuosity, plaque, and localized dissection or pseudoaneurysm from previous catheterization site
Common femoral and superficial femoral artery	Identify bifurcation and location for site choice; measure common femoral artery diameter for cannulation
Venous anatomy	Rule out venous anomalies or IVC filter

Also, from CT scan may arise the presence of diffuse atherosclerotic disease, especially in femoral arteries as well as in the descending thoracic and/or abdominal aorta; in our Center these findings are not a contraindication for minimally invasive approach, since an antero-grade flow through direct cannulation of the ascending aorta or axillary artery is possible in most cases [12, 13].

3 The "Virtual Operation" Using CT Scan as a Guide

Three-dimensional reconstruction of the chest (volume rendering) gives the possibility to observe the patient's cardiac structures in their spatial arrangement. As shown in Fig. 2, the cardiac structures are well highlighted in relation to the bony structures of the rib cage; thus, it is easy to project these through the intercostal space.

It must be kept in mind that in endoscopic surgery, whether performed with a periareolar or trans-axillary approach, the incision is limited and is the focus of the surgical instruments. Good alignment with the structures of the heart, i.e., as orthogonal as possible, and the absence of con-flict or limitation with the endoscope and other components (aortic vent, field aspirators, and aortic clamp), are critical.

We generally recommend performing the surgical incision in the intercostal space where the structures of interest project, usually at the level of the anterior axillary line.

Vision is assured and facilitated through a 30° endoscope. This allows its insertion in the same space as the surgical incision or in a superior intercostal space; by orienting or rotating the head of the endoscope, it is possible to center the structure of interest and reach it with the instru-ments without creating conflict between them. In our experience, we have observed that the most commonly used intercostal space in men has been the third while in women the fourth; more recently in our case series, the third intercostal space has proven to be the universal access for the treatment of mitro-tricuspidal pathology.

An obvious caveat is that the CT scan is performed in deep inspiration with the arms facing upwards and with cardiac chambers filled. During the intraoperative phase, it can be observed that the diaphragm tends to rise more than expected due to the effect of curarization and intra-abdominal pressure, which may worsen or obliterate the vision of the structures antici-pated by the CT scan. As expressed above, even for this intra-individual anatomic variability, the third intercostal space for surgical incision has proven useful in overcoming problems related to viewing cardiac structures.

In our Center, we use direct aortic clamping, which has also demonstrated in recent meta-analysis a superiority over the intra-aortic bal-loon in terms of efficacy and safety. The CT scan

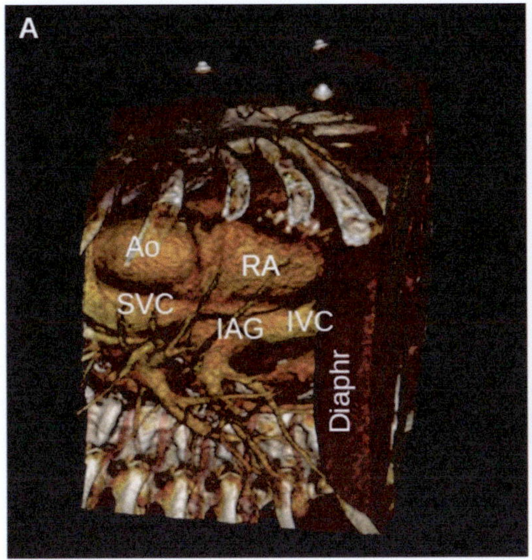

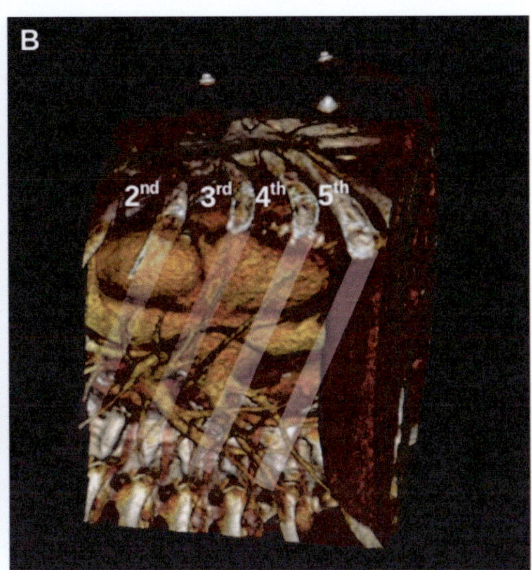

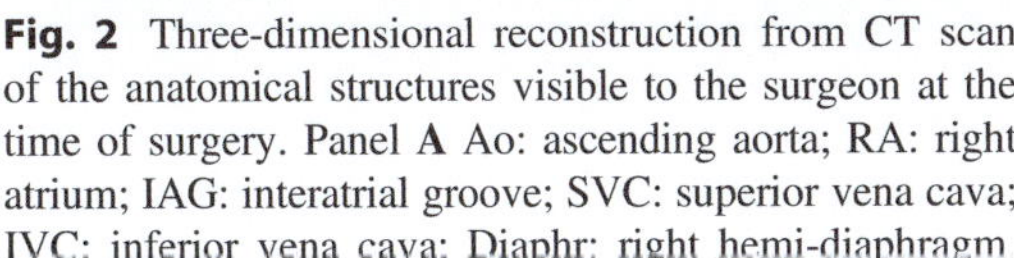

Fig. 2 Three-dimensional reconstruction from CT scan of the anatomical structures visible to the surgeon at the time of surgery. Panel **A** Ao: ascending aorta; RA: right atrium; IAG: interatrial groove; SVC: superior vena cava; IVC: inferior vena cava; Diaphr: right hemi-diaphragm Panel **B** shows the structures by opacifying the position of the ribs (intercostal space is numbered). Note how the point of entry (working port) in one space instead of another facilitates access to certain structures and makes access to others more complex

of the chest allows to visualize the ascending aorta and to plan the clamping site (usually in the *transverse sinus*), also in function of possible aortic calcifications. As we will see in the surgical setup section, external aortic clamping may involve inserting the clamp through the same surgical incision or through a higher intercostal space, depending on the instrument used.

suitable for drainage of the head and neck district is inserted using the Seldinger technique with progressive dilations. The most used cannula in our Center is 16 Fr. diameter. The cannula is then connected with a 3/8 tube and filled with saline solution after adequate flush. The tube is clamped and kept sterile for future connection to the cardio-pulmonary bypass (CPB) circuit.

4 Anesthesia and Jugular Vein Cannulation

Anesthesiologic preparation proceeds according to the standard. After induction, intubation may or may not be performed with a selective endotracheal tube. The central venous catheter is inserted under ultrasound guidance into the left internal jugular vein. Always under ultrasound guidance, the upper drainage cannula for extracorporeal circulation is inserted: after the correct insertion of the guide, 2500 IU of unfractionated heparin (UFH) is administered systemically to the patient; then the cannula with a diameter

5 Patient Positioning

The patient is positioned on the bed in supine decubitus. To expose the surgical access site, an inflatable bag is placed under the right hemithorax. The right arm moved away from the body, exposing the axilla and the anterior, middle, and posterior axillary lines. Sterile draping is done in the traditional manner, taking care to leave both groins uncovered for surgical access as well as the sternal midline for eventual surgical conversion. One endoscope holder and one atrial retractor holder are placed to the right and left of the patient, respectively.

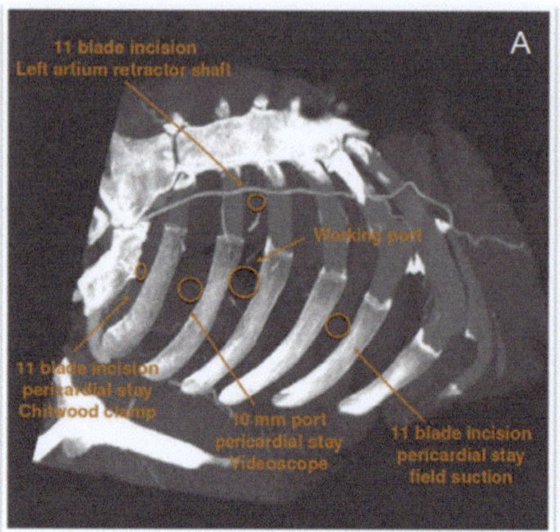

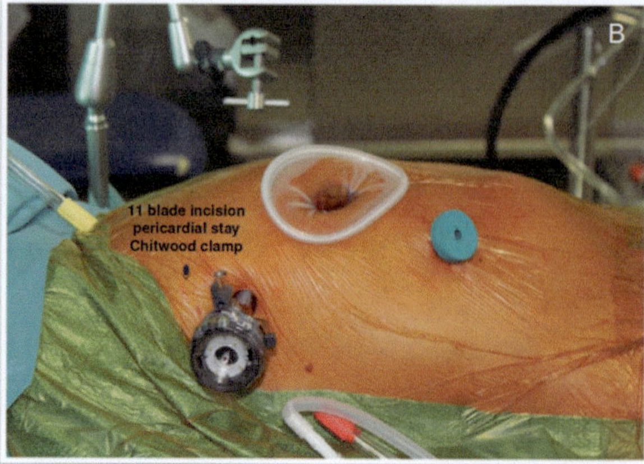

CT-scan planned Approach   Surgical Field Application of the planned approach

Fig. 3 Planned approach with CT and its transposition to the operative field

6 Surgical Access

Surgical incision is made as determined by preoperative planning with chest CT or radiography. Generally, we prefer a periareolar incision in elderly males or with poorly represented pectoral muscle; periareolar incision in women is not performed in our Center because of the need to cut the mammary gland and because of the frequent numbness of the area (up to 30% of cases in published series). We therefore recommend axillary access in most subjects.

In order to make the skin incision more aesthetic and also more functional, during the sterile draping we tend the skin toward the midline, so that the final result will be a scar that will be hidden in the axilla; doing so it is also possible an entrance in the thoracic cage some centimeters more medially to the anterior axillary line. The choice of the space is, as said, left to the planning with CT of the thorax; from the entry space comes the position of all the other instruments that constitute the surgical setup. In order to avoid a conflict between instruments, we prefer to insert a 5 or 10 mm port for the 30° endoscope in one intercostal space above and perform a small skin incision two intercostal spaces below to insert a field aspirator; the clamp will finally be inserted from a minimal incision two spaces

above the surgical access. To give an example, as shown in Fig. 3, for a 4th intercostal space access, the endoscope is scheduled to be inserted at the 3rd intercostal space, the aortic clamp at the 2nd space, and the field suction line at the 6th space. After the incision has been made and the technical feasibility has been verified (exclusion of adhesions or lysis of any adhesions), the femoral vessels are isolated.

7 Cardiopulmonary Bypass Setup

The CPB is set up, in case of isolated or associated tricuspid surgery, with a double cannulation, i.e., with a femoral-jugular venous drainage. We have already described the neck cannulation part; as for femoral vessel cannulation, this is performed through a minimal inguinal incision, sparing lymph node packages and exposing only the anterior surface of the artery and vein. UFH is then administered at the final dose required. A purse-string of polypropylene 5/0 is used to secure the cannulas. The circuit for CPB is split with a Y-connector (3/8" × 3/8" × 3/8") for the jugular and femoral venous drainage. Under transesophageal echocardiographic (TEE) guidance, the vein is cannulated on Seldinger technique guidance. The tip of the venous cannula is advanced to the inferior cavo-atrial junction. The femoral artery is cannulated in the same manner with advanced guidance always under TEE guidance in descending thoracic aorta. The cannula of the chosen diameter is advanced approximately 7 cm into the femoral artery. The cannulas are then secured with tourniquets and connected to the circuit. When the activated clotting time reaches 480 s, CPB is initiated.

8 Exposure of the Surgical Field

Once CPB is initiated, cardiac structures are detended. The lung is deflated and the pericardium opened; stapling the pericardium above the ascending aorta provides a safe spot so that the electrocautery does not injure the underlying structures. The incision is maintained craniocaudally parallel to the phrenic nerve at least 4 cm from it. The two parts of the pericardium are then separated by sutures. The upper part is through 3 points of polypropylene 3/0 that are extruded from the main surgical access (working port). In the lower part, three silk sutures are placed at the level of the superior vena cava, half of the pericardium and the lower end, respectively; these in turn are passed through the clamp port, the endoscope port, and the lower service port. By placing them in traction, these expose the superior vena cava, transverse sulcus, right atrium, and Sondergaard's sulcus, as well as pulling the diaphragm downward and enhancing complete vision; a possible "trap" in this approach is to place a stitch in the tendinuous part of diaphragm, as this may lead to injury of the liver and copious intra-abdominal bleeding, especially in elderly patients with fragile tissue. The oblique sinus is opened by blunt grinding. Two umbilical slices are passed to surround the superior and inferior vena cava. A tip to perform this procedure more quickly is to mount the umbilical webbing on an angled instrument and then pass it to encircle the vena cava in a bottom-up motion. A 4/0 polypropylene purse-string with a pledget is placed on the ascending aorta to insert the cardioplegia line and aortic vent. Finally, the ascending aorta is clamped, in our Center by external clamping with Chitwood

Clamp, and anterograde cold crystalloid cardioplegia is administered at a dose of 25 ml/kg. Both umbilical tapes are tightened, the right atrium is opened, and cardioplegia refluxed from the coronary sinus is suctioned to avoid volume overload and electrolyte alterations. The procedure then proceeds first with mitral surgery through the opening of the interatrial groove, if provided, and then with tricuspid valve surgery.

9 Operative Phase

The incision of the right atrium continues along the *sulcus terminalis*, taking care not to sever it because of the arrhythmogenic potential of the scar. The atrial retractor shaft is inserted from the anterior surface of the chest, taking care to pass it more laterally to the course of the right internal mammary artery, so as not to injure it. The retractor is usually inserted in the same intercostal space as the working port. Placement of the retractor paddle in the right atrium is sufficient to properly expose the tricuspid valve (Fig. 4, panel A). Vision is provided by the endoscope arriving obliquely from above; the chamber head is rotated in order to compensate for the oblique position and provide an orthogonal view of the valve.

The first stitch for tricuspid annuloplasty is positioned on the septal leaflet (reverse). This point improves the exposure of the valve. Subsequent stitches are placed reverse and counterclockwise to the posterior leaflet, where they are placed straight and, finally, again counterclockwise backward to complete the commissure between the septal leaflet and anterior leaflet. Gently pulling a stitch in the opposite direction to the next stitch increases the exposure and accuracy of the stitch to be placed. The procedure is depicted in Fig. 4, panel B. The tricuspid ring is then positioned in a standard manner; in our Center the stitches are secured by a system of titanium fasteners (Fig. 5).

In the case of tricuspid valve replacement, the points with pledgets on the atrial side are positioned in the same way and with the same counterclockwise direction. In order to minimize the risk of injury to the penetrating branch of the

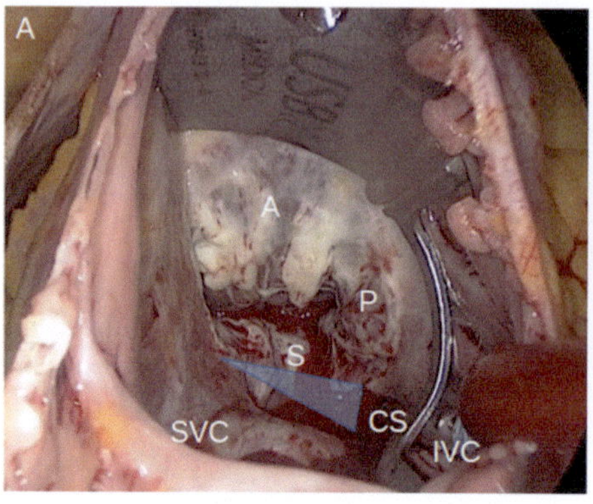
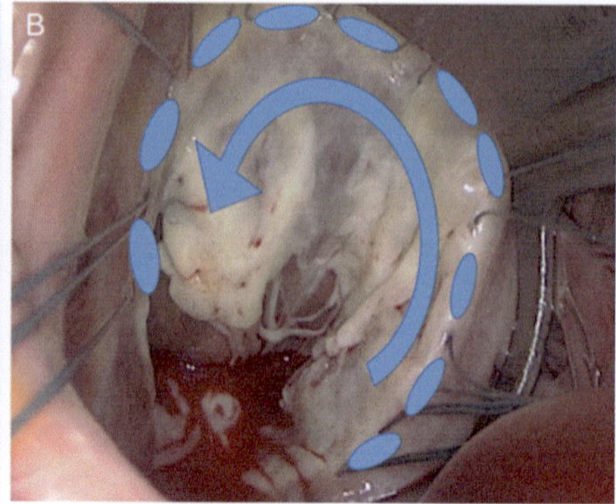

Fig. 4 Panel A: view of the right atrium after atriotomy. Note how the terminal ridge is left intact. The retractor in this case is already sufficient for optimal valve exposure. A: anterior leaflet; P: posterior leaflet; S: septal leaflet; CS: coronary sinus; IVC: inferior vena cava; SVC: superior vena cava. Koch's triangle is drawn in transparency. Panel B: sequence of annuloplasty points in counterclockwise direction

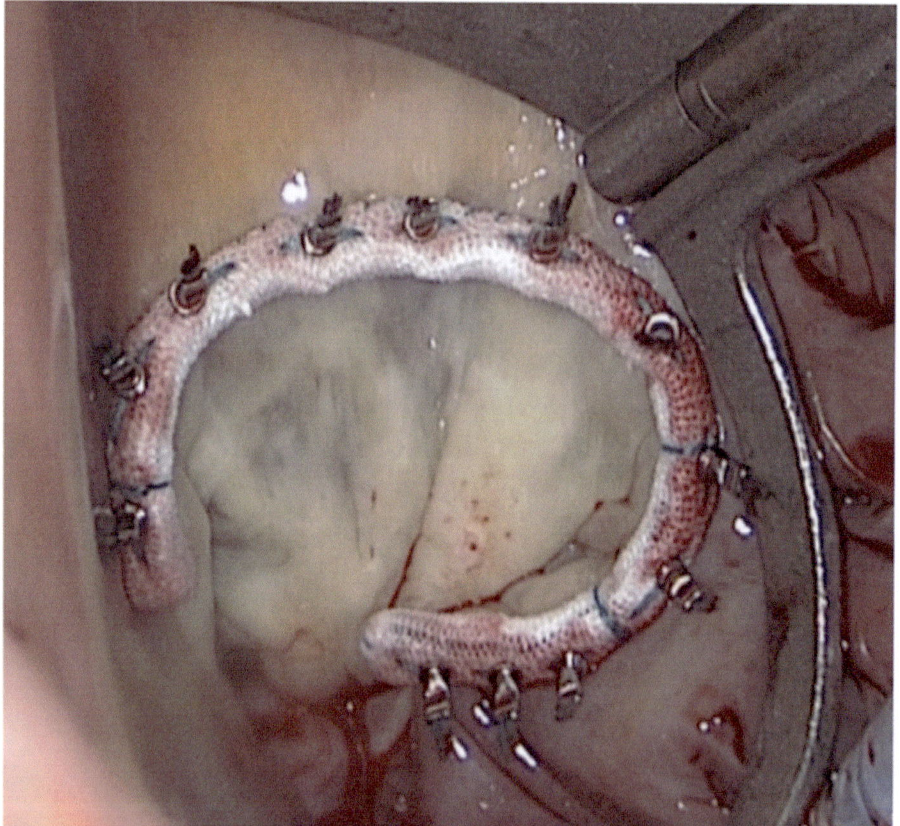

Fig. 5 Final view of the tricuspid annuloplasty ring. To be noted the titanium fastners to secure the ring to the annulus.

bundle of His, the points at the apex of the Koch triangle are positioned directly in the leaflet rather than in the tricuspid valve ring, which as we know is a virtual structure formed by the passage and intersection of fibers of the atrial and ventricular myocardium together with the extracellular matrix. The policy of our Center, corroborated by international experience, is to use biological prostheses. In the endoscopic approach an important "caveat" is the bulk of the prosthesis compared to the working port, as often the prosthesis is much larger than it. The prosthesis, if forced in the passage, could distort or fracture. We prefer a prosthesis that has the possibility of a "cincing", which reduces the size and facilitates the passage in the working port.

10 Special Considerations—Redo and Beating Heart Operative Tricuspid Valve Surgery

In reinterventions targeting the tricuspid valve, the setup presented above can be easily used without modification. The focal points, whether previous surgeries have been sternotomy or mini-thoracotomy, are pulmonary adhesions between the ascending aorta and adjacent structures. Once the adhesions have been smoothed, the procedure proceeds with cannulation, preferably peripheral (femoral artery and femoral vein in addition to the jugular venous drainage cannula) and with the initiation of extracorporeal circulation. The intervention can be performed with a beating heart by the direct opening of the right atrium, without freeing the pericardium above; thanks to the vacuum-assisted venous drainage, it is possible to perform the intervention without placing snares around the superior and inferior vena cava [8, 9]. This approach is particularly effective in cases of simple annuloplasty. All the layers are then closed in standard fashion. A possible treatment is the effective LV de-airing and the venous blood return from coronary sinus that can interfere with an optimal vision of the surgical field; this issue can be solved by lowering the CPB flow according to the temperature and placing a suction line in the coronary sinus.

A recent international multicenter study (SUR-TRI) outlined that isolated tricuspid valve surgery performed with a beating heart strategy is a safe option and resulted in a trend of increased long-term survival [14].

If feasible, the ascending aorta can be freed from adhesions and clamped directly; this also allows the placement of an aortic venting line, to ensure de-airing. Carbon dioxide flooding of the surgical field improves the de-airing in these patients. A final aspect may be the use of the endo-balloon; however, this requires close collaboration and experience of the surgical and especially anesthesiologic team for its placement. In our Center, this approach has been abandoned a long time ago, after proving to be not superior to direct cross-clamping. A recent meta-analysis showed instead a lower risk profile for the direct aortic cross-clamp [15].

11 Adjunctive Techniques and Adult Congenital Heart Disease

The endoscopic approach does not preclude the use of additional techniques such as anterior leaflet augmentation or bicuspidalization or the "edge-to-edge" also known as "Clover technique" [16].

Cannulation of the superior and inferior vena cava separately allows a better and more bloodless exposure of the surgical field as well as favoring the use of this approach in Adult Congenital Heart Disease (ACHD) patients with atrial septal defects (ASD) associated or not with partial anomalous pulmonary venous return (PAPVR). In these cases, very high superior cava snaring is required, after identification and isolation of the abnormal venous returns, above them. Therefore, the intervention will include first the packing of the atrial baffle to redirect the venous return in the left atrium, taking care not to include in it either the coronary sinus or the outlet of the superior or inferior vena cava. The same applies to ASDs in case of direct or patch closure. A simple trick to check that you have not included the inferior vena cava in the suture is to loosen the inferior snaring and advance the vein pushing it from the femoral vein; you will see it emerge in the surgical field; likewise, introducing a field aspirator in the coronary sinus helps to keep it well identified throughout the procedure. We will then proceed with the annuloplasty or tricuspid replacement.

12 End of Procedure

The right atriotomy is closed using a double suture of polypropylene 5/0. Upon completion of the first suture, the inferior cava snare is loosened, the atrium is filled, and de-airing is performed. The cross-clamp is removed, and the second run of overlap suture is completed. The operation is then carried out in standard fashion until complete weaning from CPB. Protamine is then administered, and hemostasis is done. The pericardium is then closed using the three polypropylene stitches positioned at the beginning of the procedure over a 24 Fr chest tube. The chest is closed by anatomical layers.

13 Conclusions and Future Development

As illustrated in the preceding paragraphs, the endoscopic framework allows tricuspid surgery to be performed safely and reproducibly. Furthermore, this approach to surgery is well transferable to trainee surgeons. Finally, this approach is well suited to difficult situations such as reinterventions and ACHD patients.

In the future, we propose that this type of approach will become of choice in surgery not only of the tricuspid valve but also of left heart valves, especially with an axillary approach.

Further refinements to this surgery will be the implementation of artificial intelligence and deep learning for planning and augmented reality for teaching and performing surgery. These should be followed by a further engineering revolution for the miniaturization of devices that can make surgery micro-invasive without sacrificing the completeness, efficacy, and reproducibility of the surgical gesture (See Video 1).

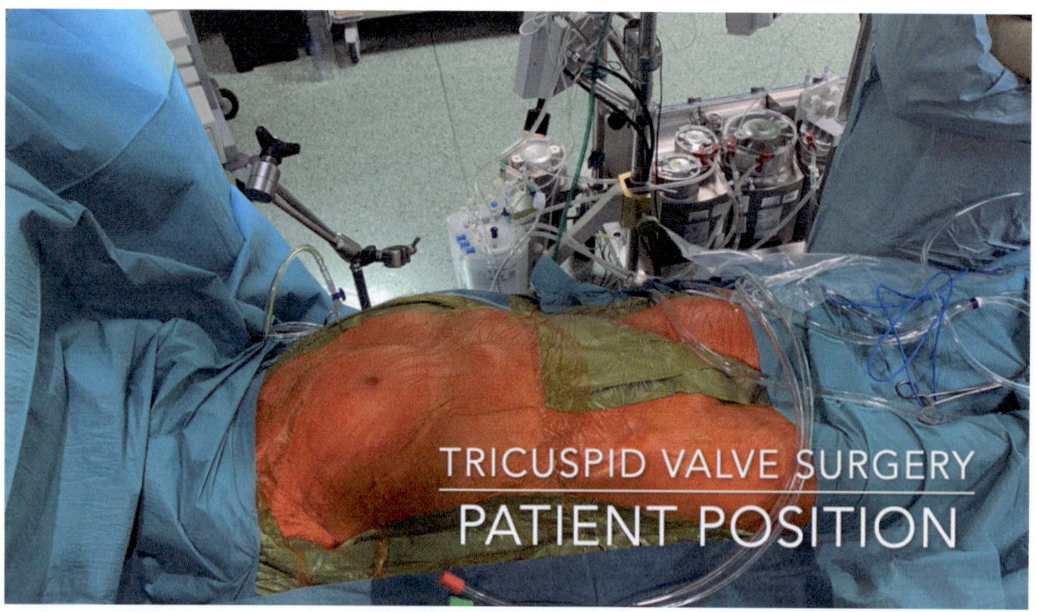

Video 1 Operative setup for tricuspid surgery, from patient positioning to exposure maneuvers and performing surgery (▶ https://doi.org/10.1007/000-a7s)

References

1. Gulielmos V, Dangel M, Solowjowa N, Wagner FM, Karbalai P, Schmidt V, et al. Clinical experiences with minimally invasive mitral valve surgery using a simplified Port Access technique. Eur J Cardio-Thorac Surg Off J Eur Assoc Cardio-Thorac Surg. agosto 1998;14(2):141–7.
2. Mohr FW, Falk V, Diegeler A, Walther T, van Son JA, Autschbach R. Minimally invasive port-access mitral valve surgery. J Thorac Cardiovasc Surg. marzo 1998;115(3):567–74; discussion 574–576.
3. Daemen JHT, Heuts S, Olsthoorn JR, Maessen JG, Sardari Nia P. Right minithoracotomy versus median sternotomy for reoperative mitral valve surgery: a systematic review and meta-analysis of observational studies. Eur J Cardio-Thorac Surg Off J Eur Assoc Cardio-Thorac Surg. 1 novembre 2018;54(5):817–25.
4. Ding C, Jiang D, Tao K, Duan Q, Li J, Kong M, et al. Anterolateral minithoracotomy versus median sternotomy for mitral valve disease: a meta-analysis. J Zhejiang Univ Sci B. 2014;15(6):522–32.
5. Kastengren M, Svenarud P, Ahlsson A, Dalén M. Minimally invasive mitral valve surgery is associated with a low rate of complications. J Intern Med. 2019;286(6):614–26.
6. Santana O, Larrauri-Reyes M, Zamora C, Mihos CG. Is a minimally invasive approach for mitral valve surgery more cost-effective than median sternotomy? Interact Cardiovasc Thorac Surg. 2016;22(1):97–100.
7. Botta L, Cannata A, Bruschi G, Fratto P, Taglieri C, Russo CF, et al. Minimally invasive approach for redo mitral valve surgery. J Thorac Dis. 2013;5 (Suppl 6):S686-693.
8. Färber G, Tkebuchava S, Dawson RS, Kirov H, Diab M, Schlattmann P, et al. Minimally Invasive, Isolated Tricuspid Valve Redo Surgery: A Safety and Outcome Analysis. Thorac Cardiovasc Surg. 2018;66 (7):564–71.
9. Lu S, Song K, Yao W, Xia L, Dong L, Sun Y, et al. Simplified, minimally invasive, beating-heart technique for redo isolated tricuspid valve surgery. J Cardiothorac Surg. 18 giugno 2020;15(1):146.
10. Murzi M, Miceli A, Di Stefano G, Cerillo AG, Farneti P, Solinas M, et al. Minimally invasive right thoracotomy approach for mitral valve surgery in patients with previous sternotomy: a single institution experience with 173 patients. J Thorac Cardiovasc Surg. 2014;148(6):2763–8.
11. Vallabhajosyula P, Wallen T, Pulsipher A, Pitkin E, Solometo LP, Musthaq S, et al. Minimally Invasive Port Access Approach for Reoperations on the Mitral Valve. Ann Thorac Surg. 2015;100(1):68–73.
12. Glauber M, Murzi M, Solinas M. Central aortic cannulation for minimally invasive mitral valve surgery through right minithoracotomy. Ann Cardio-thorac Surg. 2013;2(6):839–40.
13. Glauber M, Miceli A, Canarutto D, Lio A, Murzi M, Gilmanov D, et al. Early and long-term outcomes of minimally invasive mitral valve surgery through right minithoracotomy: a 10-year experience in 1604 patients. J Cardiothorac Surg. 7 dicembre 2015;10:181.
14. Russo M, Di Mauro M, Saitto G, Lio A, Berretta P, Taramasso M, et al. Beating vs arrested heart isolated tricuspid valve surgery: long-term outcomes. Ann Thorac Surg. 5 aprile 2021.
15. Rival PM, Moore THM, McAleenan A, Hamilton H, Du Toit Z, Akowuah E, et al. Transthoracic clamp versus endoaortic balloon occlusion in minimally invasive mitral valve surgery: a systematic review and meta-analysis. Eur J Cardio-Thorac Surg Off J Eur Assoc Cardio-Thorac Surg. 1 ottobre 2019;56 (4):643–53.
16. Raja SG, Dreyfus GD. Surgery for functional tricuspid regurgitation: current techniques, outcomes and emerging concepts. Expert Rev Cardiovasc Ther gennaio. 2009;7(1):73–84.

Minimally Invasive Endoscopic Maze Procedure for Atrial Fibrillation Through Right Mini-thoracotomy

Manuel Castella and Jesús Ruíz

Abstract

The burden of atrial fibrillation is large in society. There are many ways to deal with this condition which range from percutaneous to sternotomy to bilateral thoracoscopic to an on pump endoscopic approach. This chapter describes the procedure undertaken on bypass through a right mini thoracotomy with excellent results. The authors are well recognised for their commitment to collecting results and training in this approach. This approach is particularly useful in patients who have already had multiple percutaneous attempts or those patients with pre existing clots in the left atrium.

Keywords

Endoscopic atrial fibrillation ablation · Left atrial appendage clipping · Right minithoracotomy approach to atrial fibrillation

Supplementary Information The online version contains supplementary material available at https://doi.org/10.1007/978-3-031-21104-1_11. The videos can be accessed individually by clicking the DOI link in the accompanying figure caption or by scanning this link with the SN More Media App.

M. Castella (✉) · J. Ruíz
Department of Cardiovascular Surgery, Hospital Clínic, University of Barcelona, Barcelona, Spain
e-mail: mcaste@clinic.cat

Currently there are many different methodologies to surgically treat atrial fibrillation (AF) in a minimally invasive fashion. Among them, epicardial atrial ablation has been described through totally thoracoscopic right, left, right and left or subxiphoid approaches. These techniques have really made AF surgery minimally invasive in the beating heart with no need of extracorporeal circulation and have shown great results in large series. The limitation of all these approaches is that ablation is epicardial, that is, applying the energy to ablate from outside-in. We know that some important lines to complete the Cox-Maze pattern, as the mitral and the tricuspid lines, cannot be performed unless the energy is applied from the endocardium (Fig. 1). In most cases, these two lines are not so important in patients with paroxysmal or persistent AF and therefore, these approaches are perfectly adequate. Even in long-standing persistent patients, the thoracoscopic approaches have shown better results than percutaneous ablation. In fact, the so-called hybrid ablation is to combine thoracoscopic and percutaneous ablation to get the best results possible with minimal invasiveness and it is probably one of the most effective ways to address symptomatic patients with persistent or long-standing persistent AF [1]. In this chapter we will address a slightly more aggressive way to approach AF surgically, with the objective to perform a full Cox-Maze pattern, that can be

J. Zacharias (ed.), *Endoscopic Cardiac Surgery*,
https://doi.org/10.1007/978-3-031-21104-1_11

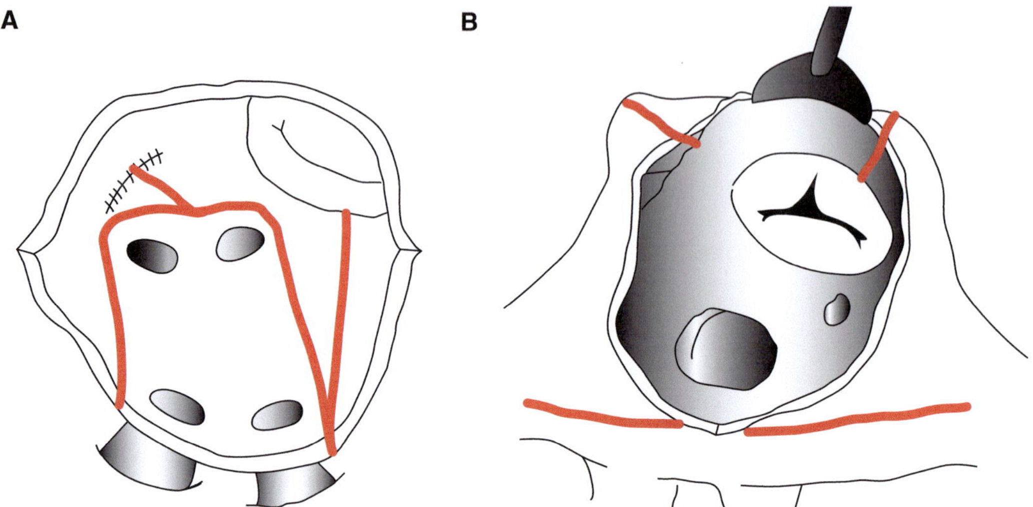

Fig. 1 **A** Lesion pattern in the left atrium, including the Box lesion and lesions towards the mitral annulus and the left appendage. **B** Lesion pattern in the right atrium including lines to the tricuspid annulus, right appendage and both venae cavae

used both for isolated persistent or long-standing persistent AF as well as for patients with mitral and/or tricuspid disease with concomitant AF.

1 Technique

1.1 General Considerations

Our technique for AF ablation is based in cryo-thermy lines performed endocardially through an 8 cm right mini-thoracotomy with the help of extracorporeal circulation by femoral cannulation.

The patient is placed in a supine position, with a small bean bag underneath his/her right chest, so the body is slightly tilted to the left. Both arms are joined to the body, being the right arm slightly lower to the chest, allowing full exposure of the right side of the thorax. Surgical draping allows access to the right thoracic wall as well as sternotomy.

It is our suggestion not to use selective bronchial cannulation with a specific orotracheal tube and to use a normal oro-tracheal tube with right bronchial blocker when needed. We strongly recommend full ventilation of both lungs as much as possible, but mostly important coming off bypass, to prevent right lung oedema.

1.2 Cannulation

Cannulation is performed by a 2–3 cm incision over following the right inguinal ligament. Femoral artery and vein are dissected only in the anterior side where cannulae are inserted by Seldinger technique through a previous 5/0 polypropylene purse string sutures. The most used arterial cannulae sizes are 17 and the 19Fr. For venous cannulation we always use the 25Fr Medtronic multiperforated cannula that it is advanced to the entrance of the superior vena cavae under echocardiographic supervision. If the right atrium is to be opened to perform the right-side lesions of the Cox-Maze, this cannula is advanced up to the diaphragm and another 19Fr venous cannula is placed in the superior vena cava by percutaneous jugular puncture.

1.3 Access to the Chest

While cannulation is performed by the first and second assistant, the surgeon places a trocar port on the third intercostal space on the anterior axillary line. If a 2D 30° camera technology is going to be used, the trocar can be a 5 mm and be the camera access to the chest. If a 3D view system is going to be used, this trocar will be a working port for needle-holders or pick-ups. In either case, this port is the first one to place in order to insufflate CO2 in the thoracic cavity and help to collapse the right lung. The next step is to perform a small (5 to 8 cm) right lateral thoracotomy through the fourth intercostal space over the anterior axillary line and places a soft tissue retractor. If a 3D camera is used, this will be a working port as well as the camera port.

After heparinization and full extracorporeal circulation is achieved, the pericardium is opened with cautery 2 cm anteriorly to the phrenic nerve, from the ascending aorta to the diaphragm. Two to three retractor stitches are placed from the inferior side of the pericardium and pulled through the chest wall with the help of Endo-close™ (Covidien™).

1.4 Myocardial Preservation

A small purse string suture is placed on the right side of the ascending aorta in order to fix the cardioplegia line. We have changed from a 4/0 polypropylene to a 2/0 tycron suture leaned on pledgets because at the end of the procedure it can be closed with a Cor-knot®(ISI Solutions®). This line will also be used for suction and venting before coming off extracorporeal circulation. It is not so important that this is not in the anterior side of the ascending aorta because the thoracic cavity is so filled with CO_2 that the chances of air embolism in the right coronary or carotids are slim. Once the cardioplegic line is in place and coming off the chest through the working port, the ascending aorta is cross-clamped with a Chitwood clamp. This clamp is placed through a new thoracic access, by a 5 mm incision on the anterior or mid axillary line at the second or third intercostal space. In order to find the best spot, an imaginary line need to be drawn from the proper place of the aorta to the chest. Cardioplegia is given as a routine case by the hospital protocol (Video 1).

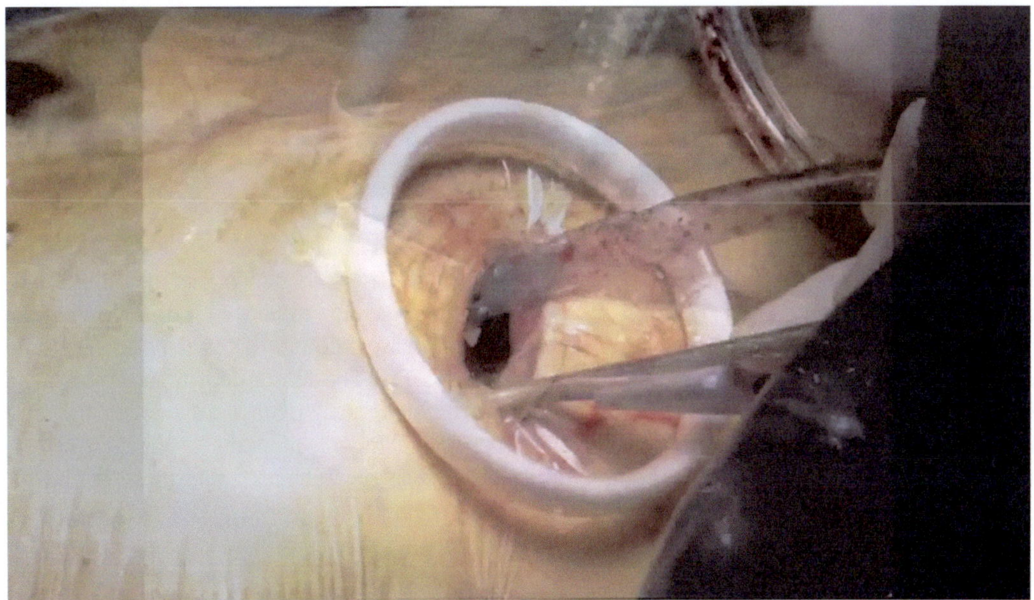

Video 1 Thoracic working port through the fourth intercostal space (▶ https://doi.org/10.1007/000-a7z)

1.5 Access to the Left Atrium and Left-Sided Lesions

As soon as cardioplegia is administered, the left atrium is open through the interatrial groove. An atrial retractor is placed through a new 2 mm incision on the fourth intercostal space one cm lateral to the right mammary artery. In order to visualize the coronary sinus, it is important to dissect in between the left inferior pulmonary vein and the inferior vena cava to reach the oblique sinus. A vent is placed in the left pulmonary veins through a new 1 cm port on the sixth intercostal space over the anterior axillary line. This port will be used aftermath to place the pleural drainage.

The ablation line set follows the pattern described by Jim Cox [2]. Basically, it follows three principles. First, to isolate the pulmonary veins and the posterior wall of the left atrium in what is called "the box line". Second, to perform a line that reaches all the different round structures of the atria to prevent macro re-entrant circuits around them. These are lines to the mitral annulus and to the left appendage, and in the right side to the tricuspid annulus, right appendage and both venae cavae. Third, AF surgery lowers the possibility of cardiogenic thromboembolism by closing the left appendage. On the left side all ablation lines need to be performed from the endocardial side, where the atrial muscle is, except of the mitral line. The target of this line is not only the atrial tissue but also the muscular fibers within the venous wall of the coronary sinus behind. Since it is most possible that cryothermy applied on the endocardial side may not freeze the coronary sinus, it is suggested to perform this line also from the epicardial side.

Ablations lines will be of 3 min of duration to ensure transmurality. To avoid gaps in the lines, it is fundamental to press the tissue with the cryothermy probe in order to span the tissue and avoid folds. It important to notice that while the probe defrost fast, the tissue will take some minutes to defrost. Therefore, it is best alternate the ablation lines from inferior to superior to allow defreezing of previous lines. Once the heart is arrested and the left atrium opened, we suggest to start ablating the mitral line on the epicardial side, paying attention to reach the coronary sinus. Since we will have to repeat this line from the endocardial side, we stain this line with metycilin blue to make sure both epi and endocardial lines are superposed (Video 2). To allow de-freezing of this first line, the second line is the superior part of the box lesion. This line runs from the superior corner of the atrial incision to the midpart of the ridge between the left pulmonary veins and the left appendage (Video 3). This line is followed by the inferior part of the box lesion, which goes from the inferior corner of the left atrial incision to the same ridge, overlapping with the previous lesion and therefore encircling all pulmonary veins and the posterior wall of the left atrium (Video 4). Next is a short line from the box lesion to the left atrial appendage (Video 5). Last line in the left side is to repeat the mitral line from the left corner of the atrial incision towards the posterior annulus of the mitral valve, making sure we reach the valve, and on top of the previously stained line (Video 6). The left appendage can be closed by a double running polypropylene suture or by placing a clip through the transverse sinus. If this is the case, we suggest the use of the Pro-2 Atriclip (Atricure inc, USA). To facilitate placing the clip, the aorta must remain cross-clamped and a 5/0 polypropylene suture can be placed in the tip of the appendage to facilitate traction towards the clip. The left atrium is closed with a 4/0 polypropylene suture starting at both ends.

1.6 Right-Sided Lesions

Right sided lesions add higher possibilities for maintaining sinus rhythm in long follow-up, but also increases the rate for pacemaker need after ablation [3]. The reasons for this are unknown, but probably deal more by damaging the sinus node than for affecting the conduction system, since none of the lines come close to the AV node of the Purkinge system. Indeed, cryothermy produce wide lines of frosted tissue that can get close not only at the superior vena cava-right atrium ridge where the sinus node is described but other zones of the free wall of the right

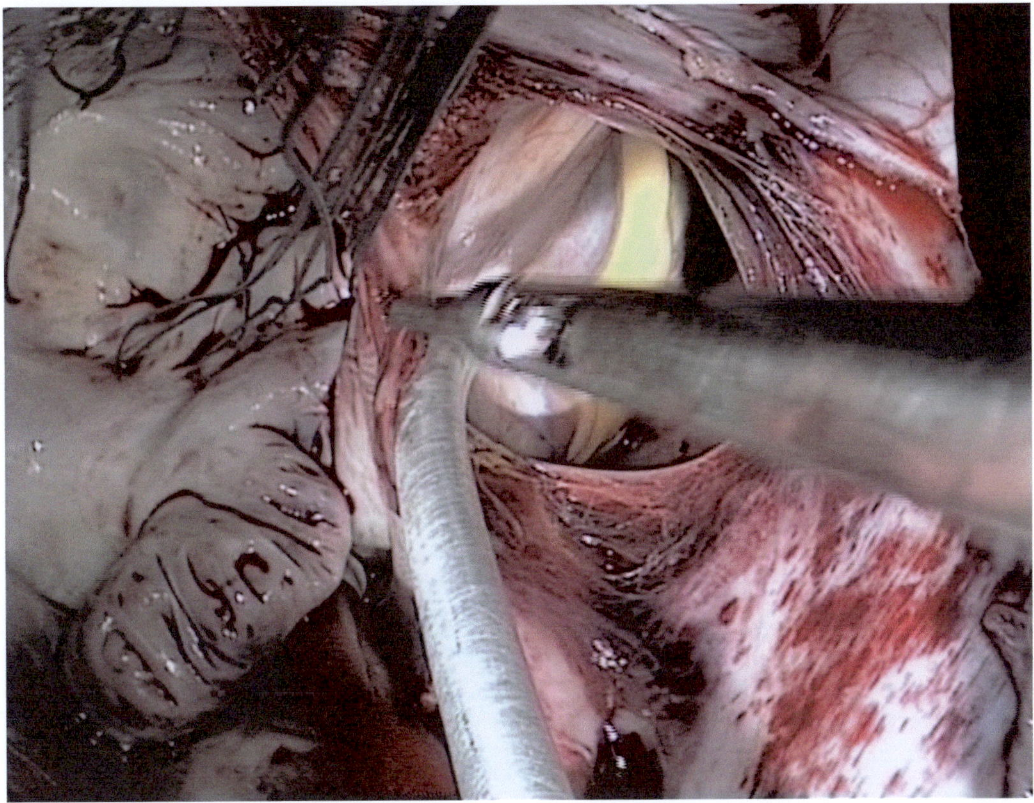

Video 2 Coronary sinus line which needs to be overlapped with the mitral line from the endocardium (Video 6) (▶ https://doi.org/10.1007/000-a7v)

atrium which may be responsible to rapid pacing during exercise [4].

To perform the right atrial lesions the right atrium must be opened. A venous line must be previously placed in the right jugular vein and the femoral cannula must be at the level of the diaphragm. The superior vena cava can be closed with a metal bulldog while it is better to encircle the inferior vena cava with a wide vessel loop. We suggest to open the right atrium with a small (5 cm) incision from the *Cresta Terminallis* towards the tricuspid annulus.

Despite all the lines except the one to the tricuspid annulus can be performed on the epicardial side, doing them from the endocardium makes it easier. The first line is to the tricuspid annulus from the upper corner of the atrial incision (Videos 7 and 8) making sure the probe reaches the anterior leaflet. So far, there is no evidence of coronary lesions by cryothermy [5]. The second line is towards the right appendage from the upper corner of the incision (Video 9). Attention must be taken to do it from the upper part of the incision to avoid freezing in the midpart of the free wall of the right atrium, that might be responsible for tachy-cardization during exercise. The third line is from the posterior corner of the atrial incision to the posterior wall of the superior vena cava, parallel to the *Cresta Terminallis*. Be careful that 3 min of freezing will span the lesion very close to the sinus node zone. Finally, a line is performed from the posterior corner of the atrial incision towards the inferior vena cava (Video 10). The right atrium is closed in the usual manner.

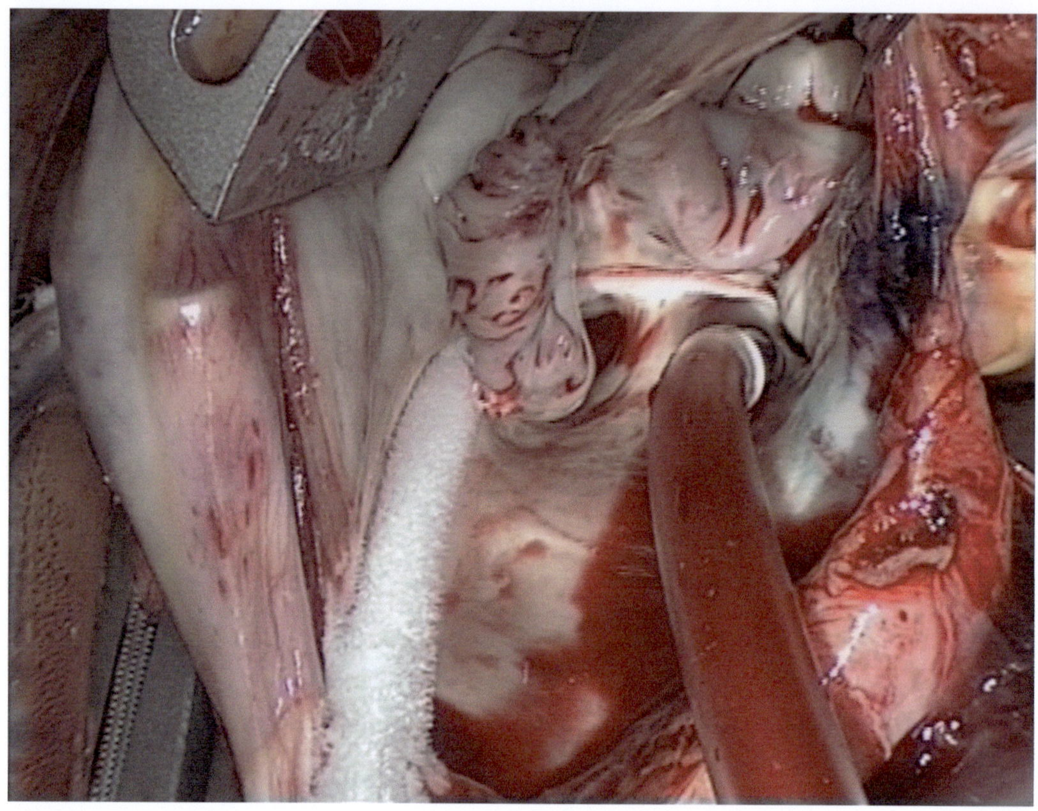

Video 3 Box lesion at the superior side. Together with the inferior line (video 4) there is complete isolation of the pulmonary veins and the posterior wall of the left atrium (▶ https://doi.org/10.1007/000-a7w)

2 Results

Surgical ablation for atrial fibrillation has demonstrated to be the most effective therapy to maintain sinus rhythm in the long term [6]. Furthermore, a recent randomized trial showed a decreased risk in stroke at 5 years follow-up [7]. and some non-randomized personal series have described benefits in mortality at 10 years [8]. In 2015 a meta-analysis by the Cochrane Foundation showed significant benefits in sinus rhythm maintenance while no difference of adding a concomitant AF ablation in regards to mortality, neurologic or thromboembolic events, cardiovascular events [9]. The most important complication described in most meta-analyses is the increased need for pacemaker after a Cox-Maze ablation [9]. A recent meta-analysis showed that the higher incidence of pacemaker happens when the right lesions are performed, but that no significant pacemaker incidence is described by left lesions only [3]. In our opinion, since none of the left or right lesions come close to the AV node or the Purkinge system, the higher incidence of pacemaker may be due to damage of the sinus node or its surrounding areas, responsible for tachycardization.

Results of a Cox-Maze with cryothermy through mini-thoracotomy as described in this chapter have been published in non-randomized series, showing a 73% of patients with maintained sinus rhythm at 5 years without the need of antiarrhythmic drugs or further ablations, 79% off antiarrhythmic drugs, or 90% allowing medication or a subsequent catheter ablation [10]. Results from mini-sternotomy have shown to be as through sternotomy [11] There are important

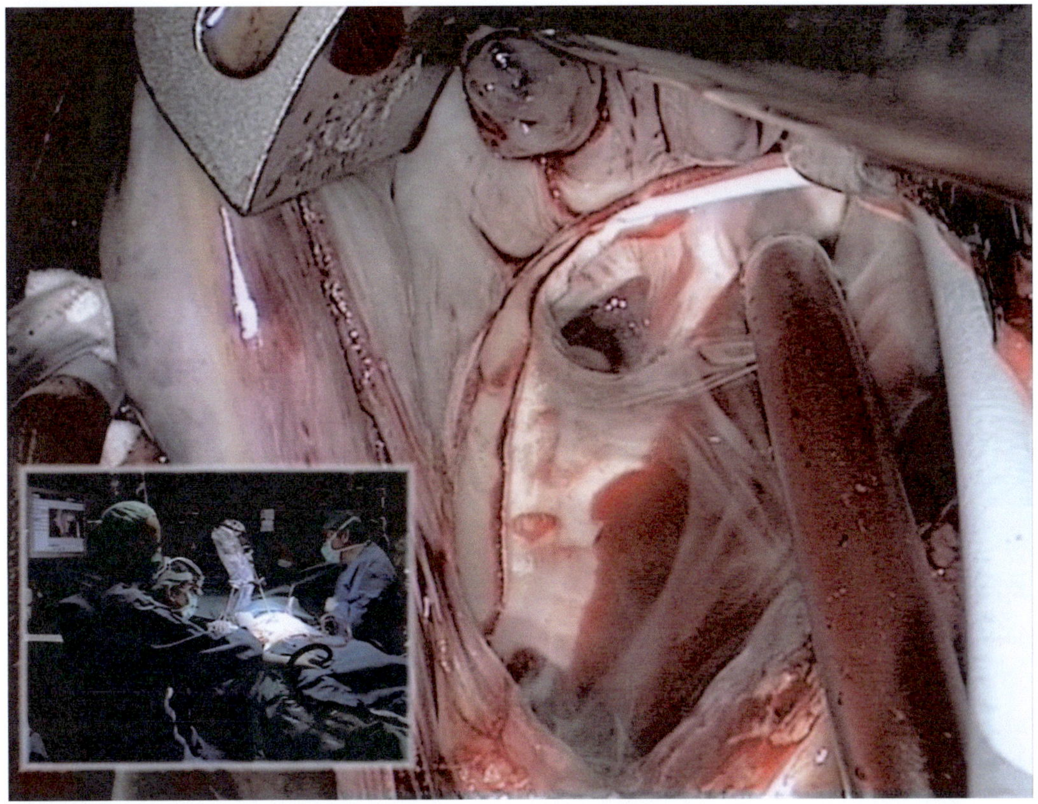

Video 4 Inferior line of the Box lesion (▶ https://doi.org/10.1007/000-a7x)

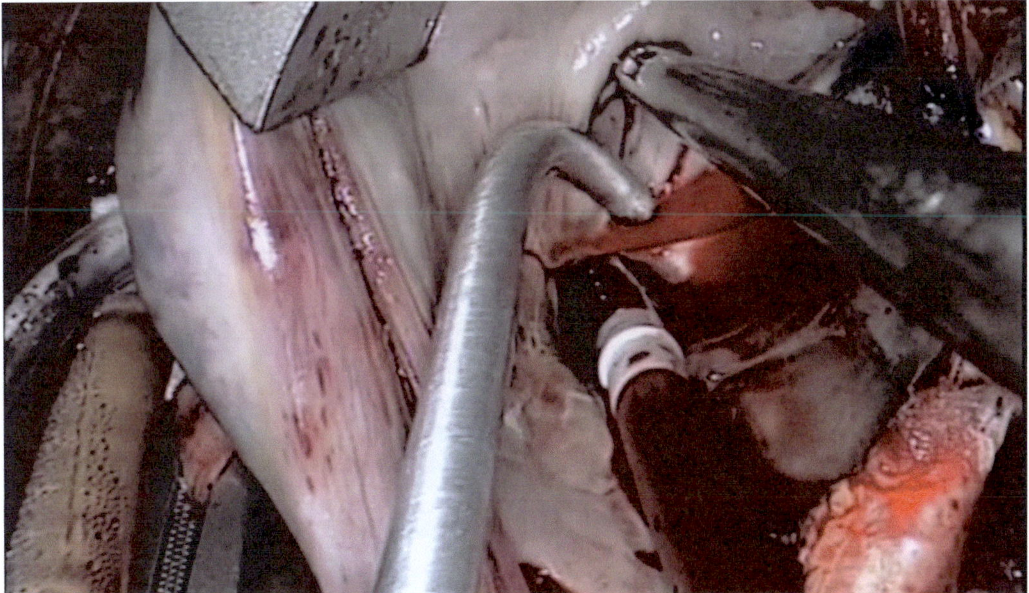

Video 5 Line from the box lesion to the entrance of the left atrial appendage (▶ https://doi.org/10.1007/000-a7y)

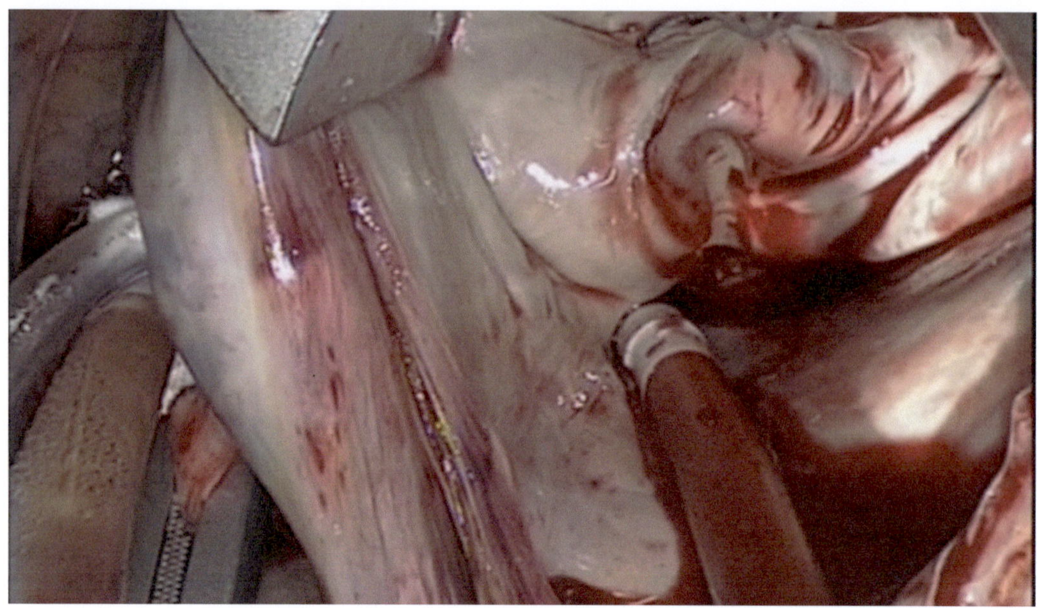

Video 6 Line to the mitral annulus on top of the coronary sinus line (Video 2) (▶ https://doi.org/10.1007/000-a7t)

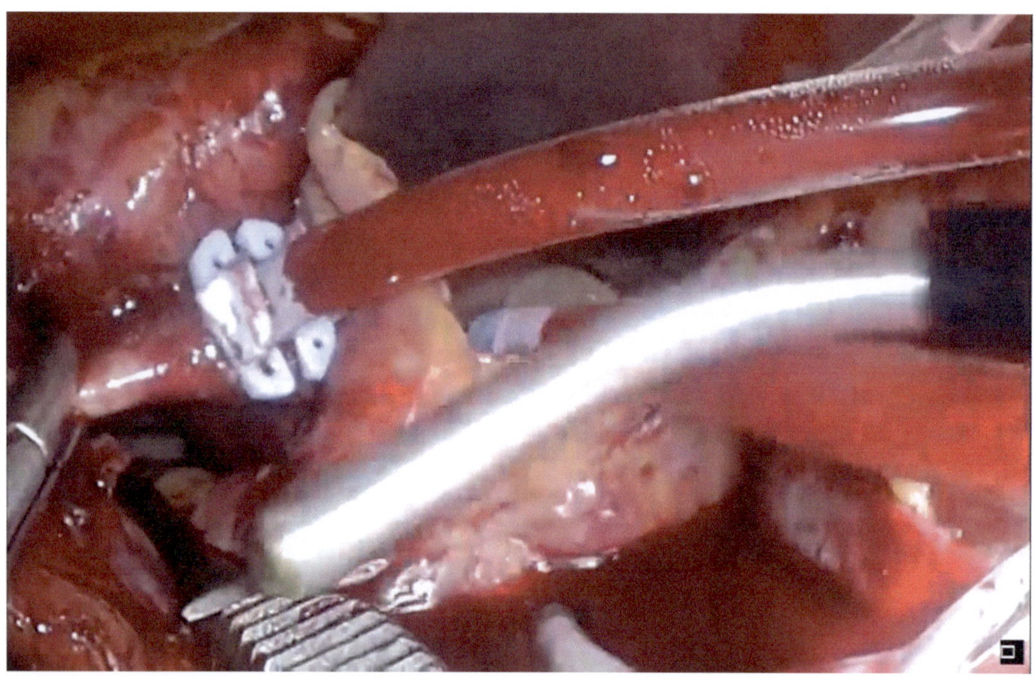

Video 7 Line to the tricuspid annulus (▶ https://doi.org/10.1007/000-a80)

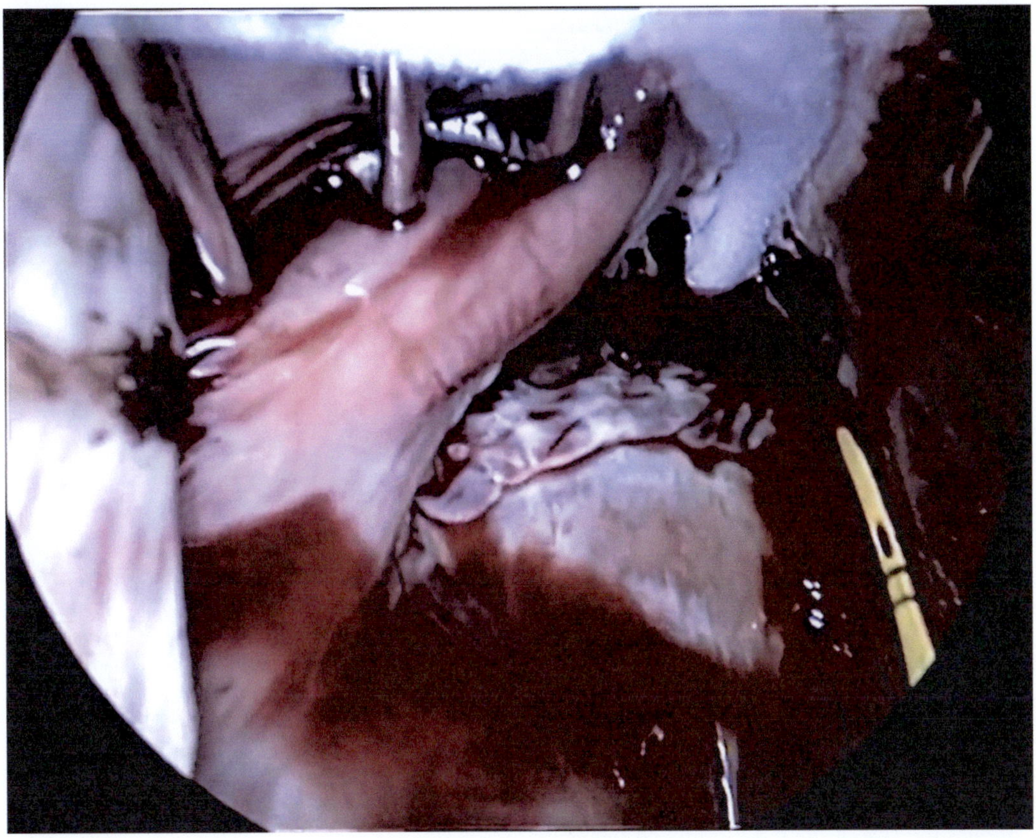

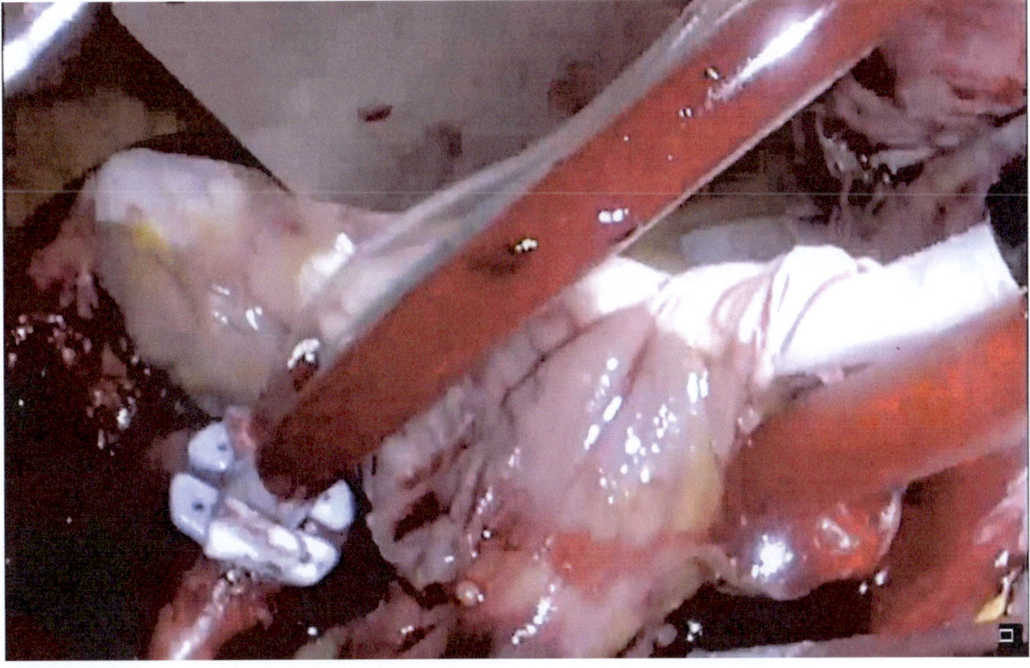

Video 8 Line to the right appendage (▶ https://doi.org/10.1007/000-a81)

Video 9 Line to the superior venae cavae (▶ https://doi.org/10.1007/000-a82)

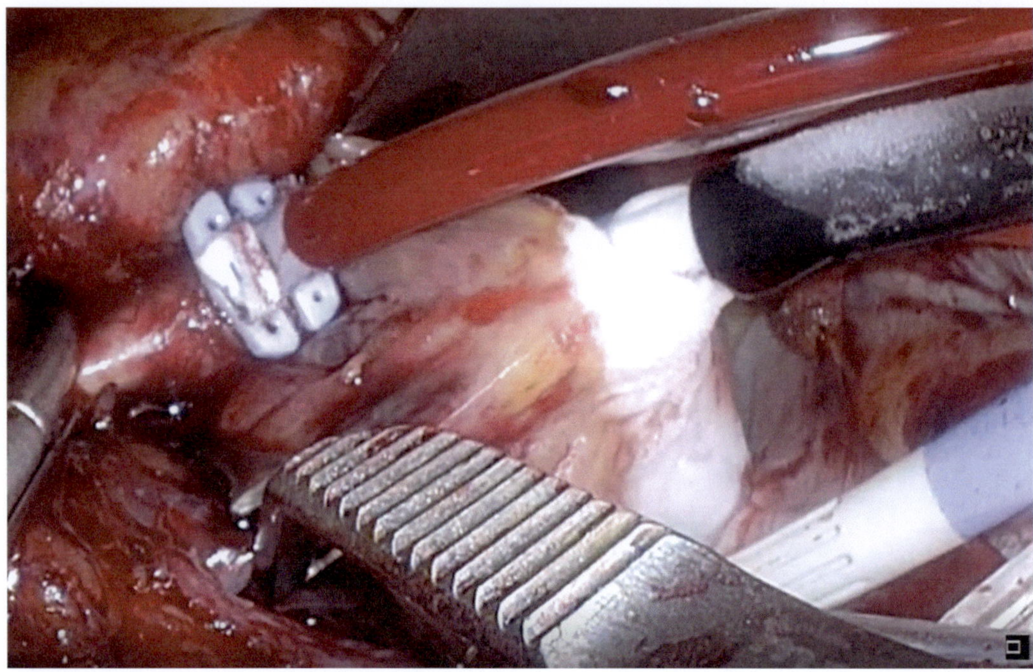

Video 10 Line to the inferior venae cavae (▶ https://doi.org/10.1007/000-a83)

factors that limit results, being the most important ones the size of the left atrium and the years in atrial fibrillation [12].

3 Conclusion

In summary, atrial fibrillation surgery is a reasonably effective therapy and can be indicated both in symptomatic patients with isolated AF which are refractory to antiarrhythmic medication or percutaneous ablation and patients with AF concomitant to other surgical disease. The technique described is one of the most effective due to the possibility of performing a full Cox-Maze lesion set while being minimally invasive.

References

1. de Asmundis C, Varnavas V, Sieira J, Ströker E, Coutiño HE, Terasawa M, Abugattas JP, Salghetti F, Maj R, Guimarães OT, Iacopino S, Umbrain V, Poelaert J, Brugada P, Gelsomino S, Chierchia GB, La Meir M. Two-year follow-up of one-stage left unilateral thoracoscopic epicardial and transcatheter endocardial ablation for persistent and long-standing persistent atrial fibrillation. J Interv Card Electrophysiol. 2020;58(3):333–343. https://doi.org/10.1007/s10840-019-00616-w. Epub 2019 Sep 13. Erratum in: J Interv Card Electrophysiol. 2020 Jan 17;: PMID: 31520292.
2. Cox JL, Schuessler RB, D'Agostino HJ Jr, Stone CM, Chang BC, Cain ME, Corr PB, Boineau JP. The surgical treatment of atrial fibrillation III development of a definitive surgical procedure. J Thorac Cardiovasc Surg. 1991;101(4):569–83. PMID: 2008095.

3. McClure GR, Belley-Cote EP, Jaffer IH, Dvirnik N, An KR, Fortin G, Spence J, Healey J, Singal RK, Whitlock RP. Surgical ablation of atrial fibrillation: a systematic review and meta-analysis of randomized controlled trials. Europace. 2018;20(9):1442–50. https://doi.org/10.1093/europace/eux336. PMID: 29186407.

4. Kawashima T, Sato F. First in situ 3D visualization of the human cardiac conduction system and its transformation associated with heart contour and inclination. Sci Rep. 2021;11(1):8636. https://doi.org/10.1038/s41598-021-88109-7.PMID:33883659; PMCID:PMC8060315.

5. Cheema FH, Pervez MB, Mehmood M, Younus MJ, Munir MB, Bisleri G, Barili F, Ayala IL, Ad N, Cox JL, Roberts HG Jr. Does cryomaze injure the circumflex artery?: a preliminary search for occult postprocedure stenoses. Innovations (Phila). 2013;8 (1):56–66. https://doi.org/10.1097/IMI. 0b013e31828e5267. PMID: 23571795.

6. Khiabani AJ, MacGregor RM, Bakir NH, Manghelli JL, Sinn LA, Maniar HS, Moon MR, Schuessler RB, Melby SJ, Damiano RJ Jr. The long-term outcomes and durability of the Cox-Maze IV procedure for atrial fibrillation. J Thorac Cardiovasc Surg. 2020:S0022–5223(20)31065–5. https://doi.org/10.1016/j.jtcvs.2020.04.100. Epub ahead of print. PMID: 32563577.

7. Osmancik P, Budera P, Talavera D, Hlavicka J, Herman D, Holy J, Cervinka P, Smid J, Hanak P, Hatala R, Widimsky P. Five-year outcomes in cardiac surgery patients with atrial fibrillation undergoing concomitant surgical ablation versus no ablation: the long-term follow-up of the PRAGUE-12 Study. Heart Rhythm. 2019;16(9):1334–1340. https://doi.org/10.1016/j.hrthm.2019.05.001. Epub 2019 May 10. PMID: 31082538.

8. Musharbash FN, Schill MR, Sinn LA, Schuessler RB, Maniar HS, Moon MR, Melby SJ, Damiano RJ Jr. Performance of the Cox-maze IV procedure is associated with improved long-term survival in patients with atrial fibrillation undergoing cardiac surgery. J Thorac Cardiovasc Surg. 2018;155 (1):159–170. https://doi.org/10.1016/j.jtcvs.2017.09. 095. Epub 2017 Sep 27. PMID: 29056264; PMCID: PMC5732870.

9. Huffman MD, Karmali KN, Berendsen MA, Andrei AC, Kruse J, McCarthy PM, Malaisrie SC. Concomitant atrial fibrillation surgery for people undergoing cardiac surgery. Cochrane Database Syst Rev. 2016;2016(8):CD011814. https://doi.org/10. 1002/14651858.CD011814.pub2. PMID: 27551927; PMCID: PMC5046840.

10. Ad N, Holmes SD, Friehling T. Minimally invasive stand-alone cox maze procedure for persistent and long-standing persistent atrial fibrillation: perioperative safety and 5-year outcomes. Circ Arrhythm Electrophysiol. 2017;10(11): e005352. https://doi.org/10.1161/CIRCEP.117.005352. PMID: 29138143.

11. Schill MR, Sinn LA, Greenberg JW, Henn MC, Lancaster TS, Schuessler RB, Maniar HS, Damiano RJ Jr. A minimally invasive stand-alone cox-maze procedure is as effective as median sternotomy approach. Innovations (Phila). 2017;12(3):186–191. https://doi.org/10.1097/IMI.0000000000000374. PMID: 28549027; PMCID: PMC5546149.

12. Ad N, Holmes SD. Prediction of sinus rhythm in patients undergoing concomitant Cox maze procedure through a median sternotomy. J Thorac Cardiovasc Surg. 2014;148(3):881–6; discussion 886–7. https://doi.org/10.1016/j.jtcvs.2014.04.050. Epub 2014 May 16. PMID: 25043863.

Totally 3D-Endoscopic Aortic Valve Replacement

Soh Hosoba and Toshiaki Ito

Abstract

Minimally invasive cardiac surgery (MICS) has evolved over the last 25 years. In aortic valve disease, MICS has been used commonly to treat both aortic stenosis and regurgitation, although the common approach relies on direct visualization via thoracotomy, often with rib spreading. In mitral valve surgery, totally endoscopic surgery with or without robotic assists has been evolving for over twenty years. Without rib spreading or longer incision, this endoscopic approach has emerged as an attractive procedure and is widely performed. We describe our approach to performing totally endoscopic aortic valve replacement, which we have refined over the years with cumulative experience of 131 cases.

Supplementary Information The online version contains supplementary material available at https://doi.org/10.1007/978-3-031-21104-1_12. The videos can be accessed individually by clicking the DOI link in the accompanying figure caption or by scanning this link with the SN More Media App.

S. Hosoba (✉) · T. Ito
Department of Cardiovascular Surgery, Japanese Red Cross Nagoya First Hospital, Nagoya, Japan
e-mail: soh.hosoba@gmail.com

Keywords

Minimally invasive cardiac surgery · Endoscopy · Aortic valve replacement · Three-dimensional endoscope · Totally endoscopic

1 Introduction

The first minimally invasive aortic valve surgery was reported through a mini sternotomy or right anterior thoracotomy in the early 1990s [1–3]. Since then, the mini-sternotomy approach gained popularity. It has been the mainstay of minimally invasive aortic valve replacement (AVR) at many centers over the world. On the other hand, AVR through right anterior thoracotomy (RAT) has also been reported [4–6]. The RAT approach usually does not require an endoscopic vison, but when it is used, it is only to assist with visualization. Twenty percent has been performed in thoracotomy approach in the recent Society of Thoracic Surgeons (STS) Adult Cardiac Surgery database report, [7].

In modern area, rapid deployment valves (RDV) have also played an important role in AVR, and the results have been favorable [8, 9]. RDV may accelerate the current momentum of mini-thoracotomy AVR.

Carpentier et at reported their first experience in endoscope-assisted surgery for valves [10]. Totally endoscopic cardiac surgery for mitral valve was also reported [11, 12]. A totally endoscopic platform has been reported in many countries with or without robotic assistance, since then [13–15].

However, the reported experience has represented only a small fraction of the actual totally endoscopic aortic valve treatment to date [16–18].

Our experience in MICS AVR started in 2011 with the right anterior thoracotomy (RAT) approach and we have modified it to trans-axillary minimally invasive AVR [19]. We switched our platform to a total endoscopic platform for AVR in 2015 after we gained expertise in 3D-endoscope for the mitral procedure [20]. We reported our initial experience for totally endoscopic AVR [21]. We subsequently broadened our application to double valve procedure [22]. We, herein, describe our approaches and results for totally endoscopic AVR in more than 130 patients.

2 Operative Technique

2.1 The Set Up: Patient Positioning, 3D Endoscope, and Monitor

We initiate the operation under general anesthesia. For single-lung ventilation, a double-lumen endotracheal tube or a bronchial blocker is used. The patient is placed in a 30-degree left lateral decubitus position with the right arm fixed over the head (Fig. 1). We place a large pillow beneath the axilla to vent over the right lateral chest. All

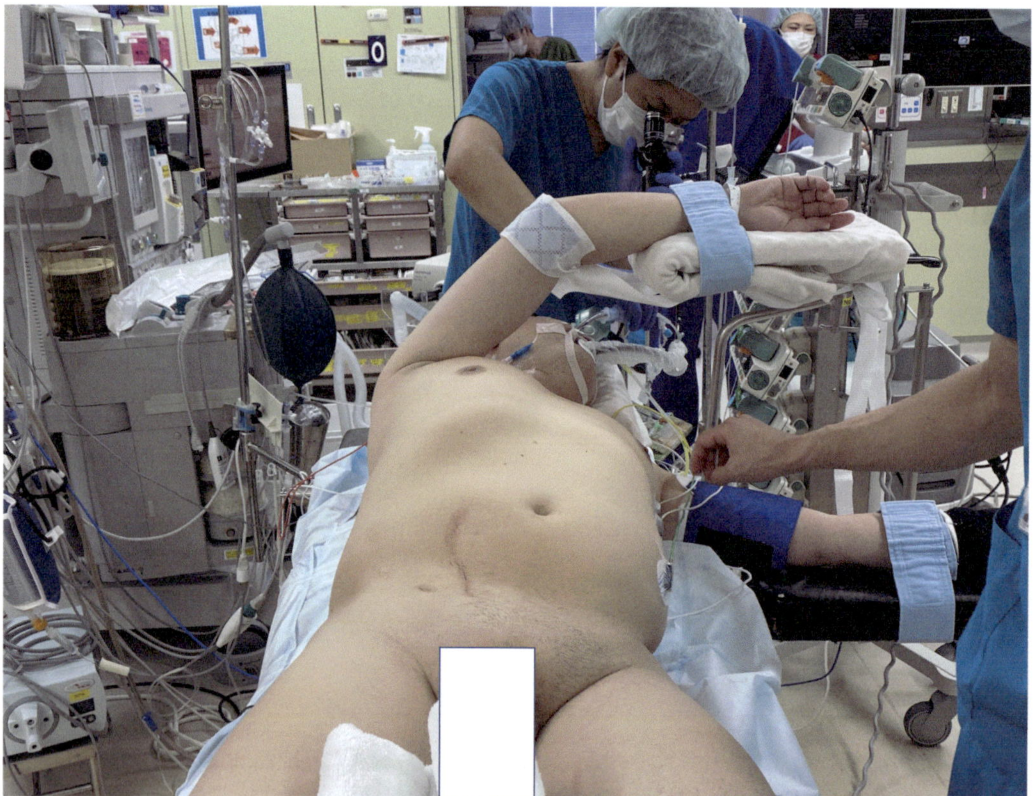

Fig. 1 The figure shows position of the patient

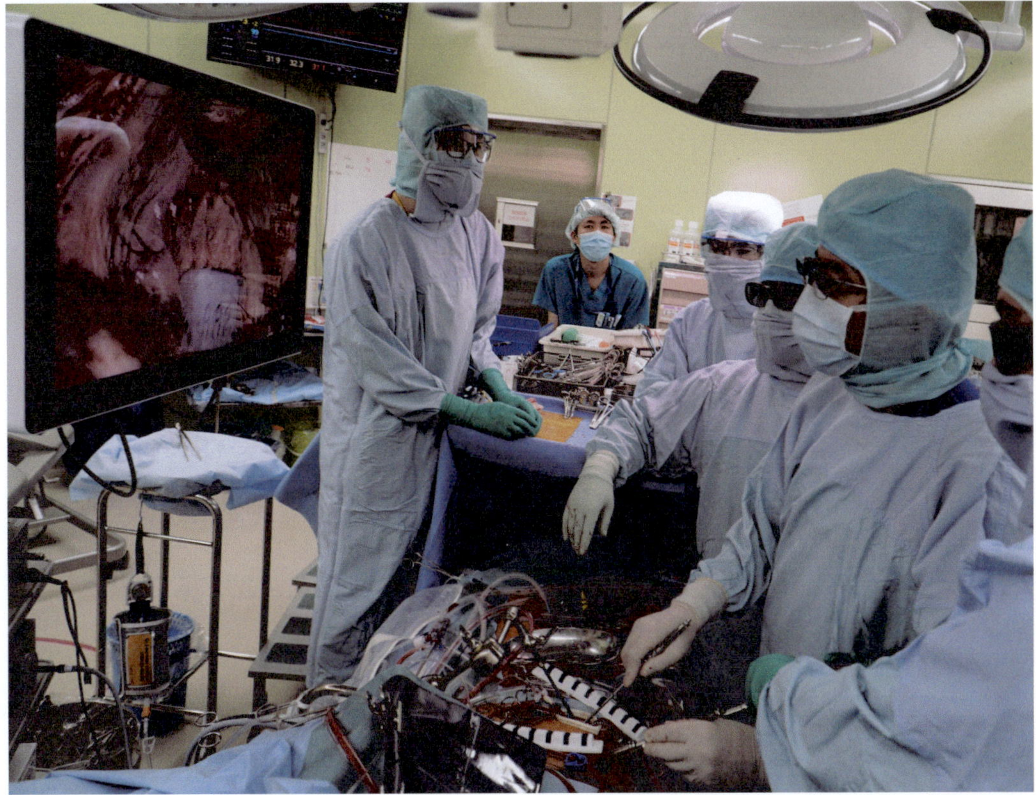

Fig. 2 OR set up for endoscopic aortic valve replacement

intracardiac component of the procedure is performed by looking at the monitor. The first assistant stands on the right side of the surgeon. The second assistant holds the 3D endoscope and stands at the left side of the surgeons (Fig. 2). The surgeon and assistants wear polarized glasses to view objects stereophonically. We make sure the monitor is placed at the correct height.

2.2 The Three-Port Technique (Video1)

We insert a 10-mm trocar for a 3D endoscope (Karl Storz, Tuttlingen, Germany) through the fourth intercostal space on the right mid-axillary line. A main 4.0 cm incision is made at the fourth intercostal space. Depending on the patients' anatomy, sometimes the 3rd or 5th intercostal space is used. The intercostal space is opened without a rib-spreader. A 5-mm port for left-handed instruments is placed at the second or third intercostal space on the right anterior axillary line. A soft tissue retractor is applied to the main port ("The three-port system" Fig. 3). The surgeon drives forceps with the left hand and needle-driver with the right hand. A 3D endoscope is placed in between the right- and left-hand ports, equidistance from each port.

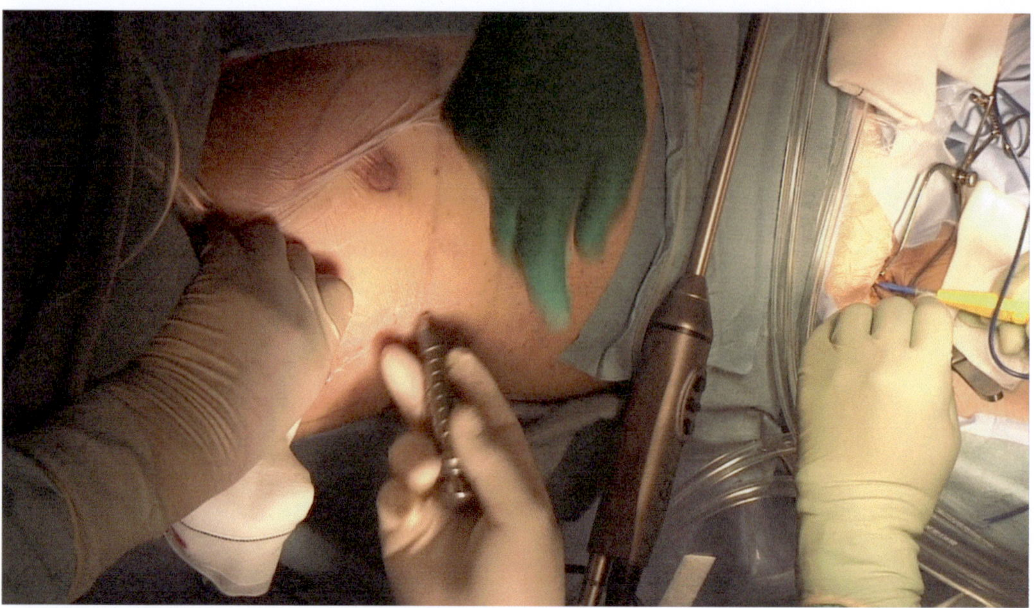

Video 1 The three-port technique and (▶ https://doi.org/10.1007/000-a85)

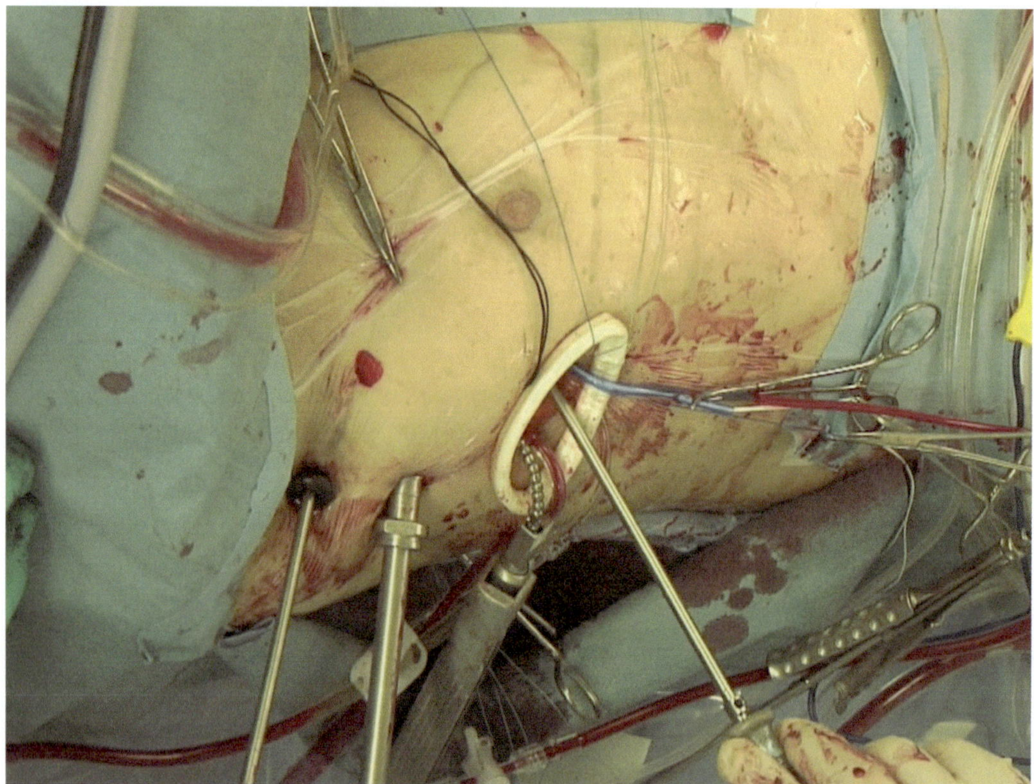

Fig. 3 Our setup of three port method for totally 3D endoscopic right mini-thoracotomy approach. The main, second, and camera ports were made at the fourth, the third, and the fourth intercostal spaces, respectively

3 Cardiopulmonary Bypass to Cross-Clamp

A cardiopulmonary bypass is established through the right femoral artery and vein for most cases. The pericardium is opened after initiating cardiopulmonary bypass. Four pericardial stay sutures are placed. The left upper suture is pulled through the right anterior chest wall using the crochet hook (Video). The lower two sutures are retracted to the outside of the chest wall utilizing a crochet hook, 5 cm below the camera port. An antegrade cardioplegia line are inserted through the main port. The inferior vena cava (IVC) is snared with CV-0 (W.L. Gore & Associates, Flagstaff, U.S.A.) to facilitate venous drainage for any valve cases. The left ventricular vent tube is inserted through the right superior pulmonary vein. Simultaneously, the patient is cooled systemically to 32C.

The ascending aorta is cross-clamped with a flexible clamp through the main port. Cardiac arrest is achieved with antegrade (and retrograde when needed) cardioplegia (Fig. 3). In cases of severe aortic regurgitation, we open the aorta and cannulate the coronary ostia directly. In concomitant mitral valve cases, we open the right atrium and inject retrograde cardioplegia directly into the coronary sinus.

Aortic valve replacement (Video 2)

An aortotomy is extended towards the left-non commissure. Two polypropylene stay sutures are placed at the right-left and right-non commissure. The aortic valve leaflets are excised, and annular calcium is debrided carefully. Everting mattress stitches are placed at each commissure. Three to four single interrupted stitches are placed between commissures. A standard pericardial stented valve is used for AVR. The pericardial valve is seated in the annulus through the 4 cm incision. The valve stiches are tied with a knot pusher with diamond like carbon coated-head (EMI Factory Co., Nagano, Japan) (Fig. 4). The aortotomy is closed with two-layer 4–0 polypropylene sutures. The cardiopulmonary bypass is weaned after meticulous hemostasis.

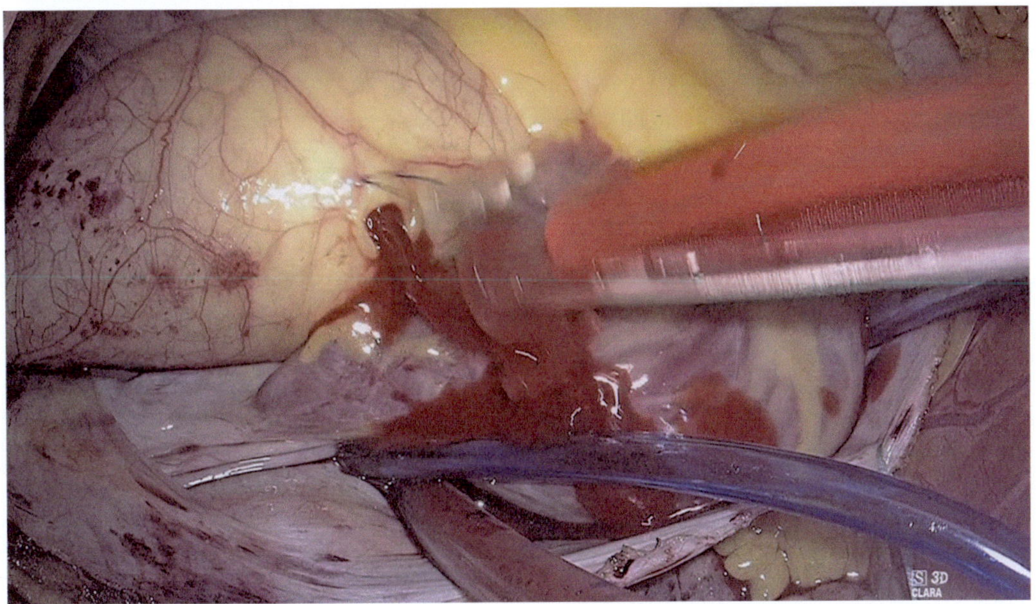

Video 2 Aortic valve replacement (▶ https://doi.org/10.1007/000-a84)

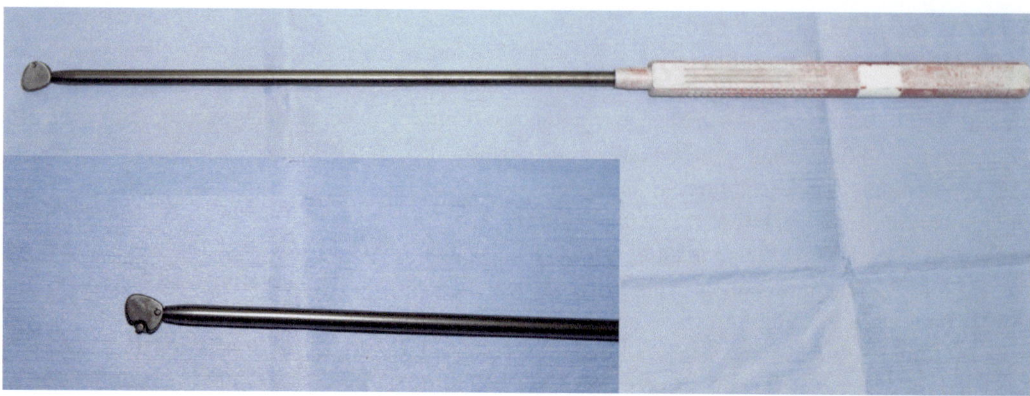

Fig. 4 Knot-pusher designed for endoscopic cardiac surgery. (EMI Factory Co., Nagano, Japan)

4 Summary

Minimally invasive cardiac surgery has evolved over the past two decades and has changed the fundamental approaches for valve treatments. In mitral surgery, endoscopic mitral valve treatment is currently considered a gold standard treatment for its minimal invasiveness. While there are extremely limited reports of totally endoscopic AVR, we believe, with our experience, that totally endoscopic AVR can be accomplished if a surgeon is well-trained in the endoscopic mitral procedure. Also, after the learning curve, the double valve procedure under the totally endoscopic vision can be safely performed in our experience.

For example, from June 2017 to December 2020, 131 patients with 72 ± 11 years of age underwent totally endoscopic aortic valve replacement at our institution using the described technique. Two patients (1.4%) underwent aortic valve repair, and the other 129 (99%) patients underwent AVR. 10 patients (7.6%) had aortic valve replacement with a mechanical valve, and 121 (92%) patients had a tissue valve replacement. Mitral valve repair and replacement were simultaneously performed in 14 (11%) and 3 (2.2%) patients respectively, and no failure in repair was noted. There was one (0.7%) 30-day mortality. Conversion to sternotomy was required in 3 (2.2%) patients and after the learning curve, total operation time shortened to less than three hours routinely.

In conclusion, totally 3D-endoscopic for aortic valve utilizing 'three-port' technique is a feasible technique for patients who required AVR.

Conflict of Interest Statement The authors have no conflicts of interest to declare.

References

1. Rao PN, Kumar AS. Aortic valve replacement through right thoracotomy. Texas Heart Inst J. 1993;20:307–8.
2. Cosgrove DM, Sabik JF. Minimally invasive approach for aortic valve operations. Ann Thorac Surg. 1996;62:596–7.
3. Cohn LH, Adams DH, Couper GS, Bichell DP, Rosborough DM, Sears SP, Aranki SF. Minimally invasive cardiac valve surgery improves patient satisfaction while reducing costs of cardiac valve replacement and repair. Ann Surg. 1997 Oct; 226(4): 421–428.
4. Lamelas J, Sarria A, Santana O, Pineda AM, et al. Outcomes of minimally invasive valve surgery versus median sternotomy in patients age 75 years or greater
5. Glauber M, Fareneti A, Solinas M, Karimov J. Aortic valve replacement through a right. Multimed Man Cardiothorac Surg. 2006;2006(1110):mmcts.2005.0 01826.
6. Glauber M, Ferrarini M, Miceli A. Minimally invasive aortic valve surgery: state of the art and future directions. Ann Cardiothorac Surg. 2015;4:26–32.

7. Ghoreishi M, Thourani V, Badhwar V et al. Less-invasive aortic valve replacement: trends and outcomes from the society of thoracic surgeons database. Ann Thorac Surg. 2021;111(4):1216–1223.

8. Glauber M, Bacco L, Cuenca J. Minimally invasive aortic valve replacement with sutureless valves: results from an international prospective registry innovations (Phila). 2020;15(2):120–30.

9. Berretta P, Andreas M, Carrel T. Minimally invasive aortic valve replacement with sutureless and rapid deployment valves: a report from an international registry (Sutureless and Rapid Deployment International Registry) Eur J Cardiothorac Surg. 2019;56 (4):793–799.

10. Carpentier A, Loulmet D, Carpentier A, et al. Open heart operation under videosurgery and minithoracotomy. First case (mitral valvulo- plasty) operated with success. C R Acad Sci III 1996. 319(3):219–223

11. Casselman FP, Van Slycke S, Wellens F, et al: Mitral valve surgery can now routinely be performed endoscopically. Circulation 2003. 108 (suppl 1): II-48-II-54

12. Casselman FP, Van Slycke S, Dom H, Lambrechts DL, Vermeulen Y, Vanermen H.J Endoscopic mitral valve repair: feasible, reproducible, and durable. Thorac Cardiovasc Surg. 2003;125 (2):273–82. https://doi.org/10.1067/mtc.2003.19. PMID: 12579095

13. Falk V, Walther T, Autschbach R et al. Robot-assisted minimally invasive solo mitral valve operation. J Thorac Cardiovasc Surg. 1998;115 470–471

14. Carpentier A, Loulmet D, Aupècle B, et al. Computer assisted open heart surgery. first case operated on with success. CR Acad SciIII. 1998;321:437–442.

15. Murphy DA, Moss E, Binongo J, et al. The expanding role of endoscopic robotics in mitral valve surgery: 1,257 consecutive procedures. Ann Thorac Surg. 2015;100(5):1675–81.

16. Badhwar V, Wei L, Cook C, et al. Robotic aortic valve replacement. J Thorac Cardiovasc Surg. 2021;161(5):1753–9.

17. Pitsis A, Boudoulas H, Boudoulas K. Operative steps of totally endoscopic aortic valve replacement. Interact Cardiovasc Thorac Surg. 2020;31(3):424. https://doi.org/10.1093/icvts/ivaa102.

18. Cresce GD, Sella M, Hinna Danesi T, Favaro A, Salvador L, Minimally invasive endoscopic aortic valve replacement: operative results. Semin Thorac Cardiovasc Surg. 2020 Autumn;32(3):416–423. https://doi.org/10.1053/j.semtcvs.2020.01.002. Epub 2020 Jan 21.

19. Ito T, Maekawa A, Hoshino S. Hayashi right infraaxillary thoracotomy for minimally invasive aortic valve replacement. Ann Thorac Surg. 2013;96(2):715–7. https://doi.org/10.1016/j.athoracsur.2013.03.003.

20. Ito T, Maekawa A, Hoshino S, et al. Three-port (one incision plus two-port) endoscopic mitral valve surgery without robotic assistance. Eur J Cardiothorac Surg. 2017;51:913–8.

21. Tokoro M, Sawaki S, Ozeki T, et al. Totally endoscopic aortic valve replacement via an anterolateral approach using a standard prosthesis. Interact Cardiovasc Thorac Surg. 2020;30(3):424–30.

22. Hosoba S, Ito T, Orii M. 3D-endoscopic concomitant mitral and aortic valve surgery. Ann Thorac Surg. 2021; S0003–4975(21)01915–9.

Totally Endoscopic Aortic Valve Replacement

Antonios A. Pitsis
and Aikaterini N. Visouli

Abstract

The replacement of the aortic valve is one of cardiac surgery's great successes and provides both life saving and life enhancing benefits. The median sternotomy and Hemi sternotomy are the preferred approaches with an anterior right mini thoracotomy gaining popularity. An endoscopic approach to aortic valve replacement has been adopted sporadically but is now gaining interest. In this chapter a step by step approach is taken to cover all the indications and contraindications to considering this approach. The authors are experts at using the automated suturing device (RAM) and describe their experience with this.

Keywords

Micro aortic valve replacement · Automated aortic valve suturing devices · Totally endoscopic surgery

Supplementary Information The online version contains supplementary material available at https://doi.org/10.1007/978-3-031-21104-1_13. The videos can be accessed individually by clicking the DOI link in the accompanying figure caption or by scanning this link with the SN More Media App.

A. A. Pitsis (✉) · A. N. Visouli
1st Cardiac Surgery Department, European Interbalkan Medical Center, Thessaloniki, Greece
e-mail: apitsis@otenet.gr

1 Introduction

"Primum non nocere".

"First do no harm" is a fundamental principal of bioethics, universally established, and accepted by the medical community. The principle of nonmaleficence supports several moral rules, including the obligation not to cause pain or suffering.

In medical ethics, nonmaleficence is the duty to cause no harm intentionally, or inflict the least harm to reach a beneficial result.

Conventional surgery is associated with significant surgical trauma, a harm considered inevitable and inherently associated with the beneficial results of restoring intracorporeal pathology, being viewed for decades as a fair tradeoff.

Advancements in technology allowed minimization of the surgical trauma without compromising the beneficial results of surgery.

Although with a latency compared to other surgical specialties, cardiac surgery evolved, incorporating since the mid-1990s minimally invasive techniques, involving smaller thoracic incisions, other than the full sternotomy.

The main approaches for surgical Minimally Invasive Aortic Valve Replacement (MIAVR) are the mini-sternotomy and the right anterior mini-thoracotomy, although several other approaches have been tried. Many potential advantages of the MIAVR have been reported, including decreased postoperative pain, reduced blood loss and transfusion requirement, better preservation of the lung function, reduced ventilation time, shorter Intensive Care Unit (ICU) and hospital stay, earlier return to work, social life, and regular activity, better patient satisfaction, and cosmetic results.

While there is demand for further investigation and robust evidence regarding the potential advantages of MIAVR, cardiac surgery continues to evolve, seeking to further minimize the surgical trauma with the aid of advanced technology, incorporating totally endoscopic and robotically assisted techniques.

In this chapter we describe the surgical technique of a Totally Endoscopic Aortic Valve Replacement (TEAVR), performed under stereoscopic screen vision, through a micro invasive approach leaving intact the sternum, the ribs, the cartilages, and the internal thoracic artery, achieved with enabling technology that allows aortic valve excision and surgical replacement with conventional, durable bioprosthetic or mechanical valves, applied for Aortic Stenosis (AS), Aortic Regurgitation (AR), mixed aortic valve disease, and a range of combined operations (Fig. 1) [1–8].

2 General Overview

Despite the micro invasive approach, TEAVR has a technical end-result largely similar to the that of a conventional full sternotomy AVR, as far as the valve replacement is concerned. TEAVR allows surgical excision of abnormal aortic valves (of any pathology, including bicuspid valves), annular decalcification/debridement as required, and replacement with a conventional biological or mechanical prosthesis, thus prosthetic valves with proven durability. Certainly, sutureless valves can be implanted if appropriate.

Furthermore, edge to edge mitral valve repair for secondary mitral insufficiency, chordal replacement for primary mitral insufficiency, myectomy for hypertrophic obstructive

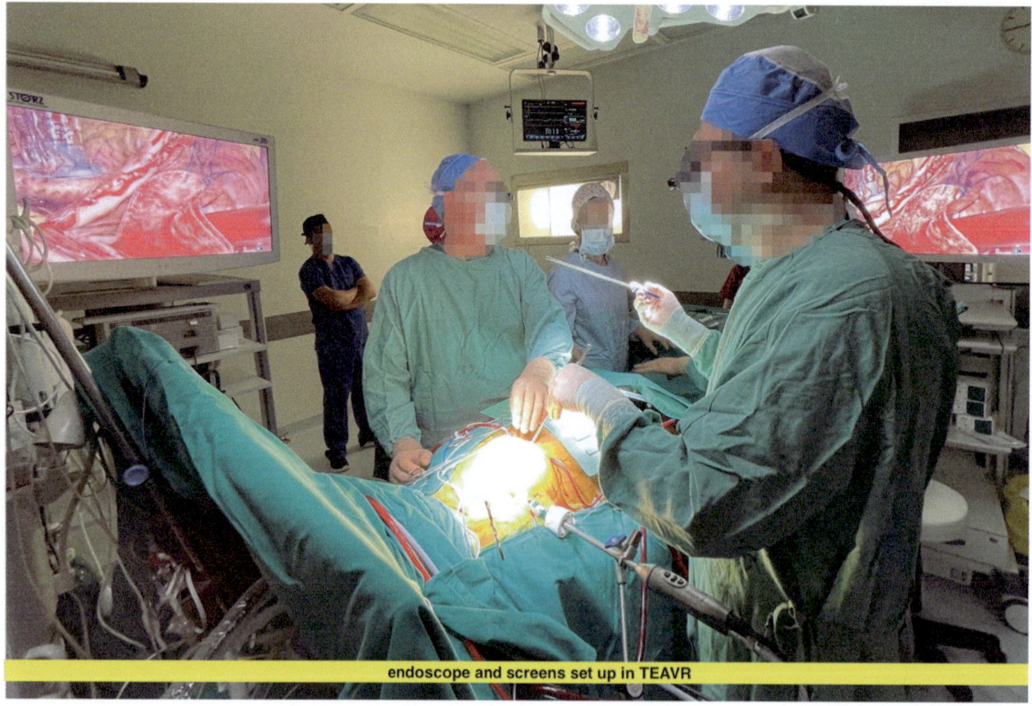

Fig. 1 Theatre setup for endoscopic aortic valve replacement

cardiomyopathy, and aortic root enlargement can be performed in combination with the TEAVR.

The operation takes place through a 3 cm right anterior micro (µ) thoracotomy, sparing the right internal thoracic artery, the sternum, the ribs and the cartilages, without any division, dislocation or application of any kind of rib spreading, and ensuring minimal surgical trauma to the intercostal nerves and the soft tissues (Fig. 2).

This working incision does not allow direct vision of the operative field, or any kind of manual activity within the thorax. The operation is mainly performed under stereoscopic (3D) screen vision, provided by a 3D endoscope inserted in the right hemithorax, and is significantly facilitated by specially designed instruments and devices, including automated suturing, sewing, and suture fastening devices.

The operation is performed under general anaesthesia, with a double lumen endotracheal tube, and the use of intraoperative Transoesophageal Echocardiography (TOE), on femoro-femoral vacuum assisted Cardiopulmonary Bypass (CPB), and cardioplegic arrest.

Further to the 3 cm right anterior micro-thoracotomy, three more thoracic microincisions (~0.4–1 cm) are necessary for the insertion of 1. the 3D endoscope (2nd intercostal space, laterally to the micro-thoracotomy working incision), 2. the aortic cross clamp (1st intercostal space, at a safe distance from the endoscope), while 3. a 4th intercostal space stamp wound microincision is used for multiple purposes (insertion of surgical instruments to dissect free and open the pericardium, insertion of a sump sucker that is also used as a right superior pulmonary vein

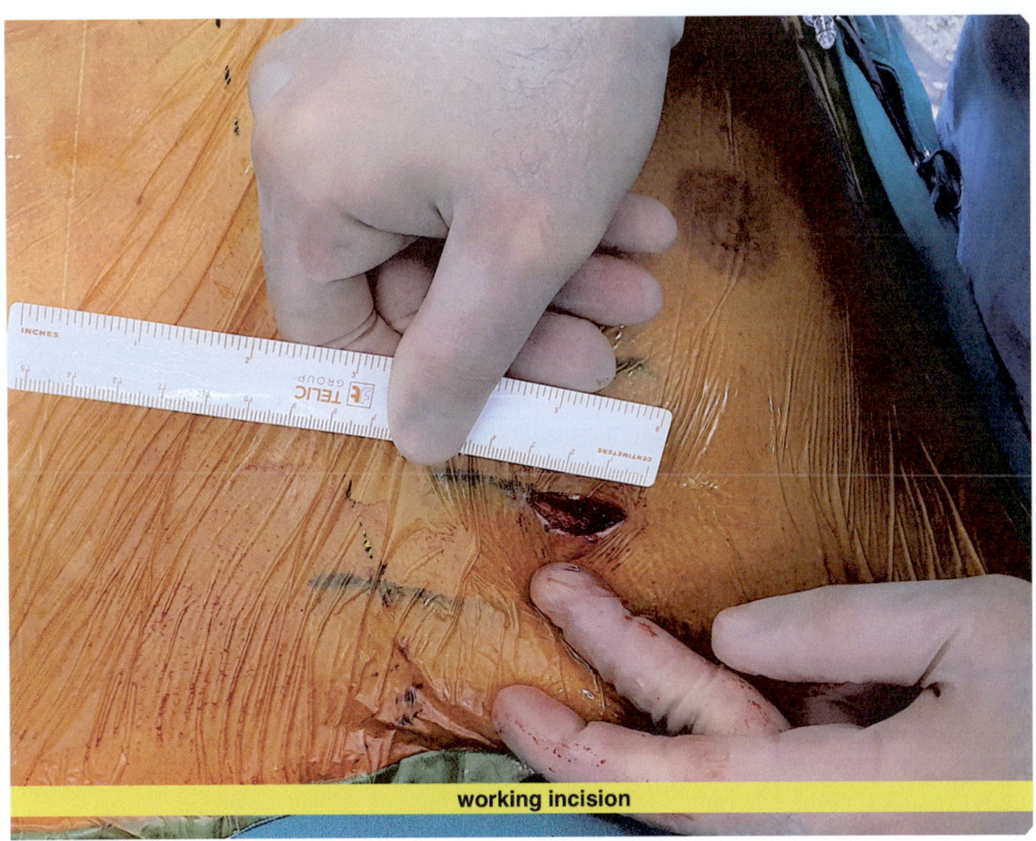

Fig. 2 Working incision

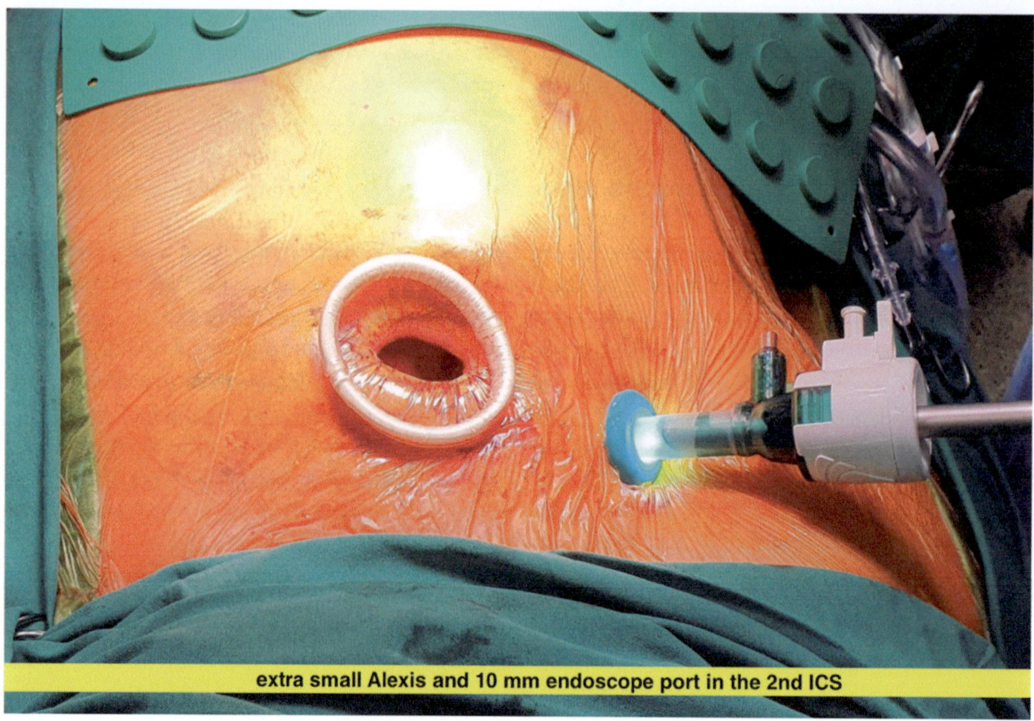

Fig. 3 Extra small retractor and endoscope port in the second intercostal space

vent, and placement of a pericardial drain at the end of the procedure) (Fig. 3).

The preoperative evaluation involves all standard surgical AVR protocols, including preoperative TOE, plus a thoracic Computed Tomography (CT) scan, to evaluate the position of the aortic valve in relation to the bones of the thoracic cage, the size, shape, position, and angulation of the ascending aorta, its distance from the sternum, the presence of calcified aortic plaques, particularly at the distal ascending aorta (which is the site of the cross-clamp placement), but also the sites of the transverse aortotomy, and the cardioplegia catheter insertion. The right hemithorax is also checked for the presence of dense adhesions or other significant pathology/ deformity. Certainly, all CT findings (including the random) are considered and evaluated. Furthermore, both femoral arteries are palpated, to ensure vigorous pulse bilaterally. In case of suspicion of peripheral vascular disease further investigation is required. The patient is positioned supine on the operating table, with his

right hemithorax elevated by 30 degrees with the aid of a pillow under his right shoulder, while external defibrillation pads are placed on his left hemithorax. The surgeons stand up during the whole procedure.

The general set-up of the operating room (OR) is the same as in conventional cardiac procedures, with the addition of a 3D endoscopic system, suturing, sewing, suture fastening devices, accessories, and elongated endoscopic surgical instruments.

The operative field is visualized on two screens, set in the operating room:

a. A 3D screen at the patient's left side, viewed by the surgeon (standing at the patient's right side), and the perfusionist (seating behind the surgeon). In order to have 3 D vision the surgeon wears 3D glasses. This system offers a good quality image, with a high degree of depth and spatial perception.

b. A 2D screen at the patient's right side, seen by the 1st assistant and the scrub nurse (Fig. 1).

Table 1 Operative steps of the TEAVR:

1. Right anterior micro-Thoracotomy (3 cm, 2nd intercostal)/3D scope placement
2. Groin cannulation for Cardiopulmonary Bypass (CPB)
3. Aortic cross clamping/antegrade cardioplegia
4. Aortotomy/aortic valve excision/debridement
5. Annular sizing/enhancing exposure of the annulus
6. RAM annular suturing
7. SEW EASY cassette loading/Prosthetic valve sewing cuff suturing
8. Valve Parachuting/Valve securing with COR-KNOT titanium fastener
9. Two-layer aortotomy closure/deairing/removal of aortic cross clamp
10. Pacing wire insertion/pericardial drain insertion
11. Hemostasis/pericardial closure
12. Weaning from CBP/CPB cannulae removal/pleural drain/wound closure

Table 2 Devices, instruments and accessories required for the TEAVR

1. TIPCAM®1 RUBINA™ 3D 30-degree Karl Storz endoscope, (KARL STORZ SE & Co. KG, Germany)
2. Endoscopic port with built-in CO_2 side line, endoscope holder
3. IMAGE 1S™ RUBINA 32″ 3D 4 K screen (3D glasses), 2D screen, (KARL STORZ SE & Co. KG, Germany)
4. Extra small Alexis wound protector/retractor*, (Applied Medical Corp., CA, USA)
5. RAM® Suturing Device (3.5 or 5.0)*, LSI Solutions
6. RAM® COR-SUTURE® QUICK LOAD® surgical suture (3.5 or 5.0 mm)*, LSI Solutions
7. RAM® RACK Suture Management System* (Suture organizer), LSI Solutions
8. SEW-EASY® Cassette*, LSI Solutions
9. SEW-EASY® DEVICE (3.5 or 5.0)*, LSI Solutions
10. COR-KNOT® DEVICE*, (COR-KNOT® MINI®), LSI Solutions
11. COR-KNOT® QUICK LOAD® UNIT (COR-KNOT fastener, loading unit)*, LSI Solutions
12. Chitwood clamp (Geister, Tuttlingen, Germany), Endoscopic surgical instruments
*Sterilized, single use
13. Endo Close™ device (Medtronic, USA)

The anesthetist can see either screen. Thus, the whole team, as well as other professionals present in the OR (cardiologists, trainees) share the surgeon's view. The procedure is interactive, and the videos can be used for educational and training purposes. The main operative steps of the TEAVR are included in Table 1.

The devices and surgical instruments used for the TEAVR are included in Table 2.

3 Steps of the Operative Technique of the TEAVR

We describe the operative procedure step by step, as it has evolved and standardized after performance of about 250 cases. The steps are largely the same as in conventional open surgical AVR, the main differences are the significantly limited access and the use of enabling technology (devices and instruments).

1. Right anterior micro-Thoracotomy/3D endoscope placement

The working incision is a 3 cm, horizontal, parasternal, right anterior micro-thoracotomy, in the second (2nd) intercostal space, 2–3 cm laterally to the right sternal border, sparing the right internal thoracic artery, and leaving intact the ribs, the cartilages and the sternum. A length of 3 cm is required to pass most conventional mechanical or biological valves through the working incision. (Three centimeters are required for a 25 mm mechanical prosthesis, while up to 4 cm may be required for a 29 mm conventional bioprostheses.)

After entering the pleura, an extra small Alexis soft tissue protector/retractor is placed in the working incision. The Alexis tissue protector provides gentle soft tissue retraction, and seals the wound, preserving moisture and minimizing blood loss, without spreading the ribs at all. No other kind of retraction is used, in order to protect the ribs from fracture or dislocation, and the soft tissues from tension, ischaemia, and blunt trauma, while vision is ensured by the endoscope.

The right lung is left to collapse, and a 10 mm endoscopic port is placed about 4 cm laterally to the working incision, in the same intercostal space (2nd intercostal space, a few finger breaths laterally to the working incision, on the anterior axillary line). A three-dimensional 30-degree (3D 4 K) Karl Storz endoscope is inserted through the endoscopic port to provide stereoscopic vision of the operative field. In the early learning period (first 30 cases), two endoscopic ports had been used, one in the 3rd intercostal space, to facilitate dissection and opening of the pericardium, as well as opening and closure of the aortotomy, and another endoscopic port in the 2nd intercostal space, to facilitate the aortic valve replacement.

The endoscopic port has a built-in side arm for the carbon dioxide (CO_2) line, so that no additional microincision is required for its insertion. Continuous CO_2 insufflation (at a flow of 0.5–1.0 l/min to flood the surgical field) is a preventive measure of air embolism, since de-airing of the heart is more challenging than in open procedures (Fig. 3).

The endoscope is stabilized by the endoscope holder (set laterally and anteriorly to the patient's right hemithorax, below and behind the surgeons left arm).

A 4th intercostal space stamp wound microincision, at the anterior axillary line (about 3 finger breaths below the nipple in men) is used for insertion of the right-hand instruments to dissect free and open the pericardium.

The pericardium is dissected free from the mediastinal tissue, the right phrenic nerve is identified, and the pericardium is opened longitudinally, 3–4 cm anterior to the right phrenic nerve, on CO_2 insufflation. Three pericardial stay sutures are placed: the left pericardial stay suture is exteriorized through the working incision to the left and the two right pericardial stay sutures are exteriorized through the skin to the right

(using the Endo Close™ device (Medtronic) to retract the right sided margin of the pericardium and the heart towards the endoscope, being externalized in the first and third intercostal spaces in the right anterior and mid axillary lines respectively.

After suspension of the pericardium, a sump sucker is inserted inside the pericardial cavity through the 4th intercostal microincision (the same one used for insertion of the surgical instruments to open the pericardium). The sump sucker line will be used at a later stage as a left atrial vent.

2. Groin cannulation for Cardiopulmonary Bypass (CPB)

Peripheral femoro-femoral cannulation takes place, through a 3 cm oblique inguinal incision, usually on the right side. In order to avoid lymphatic disruption and leakage, minimal subcutaneous tissue dissection is performed, adequate to expose only the anterior wall of the common femoral vessels, at a length of about 1,5 cm just below the inguinal ligament. After full heparinization, the Seldinger technique is applied under TOE guidance, for wire insertion and long cannula placement, through double pledgeted 4–0 prolene purse string sutures, placed on the anterior wall of the common femoral vessels.

An 18 Fr arterial cannula is inserted into the common femoral artery in patients with Body Surface Area (BSA) <2.2 m^2, while a 20 Fr arterial cannula is inserted in patients with a BSA ≥ 2.2 m^2. The tip of the arterial cannula is placed in the abdominal aorta.

A 25 Fr venous cannula is inserted through the common femoral vein and advanced into the right atrium with its tip placed at the superior vena cava (SVC), 3–5 cm above its junction to the right atrium. The venous cannula is usually inserted first. It is important to ensure by TOE performed by the anaesthetist that the guidewire has entered the SVC before inserting the venous cannula, to prevent penetration of the right ventricular free wall, the interventricular septum, the interatrial septum or the right atrial wall by the cannula tip.

Tension is applied to the tourniquets of the purse string sutures around the inserted cannulae, which are further secured in place.

Full, normothermic or mildly hypothermic CPB, with active venous drainage (vacuum assisted) is initiated.

3. Aortic cross clamping/antegrade cardioplegia

On CPB, the aorta is dissected free from the right pulmonary artery, to allow placement of the aortic cross clamp at the distal ascending aorta. A double pledgeted polypropylene 4–0 purse string suture is placed on the anterior wall of the ascending aorta about 2 cm distal to the fat pad (concato preaortic rim), and the cardioplegia catheter is inserted through it.

A Chitwood clamp, used for aortic cross clamping, is inserted through a separate stab wound microincision in the 1st intercostal space lateral to the midclavicular line, superiorly to the endoscope to avoid any conflict (Fig. 4). The aim is to place the cross clamp to the distal ascending aorta as cephalad as possible to allow a large operative field, but also place the clamp in a way that it rests on the aorta without tension or traction. The jaws of the Chitwood clamp must be facing the head of the patient to avoid injury of the pulmonary artery.

On CPB, the distal ascending aorta is cross clamped, and antegrade, cold, crystalloid cardioplegia (Custodiol, Koehler Chemie, Alsbach-Haenlein, Germany) or cold blood cardioplegia (DelNido) is administered. If there is no aortic regurgitation, the whole dose of the cardioplegic solution is administered in a single shot. In the presence of aortic regurgitation, half of the cardioplegia dose is administered during this step, while the other half is administered directly to the

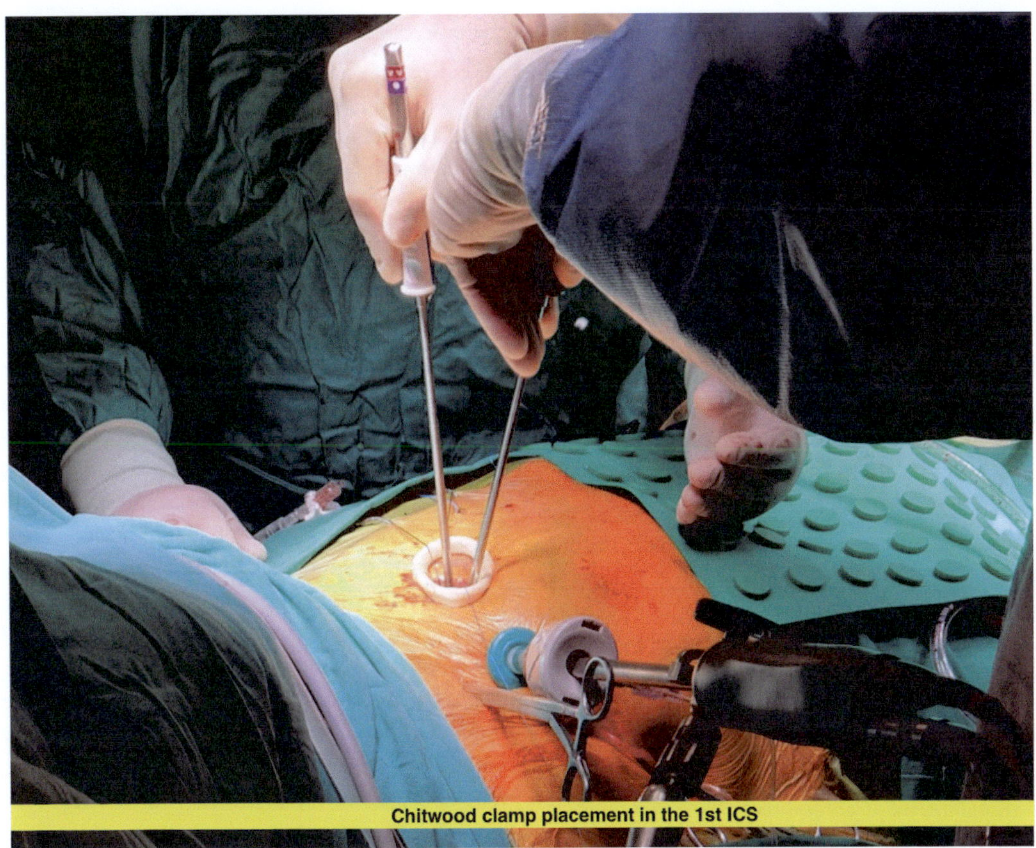

Fig. 4 External clamp placement in the first intercostal space

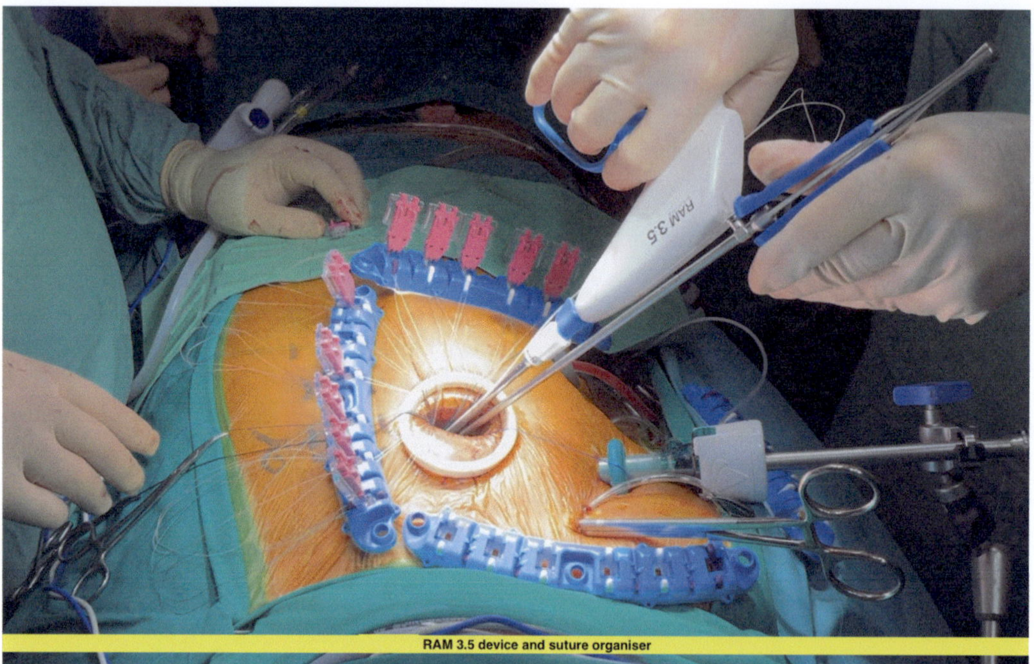

Fig. 5 RAM device use and suture organiser

coronary ostia after opening of the aorta (in the next step) (Fig. 5).

As soon as the heart is arrested (before administration of the whole dose of the cardioplegia), a left atrial vent is placed to prevent distension of the left ventricle. The sump sucker line is used as a vent, inserted though the right superior pulmonary vein, via a small transverse incision made with a scalpel.

4. Aortotomy/aortic valve debridement

After cardiac arrest and discontinuation of root cardioplegia, suction is applied on the cardioplegia catheter and the left atrial vent, on continuous CO_2 insufflation.

The aorta is opened through a transverse aortotomy, performed just proximal to the fat pad of the ascending aorta (i.e., about 3 cm distal to the right coronary ostium or about 2 cm distal to the sinotubular junction). It is important not to go through a hockey stick incision, unless aortic root enlargement is required.

The aortic root is stabilised with three horizontal mattress, Teflon buttressed sutures (two for the proximal part and one for the distal part of the aortotomy). The aortotomy stay sutures are placed in such a way so the aortic root remains stable and the endoscope is perpendicular to the aortic annulus.

In case of implantation of a rapid deployment valve (e.g., during the early learning period, in order to reduce the aortic cross clamp and CBP times), the transverse aortotomy may be performed just distal to the aortic fat pad (particularly in patients with a short ascending aorta), to provide space for the high profile sutureless valve.

The cardioplegia catheter is removed and the purse string suture is passed under the aortic cross clamp in order to retract the distal part of the aorta and facilitate exposure.

In the presence of aortic regurgitation, the remaining half dose of the cardioplegia is directly administered into the coronary ostia, first to the left, and then to the right ostium, facilitated by the endoscope which provides an excellent 3D 4 K view of the aortic root.

Under stereoscopic screen view, the aortic valve is excised, and the annulus is decalcified and debrided as required (usually in aortic stenosis), with the use of long-shafted instruments (scissors, rongeurs). Suction is applied to remove any remaining debris, while the magnification provided by the 3D screen helps in detection of tiny debris, offering an added protection from embolism. Although this is not included in our routine, in case of heavy calcification, a small gauze may be placed below the annulus at the left ventricular outflow tract (LVOT) to prevent debris spilling into the left ventricle. After completion of cusp excision and annular decalcification, the annulus, the aortic root, and the LVOT are washed with cold normal saline.

Thus, aortotomy, excision of the abnormal aortic valve, debridement, annular decalcification if required, and irrigation followed by suction, are performed as in conventional open surgery, the only differences being that there is no direct vision (but 3D screen vision), and long shafted instruments are passed through a 3 cm working incision.

5. Annular sizing/enhancing exposure of the annulus

Direct sizing of the aortic annulus is performed, with the use of the sizers of the chosen biological or mechanical prosthesis, as in conventional open surgery. The diameter of the annulus as measured intraoperatively by the sizers of the prosthetic valve is generally a little ($\sim$ 1–2 mm) larger than the TOE estimation. Annular decalcification and debridement result in increased compliance of the annulus that can usually accommodate a slightly larger prosthesis at a supra-annular position.

After excision of the aortic valve and debridement, the aortic root collapses, particularly in younger patients without atherosclerotic disease.

Three more stay sutures are placed to the ascending aorta, 2 proximal to the aortotomy and 1 the distal to it, in order to keep open the aortic incision.

To further facilitate the placement of the annular sutures, a cylindrical, self-expanding iron net is inserted into the aortic root to keep it open and increase its volume, providing a sort of an internal scaffolding and enhancing exposure of the annulus.

In order to facilitate the handling of the annular sutures after being passed through the aortic annulus (as described in the next step), a suture organizer, comprised by 3 separate racks, corresponding to the 3 aortic cusps (RAM® RACK Suture Management System) is attached on the draped anterior wall of the patient's right hemithorax, at an open triangular configuration, around the working incision (an inverted open Δ or Π configuration as seen by the surgeon). The suture organizer is very useful to prevent tangling of the sutures, which is particularly important, as the whole length of the suture (inside and outside the thorax) cannot be seen in one go (Fig. 6).

6. RAM annular suturing

The annular suturing takes place with the RAM® DEVICE, an automated, dual curved-needle, annular suturing device, that places a horizontal mattress stich in one squeeze.

The RAM device is used in conjunction with the RAM® COR-SUTURE® QUICK LOAD® surgical sutures, which are 2–0, non-absorbable, braided polyester, annular sutures, available in 3 colors (white, green, and striped), optionally pledgeted (polytetrafluoroethylene (PTFE) buttressed sutures), similar, in these respects, to the annular sutures used in conventional open AVR. We place the annular sutures in alternating colors (green and white) and opt to use pledgeted sutures, as in conventional AVR routine.

Both, conventional and RAM annular sutures are double armed, the only difference being that unlike the conventional annular sutures which are attached to needles, the RAM sutures are attached to short stainless-steel tubing: the "needle caps".

The pledgeted RAM suture is loaded to the RAM device, with the needle caps placed at the tip jaw (opposite to the retracted needles).

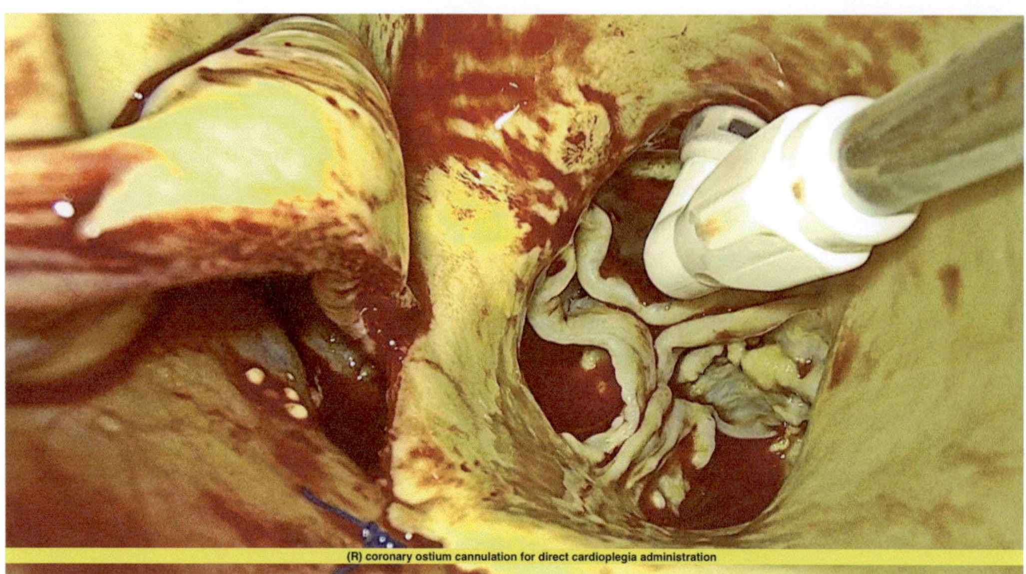

Fig. 6 Right coronary osmium cannulation for cardioplegia delivery

The RAM device is positioned so that the jaws of its tip embrace the annulus at a selected site and depth. After a single squeeze on the lever of the RAM device, the two curved needles simultaneously deliver both arms of the suture through the annulus. The pledget stays at the ventricular aspect of the annulus, while the 2 arms of the suture are passed through the annulus, from the ventricular side to its aortic side. Thus, RAM annular suturing has an end-result similar to that of conventional annular suturing, leading to supra-annular placement of the prosthetic valve, similar to the established routine in open aortic valve surgery.

The RAM device facilitates proper positioning of its blue suturing tip, which can be adjusted to the desired orientation (using the articulation and/or the rotational knob), so as to embrace the annular tissue at a specific position and depth, without the need for awkward positions of the surgeon's hand.

Details of RAM annular suturing:

The pledgeted RAM suture is loaded to the RAM device: the needle caps are placed to the respective compartments of the tip jaw, opposite to the (retracted) needles of the device.

The blue tip of the RAM device is positioned so that its jaws embrace the selected part of the aortic annulus, at the desired location and depth (or in other words, the annular tissue is placed within the tissue gap of the blue tip of the device).

The tip jaw containing the needle caps is placed underneath the aortic annulus (at its ventricular side), the jaw close to the retracted needles is placed above the annulus (at its aortic side).

By squeezing the blue lever, the two curved needles are simultaneously advanced (moving towards the needle caps), passing through the annulus placed in the tissue gap, penetrating from the aortic side to the ventricular side of the annulus, at right angles (if properly positioned). The device provides full control of the needles that can be seen being advanced towards and through the aortic annulus.

After a full squeeze of the blue lever, the needles of the RAM device become engaged to the needle caps located at the tip jaw and attached to the 2 arms of the annular suture.

After releasing the blue lever, the needles are simultaneously retracted back, pulling the needle caps and thus the 2 arms of the annular suture through the aortic annulus, passing them from the ventricular side to the aortic side of the annulus.

After placing each suture through the annulus and when the needles are fully retracted back, the RAM device is pulled out of the thorax, pulling out the two arms of the suture that remain attached to its tip. Each suture is manually loaded on a SEW-EASY® cassette (pink in color), which is then orderly placed into the appropriate slot of the corresponding rack of the suture organizer (Figs. 6 and 7).

The RAM device is available in two sizes: 3.5 and 5.0, that accordingly provide 3.5 mm and 5.0 mm suture spacing (i.e., the distance between the two needles of the device, and thus the distance between the 2 arms of the suture of each horizontal mattress stich). The pledgeted sutures are also available in two sizes for suture spacings: 3.5 mm and 5.0 mm (used in conjunction with the RAM® DEVICE 3.5 and 5.0, respectively).

Generally, we use the RAM 3.5 in cases with an aortic annulus diameter of up to 22 mm ($\leq$ 22 mm) measured by TOE, and a RAM 5 in cases with an aortic annulus diameter of 23 mm or more ($\geq$ 23 mm) measured by TOE. The TOE "underestimates" the annulus diameter, and we can usually insert one size larger valve, supra-annularly (e.g., when the aortic annulus diameter measured by TOE is 23 mm, we can usually implant a 25 mm valve).

Usually, 5 sutures are placed at each third of the annulus, making a total of 15 annular sutures.

First, annular sutures are placed at the right-coronary part of the annulus (which represents the most difficult part, regarding visualization and working angles), then sutures are place at the non-coronary part, and finally at the left-coronary part of the annulus (which is the least technically demanding part).

Suture placement may start from the commissure between the left and the right coronary cusp and proceed clock-wise to the right and the non-coronary part of the annulus, and anti-clock wise to the left-coronary part. Alternatively, it is useful to start at the nadir of each cusp and then

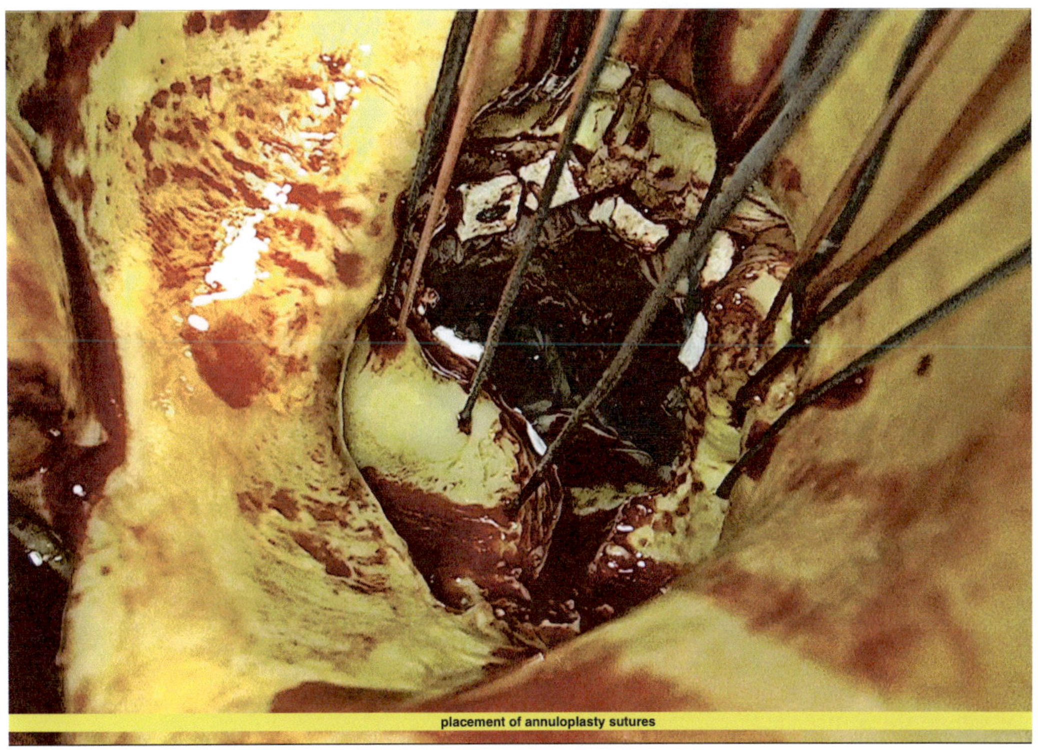

Fig. 7 Placement of sutures into the aortic annulus

proceed towards the commissures, as each suture facilitates the placement of the adjacent suture.

7. SEW EASY Cassette loading/Sewing cuff suturing

When all the (usually 15) annular sutures are placed through the aortic annulus with the use of RAM® device, the SEW-EASY® device is used to place the sutures through the sewing cuff of the prosthetic valve (bioprosthetic or mechanical). This step is performed outside the thorax under direct vision.

The SEW-EASY® Cassette is loaded from the rack of the suture organizer to the receiver located at the tip of the SEW-EASY® device, which works with a mechanism similar to that of the RAM device. By a single squeeze of the pink lever of the properly positioned SEW-EASY® device, a double bite is delivered, and both arms of the annular suture are passed through the sewing cuff (from the ventricular side to the aortic side of the cuff).

Details of the SEW EASY sewing cuff suturing: The SEW-EASY® Cassette (containing the double armed annular suture) is loaded to the receiver located at the tip of the SEW-EASY® device. The SEW-EASY® device is positioned so that the jaw of the cassette tip is placed at the ventricular side of the selected part of the sewing cuff, and the (retracted) needles of the device are positioned at the corresponding part of the aortic side of the sewing cuff. By squeezing the pink lever, the needles are simultaneously advanced, penetrating through the prosthetic material of the sewing cuff from its aortic side to its ventricular side, at right angles (if properly positioned). After a full squeeze of the pink lever, the needles of the SEW-EASY® device become engaged to the needle caps located at the cassette tip and attached to the 2 arms of the annular suture. After releasing the pink lever, the needles are simultaneously retracted back, pulling the needle caps and thus the 2 arms of the annular suture through the sewing cuff, passing them from the ventricular side to the aortic side of the sewing cuff.

In order to place the annular sutures through the sewing cuff, the surgeon holds the prosthetic valve with his/her non dominant hand, with the aid of a streamlined valve holder, so that he/she faces the aortic aspect of the valve. In some valves, particularly mechanical valves, the holder is in close proximity to the sewing cuff, thus interfering with the SEW-EASY® device. In these cases, the valve holder is removed, and the valve is held with a clean gloved hand.

When each double armed RAM annular suture is passed through the sewing cuff of the prosthetic valve and the device's needles are fully retracted back, the SEW-EASY® device is pulled away from the prosthesis, pulling the sutures away from the sewing cuff. The cassette is unloaded from the SEW-EASY® device, which is then ready to receive the next cassette with loaded suture. By repeating the same procedure, all the double armed annular sutures are orderly passed through the sewing cuff of the prosthetic valve.

The SEW-EASY® device is available in two sizes: 3.5 and 5.0, used in conjunction with the 3.5 or 5.0 RAM® DEVICE, and the 3.5 mm or 5.0 mm RAM® COR-SUTURE ® QUICK LOAD ® annular surgical sutures, respectively.

8. Valve Parachuting/Valve securing with COR-KNOT titanium fastener

When all sutures have been passed through the sewing cuff, the prosthetic valve is parachuted down to the aortic root (Fig. 8).

The procedure of lowering the prosthetic valve from an extracorporeal to an intrathoracic position through the 3 cm working incision is somewhat different for mechanical and conventional biological prosthetic valves.

a. Mechanical prostheses have a low profile, and can be tilted and easily passed through the incision like a coin in a slot.

b. Conventional bioprosthetic valves have a higher profile, posing increased difficulty to the passage through the working incision.

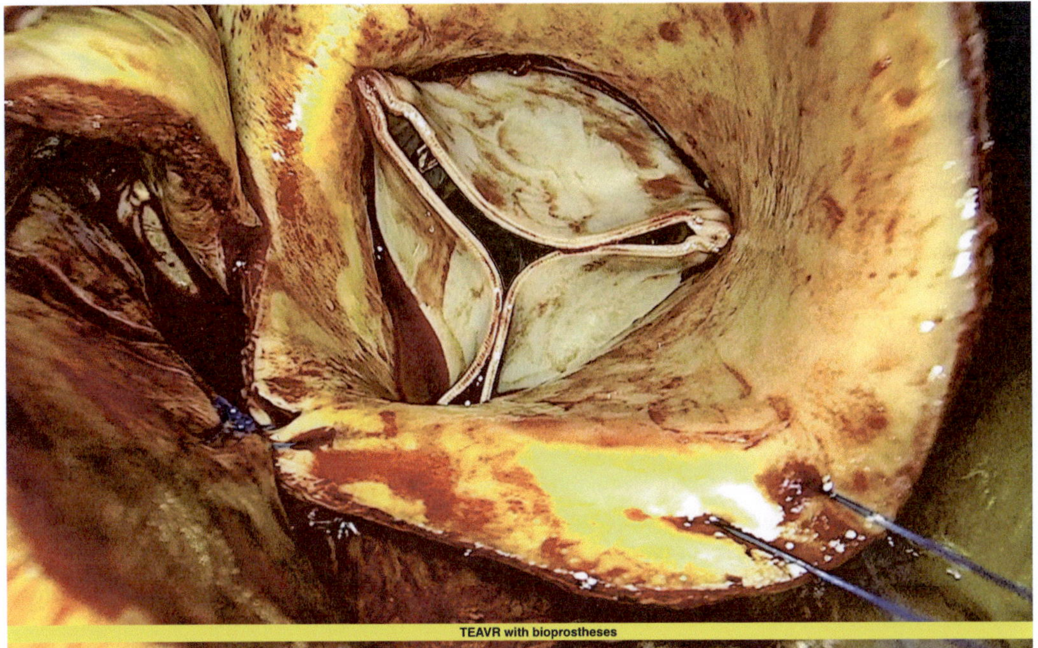

Fig. 8 Endoscopic bio-prosthetic aortic valve replacement

In order to ease the parachuting of bioprosthetic valves that have synthetic material (polymer frame) at the commissural posts (e.g., the Avalus, Medtronic), a 4–0 prolene suture is used, passed twice around, and through the commissural posts, to cinch them together. This cinching suture is cut and removed after all annular sutures have been fastened.

Bioprostheses without synthetic material at the commissural posts (e.g., the Trifecta, Abbott) are not amenable to this maneuver. The VALVEVAULT is a new stainless-steel surgical instrument, specially designed to protect these valves while been passed through the working incision. The VALVEVAULT container/protector resembles to a double-bowl spoon, having a central handle and 2 valve containers (cases) one at each end, plus a removable flattened cover. There are three sizes of the VALVEVAULT surgical instrument, each one having two valve containers (Extra Small and Small, Medium and Medium/Large, Large and Extra Large). The bioprosthetic valve is placed in the appropriately sized container, the flat cover is put

in place, and the VALVEVAULT instrument containing and protecting the valve is lowered into the surgical field, been passed through the working incision. The flat cover is removed manually, releasing the valve near the aorta.

When the prosthetic valve is parachuted and seated on the native aortic annulus, the annular sutures are secured with the aid of the COR-KNOT® DEVICE, an automated suture-fastening device. This technique is alternative to tying down the sutures, by making surgical knots as is routinely done in conventional open surgery. The two arms of each annular suture are fastened together by placement of a COR-KNOT® FASTENER, which is a specially designed clip (a medical-grade titanium, inverted-mushroom shaped hollow sleeve) that is crimped by the COR-KNOT® DEVICE, which secures the sutures, and also trims them close to the crimped titanium fastener.

There are two sizes of the COR-KNOT® DEVICE, the COR-KNOT MINI® (with a 4 mm shaft diameter, and 17 mm shaft length) and the COR-KNOT® MIS (with a 5 mm shaft diameter, and 31 mm shaft length). We use the shorter device for endoscopic aortic valve surgery, and the long one for endoscopic mitral and tricuspid valve surgery, repair of atrial septal defects, ventricular septal defects, etc. [1–8].

9. Two-layer aortotomy closure/deairing

The aortotomy is closed in two layers, first a continuous horizontal mattress suture, and then an over and over running suture (the same as in open surgery routine). A perfectly haemostatic closure is imperative, because the limited access poses increased difficulty in placing additional sutures after removal of the aortic cross clamp (Fig. 9).

A purse string suture is placed around the insertion site of the right superior pulmonary vein vent, and tied down when the vent is removed.

The heart is deaired through the site of insertion of the cardioplegia catheter, after loosening of the purse string suture. Completeness of deairing is check by TOE. Left table tilting may be used to remove residual "air" bubbles in the left ventricle, although the CO_2 insufflation reduces the risk of trapped bubbles that may cause embolism.

A bipolar pacing wire is passed through the right ventricular myocardium before removing the aortic cross clamp, because when the heart is beating, wire placement becomes more challenging.

After deairing and pacing wire insertion, the aorta cross-clamp is removed.

Hemostasis, pericardial drain placement and closure of the pericardium is done on CPB.

10. Weaning from CBP /cannulae removal/ pleural drain placement/wound closure

The patient is weaned from CPB, and the function of the prosthetic valve is evaluated by TOE. The CBP cannulae are removed and heparin is reversed with protamine.

Haemostasis is secured, a pericardial drainage tube is placed, inserted through the multipurpose 5th intercostal microincision.

We prefer to close the pericardium whenever feasible, to minimize adhesion formation. Nevertheless, pericardial closure increases the risk of tamponade, and takes place to the extent that no excessive tension is exerted.

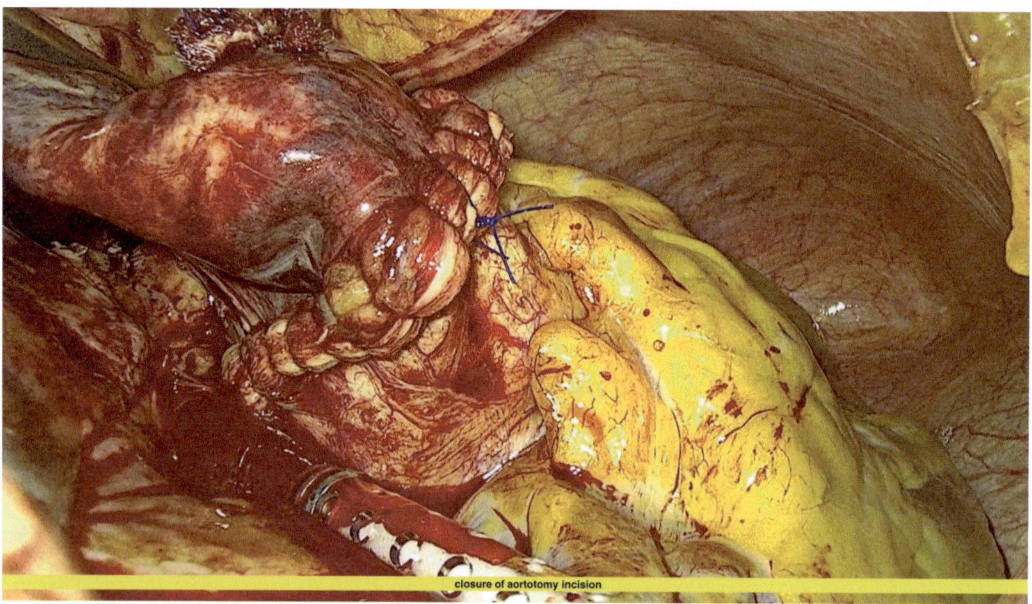

Fig. 9 Closure of Aortic incision

The endoscope and the endoscopic port are removed. A right pleural drainage tube is inserted through the second intercostal microincision previously used for the insertion of the endoscopic port/endoscope. The right lung is inflated.

The working incision is closed in layers, the thoracic micro-incisions and the inguinal incision are closed with subcutaneous tissue and skin approximation.

4 Patient Selection

The patient selection criteria are evolving along with the evolution of the technique, becoming less strict as experience is accumulated.

Currently, we consider all patients with significant aortic valve disease, including aortic stenosis (AS), aortic regurgitation (AR) or mixed aortic valve disease, as potential candidates for the TEAVR, unless they meet the following contraindications: ascending aortic root aneurysm requiring replacement, significant Coronary Artery Disease (CAD) requiring Coronary Artery Bypass Grafting (CABG), dense adhesions in the right hemithorax, porcelain ascending aorta, or significant aortoiliac disease not allowing distal cannulation (Tables 3 and 4).

The presence of bicuspid aortic valve is not a contraindication, obesity puts some additional difficulty (which applies for all operations and interventions) and is not a contraindication. Reoperation can be challenging, but is not an absolute contraindication. Concomitant severe secondary mitral insufficiency (3–4+), Hypertrophic Obstructive cardiomyopathy (HOCM), or narrow aortic root are not contraindications, as TEAVR can be performed combined with edge-to-edge mitral valve repair, Morrow myectomy, or aortic root patch-enlargement (Table 3).

The patient selection process should be individualized, and shared decision making is encouraged after discussion session(s) with fully informed patients, taking into consideration the patient's values, life-style, expectations, and preferences.

5 Brief Presentation of Our Experience in TEAVR

Between January 2019 and May 2020, 90 consecutive patients with Aortic Stenosis (AS) and/or Aortic Insufficiency (AI) (all comers) were treated with Totally Endoscopic Aortic Valve Replacement. The first 60 patients (January 2019–October 2019) were operated without the use of RAM annular suturing device, the last 30 patients (November 201–May 2020) were operated with the use of the RAM device. In all

Table 3 Indications for TEAVR

All patients with significant aortic valve disease, including AS, AR or mixed aortic valve disease may be evaluated for the TEAVR, if they do not have contraindications listed in Table 4

    Obesity is not an absolute contraindication

    Redo surgery is not an absolute contraindication

    Patients with significant aortic valve disease and severe secondary mitral regurgitation (3–4+) can have transaortic edge to edge mitral valve repair combined with the TEAVR

    Patients with hypertrophic obstructive cardiomyopathy (HCOM) can have Morrow myectomy combined with TEAVR

    Patients requiring aortic root enlargement can have combined TEAVR and patch aortic root enlargement

Table 4 Contraindications for TEAVR

The TEAVR is NOT indicated in the presence of significant aortic valve disease and one or more of the following comorbidities:
    Ascending aortic or root aneurysm, when aortic replacement is indicated
    (Mini-sternotomy is preferred)
    Significant Coronary Artery Disease (CAD) requiring Coronary Artery Bypass Grafting (CABG)
    (Full sternotomy is preferred)
    Porcelain ascending aorta
    (Transcatheter Aortic Valve Implantation (TAVI) is preferred)
    Dense adhesions in the right hemithorax (previous lobectomy, empyema, decortication, etc.)
    (Mini-sternotomy is preferred)
    Significant aortoiliac disease not allowing distal cannulation
    (Mini-sternotomy is preferred)

patients the COR-KNOT device was used for suture fastening.

The mean age of the 90 patients was 68.9 years (range 26–90, median 73), the mean EuroSCORE 2 was 3.07 (range 0.9–12.01, median 1.99). All patients were implanted with conventional aortic valve prostheses (the same as those used in open valve surgery): about 84% of patients received a stented bioprosthesis, while about 16% received a mechanical prosthesis; 2 patients (2.2%) underwent reoperation, 5 patients (5.55%) underwent combined transaortic edge to edge mitral valve repair for secondary severe (3–4+) mitral valve insufficiency, 1 patient (1.1%) underwent combined transaortic Morrow myectomy for concomitant Hypertrophic Obstructive Cardiomyopathy (HOCM), and 1 patient (1.1%) underwent combined aortic root patch enlargement.

The mean CPB time was 118.4 min, the mean aortic cross clamp time was 78.5 min.

The mean size of the prostheses was 23.6 mm (range 19–29, median 23). The mean peak gradient of prostheses (postoperatively) was 13.7 mmHg.

There was no in-hospital or 30-day mortality, no myocardial infarction, no life-threatening arrhythmias, no pacemaker insertion, no reopening for bleeding, no peripheral vascular complications, no wound complications. Conversion to full sternotomy was not required. One patient had a mild (1+) paravalvular leak (early period, without the use of RAM), and one patient suffered cerebrovascular accident (in the same period) (Table 5).

Excellent wound healing was observed in all patients, with minimal wound care. The cosmetic results were excellent, and contributed to patient satisfaction, while early return to regular activity was impressive, particularly in younger patients.

The absence of peripheral vascular complications associated with the groin cannulation (no limb ischaemia, arteriovenous fistula, pseudoaneurysm, haematoma, lymphatic leak, etc.) (Table 5) is at least partially attributed to the adoption of the hybrid cannulation technique with minimally invasive surgical access and cannulae insertion in the common femoral vessels with the Seldinger technique (surgical exposure of a small area of the common femoral vessels' anterior wall, and guide-wire cannulae insertion as in percutaneous cannulation). The hybrid femoral cannulation technique combines the advantages of the two (open and percutaneous) approaches: direct vision and identification of the inguinal ligament to ensure cannulae insertion into the common femoral vessels, accurate size evaluation of the two vessels, palpation of the common femoral artery for atherosclerotic plaque detection, cannulae insertion and removal under direct vision through purse string sutures, complete haemostasis achieved via purse string suture closure and direct visual inspection, and minimal vascular, soft tissue, and lymphatic trauma. TOE guidance is a must, to prevent misplacement of the venous cannula (Table 6).

Introduction of the RAM device facilitated annular suturing. Although development of the totally endoscopic procedure required a long

Table 5 Results of the Totally Endoscopic micro Aortic Valve Replacement (pre and post RAM)

Period Number of patients	Pre-RAM Jan 2019–Oct 2019 N = 60	Post-RAM Nov 2019–May 2020 N = 30	Total Jan 2019–May 2020 N = 90
In-hospital/30-day mortality	0	0	0
Myocardial infarction	0	0	0
Life threatening arrhythmia	0	0	0
Cerebrovascular accident	1/60 (1.6%)	0/30 (0%)	1/90 (1.1%)
Conversion to sternotomy	0	0	0
Reopening for bleeding	0	0	0
Wound complications	0	0	0
Vascular complications	0	0	0
Paravalvular leak (mild, 1+)	1/60 (1.6%)	0/30 (0%)	1/90 (1.1%)
Pacemaker insertion	0	0	0

learning curve, the learning curve of the RAM suturing (introduced after significant experience in the totally endoscopic technique) was rather fast: after the first 2 or 3 cases, the ease was increased and the suturing time was progressively decreased.

RAM annular suturing and SEW EASY sewing cuff suturing ensure absolute accuracy of the suture spacing (distance between the two arms of the annular suture of each horizontal mattress stich placed through the native aortic valve annulus, and subsequently through the sewing cuff). Usually 15 annular sutures were placed (5 in each third of the annulus). The RAM 3.5 was used for annular diameter up to 22 cm, and the RAM 5.0 for annular diameter 23 or more measured by TOE (Table 6).

The size of the valves implanted was very satisfying with very good patient-prosthesis match, as indicated not only by the mean and median valve sizes (23.6 and 23 respectively), but also by the low postoperative mean peak gradient of the prosthetic valves (13.7 mmHg). This is at least partially attributed to excision of the native valve, debridement and decalcification if required, and supra-annular valve placement,

an end-result similar to that achieved in conventional open valve surgery.

Regarding the thoracic wall trauma, it is self-evident that the structural end-result at the end of the operation is superior to that demonstrated not only with full or mini-sternotomy, but also with the mini-thoracotomy. The totally endoscopic technique is the only described technique that leaves intact all the bony structures of the thoracic cage, spares the Right Internal Mammary Artery (RITA), and causes minimal soft tissue trauma (Table 6).

Conclusively, we have applied the TEAVR (with and without the RAM device) in low-, intermediate- and high-risk patients of both genders, and all ages, from young athletes to fragile nonagenarians, with excellent results, regarding mortality and morbidity. Valves with proven durability were implanted (the same valves used in conventional AVR), and excellent valve performance was documented.

This small size (n = 90), single center, single surgeon (A.P.), preliminary, observational study has several limitations and does not provide evidence on the comparative outcomes of the TE μAVR versus other treatment options (full

Table 6 Key points

Feasibility of the totally endoscopic (RAM) micro AVR
    Feasibility based on technology (endoscopic system)
    Facilitated by technology (suturing, sewing, suture fastening devices)

Evidence of safety of the TE RAM AVR (low morbidity and mortality)
Use of automated devices is feasible in all cases, facilitates operation, helps in standardization

Use:
    RAM 3.5 when aortic annulus diameter ≤ 22 mm measured by TOE
    RAM 5.0 when aortic annulus diameter ≥ 23 mm measured by TOE

Use:
    RAM 3.5 for annular suturing in conjunction with SEW EASY 3.5 for sewing cuff suturing
    RAM 5.0 for annular suturing in conjunction with SEW EASY 5.0 for sewing cuff suturing

Use:
    Pledgeted RAM sutures 3.5 and 5.0, respectively
    Usually 15 sutures are placed (5 in each third of the annulus)

Peripheral hybrid femoro-femoral cannulation (vacuum assisted CPB)
    Minimal surgical exposure
    Seldinger technique
    TOE guidance for wire and long venous cannula insertion

TEAVR characteristics
    Feasibility of application in Aortic Stenosis, Aortic Regurgitation, and mixed aortic valve disease
    Excision of the native valve, debridement, decalcification if required
    Implantation of conventional bioprosthetic or mechanical valves, with proven durability
    Excellent patient-valve match, valve size mean: 23.6, median: 23, mean peak gradient: 12.7 mmHg
    Some combined operations may be performed
    Truly minimized surgical trauma (intact all bony structures)[a]
    Absence of sternal wound complications and related morbidity/mortality[a]
    Better cosmetic results[a]

[a] Self-evident advantages

sternotomy AVR, mini-sternotomy AVR, mini-thoracotomy AVR or TAVI), nor does it allow generalization of the results. Furthermore, it does not provide evidence about the large-scale reproducibility of the technique (Table 6).

Nevertheless, it certainly shows the feasibility of the TEAVR with or without the RAM device, and provides very encouraging results regarding the safety of the procedure (mortality 0/90, major morbidity 1/90) when performed by experienced and properly trained surgeons, in high volume centers. Standardization of the technique may facilitate adoption and reproducibility (Tables 5 and 6).

It is self-evident that the cosmetic results are better than in conventional or the minimal invasive AVR, and that sternal wound complications, and the associated morbidity and mortality are no longer applicable with the TEAVR. Further investigation is required to produce robust evidence on the other potential advantages of this micro invasive technique compared with the conventional or minimal invasive AVR, as well as the transcatheter approaches (Table 6).

Challenging and technically demanding technique with a long learning curve

Strong background, high volume center, proper team training required

The nature of this preliminary study does not allow generalization.

Single center, single surgeon, observational study, thus low quality of evidence

The results regarding safety must be interpreted with caution

Further studies required to document potential advantages further to the self-evident

Technology, standardization, and training may facilitate dissemination and reproducibility.

6 Discussion

The rationale of the TEAVR is preservation of the benefits of conventional full sternotomy AVR and augmentation of the benefits of minimal invasiveness, progressing to a micro-invasive technique [1–4].

Full median sternotomy AVR provides proven and excellent short and long-term results and remains the mainstay of treatment to which all recent treatment options including TAVI and minimally invasive AVR are compared [9–11].

TAVI is gaining acceptance, adoption, and guideline driven indications extending from high risk to intermediate risk patients with Aortic Stenosis and indication for biological valve placement. The gradual establishment of TAVI is based on high quality evidence produced mainly by Randomized Controlled Trials (RCT) and their meta-analyses, that mainly compare TAVI versus conventional full sternotomy AVR [11–25].

Minimally invasive AVR (mainly ministernotomy or mini-thoracotomy AVR) is also evolving [26–57]. While safety of the minimally invasive AVR is uniformly demonstrated, the potential advantages of the minimally invasive approach (decreased: pain, blood loss, transfusions, ventilation time, ICU/hospital stay; preservation of lung function, faster return to regular activity, etc.) are less well documented [26–57].

The small sample size of the RCTs, which, furthermore, demonstrated contradictory results [42–52], the inadequate statistical power and the heterogeneity within and between studies (characterising not only observational studies but also RCTs), including application of several techniques and variations, led to inconclusive results and thus uncertainty regarding the potential advantages of the minimally invasive techniques, even when the data was pooled in systematic reviews, weighted and included in meta-analyses [53–57].

The main benefit of the conventional full sternotomy Aortic Valve Replacement (AVR) compared to the transfemoral Transcatheter Aortic Valve Implantation (TAVI) is the proven durability of the implanted valves and the excellent long-term results. Other advantages of the surgical approach include the ability to treat any kind of aortic valve disease (not only aortic stenosis), to implant not only biological but also mechanical valves, and to treat concomitant cardiac or aortic disease by combined operations.

The TEAVR largely preserves all the advantages of the conventional full sternotomy Aortic Valve Replacement, with the exception of the potential to intervene in complex aortic disease, including ascending aortic aneurysm, and type A dissection, or allow combined CABG (Tables 4, 6, 7).

Regarding valve replacement, the structural end-result at the completion of the TEAVR is similar to that achieved with the conventional full sternotomy AVR, the only difference being that instead of hand tied knots, the sutures are secured by the COR-KNOT titanium fastener (Table 7).

FS-AVR, Full Sternotomy Aortic Valve Replacement.

Aortic cross clamp placement, cardioplegia administration, and aortotomy opening and closure are largely the same as in conventional full sternotomy AVR. The aortic cross clamp and CBP

Table 7 Structural end-result of TEAVR similar to conventional full sternotomy AVR (FS-AVR), regarding valve replacement

1. Replacement feasible in all native valve pathology (AS and/or AI, bicuspid valve), as in FS-AVR
2. Native valve excision/debridement, decalcification if required, as in conventional FS-AVR (with surgical instruments similar to those used in conventional FS-AVR)
3. Replacement with conventional bioprosthetic or mechanical valves of proven durability, the same valves used in conventional FS-AVR. (Feasibility of implantation of sutureless valves)
4. Use of annular sutures similar to those used in conventional FS-AVR (2–0, polyester, pledgeted)
5. Suture placement through the native aortic valve annulus, and the sewing cuff of the prosthetic valve in the same configuration as in FS-AVR (with the aid of devices that facilitate suture placement)
6. Supra-annular prosthetic valve placement, as in conventional FS-AVR
7. Opening and closure of the aortotomy, as in conventional FS-AVR

Table 8 Structural end-result of TEAVR, regarding thoracic wall trauma

1. Intact sternum
2. Intact ribs and cartilages (no division, no dislocation, no rib spreading)
3. Intact Right Internal Thoracic Artery
4. Minimal soft tissue trauma (skin, subcutaneous tissue, intercostal nerves, etc.)
5. Smaller working incision

times are somewhat increased compared to the full sternotomy AVR, but are progressively decreasing with accumulating experience (although they will probably remain at least slightly higher, until further aid is provided by technology).

Implantation of a sutureless valve may be tried in the initial learning period to decrease aortic cross clamp and CBP times, nevertheless, implantation of a high profile sutureless valve with unproven durability confers no benefit in comparison to TAVI, except perhaps feasibility of placement of larger valves after native valve excision and partial decalcification, more accurate valve positioning, fixation and orientation, performed under stereoscopic vision.

Made possible with use of the endoscopic/3D screen vision (TEAVR), without the use of retractors, rib spreaders, etc. in order to have direct vision (minimally invasive AVR).

Regarding the thoracic wall surgical trauma, superiority of the TEAVR is self-evident when compared to full sternotomy AVR. Although less self-evident, in our opinion the TEAVR causes significantly less surgical trauma compared not only to mini-sternotomy but also to mini-thoracotomy AVR (Table 8).

In our opinion, further to the above mentioned reasons of uncertainty regarding the potential advantages of the minimally invasive AVR (small samples size, inadequate statistical power, heterogeneity, etc.), significant contributing factors are lack of standardization and occasionally the lack of true minimal invasiveness.

In our opinion, the length of the skin incision is not directly correlated to indicate the surgical trauma induced. When trying to perform a certain operation, under direct vision, using practically the same surgical instruments, through a significantly limited access, the technical difficulty is increased, the procedure becomes highly operator-dependent, while occasionally (e.g., in adverse anatomy) it may even result in actually increased surgical trauma, resulting from excessive traction, unintended rib or/and sternal fracture(s), skin, intercostal nerve, and subcutaneous tissue blunt trauma and ischaemia.

In our opinion, the main difference between the TEAVR and the mini-thoracotomy AVR, regarding the thoracic wall surgical trauma, is not the length of the skin incision (3 cm versus 6 cm), but the absence of rib and/or cartilage division/dislocation, absence or rib spreading, preservation of the Right Internal Thoracic Artery, and protection of the intercostal nerves, skin and subcutaneous tissue. The use of the endoscopic system provides feasibility without the need of rib spreaders and retractors, while the use of automated devices facilitates the procedure and contributes to standardization (Table 8).

Development of the technique was based on expertise in conventional cardiac surgery, followed by minimally invasive approaches, with progressively increasing technical difficulty. Mini-sternotomy was the first step, followed by the right anterior mini-thoracotomy under direct vision, the video assisted right-anterior mini-thoracotomy, and finally the totally endoscopic approach [1–8].

Development of the technique was further based on accumulated collective experience, starting from the pioneering cardiac surgeons who performed minimally invasive procedures in the mid-1990s [26–31] and being continued up to nowadays with innovative surgeons who perform totally endoscopic procedures [58–63].

The learning curve of the totally endoscopic approaches (TE) was long, and involved a process moving from less to more technically demanding operations (repair of ostium secundum atrial septal defect (ASD), cardiac tumor resection, mitral valve repair/replacement, tricuspid valve repair, sinus venosus and ostium primum ASD repair, reoperations, TE Aortic Valve Replacement (AVR) with sutureless prosthesis, TE AVR with conventional prosthesis, and finally totally endoscopic AVR combined with myectomy, edge to edge mitral valve repair, or aortic root enlargement) [1–8, 64].

This analytical and detailed description of the operative steps of the TE RAM µAVR aims to dissemination of our accumulated experience, in order to facilitate reproducibility. Details are always important in cardiac surgery, and become more important when the mistake margin is narrowed in parallel to the narrowed access. Furthermore, standardization of the technique may assist in decreased heterogeneity, and facilitate investigation of the comparative results.

For the time being, the full sternotomy cardiac surgery remains fundamental in the training process, and should be mastered before proceeding to minimally invasive procedures. Minimally invasive approaches and particularly the video assisted right-anterior mini-thoracotomy may represent a stepping stone to reach the totally endoscopic AVR technique.

7 Conclusions

The Totally Endoscopic Aortic Valve Replacement (TEAVR) combines the advantages of a full sternotomy Aortic Valve Replacement with the benefits of a micro invasive access, made possible with the use of enabling technology.

Our drive was to develop a micro invasive surgical technique to meet the demands of the present and the challenges of the future, aiming above all to minimize patients' suffering.

The TEAVR adds to the armamentarium of cardiac surgery the least invasive technique for surgical AVR. It should be viewed as a complementary rather than a competing treatment in relation to other treatment options, including conventional AVR, minimally invasive AVR, and TAVI.

Use of enabling technology provides feasibility (endoscopic system), facilitates the operation (automated suturing, sewing, and suture fastening devices), and contributes to standardization.

Technique standardization, as well as appropriate training and guidance, may counterbalance the increased technical difficulty, contribute to reproducibility and dissemination, and facilitate future comparative studies (Videos 1, 2, and 3).

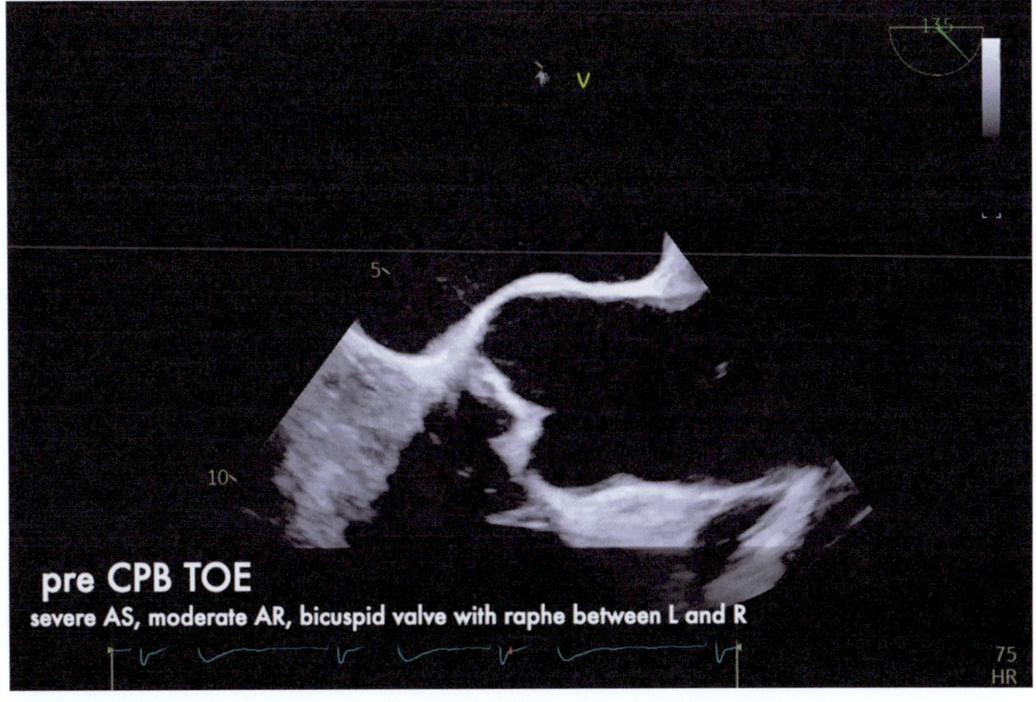

Video 1 TEAVR using an Avulus bioprosthesis (▶ https://doi.org/10.1007/000-a87)

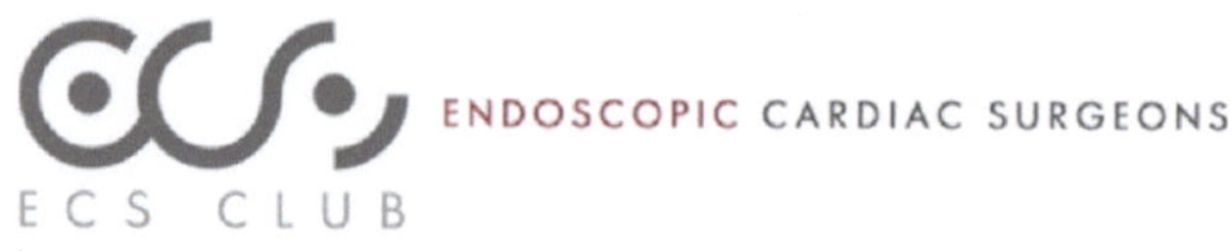

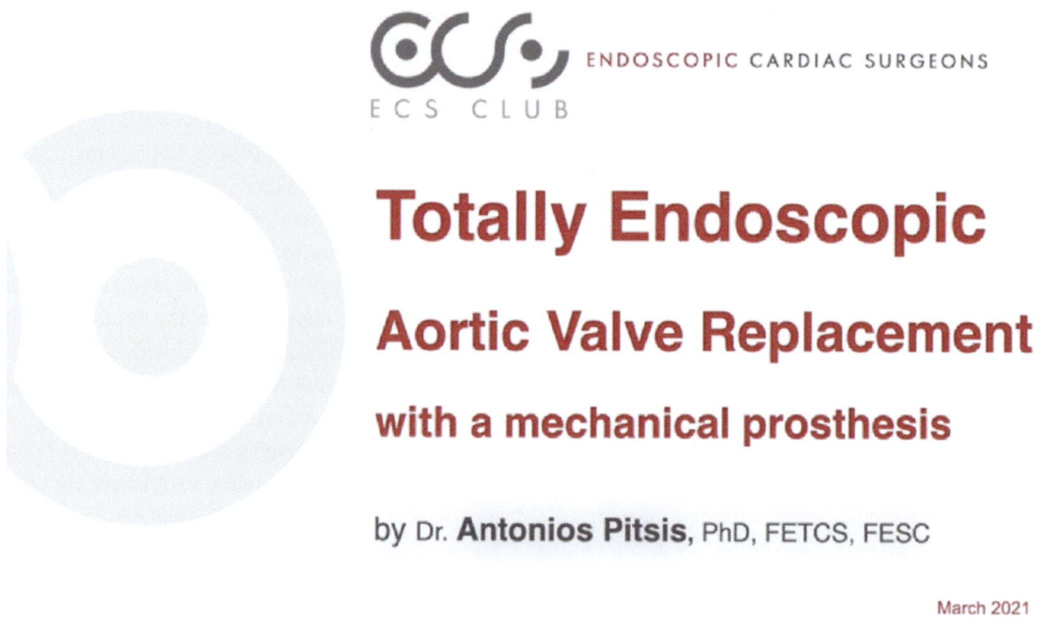
ENDOSCOPIC CARDIAC SURGEONS
ECS CLUB
Totally Endoscopic
Aortic Valve Replacement
with a mechanical prosthesis
by Dr. Antonios Pitsis, PhD, FETCS, FESC
March 2021

Video 2 TEAVR using a mechanical Onyx Prosthesis (▶ https://doi.org/10.1007/000-a86)

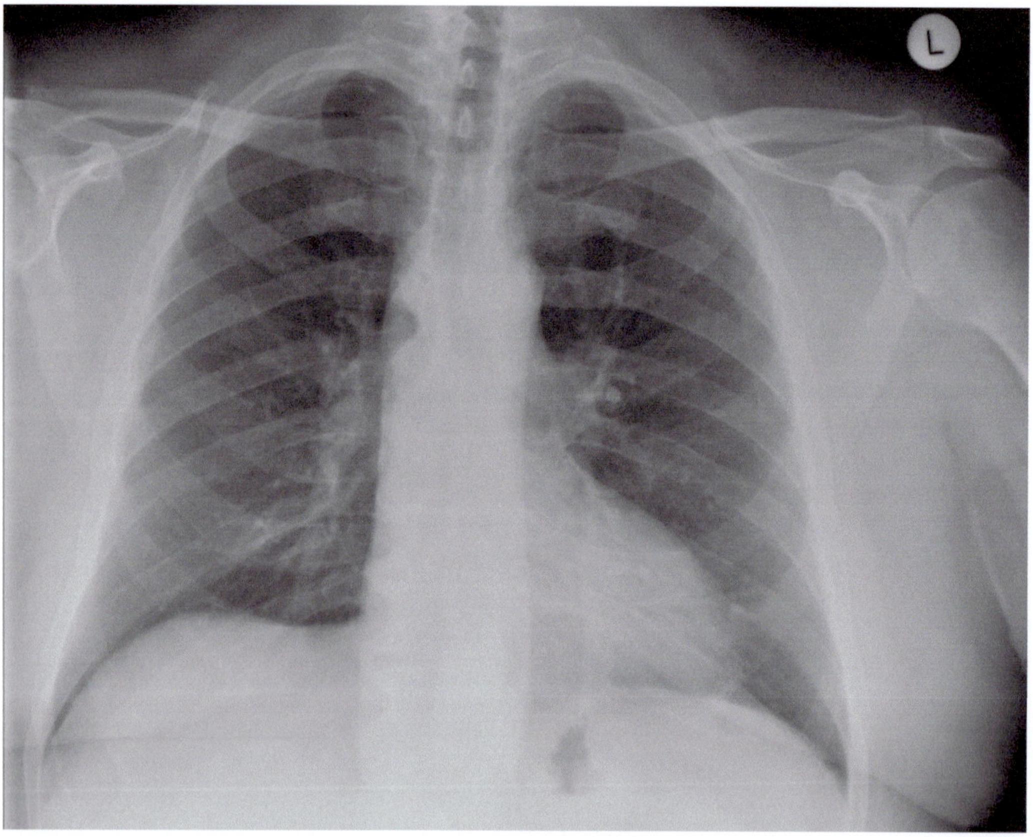
L

Video 3 TEAVR using the RAM device (▶ https://doi.org/10.1007/000-a88)

Disclosures Dr Pitsis is Consultant for teaching and training for Abbott, Medtronic, and LSI SOLUTIONS.

References

1. Pitsis A, Boudoulas H, Boudoulas KD. Operative steps of totally endoscopic aortic valve replacement. Interact Cardiovasc Thorac Surg. 2020;31(3):424. https://doi.org/10.1093/icvts/ivaa102. PMID: 32860037

2. Pitsis A, Tsotsolis N, Nikoloudakis N, et al. Totally endoscopic aortic valve replacement using an automated annular suturing device. March 2020. https://doi.org/10.25373/ctsnet.12024627.

3. Pitsis A, Tsotsolis N, Nikoloudakis N, Keremidis I, Boudoulas H, Boudoulas KD. Totally endoscopic aortic valve replacement and transaortic mitral valve repair. February 2020.https://doi.org/10.25373/ctsnet.11689443.

4. Pitsis A, Tsotsolis N, Nikoloudakis N, Kelpis T, Economopoulos V, Keremidis I. Totally endoscopic aortic valve replacement with a trifecta GT Bovine Pericardial Valve. August 2019https://doi.org/10.25373/ctsnet.9587900.

5. Pitsis A, Tsotsolis N, Nikoloudakis N, Kelpis T, Economopoulos V, Efthimiadis G. Totally endoscopic transaortic septal myectomy for hypertrophic cardiomyopathy. February 2021https://doi.org/10.25373/ctsnet.13681660.

6. Pitsis A, Tsotsolis N, Nikoloudakis N, et al. Totally endoscopic mitral valve repair with predetermined length of synthetic chordae. November 2019.https://doi.org/10.25373/ctsnet.10070126.

7. Pitsis A, Tsotsolis N, Nikoloudakis N, et al. Totally endoscopic redo tricuspid valve repair. June 2019. https://doi.org/10.25373/ctsnet.8199260.

8. Pitsis A, Nikoloudakis N, Tsotsolis N, et al. Totally endoscopic bileaflet mitral valve repair with preformed chordae loops. March 2019. https://doi.org/10.25373/ctsnet.7837853.

9. D'Agostino RS, Jacobs JP, Bardhwar V, et al. The society of thoracic surgeons adult cardiac surgery satabase: 2018 update on outcomes and quality. Ann Thorac Surg. 2018;105:15–23. https://doi.org/10.1016/j.athoracsur.2017.10.035.

10. D'Agostino RS, Jacobs JP, Badhwar V, Fernandez FG, Paone G, Wormuth DW, Shahian DM. The society of thoracic surgeons adult cardiac surgery database: 2019 update on outcomes and quality. Ann Thorac Surg. 2019;107(1):24–32. https://doi.org/10.1016/j.athoracsur.2018.10.004. Epub 2018 Nov 10 PMID: 30423335.

11. Otto CM, Nishimura RA, Bonow RO, Carabello BA, Erwin JP 3rd, Gentile F, Jneid H, Krieger EV, Mack M, McLeod C, O'Gara PT, Rigolin VH, Sundt TM 3rd, Thompson A, Toly C. 2020 ACC/AHA guideline for the management of patients with valvular heart disease: a report of the American College of Cardiology/American Heart Association joint committee on clinical practice guidelines. Circulation. 2021;143(5):e72-e227. https://doi.org/10.1161/CIR.0000000000000923. Epub 2020 Dec 17. Erratum in: Circulation. 2021;143(5):e229. PMID: 33332150.

12. Lichtenstein SV, Cheung A, Ye J, Thompson CR, Carere RG, Pasupati S, Webb JG. Transapical transcatheter aortic valve implantation in humans: initial clinical experience. Circulation. 2006;114 (6):591–6. https://doi.org/10.1161/CIRCULATION AHA.106.632927. Epub 2006 Jul 31 PMID: 1688 0325.

13. Leon MB, Smith CR, Mack M, Miller DC, Moses JW, Svensson LG, Tuzcu EM, Webb JG, Fontana GP, Makkar RR, Brown DL, Block PC, Guyton RA, Pichard AD, Bavaria JE, Herrmann HC, Douglas PS, Petersen JL, Akin JJ, Anderson WN, Wang D, Pocock S; PARTNER Trial Investigators. Transcatheter aortic-valve implantation for aortic stenosis in patients who cannot undergo surgery. N Engl J Med. 2010 Oct 21;363(17):1597–607. https://doi.org/10.1056/NEJMoa1008232. Epub 2010 Sep 22. PMID: 20961243.

14. Kodali SK, Williams MR, Smith CR, Svensson LG, Webb JG, Makkar RR, Fontana GP, Dewey TM, Thourani VH, Pichard AD, Fischbein M, Szeto WY, Lim S, Greason KL, Teirstein PS, Malaisrie SC, Douglas PS, Hahn RT, Whisenant B, Zajarias A, Wang D, Akin JJ, Anderson WN, Leon MB; PARTNER Trial Investigators. Two-year outcomes after transcatheter or surgical aortic-valve replacement. N Engl J Med. 2012;366(18):1686–95. https://doi.org/10.1056/NEJMoa1200384.

15. Adams DH, Popma JJ, Reardon MJ, Yakubov SJ, Coselli JS, Deeb GM, Gleason TG, Buchbinder M, Hermiller J Jr, Kleiman NS, Chetcuti S, Heiser J, Merhi W, Zorn G, Tadros P, Robinson N, Petrossian G, Hughes GC, Harrison JK, Conte J, Maini B, Mumtaz M, Chenoweth S, Oh JK; U.S. CoreValve Clinical Investigators. Transcatheter aortic-valve replacement with a self-expanding prosthesis. N Engl J Med. 2014;370(19):1790–8. https://doi.org/10.1056/NEJMoa1400590. Epub 2014 Mar 29. PMID: 24678937.

16. Popma JJ, Adams DH, Reardon MJ, Yakubov SJ, Kleiman NS, Heimansohn D, Hermiller J Jr, Hughes GC, Harrison JK, Coselli J, Diez J, Kafi A, Schreiber T, Gleason TG, Conte J, Buchbinder M, Deeb GM, Carabello B, Serruys PW, Chenoweth S, Oh JK; CoreValve United States Clinical Investigators. Transcatheter aortic valve replacement using a self-expanding bioprosthesis in patients with severe aortic stenosis at extreme risk for surgery. J Am Coll Cardiol. 2014;63(19):1972–81. https://doi.org/10.1016/j.jacc.2014.02.556. Epub 2014 Mar 19. PMID: 24657695.

17. Mack MJ, Leon MB, Smith CR, Miller DC, Moses JW, Tuzcu EM, Webb JG, Douglas PS, Anderson WN, Blackstone EH, Kodali SK,

Makkar RR, Fontana GP, Kapadia S, Bavaria J, Hahn RT, Thourani VH, Babaliaros V, Pichard A, Herrmann HC, Brown DL, Williams M, Akin J, Davidson MJ, Svensson LG; PARTNER 1 trial investigators. 5-year outcomes of transcatheter aortic valve replacement or surgical aortic valve replacement for high surgical risk patients with aortic stenosis (PARTNER 1): a randomised controlled trial. Lancet. 2015;385(9986):2477–84. https://doi.org/10.1016/S0140-6736(15)60308-7. Epub 2015 Mar 15. PMID: 25788234.

18. Kapadia SR, Leon MB, Makkar RR, Tuzcu EM, Svensson LG, Kodali S, Webb JG, Mack MJ, Douglas PS, Thourani VH, Babaliaros VC, Herrmann HC, Szeto WY, Pichard AD, Williams MR, Fontana GP, Miller DC, Anderson WN, Akin JJ, Davidson MJ, Smith CR; PARTNER trial investigators. 5-year outcomes of transcatheter aortic valve replacement compared with standard treatment for patients with inoperable aortic stenosis (PARTNER 1): a randomised controlled trial. Lancet. 2015;385 (9986):2485–91. https://doi.org/10.1016/S0140-6736 (15)60290-2. Epub 2015 Mar 15. PMID: 25788231.

19. Abdel-Wahab M, Neumann FJ, Mehilli J, Frerker C, Richardt D, Landt M, Jose J, Toelg R, Kuck KH, Massberg S, Robinson DR, El-Mawardy M, Richardt G; CHOICE Investigators. 1-year outcomes after transcatheter aortic valve replacement with balloon-expandable versus self-expandable valves: results from the CHOICE randomized clinical trial. J Am Coll Cardiol. 2015;66(7):791–800. https://doi.org/10.1016/j.jacc.2015.06.026. PMID: 26271061.

20. Deeb GM, Reardon MJ, Chetcuti S, Patel HJ, Grossman PM, Yakubov SJ, Kleiman NS, Coselli JS, Gleason TG, Lee JS, Hermiller JB Jr, Heiser J, Merhi W, Zorn GL 3rd, Tadros P, Robinson N, Petrossian G, Hughes GC, Harrison JK, Maini B, Mumtaz M, Conte J, Resar J, Aharonian V, Pfeffer T, Oh JK, Qiao H, Adams DH, Popma JJ; CoreValve US Clinical Investigators. 3-Year outcomes in high-risk patients who underwent surgical or transcatheter aortic valve replacement. J Am Coll Cardiol. 2016;67(22):2565–74. https://doi.org/10.1016/j.jacc.2016.03.506. Epub 2016 Apr 3. PMID: 27050187.

21. Leon MB, Smith CR, Mack MJ, Makkar RR, Svensson LG, Kodali SK, Thourani VH, Tuzcu EM, Miller DC, Herrmann HC, Doshi D, Cohen DJ, Pichard AD, Kapadia S, Dewey T, Babaliaros V, Szeto WY, Williams MR, Kereiakes D, Zajarias A, Greason KL, Whisenant BK, Hodson RW, Moses JW, Trento A, Brown DL, Fearon WF, Pibarot P, Hahn RT, Jaber WA, Anderson WN, Alu MC, Webb JG; PARTNER 2 Investigators. Transcatheter or surgical aortic-valve replacement in intermediate-risk patients. N Engl J Med. 2016;374(17):1609–20. https://doi.org/10.1056/NEJMoa1514616. Epub 2016 Apr 2. PMID: 27040324.

22. Thourani VH, Kodali S, Makkar RR, Herrmann HC, Williams M, Babaliaros V, Smalling R, Lim S, Malaisrie SC, Kapadia S, Szeto WY, Greason KL, Kereiakes D, Ailawadi G, Whisenant BK, Devireddy C, Leipsic J, Hahn RT, Pibarot P, Weissman NJ, Jaber WA, Cohen DJ, Suri R, Tuzcu EM, Svensson LG, Webb JG, Moses JW, Mack MJ, Miller DC, Smith CR, Alu MC, Parvataneni R, D'Agostino RB Jr, Leon MB. Transcatheter aortic valve replacement versus surgical valve replacement in intermediate-risk patients: a propensity score analysis. Lancet. 2016;387(10034):2218-25. https://doi.org/10.1016/S0140-6736(16)30073-3. Epub 2016 Apr 3. PMID: 27053442.

23. Siemieniuk RA, Agoritsas T, Manja V, Devji T, Chang Y, Bala MM, Thabane L, Guyatt GH. Transcatheter versus surgical aortic valve replacement in patients with severe aortic stenosis at low and intermediate risk: systematic review and meta-analysis. BMJ. 2016;354:i5130. https://doi.org/10.1136/bmj.i5130. PMID: 27683246; PMCID: PMC5040923.

24. Mack MJ, Leon MB, Thourani VH, Makkar R, Kodali SK, Russo M, Kapadia SR, Malaisrie SC, Cohen DJ, Pibarot P, Leipsic J, Hahn RT, Blanke P, Williams MR, McCabe JM, Brown DL, Babaliaros V, Goldman S, Szeto WY, Genereux P, Pershad A, Pocock SJ, Alu MC, Webb JG, Smith CR; PARTNER 3 Investigators. Transcatheter aortic-valve replacement with a balloon-expandable valve in low-risk patients. N Engl J Med. 2019;380 (18):1695–1705. https://doi.org/10.1056/NEJMoa18 14052. Epub 2019 Mar 16. PMID: 30883058.

25. Siontis GCM, Overtchouk P, Cahill TJ, Modine T, Prendergast B, Praz F,et al. Transcatheter aortic valve implantation vs. surgical aortic valve replacement for treatment of symptomatic severe aortic stenosis: an updated meta-analysis. Eur Heart J. 2019;40 (38):3143–3153. https://doi.org/10.1093/eurheartj/ehz275. PMID: 31329852.

26. Cosgrove DM 3rd, Sabik JF. Minimally invasive approach for aortic valve operations. Ann Thorac Surg. 1996;62(2):596–7 PMID: 8694642.

27. Svensson LG. Minimal-access "J" or "j" sternotomy for valvular, aortic, and coronary operations or reoperations. Ann Thorac Surg. 1997;64(5):1501–3. https://doi.org/10.1016/S0003-4975(97)00927-2. PMID: 9386741.

28. Cosgrove DM 3rd, Sabik JF, Navia JL. Minimally invasive valve operations. Ann Thorac Surg. 1998;65 (6):1535–8; discussion 1538–9. https://doi.org/10.1016/s0003-4975(98)00300-2. PMID: 9647054.

29. Tam RK, Almeida AA. Minimally invasive aortic valve replacement via partial sternotomy. Ann Thorac Surg. 1998;65(1):275–6. https://doi.org/10.1016/s0003-4975(97)01204-6. PMID: 9456142.

30. Rao PN, Kumar AS. Aortic valve replacement through right thoracotomy. Tex Heart Inst J. 1993;20(4):307–8. PMID: 8298332; PMCID: PMC325118.

31. Benetti FJ, Mariani MA, Rizzardi JL, Benetti I. Minimally invasive aortic valve replacement. J Thorac Cardiovasc Surg. 1997;113(4):806–7. https://doi.org/10.1016/S0022-5223(97)70246-0. Erratum in: J Thorac Cardiovasc Surg 1997;114(6):947. PMID: 9104997.

32. Sharony R, Grossi EA, Saunders PC, Schwartz CF, Ribakove GH, Baumann FG, Galloway AC, Colvin SB. Propensity score analysis of a six-year experience with minimally invasive isolated aortic valve replacement. J Heart Valve Dis. 2004;13 (6):887–93 PMID: 15597578.

33. Brinkman WT, Hoffman W, Dewey TM, Culica D, Prince SL, Herbert MA, Mack MJ, Ryan WH. Aortic valve replacement surgery: comparison of outcomes in matched sternotomy and PORT ACCESS groups. Ann Thorac Surg. 2010;90(1):131–5. https://doi.org/10.1016/j.athoracsur.2010.03.055. PMID: 20609763.

34. Mariscalco G, Musumeci F. The minithoracotomy approach: a safe and effective alternative for heart valve surgery. Ann Thorac Surg. 2014;97(1):356–64. https://doi.org/10.1016/j.athoracsur.2013.09.090. Epub 2013 Nov 19 PMID: 24263013.

35. Bowdish ME, Hui DS, Cleveland JD, Mack WJ, Sinha R, Ranjan R, Cohen RG, Baker CJ, Cunningham MJ, Barr ML, Starnes VA. A comparison of aortic valve replacement via an anterior right minithoracotomy with standard sternotomy: a propensity score analysis of 492 patients. Eur J Cardiothorac Surg. 2016;49(2):456–63. https://doi.org/10.1093/ejcts/ezv038. Epub 2015 Mar 6. PMID: 25750007; PMCID: PMC4711701.

36. Miceli A, Murzi M, Gilmanov D, Fugà R, Ferrarini M, Solinas M, Glauber M. Minimally invasive aortic valve replacement using right minithoracotomy is associated with better outcomes than ministernotomy. J Thorac Cardiovasc Surg. 2014;148 (1):133–7. https://doi.org/10.1016/j.jtcvs.2013.07.060. Epub 2013 Sep 13 PMID: 24035370.

37. Phan K, Xie A, Tsai YC, Black D, Di Eusanio M, Yan TD. Ministernotomy or minithoracotomy for minimally invasive aortic valve replacement: a Bayesian network meta-analysis. Ann Cardiothorac Surg. 2015;4(1):3–14. https://doi.org/10.3978/j.issn.2225-319X.2014.08.01. PMID: 25694971; PMCID: PMC4311162.

38. Fattouch K, Moscarelli M, Del Giglio M, Albertini A, Comoglio C, Coppola R, Nasso G, Speziale G. Non-sutureless minimally invasive aortic valve replacement: mini-sternotomy versus mini-thoracotomy: a series of 1130 patients. Interact Cardiovasc Thorac Surg. 2016;23(2):253–8. https://doi.org/10.1093/icvts/ivw104. Epub 2016 May 8 PMID: 27160409.

39. Semsroth S, Matteucci Gothe R, Raith YR, de Brabandere K, Hanspeter E, Kilo J, Kofler M, Müller L, Ruttman-Ulmer E, Grimm M. Comparison of two minimally invasive techniques and median sternotomy in aortic valve replacement. Ann Thorac Surg. 2017;104(3):877–83. https://doi.org/10.1016/j.athoracsur.2017.01.095. Epub 2017 Apr 20 PMID: 28433220.

40. Balmforth D, Harky A, Lall K, Uppal R. Is ministernotomy superior to right anterior minithoracotomy in minimally invasive aortic valve replacement? Interact Cardiovasc Thorac Surg. 2017;25 (5):818–21. https://doi.org/10.1093/icvts/ivx241.

41. Seitz M, Goldblatt J, Paul E, Marcus T, Larobina M, Yap CH. Minimally invasive aortic valve replacement via right anterior mini-thoracotomy: propensity matched initial experience. Heart Lung Circ. 2019;28 (2):320–6. https://doi.org/10.1016/j.hlc.2017.11.012. Epub 2017 Dec 7 PMID: 29291961.

42. Aris A, Cámara ML, Montiel J, Delgado LJ, Galán J, Litvan H. Ministernotomy versus median sternotomy for aortic valve replacement: a prospective, randomized study. Ann Thorac Surg. 1999;67(6):1583–7; discussion 1587–8. https://doi.org/10.1016/s0003-4975(99)00362-8. PMID: 10391259.

43. Mächler HE, Bergmann P, Anelli-Monti M, Dacar D, Rehak P, Knez I, Salaymeh L, Mahla E, Rigler B. Minimally invasive versus conventional aortic valve operations: a prospective study in 120 patients. Ann Thorac Surg. 1999;67(4):1001–5. https://doi.org/10.1016/s0003-4975(99)00072-7. PMID: 10320242.

44. Bonacchi M, Prifti E, Giunti G, Frati G, Sani G. Does ministernotomy improve postoperative outcome in aortic valve operation? A prospective randomized study. Ann Thorac Surg. 2002;73(2):460–5; discussion 465–6. https://doi.org/10.1016/s0003-4975(01)03402-6. PMID: 11845860.

45. Dogan S, Dzemali O, Wimmer-Greinecker G, Derra P, Doss M, Khan MF, Aybek T, Kleine P, Moritz A. Minimally invasive versus conventional aortic valve replacement: a prospective randomized trial. J Heart Valve Dis. 2003;12(1):76–80 PMID: 12578340.

46. Moustafa MA, Abdelsamad AA, Zakaria G, Omarah MM. Minimal vs median sternotomy for aortic valve replacement. Asian Cardiovasc Thorac Ann. 2007;15(6):472–5. https://doi.org/10.1177/021849230701500605. PMID: 18042770.

47. Calderon J, Richebe P, Guibaud JP, Coiffic A, Branchard O, Asselineau J, Janvier G. Prospective randomized study of early pulmonary evaluation of patients scheduled for aortic valve surgery performed by ministernotomy or total median sternotomy. J Cardiothorac Vasc Anesth. 2009;23(6):795–801. https://doi.org/10.1053/j.jvca.2009.03.011. Epub 2009 May 17 PMID: 19450991.

48. Borger MA, Moustafine V, Conradi L, Knosalla C, Richter M, Merk DR, Doenst T, Hammerschmidt R, Treede H, Dohmen P, Strauch JT. A randomized multicenter trial of minimally invasive rapid deployment versus conventional full sternotomy aortic valve replacement. Ann Thorac Surg. 2015;99 (1):17–25. https://doi.org/10.1016/j.athoracsur.2014.09.022. Epub 2014 Nov 20 PMID: 25441065.

49. Nair SK, Sudarshan CD, Thorpe BS, Singh J, Pillay T, Catarino P, Valchanov K, Codispoti M,

Dunning J, Abu-Omar Y, Moorjani N, Matthews C, Freeman CJ, Fox-Rushby JA, Sharples LD. Mini-Stern Trial: a randomized trial comparing mini-sternotomy to full median sternotomy for aortic valve replacement. J Thorac Cardiovasc Surg. 2018;156 (6):2124-2132.e31. https://doi.org/10.1016/j.jtcvs. 2018.05.057. Epub 2018 Jun 4 PMID: 30075959.

50. Vukovic PM, Milojevic P, Stojanovic I, Micovic S, Zivkovic I, Peric M, Milicic M, Milacic P, Miloje-vic M, Bojic M. The role of ministernotomy in aortic valve surgery-A prospective randomized study. J Card Surg. 2019;34(6):435–9. https://doi.org/10.1111/jocs. 14053. Epub 2019 Apr 24 PMID: 31017315.

51. Rodríguez-Caulo EA, Guijarro-Contreras A, Guzón A, Otero-Forero J, Mataró MJ, Sánchez-Espín G, Porras C, Villaescusa JM, Melero-Tejedor JM, Jiménez-Navarro M. Quality of life after minister-notomy versus full sternotomy aortic valve replace-ment. Semin Thorac Cardiovasc Surg. 2021 Summer;33(2):328–334. https://doi.org/10. 1053/j.semtcvs.2020.07.013. Epub 2020 Aug 25. PMID: 32853740.

52. Hancock HC, Maier RH, Kasim A, et al. Mini-sternotomy versus conventional sternotomy for aortic valve replacement: a randomized controlled trial. BMJ Open. 2021;11: e041398. https://doi.org/10. 1136/bmjopen-2020-041398.

53. Phan K, Xie A, Di Eusanio M, Yan TD. A meta-analysis of minimally invasive versus conventional sternotomy for aortic valve replacement. Ann Thorac Surg. 2014;98(4):1499–511. https://doi.org/10.1016/ j.athoracsur.2014.05.060. Epub 2014 Jul 24 PMID: 25064516.

54. Kirmani BH, Jones SG, Malaisrie SC, Chung DA, Williams RJ. Limited versus full sternotomy for aortic valve replacement. Cochrane Database Syst Rev. 2017;4(4):CD011793. https://doi.org/10.1002/ 14651858.CD011793.pub2. PMID: 28394022; PMCID: PMC6478148.

55. Chang Chang C, Raza S, Altarabsheh SE, Delozier S, Sharma UM, Zia A, Khan MS, Neudecker M, Markowitz AH, Sabik JF 3rd, Deo SV. Minimally invasive approaches to surgical aortic valve replace-ment: a meta-analysis. Ann Thorac Surg. 2018;106 (6):1881–9. https://doi.org/10.1016/j.athoracsur. 2018.07.018. Epub 2018 Sep 4 PMID: 30189193.

56. Jahangiri M, Hussain A, Akowuah E. Minimally invasive surgical aortic valve replacement. Heart. 2019;105(Suppl 2):s10–5. https://doi.org/10.1136/ heartjnl-2018-313512. PMID: 30846519.

57. Yousuf Salmasi M, Hamilton H, Rahman I, Chien L, Rival P, Benedetto U, Young C, Caputo M, Angelini GD, Vohra HA. Mini-sternotomy vs right anterior thoracotomy for aortic valve replacement. J Card Surg. 2020;35(7):1570–82. https://doi.org/10. 1111/jocs.14607. PMID: 32652784.

58. Vola M, Fuzellier JF, Chavent B, Duprey A. First human totally endoscopic aortic valve replacement: an early report. J Thorac Cardiovasc Surg. 2014;147 (3):1091–3. https://doi.org/10.1016/j.jtcvs.2013.10. 010. Epub 2013 Nov 27 PMID: 24290705.

59. Vola M, Fuzellier JF, Campisi S, Faure M, Bouchet JB, Sandri F, Cler M, Favre JP, Grinberg D. Totally endoscopic aortic valve replacement (TEAVR). Ann Cardiothorac Surg. 20154(2):196-7. https://doi.org/10.3978/j.issn.2225-319X.2014.09.25 . PMID: 25870819; PMCID: PMC4384263.

60. Vola M, Fuzellier JF, Campisi S, Grinberg D, Albertini JN, Morel J, Gerbay A. Total endoscopic sutureless aortic valve replacement: rationale, devel-opment, perspectives. Ann Cardiothorac Surg. 2015;4(2):170–4. https://doi.org/10.3978/j.issn. 2225-319X.2014.11.04. PMID: 25870813; PMCID: PMC4384245.

61. Hinna Danesi T, Salvador L. Minimally invasive aortic valve replacement techniques using endo-scopic surgery: 'must dos' and 'preferences'. Eur J Cardiothorac Surg. 2018 May 1;53(suppl_2):ii27-ii28. https://doi.org/10.1093/ejcts/ezy087. PMID: 29718233.

62. Cresce GD, Sella M, Hinna Danesi T, Favaro A, Salvador L. Minimally Invasive Endoscopic Aortic Valve Replacement: Operative Results. Semin Tho-rac Cardiovasc Surg. 2020 Autumn;32(3):416–423. https://doi.org/10.1053/j.semtcvs.2020.01.002. Epub 2020 Jan 21. PMID: 31972301.

63. Tokoro M, Sawaki S, Ozeki T, Orii M, Usui A, Ito T. Totally endoscopic aortic valve replacement via an anterolateral approach using a standard prosthesis. Interact Cardiovasc Thorac Surg. 2020;30(3):424–30. https://doi.org/10.1093/icvts/ivz287. PMID: 31800039.

64. Pitsis A, Tsotsolis N, Boudoulas H, Boudoulas KD. Totally endoscopic aortic valve replacement with concomitant trans-aortic mitral valve repair for mitral regurgitation. J Cardiothorac Surg. 2021;16(1):318. https://doi.org/10.1186/s13019-021-01694-6. PMID: 34717719; PMCID: PMC8557064.

Endoscopic Repair of Septal Defects

Joseph Zacharias

Abstract

Atrial septal defects were one of the first defects tackled by the pioneers in cardiac surgery some years ago and continue to be one of the most cost effective treatments in both improving a patients quality of life and their longevity. These defects were also one of the early successes of an endoscopic approach partly due to the relative ease of the procedure but also because it affects younger patients more likely to be adversely impacted by the long term cosmetic effects of a sternotomy scar. Many surgeons and teams have published excellent results with this approach and this chapter tries to capture that experience and break down the procedure to the steps that are required to safely offer this approach to patients.

Supplementary Information The online version contains supplementary material available at https://doi.org/10.1007/978-3-031-21104-1_14. The videos can be accessed individually by clicking the DOI link in the accompanying figure caption or by scanning this link with the SN More Media App.

J. Zacharias (✉)
Cardiothoracic Surgeon, Lancashire Cardiac Centre, Blackpool, England
e-mail: drjzacharias@gmail.com

Keywords

Atrial septal defects · Endoscopic surgery · Minimally invasive cardiac surgery · Adult congenital heart surgery

1 Introduction

The repair and closure of septal defects were one of the earliest challenges taken on by the early cardiac surgeons using a multitude of clever solutions like hypothermic baths, parental cross circulation, and eventually cardiac bypass [1]. Congenital heart defects continue to be a burden and affects 0.5% of births [2]. The commonest defects that affect the atrial septum take the form of ostium secundum defects and sinus venous defects. Technically these defects are very attractive to be dealt with by an endoscopic approach but as these procedures are in young and fit patients there is no acceptance of a learning curve and this should be factored in when planning to take on these patients.

As our interventional colleagues get better at closing larger defects with occluders the numbers of these cases coming to surgery are getting fewer. The long term effects of large occluders are still under study and a non sternotomy approach can help some patients decide on a surgical closure based on costs, unknown long term effects and complete closure of defects

J. Zacharias (ed.), *Endoscopic Cardiac Surgery*, https://doi.org/10.1007/978-3-031-21104-1_14

surgically. Some centres and surgeons have noticed increased referrals for surgical ASD closures after offering a endoscopic approach [3]. Most centres do not show any negative impact on outcomes with the obvious cosmetic advantages over a sternotomy approach.

In Blackpool we offered this approach to 26 adults identified with large defects that were not suitable for device closure as deemed by expert interventional cardiologists. We did not see any mortality or morbidity in this group and had some very early discharges home with excellent cosmetic outcomes as reported by the patients. Sadly as an unintended consequence of a national review all simple atrial septal defect surgical closures were moved to designated adult congenital heart defect centres in the UK, many of which do not offer an endoscopic approach, and that has prevented us offering this service until further review. The following points are both based on our experience but also drawing on experience from larger series published in the literature which we reference at the end for further reading.

2 Atrial Septal Defects

See Fig. 1.

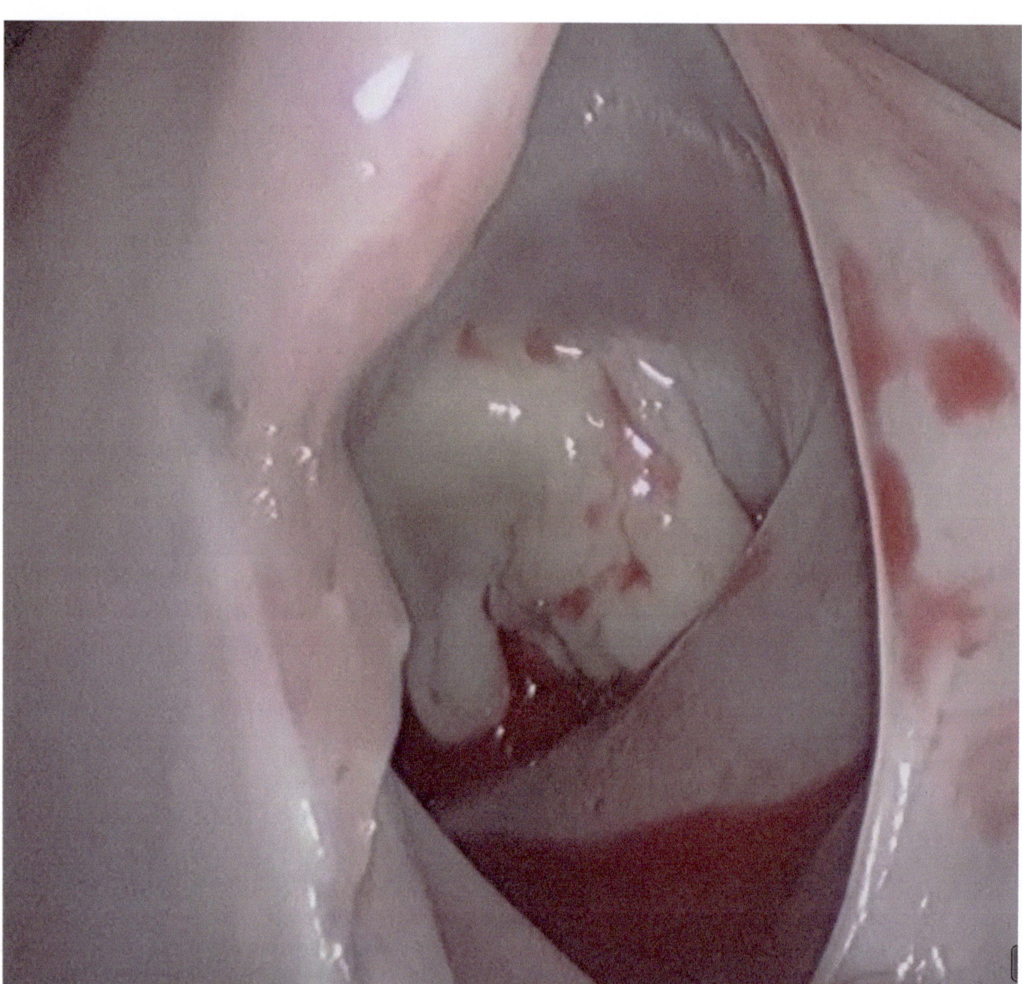

Fig. 1 The view of the mitral valve through a large atrial septal defect

Patient Selection

Most patients are picked up as an incidental finding on an echocardiogram or on auscultation with a systolic flow murmur across the pulmonary valve. Some patients present late in life either with an arrhythmia or due to the effects of tricuspid regurgitation with breathlessness or peripheral oedema. In countries with routine echo screening these defects are picked up early and the recommendation is for these defects to be closed around the age of 4–5 years. The ideal patients at the start of your experience is one with a normal body surface area but with increasing experience and more reliance on an endoscope patients with large body habits benefit most from the smaller incisions. We would recommend considering all patients with simple defects for this approach and referring patients with more complex defects to centres with bigger experience.

Echo: All patients are identified initially on a trans thoracic echo and referred to a specialist cardiologist with a background in dealing with patients with congenital heart defects. The next step is to arrange a trans oesophageal echocardiogram in order to understand the type of septal defect and clearly identify the rim of the defect. This also facilitates exact measurements in case a device is considered as a closure option. We would suggest that these images are reviewed by the surgeon and cardiologist together to agree the type and extent of the septal defect before a decision is made as to how closure is planned.

CT scans: Despite the slight increase in radiation involved with Computerised Tomogram (CT) scans we believe that this is a very useful investigation prior to embarking on an endoscopic approach. Particularly in patients with congenital abnormalities it is important to look carefully at the anatomy in order to rule out any associated changes. Particular interest should be paid to the aorta, the venous anatomy drainage both into the SVC and IVC and a final check of pulmonary venous drainage. Once again the involvement of a dedicated cardiac radiologist with a training in recognising congenital heart defects is highly recommended in order to avoid unpleasant surprises.

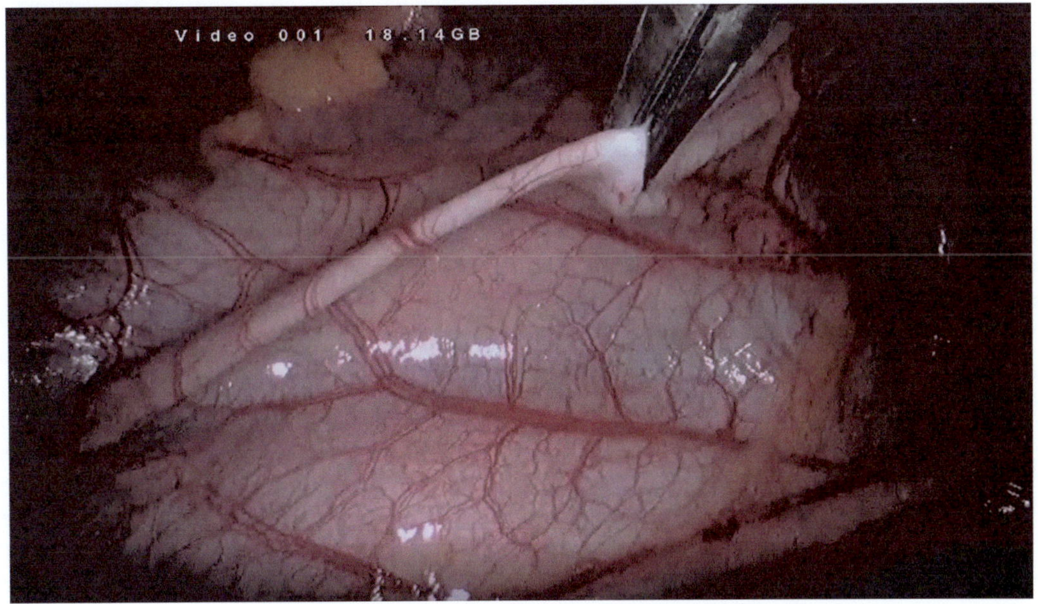

Video 1 Endoscopic repair of an atrial septal defect (▶ https://doi.org/10.1007/000-a8a)

MDT discussions: In the UK following a Adult congenital heart defect review a decision was made that all patients with heart defects should be discussed at a multi disciplinary meeting and the best treatment agreed by the group prior to planning any form of intervention. This is an excellent model and one that has many benefits and is highly recommended. Unfortunately most centres with this multi disciplinary team discussion facility do not have access to surgeons or teams with large endoscopic cardiac surgery experience and this is something that is still being discussed at local and regional centres in the UK. Despite its potential logistic problems we are very supportive of this approach and hope a patient centred decision is reached soon.

Operative planning: With the information available from the TOE and CT scan we are able to decide if the patient has isolated atrial septal defect and the potential size. From the CT scan we can also have a clear plan as to the size of the femoral vessels and the options of an external aortic clamp or an endoclamp which requires a larger femoral cannula. We also rule out any venous abnormalities both with the SVC drainage and the venous anatomy below the diaphragm. The CT scan also gives valuable detail of the possibility of calcification in the heart or the vascular tree.

Positioning: After general anaesthetic and the application of defibrillator pads on the right scapula and the left anterior axillary line, the patient is placed supine and an inflatable bag placed under the 3rd and 4th ribs on the right side. On inflating this bag there is both an elevation of the right chest away from the arm giving more space for the rigid camera and external clamp, and an element of rib spreading that reduces the trauma to intercostal nerves during the passage of instruments.

Pre-operative ultra sound scanning: After anaesthesia we use the available ultra sound machine to scan the femoral vessels and measure the internal diameter as a final check prior to deciding on the size of cannula. This is very useful as often in young patients the femoral

artery is prone to spasm once exposed and if this happens we soak the artery in a swab dipped in a solution of glycerol trinitrate to reverse the spasm prior to cannulation.

Intra operative TOE: We will recommend an experienced individual to review the intra operative TOE as a final check to decide the suitability of an endoscopic approach. In the initial part of the experience it is best to concentrate on ostium secundum defects, but with increasing experience more complicated defects can be dealt with.

Cannulation options: As these patients are often young and have a large shunt from the left to right the venous tree is well developed but the arteries can be small. The pre-operative CT scan along with ultra sound imaging helps decide the largest cannula for the best inflow. If the plan is to use a endobaloon (Intraclude[R] Edwards Lifesciences) the options are a 19fr introducer or a 21 or 23 Fr endoreturn cannula made by Edwards Lifesciences. If the plan is to go with an external aortic clamp then the options for femoral artery cannulation are extensive and the decision based on body surface area and flow characteristics of the cannula. The venous return is best dealt with by a separate cannula in the SVC and IVC in order to snare them during the procedure (See Video 1). Occasionally if there is difficulty getting a SVC cannula into place we have inserted a Biomedical Medtronic 17 fr. cannula through a separate stab incision and snared it over the cannula. This is best attempted after a larger experience with endoscopic procedures.

Myocardial protection: Despite the dilated right sided chambers a short period of cardioplegia is well tolerated by patients. We use cold crystalloid cardioplegia given through an endobaloon but in cases where we use an external cross clamp we use cold blood cardioplegia. There are surgeons and teams that has presented a large series of atrial septal defect closures with a beating heart technique [4, 5]. This needs to be practised with skilled clinicians so that air does not enter the left sided chambers of the heart. We have done all our patients with cardioplegic

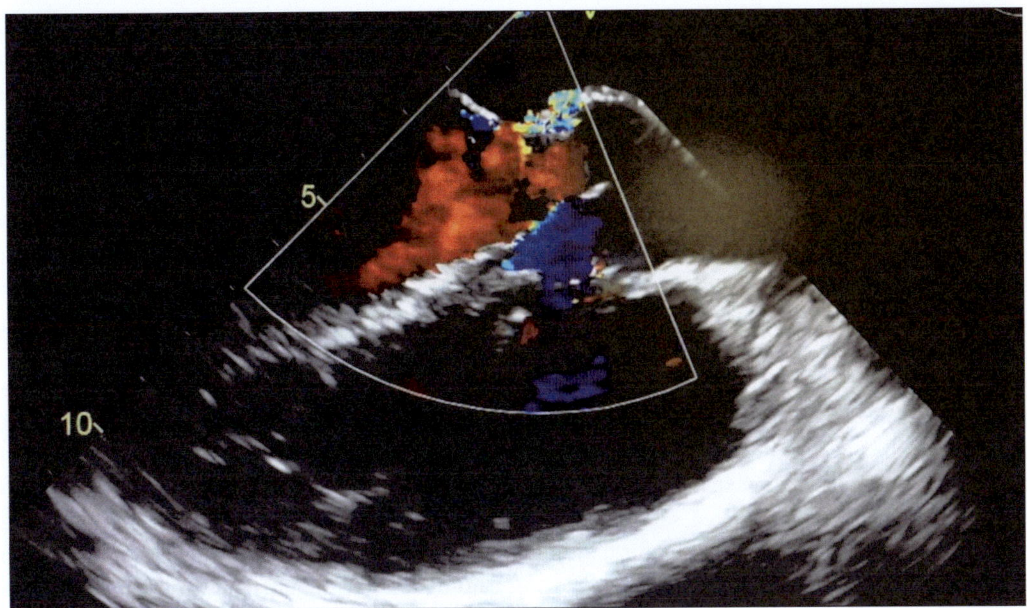

Video 2 Endoscopic repair of a superior Sinus Venosus ASD and tricuspid valve repair
(▶ https://doi.org/10.1007/000-a89)

arrest and have not needed any inotropic support post septal defect closure despite a wide age range. Generally after the completion of the patch closure the right atrium can be closed in two layers with the heart reperfusing with the clamp off. It is best to remove the naval snares so that blood from the coronary sinus can be drained from the IVC line. With increasing experience now we dont snare the IVC routinely but just pull the pipe back into the hepatic portion and this reduces the air as often the Eustachian valve closes off the IVC with vacuum assist.

Patch selection: As most smaller atrial septal; defects are closed using a percutaneous device the ones that reach a surgeon are increasingly large with poor margins and this then requires a patch in order to close the defect. We often start with four 4–0 prolene sutures at the edges of the defect and after passing them through a suitably sized patch we tie the sutures down to convert the defect into four quadrants and run the sutures towards each other leaving the inferior edge to last as this is often the easiest and best defined. There are a whole range of options of type of patch and our preferred choice is a bovine pericardium though there are increasing reports of excellent results with newer materials which are more supple and easier to handle through a small incision. (See Video 2). Once the defect is closed the left lung is bagged and any flow from left to right is looked for. Occasionally an extra mattress suture is required to control the area where flow is identified. Minor suture bleeding is accepted as these do not lead to any significant shunts. After the right atrium is closed with a continue suture technique and reinforced with a second layer we routinely fill the heart to rule out any areas that need further sutures. If the atrial tissue is thinned out pericardial reinforced sutures are used and rarely haemostat agents may be necessary to control needle point bleeding. A drain is left within the pericardium prior to using three interrupted sutures to appose the pericardium prior to weaning off the bypass machine. Both lungs are then reinflated prior to weaning off cardiopulmonary bypass as poor oxygenation is detrimental to right ventricular function and should be avoided. Once the patient is weaned off bypass the cannula are removed and the effects of Heparin are reversed with protamine. This period can be quite unnerving for surgeons who are used to watching the right ventricle and a proxy of the RV function is to watch the Central venous pressure (CVP). If there are any signs of the CVP going up and TOE shows poor RV function a period back on bypass to rest the heart is a safe strategy. If the ASD has a long history and the right ventricle is dilated and there was a need for a concomitant tricuspid valve repair then a small dose of a positive inotrope is useful to protect the right heart for the first few hours until extubation. Our preferred drug is to use dobutamine in small doses to assist the right ventricle. In our limited series we have not required any other form of assist for the right ventricle.

Post-operative pain management: We use local anaesthesia generously either into the wound or sometimes into the rib spaces in order to reduce post operative pain. We do leave a drain in the thoracic cavity through one of the port sites. Most patients have very little pain once the drains are removed and if there is very little bleeding we routinely take both drains out by the end of the first post operative day.

Management of post-operative care: The immediate post operative care of patients with large atrial septal defects needs to focus on avoiding fluid overload as they are used to high right sided filling pressures. A strict protocol for usage of colloids sparingly is important to avoid right ventricular strain with fluid overload. Some patients particularly those who have been on high dose of diuretics pre surgery will need close monitoring of pre-load and after-load of the heart in cardiac intensive care unit. The right ventricle is a very temperamental chamber and if dysfunction sets in it can be very difficult to reverse in the short term. These patients will need close and experienced input for the first 48 h post cardiac surgery. Once they are extubated and there are no concerns of hypoxia related to incision pain they can be mobilised and moved to the ward. Once on the ward we routinely do blood checks and a Chest Xray on day 3

morning. Pacing wires are removed on the third day and if the physiotherapy team are happy with the patients mobility we start to plan for discharge depending on the circumstances at home.

Once discharged we recommend that women wear a sports bra to apply gentle pressure on the right breast in order to prevent any post operative collections of fluid or blood. The sutures that held the drain in are removed on day 5 and as all other sutures are biodegradable there is no further attention to the wounds required.

Post operative follow up is required for these patients and it involves a Chest Xray and ECG at the 6 week review. If patients are self employed and want to go back to work early we arrange to see them at 3–4 weeks and sign them off if all the scars have healed well. All patients have an echo cardiogram at 3 months and if there is no residual leaks they are discharge back to routine cardiology follow up. We have had one patient with a small remnant leak from the suture line and this was easily dealt with with a percutaneous amplatzer device deployment at 1 year after the initial procedure. The group in Leipzig have published on a subgroup of patients that needed surgery after percutaneous closure [6] and these two techniques need to be seen as collaborative approaches picking the appropriate patient for the procedure.

As we see these patients in Blackpool as adults a proportion of our patients required a mitral and a tricuspid valve repair. All four patients that needed mitral valve surgery had the approach through the atrial septal defect and the view is excellent as seen in Fig. 1. The tricuspid valve is nearly always done with the heart reperfusing and as the atrial septal defect is already closed there is no danger of air bubbles being trapped into the left heart. Most often the tricuspid annulus is dilated and all that is required is an undersized annuloplasty ring.

We have dealt twice with superior sinus atrial septal defects and once recognised can be dealt with an endoscopic approach safely. The key dissection is to snare the SVC above the opening of the superior pulmonary vein and this can be tricky as the space between the azygos opening can be tight. We use a bull dog clamp to control this area (Video 2) and that fits into the narrow space easily. We use a double patch technique as recommended and use a small patch to close the atrial septal defect while baffling the blood from the superior pulmonary vein towards the left atrium and a second larger patch to widen the superior vena cava connection to the right atrium.

With increasing experience dealing with simple ventricular septal defects through the tricuspid valve can also be a rewarding approach. We have used this approach twice for remnant defects after post infarct ventricular septal defect closures. We are aware of other surgeons with a large experience of using endoscopic approaches to dealing with ventricular septal defects. (see recommended reading).

Tips:

We recommend the use of cerebral oximetry for any procedure that involves SVC cannulation in order to keep a watch on potential kinking or occlusion of the cannula causing cerebral venous congestion.

After patch closure of the ASD we always gently introduce the IVC cannula to make sure that the Eustatian valve and IVC are freely open into the right atrium.

Tricks:

If a neck cannula cannot be placed then once the snares are placed around the SVC a 15 or 17 French cannula can be passed through a small stab incision in the 2nd or 3rd space inserted into the SVC through an open atriotomy or with a Seldinger technique directly into the SVC. At the end the small entry point can be oversewn with a proline suture.

Cooling the patient and dropping the flow for 60–90 s will give enough time to put crucial sutures in case of excessive venous return obscuring visibility.

In a redo setting the tricuspid annulus hangs off the sternum and this makes most of the circumference of the tricuspid annulus visible for suturing even if the vena cavae are not snared. Sutures along the septal leaflet will need a period of reduced inflow.

Traps:

Beware other congenital abnormalities that may co exist with the septal defects. The common ones are Coarctation of the aorta, Bicuspid aortic valves, Vascular abnormalities of the aorta or venous system, Possible left SVC which should change the neck cannulation strategy.

The common femoral artery can be very likely for spasm in young patients and bypass should be established very slowly. If there is any concern with high line pressures that do not subside with vasodilator infusion, then a contralateral femoral cannula is recommended to achieve full bypass.

A left SVC will need a suction cannula placed into the lumen to deal with the venous return and possibly a purse string and snugger to prevent overflow.

We recommend a short period to identify the coronary sinus and the Eustation valve within the right atrium before closing the atrial septal defect as both these structures can get caught up in the closure and cause clinical problems later if missed.

References

1. Alexi-Meskishvili VV, Konstantinov IE. Surgery for atrial septal defect: from the first experiments to clinical practice. Ann Thorac Surg. 2003;76(1):322–7. https://doi.org/10.1016/s0003-4975(03)00508-3. PMID: 12842577.
2. Mylonas KS, Ziogas IA, Evangeliou A, Hemmati P, Schizas D, Sfyridis PG, Economopoulos KP, Bakoyiannis C, Kapelouzou A, Tzifa A, Avgerinos DV. Minimally invasive surgery vs device closure for atrial septal defects: a systematic review and meta-analysis. Pediatr Cardiol. 2020;41(5):853–61. https://doi.org/10.1007/s00246-020-02341-y. Epub 2020 Mar 11 PMID: 32162027.
3. Schneeberger Y, Schaefer A, Conradi L, Brickwedel J, Reichenspurner H, Kozlik-Feldmann R, Detter C. Minimally invasive endoscopic surgery versus catheter-based device occlusion for atrial septal defects in adults: reconsideration of the standard of care. Interact Cardiovasc Thorac Surg. 2017;24(4):603–8. https://doi.org/10.1093/icvts/ivw366.
4. Ma Z-S, Dong M-F, Yin Q-Y, Feng Z-Y, Wang L-X. Totally thoracoscopic closure for atrial septal defect on perfused beating hearts. Eur J Cardiothorac Surg. 2012;41(6):1316–9. https://doi.org/10.1093/ejcts/ezr193.

5. Dang QH, Le NT, Nguyen CH, et al. Totally endoscopic cardiac surgery for atrial septal defect repair on beating heart without robotic assistance in 25 patients. Innovations (Phila). 2017;12(6):446–52. https://doi.org/10.1097/IMI.0000000000000436.
6. Walther T, Binner C, Rastan A, Dähnert I, Doll N, Falk V, Mohr FW, Kostelka M. Surgical atrial septal defect closure after interventional occluder placement: incidence and outcome. J Thorac Cardiovasc Surg. 2007;134(3):731–7. https://doi.org/10.1016/j.jtcvs.2007.04.041. Epub 2007 Jul 20 PMID: 17723825.

Further Recommended Viewing

7. Abdelbar A, Laswaski G, Zacharias J. An endoscopic solution to a residual postinfarct ventricular septal defect. December 2019https://doi.org/10.25373/ctsnet.11310929.
8. ECSClub Youtube channel: https://www.youtube.com/watch?v=jDS84IfbN6M.

Multi-vessel Endoscopic Coronary Artery Bypass Grafting

Alaaddin Yilmaz, Jade Claessens, and Abdullah Kaya

Abstract

Coronary artery bypass grafting (CABG) is the most commonly performed cardiac surgery since its introduction in 1968. In the years that followed, research focused on reducing the surgical trauma caused by the median sternotomy. To make the surgery less invasive, smaller incisions in the chest were used, eventually leading to totally endoscopic surgery. In this case, the entire procedure is performed through endoscopic ports. The most common way to perform totally endoscopic CABG is robotically assisted surgery which is more expensive and time-consuming that other types of minimally invasive cardiac surgery. An alternative technique is using endoscopic instruments to perform CABG which is called endo-CABG. This technique is proven to be a safe and effective procedure for multi-vessel coronary artery disease without patient selection. During endo-CABG, the mammary arteries are chosen as conduits for grafting to avoid the need for proximal anastomoses. In this way, no manipulation of the ascending aorta is needed (no touch). The mammary arteries are harvested using three endoscopic ports in a triangular configuration. Additionally, a utility port of 3–4 cm is made to perform the anastomosis. When the patient has three vessel disease, a Y-graft construction is created intrathoracically by performing an end to side anastomosis of the free right internal mammary artery to the in situ left internal mammary artery. An overview of multi-vessel coronary bypass grafting using endoscopic instruments is explained in this chapter, including a step-by-step explanation.

Keywords

Endoscopic on pump CABG · Bilateral mammary artery harvesting · No touch CABG · Total arterial endo grafting

Supplementary Information The online version contains supplementary material available at https://doi.org/10.1007/978-3-031-21104-1_15. The videos can be accessed individually by clicking the DOI link in the accompanying figure caption or by scanning this link with the SN More Media App.

A. Yilmaz (✉) · J. Claessens · A. Kaya
Jessa Hospital, Stadsomvaart 11, Hasselt, Belgium
e-mail: alaaddin.Yilmaz@jessazh.be

J. Claessens · A. Kaya
UHasselt - Hasselt University, Martelarenlaan 42, 3500 Hasselt, Belgium

Since the introduction in the 1960s, coronary artery bypass grafting (CABG) is the most commonly performed cardiac surgery [1]. In 1964, Vasilli I. Kolesov performed the first sutured internal mammary artery coronary anastomosis through a median sternotomy [2]. After this surgery, the symptoms of coronary artery disease, chest pain and shortness of breath, were relieved in these patients [3]. However, according to the European Association for Cardio-Thoracic Surgeons (EACTS) database, several procedural risks such as atrial fibrillation, cerebrovascular accidents (CVA) and myocardial infarction after CABG can occur [1]. Due to morbidity and mortality of the median sternotomy, the focus on research in the field of cardiac surgery was to reduce the surgical trauma by using smaller incisions in the chest and, in this way, making the surgery less invasive. Starting from 1994, some centres performed minimally invasive CABG through a left mini-thoracotomy using video-assisted left internal mammary artery (LIMA) harvesting, also called minimally invasive direct coronary artery bypass (MIDCAB) [4, 5].

The surgical trauma was reduced even more by the use of totally endoscopic surgery [6]. In totally endoscopic CABG (TECAB), the entire procedure is performed without any surgical incision, only using access through endoscopic ports. Robotically assisted TECAB is the most common way to perform a TECAB nowadays, but it is more expensive and time-consuming than other types of minimally invasive cardiac surgery [7].

Some centres use endoscopic instruments to perform CABG. This alternative technique has the advantage of being less expensive but is technically more challenging with a steep learning curve. Generally, TECAB is proven to have an acceptably low operative risk. The pooled event rate for operative mortality in 16 studies was 0.80% [8]. Recently, Yilmaz et al. introduced a newly developed endoscopic CABG (endo-CABG) method, using endoscopic instruments [9]. The results showed that endo-CABG is a safe and effective procedure for treating single- and multi-vessel coronary artery disease without patient selection. In this chapter, the multi-vessel endo-CABG technique will be explained step-by-step.

1 Anesthesiological Preparation

The patient is placed in a supine position on the operating table. All patients receive external defibrillating pads, as well as diathermy and electrocardiogram pads. Like a conventional CABG procedure, the patient is lined up with a peripheral intravenous line, a radial artery line, and after induction of general anesthesia, a single lumen intratracheal tube, a urinary catheter and an internal jugular vein line is introduced. Also, near-infrared oxygenation monitoring pads (NIRO) are placed at the frontal area of the head of the patient, and a transesophageal echocardiography (TEE) probe is inserted (Fig. 1).

2 Position of the Endoscopic ports

Arrangement of the access ports is crucial for endoscopic surgery. The 2nd, 3rd and 4th intercostal spaces are used to introduce the 5 mm endoscopic ports. The first port is introduced approximately 2 cm below the anterior axillary line in the 3rd intercostal space and is used for the 0-degree endoscope (5 mm, Karl Storz, Tuttlingen, Germany). During the introduction of this initial port, the ventilation is stopped for a short moment, the port is introduced, and CO2 is insufflated through the side-port of this endoscopic port and ventilation is restarted. To create an adequate working space and avoid selective lung ventilation, a CO_2-induced controlled pneumothorax (6–8 mmHg) is applied. The other ports are introduced approximately 2 cm *above* the anterior axillary line in the 2nd and 4th intercostal spaces and are the working ports. These three ports form a triangular configuration (Fig. 2).

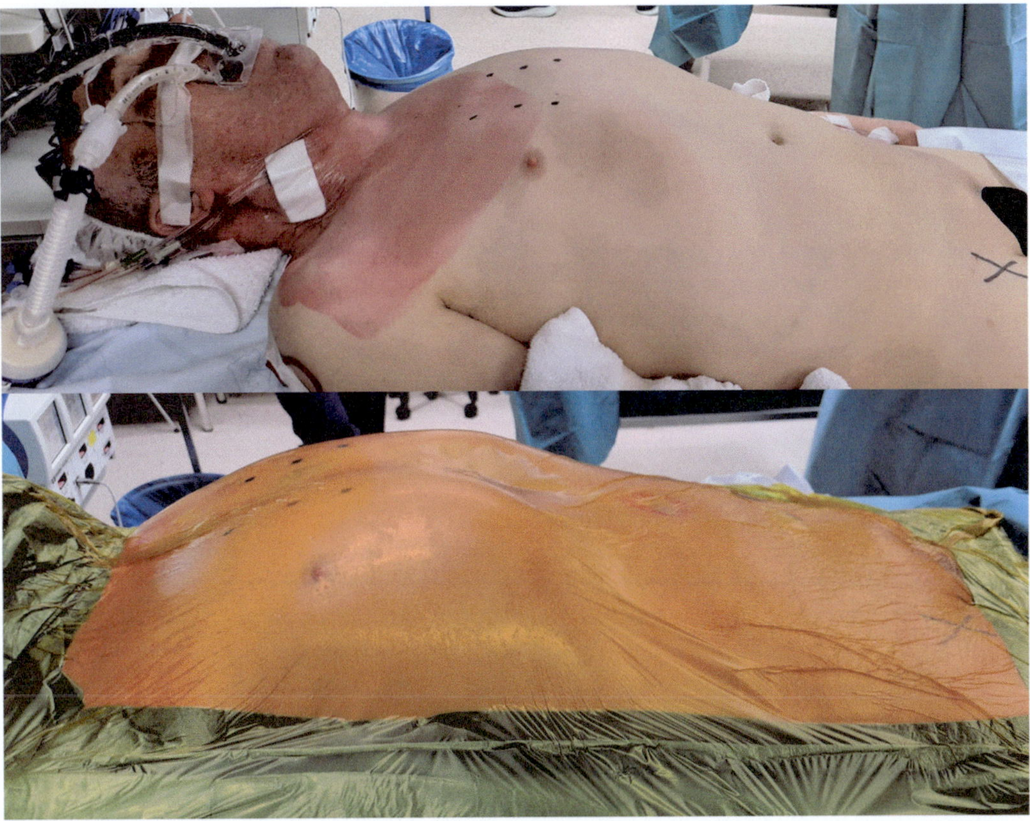

Fig. 1 Supine position of the patient on the operating table before and after sterile drapes

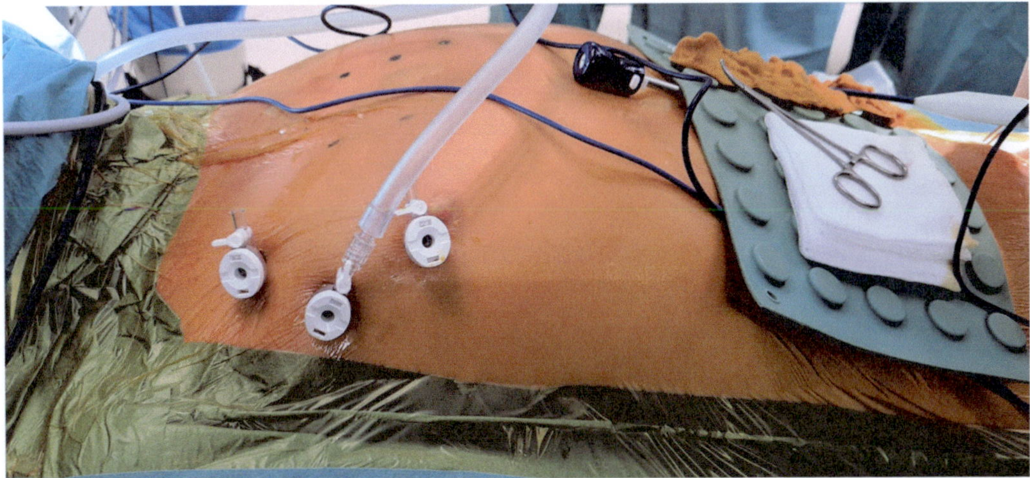

Fig. 2 Position of the endoscopic ports

3 Endoscopic Mammary Artery Harvesting

The 3 endoscopic ports and CO_2 insufflation provide enough working space in the pleural cavity. When the right internal mammary artery (RIMA) is needed as a graft, the three endoscopic ports are placed on the right thoracic side, as described above. Long-shafted instruments are used like an endo grasping forceps and a 34-cm long-shafted diathermia (Fig. 3). Initially, the right phrenic nerve is identified and preserved. The pericardium is opened diathermically in a vertical fashion to get full exposure of the ascending aorta. Consecutively, the fascia on the RIMA is opened in full length and admission of gentle traction and short diathermia use facilitates harvesting the RIMA with its pedicle (Fig. 4). Side branches of the RIMA are clipped with a small endoscopic clip-applicator (Fig. 5). Harvesting the RIMA or LIMA endoscopically is preferred pedicled to prevent damage or severe spasm to the mammary artery. Next, the anterior mediastinum is opened to the left pleural space. On the left thoracic side three endoscopic ports are introduced, as described above. Again, the left phrenic nerve is identified and preserved. Any major fat pads on the left-sided pericardium are removed, and the pericardium is opened in full length 2–3 cm above the phrenic nerve. The LIMA is harvested as described above for the RIMA. After completing the dissection, heparin is given to the patient (300 IU/kg), and the LIMA is clipped and transected after its distal bifurcation. It is important to fixate the LIMA and/or the RIMA to the pericardium with a clip to prevent torsion of it.

4 Groin Vessel Cannulation

While harvesting the mammary arteries, the groin vessels can be prepared for cannulation. We prefer the left groin vessels because of the position of the heart–lung machine. A 2–3 cm oblique skin incision below the inguinal ligament is made in the left groin. De common femoral artery and vein are exposed using forceps and diathermia. It is important to dissect the vessels lengthwise to avoid excessive lymph node/vessel damage and postoperative lymphedema. With digital palpation, we detect any calcification of the left common femoral artery. A purse-string with a prolene 5–0 is placed on each vessel. After heparin administration, the Seldinger method is used to cannulate. The artery is punctured with a needle, and a guidewire is advanced in the thoracic aorta and confirmed on TEE. After pre dilatation, a 17–21 Fr arterial cannula (Bio-medicus, Medtronic Inc., Minneapolis, MN, USA), depending on the patient's size and thus on the magnitude of ECC flow needed, is inserted. The common femoral vein is thereafter punctured with a needle, and the guidewire is advanced in the superior caval vein and confirmed on TEE, and a 21–25 Fr multi-stage drainage venous cannula (Bio-medicus, Medtronic Inc., Minneapolis, MN, USA) is introduced (Fig. 6). Cardiopulmonary bypass (CPB) with retrograde perfusion is achieved using a minimally invasive ECC system [the mini-Inspire JESSA MiECC (Sorin S.p.A., Mirandola, Italy)] [10]. In case of severe calcification of the common femoral arteries or the iliac arteries, we prefer to cannulate the right subclavian artery.

5 Mini-Thoracotomy

The selection of the exact intercostal space for the mini-thoracotomy is based on the location of the target coronary vessel. This is achieved by simple transthoracic needle insertion through the selected space under endoscopic vision (Fig. 7). The 2nd and 3rd intercostal spaces close to the midline are mainly selected. A final 5 mm endoscopic port is inserted subxyphoidal under endoscopic vision and is necessary in a later phase of the operation. A 3–4 cm skin incision is made through the selected intercostal space, the pectoral muscle is divided in line of the muscle fibres and a soft tissue retractor (Shanghai International Holding Corporation GmbH,

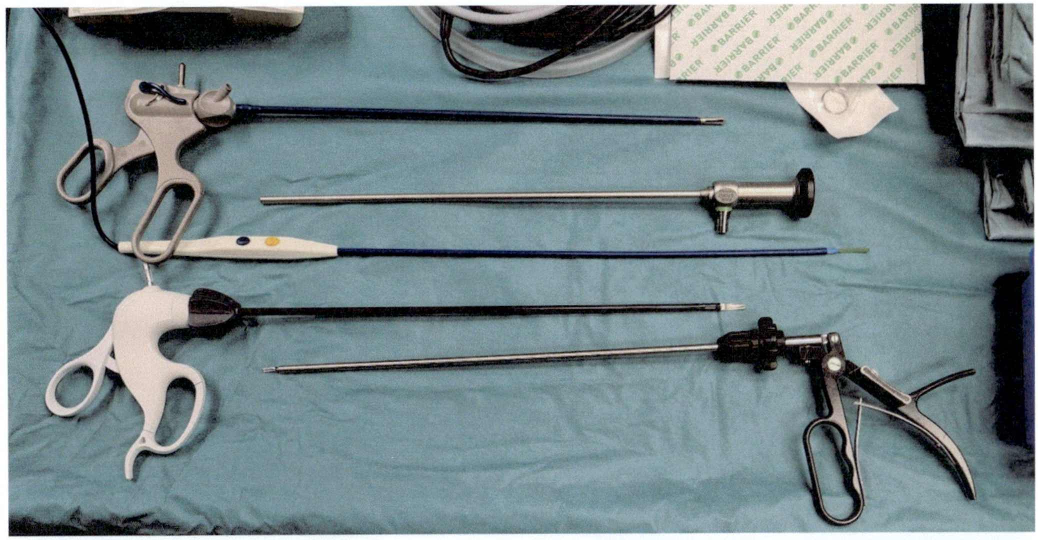

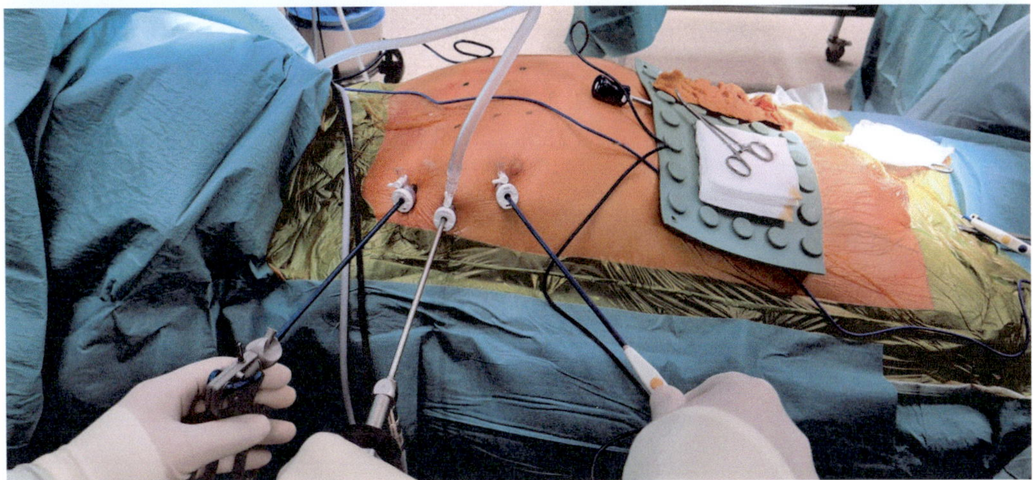

Fig. 3 Long-shafted instruments from top till down: endo grasping forceps, 0-degree endoscopic lens, long-shafted diathermia, endo scissors, a small endoscopic clip-applicator and their positions through the ports

Hamburg, Germany) is placed to enable a sufficient view of the heart (Fig. 8). In case of a large intercostal space (thickness digit 2 of the operator), no rib spreader is necessary. In all other cases, a low profile rib spreader (Mini-access retractor, Delacroix-Chevalier, Paris, France) is used (Fig. 9). Subsequently, the transected end of the mammary artery is brought extracorporeal through the mini-thoracotomy and injected intraluminal with papaverine fluid. Care is specially taken not to twist the pedicle, and this can be realised by marking the correct side of the pedicle with a prolene 6–0 (Fig. 10).

6 Cardioplegia Catheter

Patients undergoing single vessel LIMA to the left anterior descending (LAD) artery bypass are placed on MiECC CPB to decompress the heart but do not receive cardioplegia. All multi-vessel endo-CABG's are done under cardioplegic arrest of the heart. The three ports on the right thoracic wall and the mini-thoracotomy is used to place a pledged ticron 2–0 purse-string suture for antegrade cardioplegia. The location of this suture is near the fat rim of the ascending aorta. An

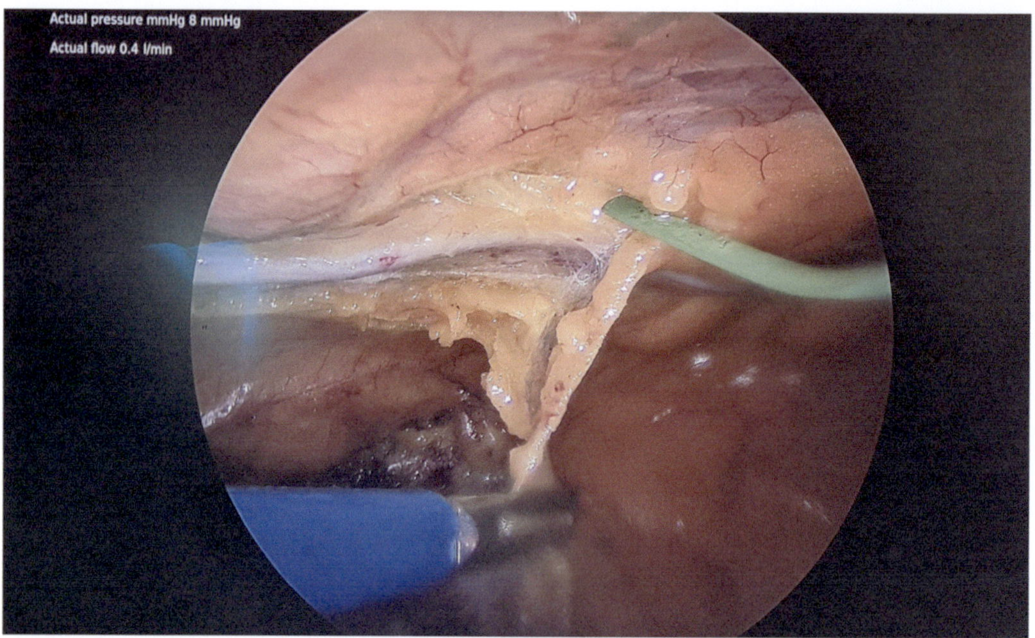

Fig. 4 Opening the fascia on the RIMA in full length

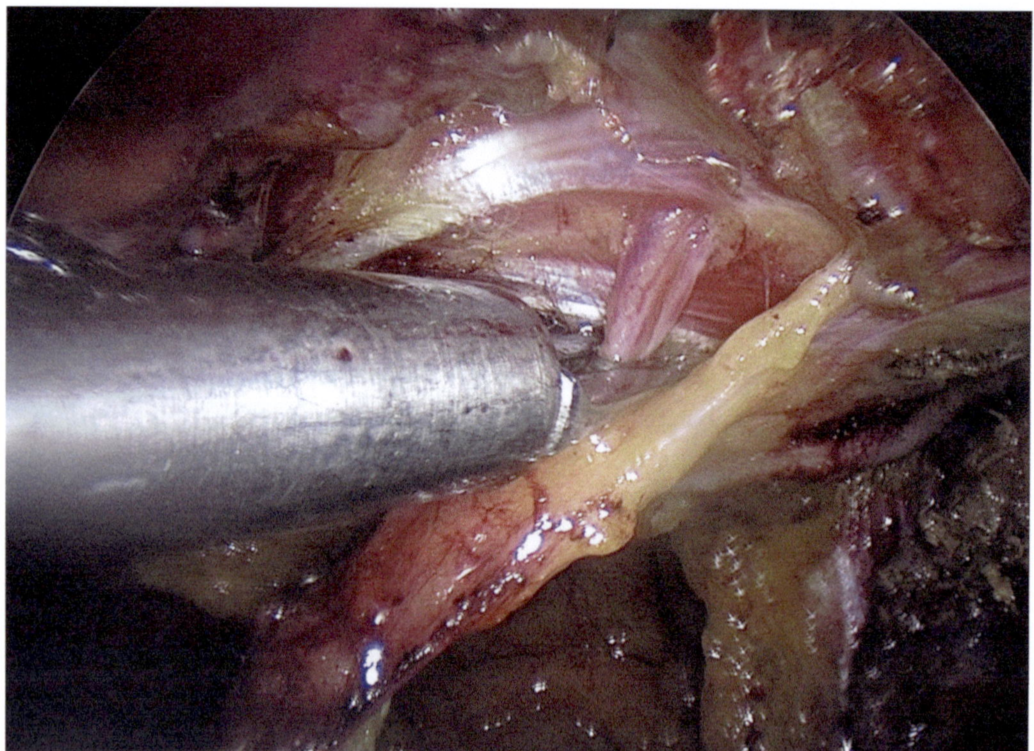

Fig. 5 Clipping a side branche of the RIMA with a small endoscopic clip-applicator

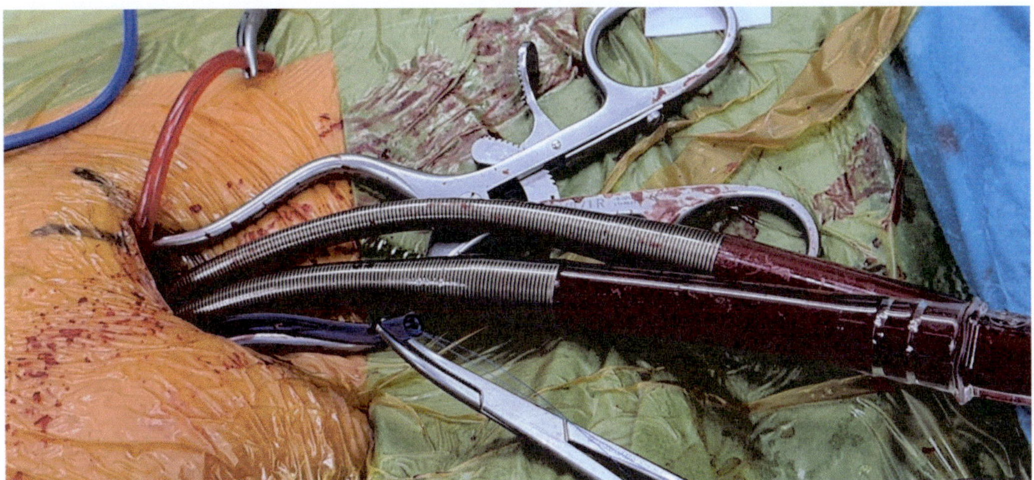

Fig. 6 Cannulated left groin vessels with on top the arterial cannula

endoscopic grasping forceps and an endoscopic needle holder is used to perform this (Fig. 11). To select the correct intercostal space for the transthoracic cardioplegia catheter (14G Argon Secalon-TTM, Singapore, Pte. Ltd., Singapore) is, again, by simple transthoracic needle insertion under endoscopic vision. The cardioplegia catheter is positioned transthoracic but not yet inserted in the aorta. After removing the port in the 2nd intercostal space, the transthoracic aortic clamp is introduced. By gentle manipulation of the aorta with a blunt endoscopic suction device, the transthoracic aortic clamp is placed fully over the distal ascending aorta, and the cardioplegia catheter is inserted in the aorta in the middle of the purse-string (Fig. 12). Cardioplegia is infused, and the heart is arrested. We prefer a single shot of cold (8°Celsius) mixed blood cardioplegia (blood:crystalloid 3:1, Fresenius Kabi, Schelle, Belgium). Afterwards, this cardioplegia catheter is used for venting the aortic root, achieving a totally empty heart.

7 Mobilising the Heart

All target coronary vessels, including the right coronary artery, can be visualized and reached by gentle manipulation of the empty heart by a subxyphoid introduced endoscopic clamp holding a peanut gauze and a clamp with a peanut used through the mini-thoracotomy (Fig. 13). With gentle movements, the heart can be mobilised towards the mini-thoracotomy with these two atraumatic instruments. It is essential to have already opened the pericardium on the left side in full length for comfortable manipulation of the heart. After positioning the heart in the way that the target vessel is fully exposed via the mini-thoracotomy, the subxyphoid endoscopic clamp is fixed in that position with an instrument holder attached to the operating table (Fig. 14). Additional epicardial stay sutures with prolene 6–0 laterally to the target vessels are used when necessary. To visualize and anastomose target vessels on the anterior wall, the heart has to be gently pushed cranially. For the lateral wall, the empty heart has to be pushed up and tilted to the midline. When the posterior descending artery needs to be anastomosed, the inferior wall of the empty heart has to be pushed cranially.

8 Coronary Artery Anastomosis Technique

Anastomoses with LIMA and/or RIMA are performed through the mini-thoracotomy in a typical fashion using a normal Castroviejo needle-holder and forceps. The suturing technique is the

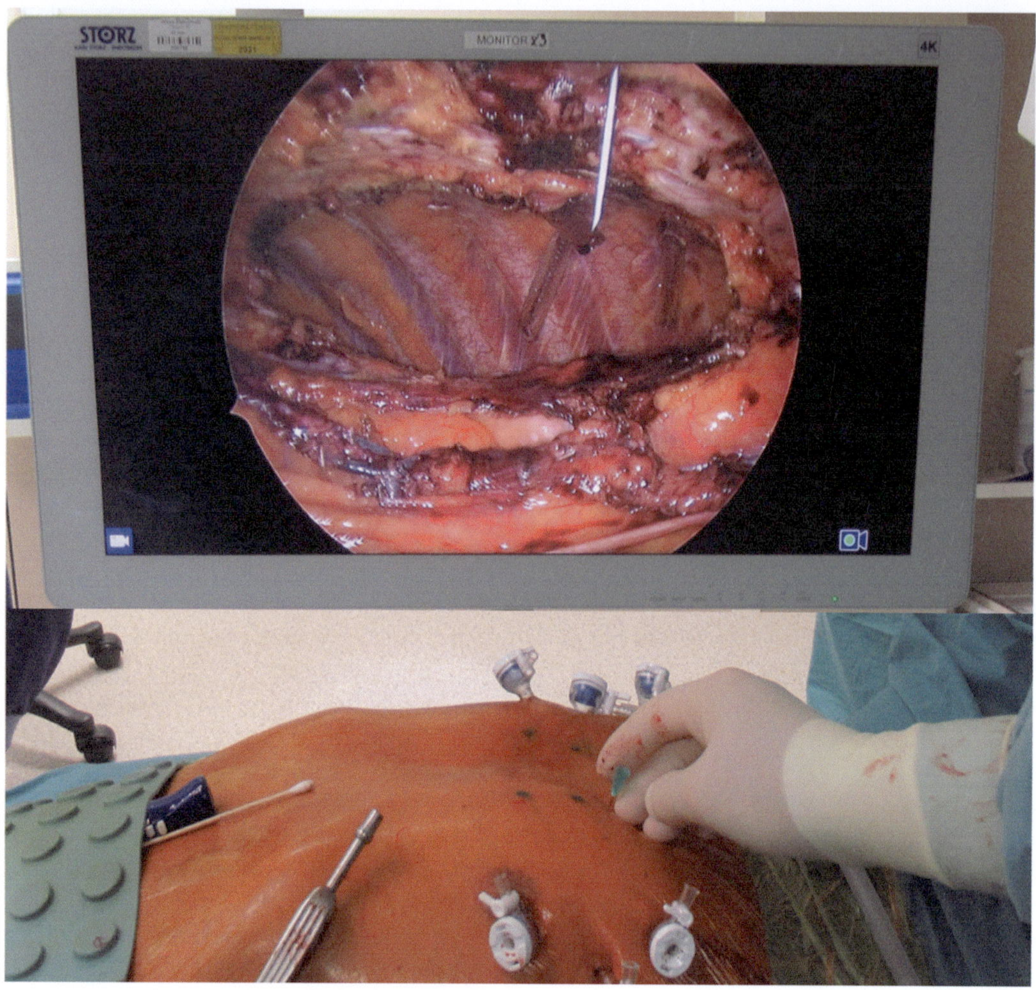

Fig. 7 Selection of the exact intercostal space for the mini-thoracotomy is by simple transthoracic needle insertion through the selected space under endoscopic vision

same as in open surgery, namely a running 8–0 suture (Fig. 15). When necessary, a Y-graft construction is created intrathoracically by performing an end to side anastomosis of free RIMA to in situ LIMA through the mini-thoracotomy utility port (Fig. 16). An intracoronary shunt can be used to create a blood-free operative field in case of back bleeding. After completing the anastomoses, the temporary clamp on the LIMA and/or RIMA is released, and the grafts are checked for leakage or possible twists or distensions. When this is not the case, the heart is returned to its natural position in the pericardium. Care is taken that the LIMA or RIMA does not get caught at the edge of the pericardial opening while descending the heart intrapericardial by pulling the pericardium laterally with a forceps. Subsequently, the aortic clamp is released and the cardioplegia catheter removed, and its suture tied down with an automated fastener device (Cor-knot®, LSI Solutions, NY, USA) (Fig. 17). The pericardium on the left side is always closed by separated sutures, leaving only the entrance space for the LIMA or RIMA.

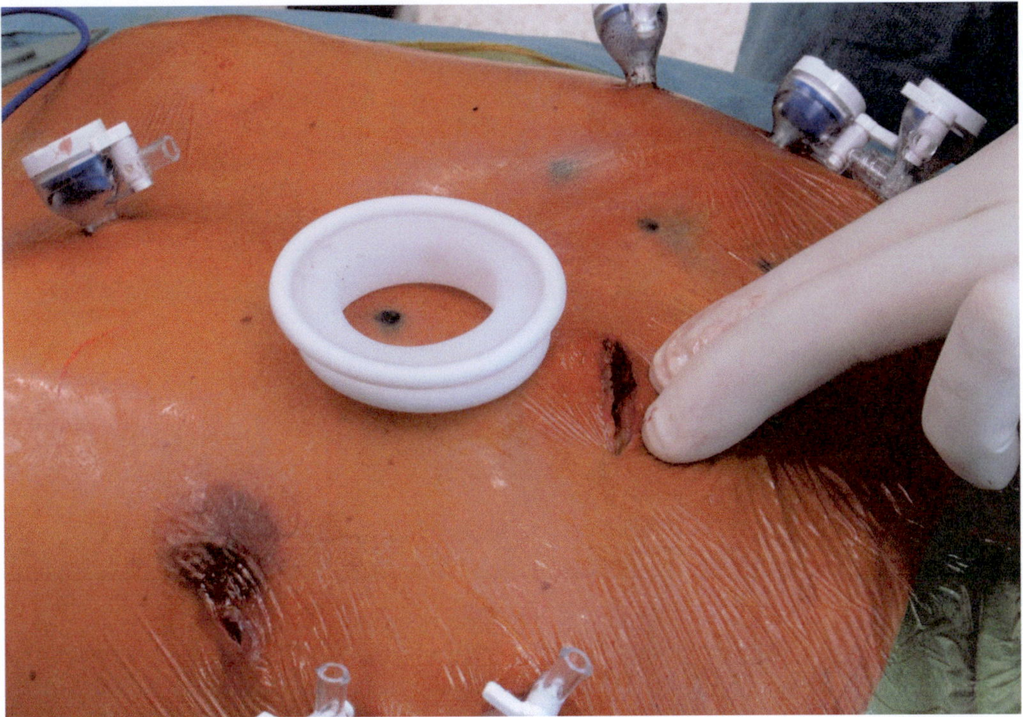

Fig. 8 Left sided mini-thoracotomy skin incision with a soft tissue retractor

9 Weaning from CPB

While the heart is regaining its rhythm, the thoracic port wounds are coagulated for haemostasis. Pericardial drainage is only used when necessary. Chest tubes are placed in both thoracic cavities with negative suction (−15 cm water). When a retractor is used, a local pain catheter (Pajunk SonoLong Echo NanoLine® 19G x 60 mm, Geisingen, Germany) is inserted in the same intercostal space and Ropivacaine (2 mg/ml, Fresenius Kabi, Schelle, Belgium) is infused postoperatively (Fig. 18). The ventilation is restarted, and the patient is weaned from cardiopulmonary bypass, and an appropriate dose of protamine is administered. Surgical wounds are closed with uninterrupted intradermal sutures and simple stitches (Fig. 19).

10 Graft Construction

In our centre, there is a strong conviction that mammary arteries are superior as grafting material compared to all other available conduits, especially in-situ mammary arteries. We reach a near 100% totally mammary artery grafting in our endo-CABG group. By using the mammary arteries, proximal anastomoses (with venous graft or radial artery) are avoided, and the transthoracic aortic clamping with the cardioplegia line are the only manipulations of the ascending aorta that is needed.

Obviously, in single-vessel coronary artery disease, we look for solutions with in situ mammary arteries, like LIMA to the LAD or LIMA to the obtuse marginal (OM) branch of the circumflex artery (Cx). An in situ RIMA to the

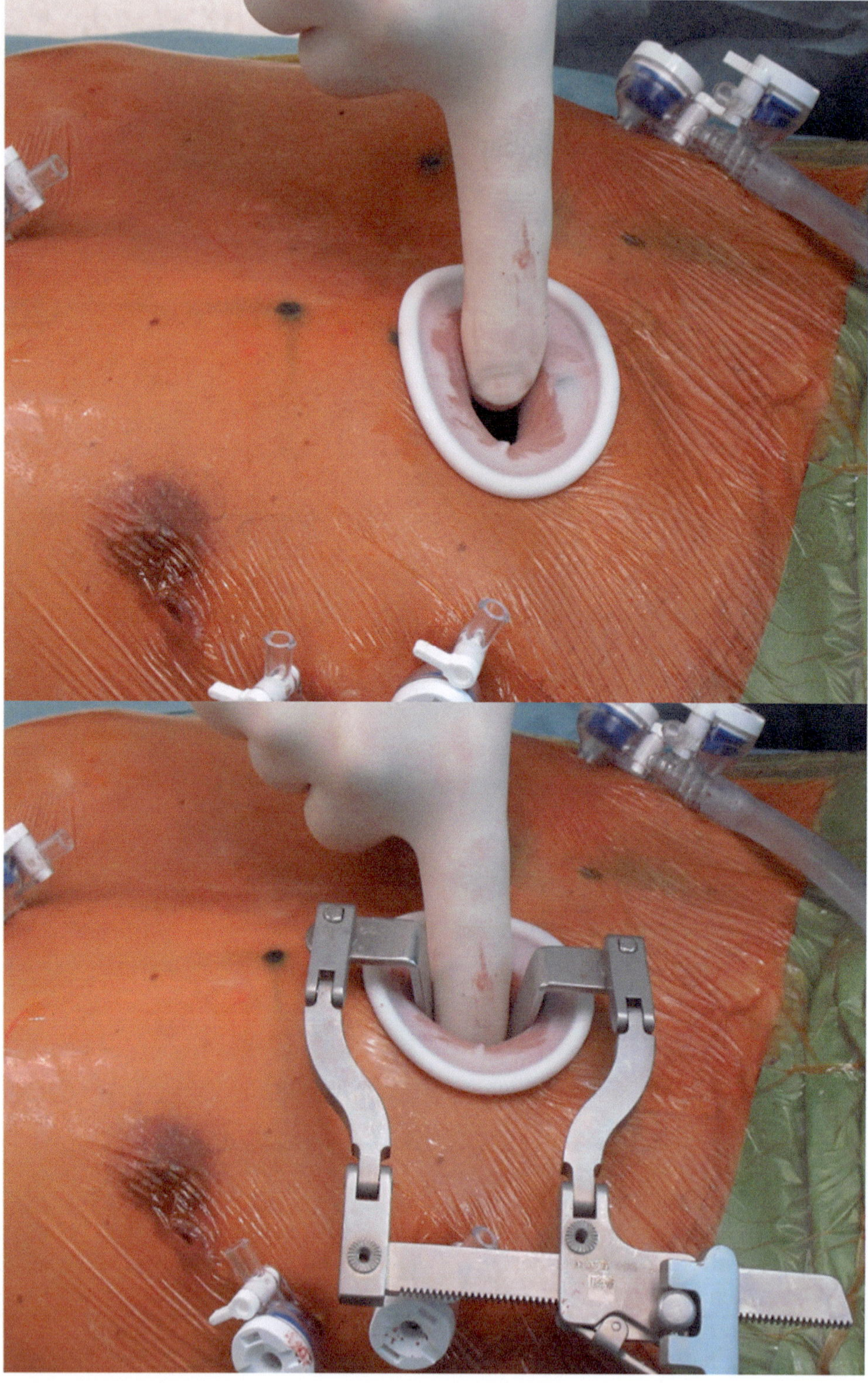

Fig. 9 Left sided mini-thoracotomy with a soft tissue retractor and with a low profile rib spreader

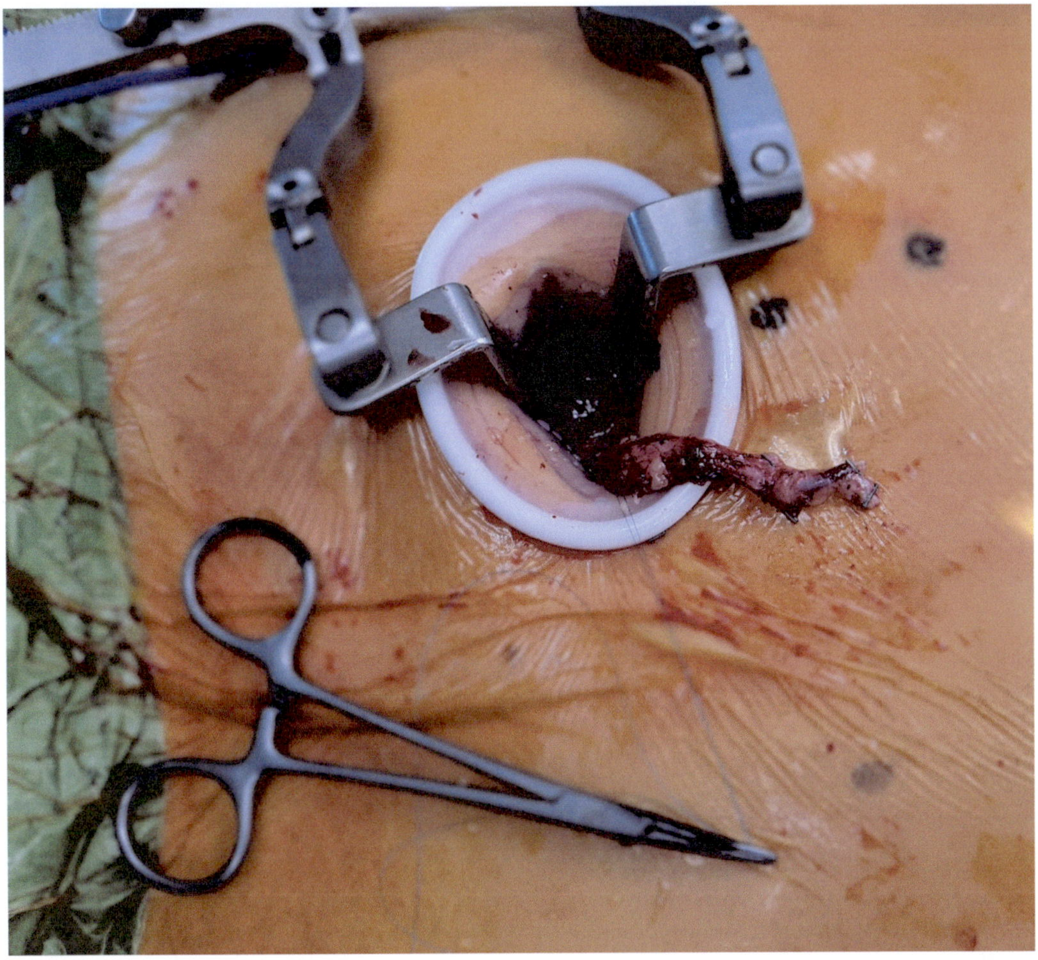

Fig. 10 Marking the correct side of the pedicle with a prolene 6–0

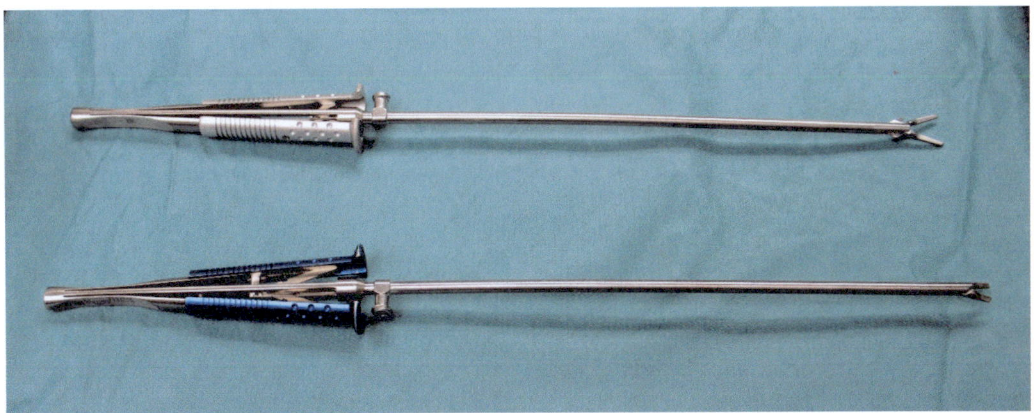

Fig. 11 An endoscopic grasping forceps and an endoscopic needle holder

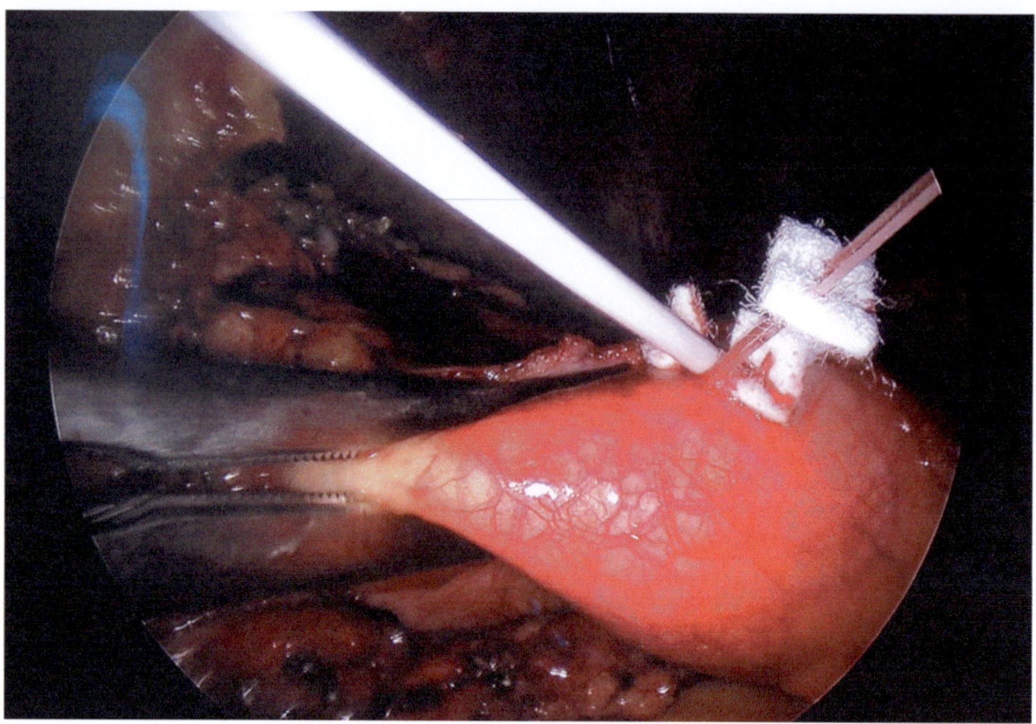

Fig. 12 The transthoracic aortic clamp is placed fully over the distal ascending aorta, and the cardioplegia catheter is inserted in the aorta

RCA can be realized through a right mini-thoracotomy as far as the crux of the RCA.

For multi-vessel coronary artery disease, the in situ mammary artery usage is applied *as much as possible*. For example, in case of a left main (LM) stem disease or a proximal LAD and Cx coronary artery disease, the in situ LIMA is used to the OM branch and the in situ RIMA to the LAD (Fig. 20). If only the proximal LAD and the proximal RCA is significantly calcified, then the in situ LIMA is used for the LAD through a left mini-thoracotomy and the in situ RIMA for the RCA via a right mini-thoracotomy (Fig. 21). In case a diagonal branch of the LAD is needed to be bypassed together with the LAD and the OM branch, then the in situ LIMA is used as a jump graft to the diagonal and LAD and the in situ RIMA is brought to the OM branch via the transverse pericardial sinus (Fig. 22). This last aspect is done as the operator is standing on the left side of the patient. The RIMA is clipped and

transected after its distal bifurcation and hold in the left hand with an endoscopic grasping forceps. Next, the right hand holds another endoscopic grasping forceps, and this instrument *and* the endoscope enter the transverse pericardial sinus on the left side and exit the sinus on the right side. The in situ RIMA is cautiously handed over from the left hand to the right hand endoscopic grasping forceps. The endoscope is pulled back, and the right hand endoscopic forceps is also pulled back gently with the in situ RIMA in it. The in situ RIMA is fixed to the edge of the pericardium with a clip to prevent torsion.

When the patient has three vessel disease, a Y-graft construction is needed as described above. If the postero-lateral branch of the Cx (PLCx) or the RCA (PLR) needs to be bypassed, then a Y-graft construction is also necessary.

In conclusion, with the in situ LIMA, the anterior wall and the OM region can be reached. With the in situ RIMA, the RCA as far as the

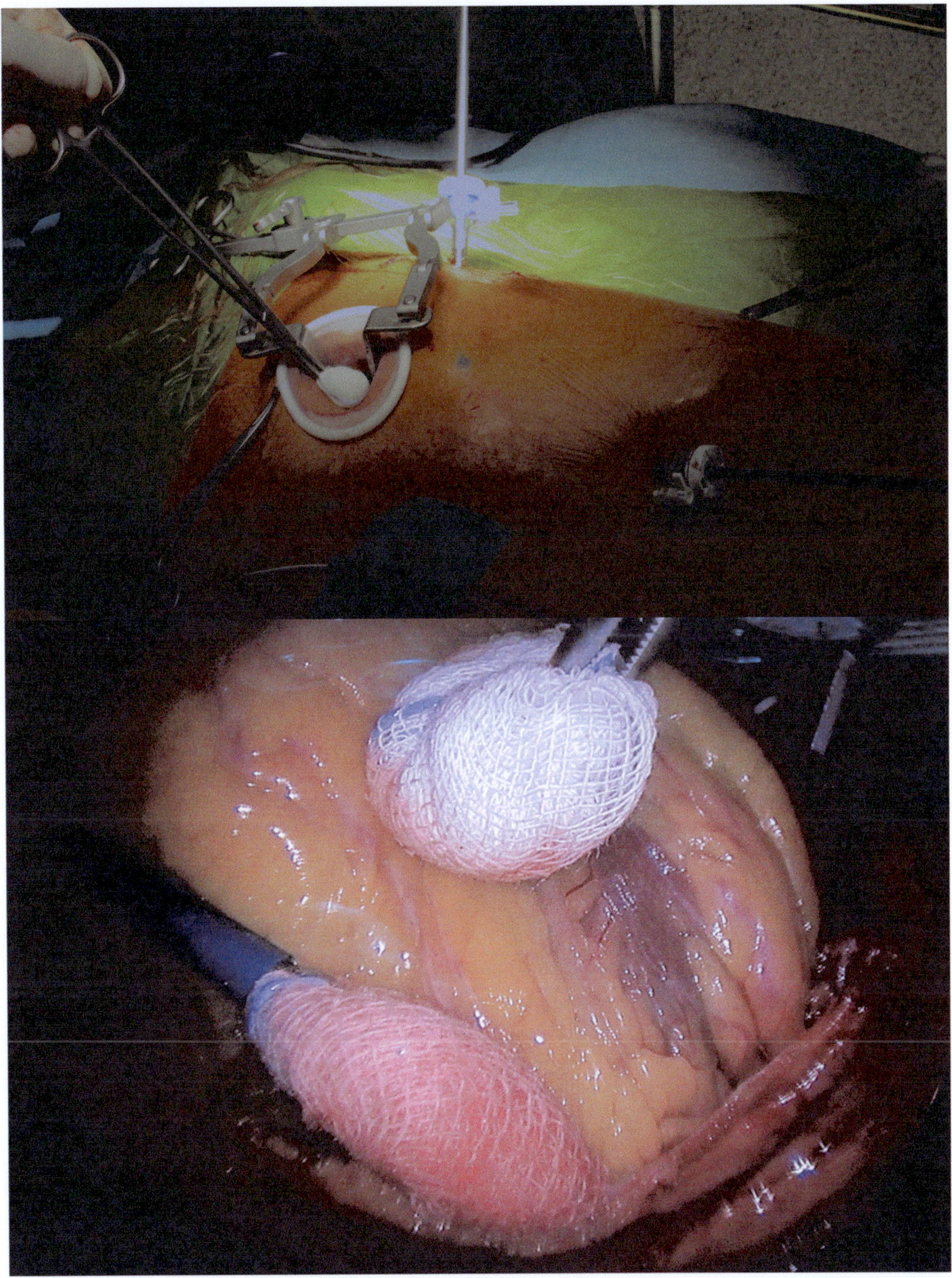

Fig. 13 A subxyphoid introduced endoscopic clamp holding a peanut gauze and a clamp with a peanut used through the mini-thoracotomy

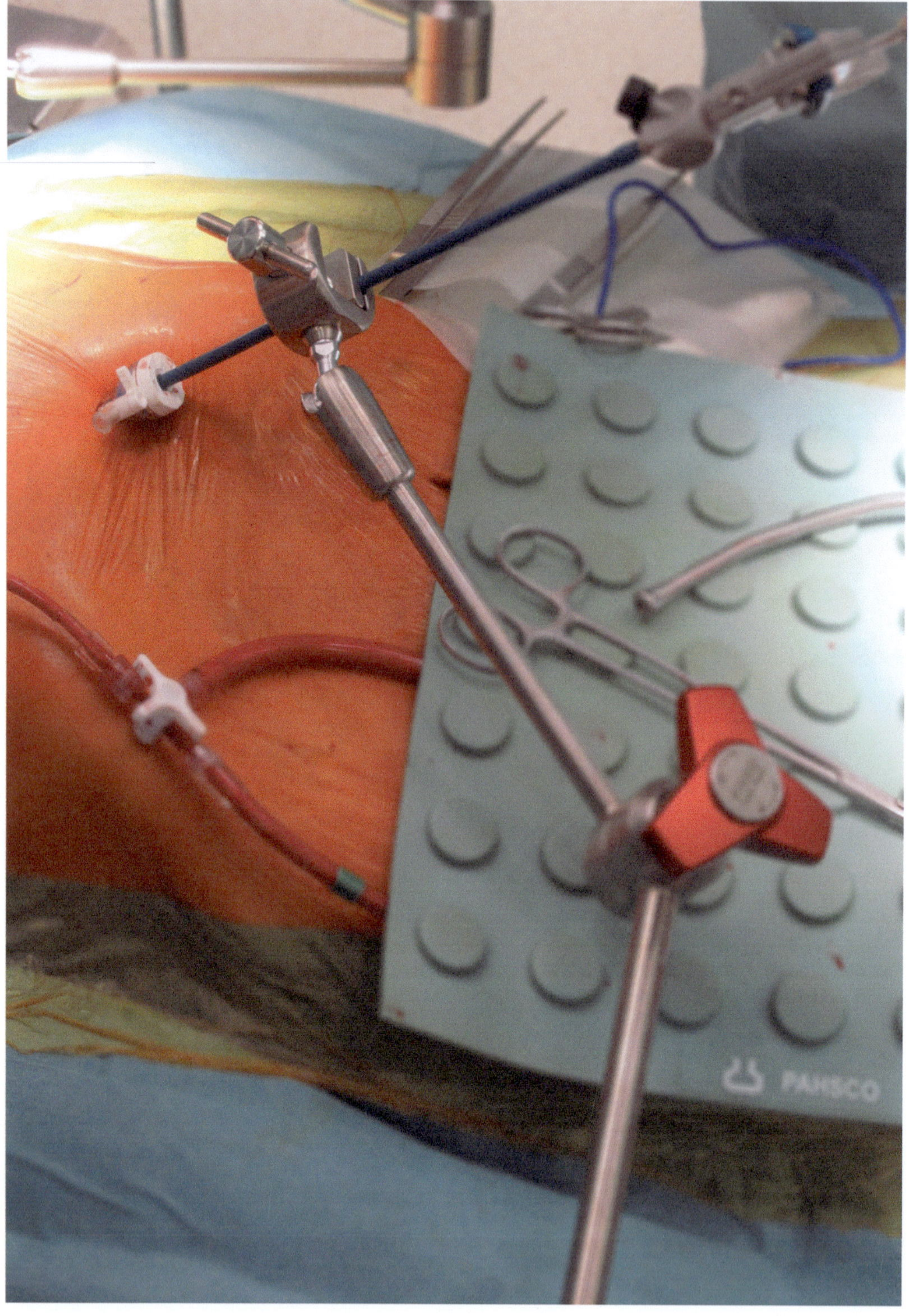

Fig. 14 An instrument holder attached to the operating table

crux of the RCA and the OM region, via the transverse pericardial sinus, can be achieved. In all other situations a Y-graft construction is required (Video 1).

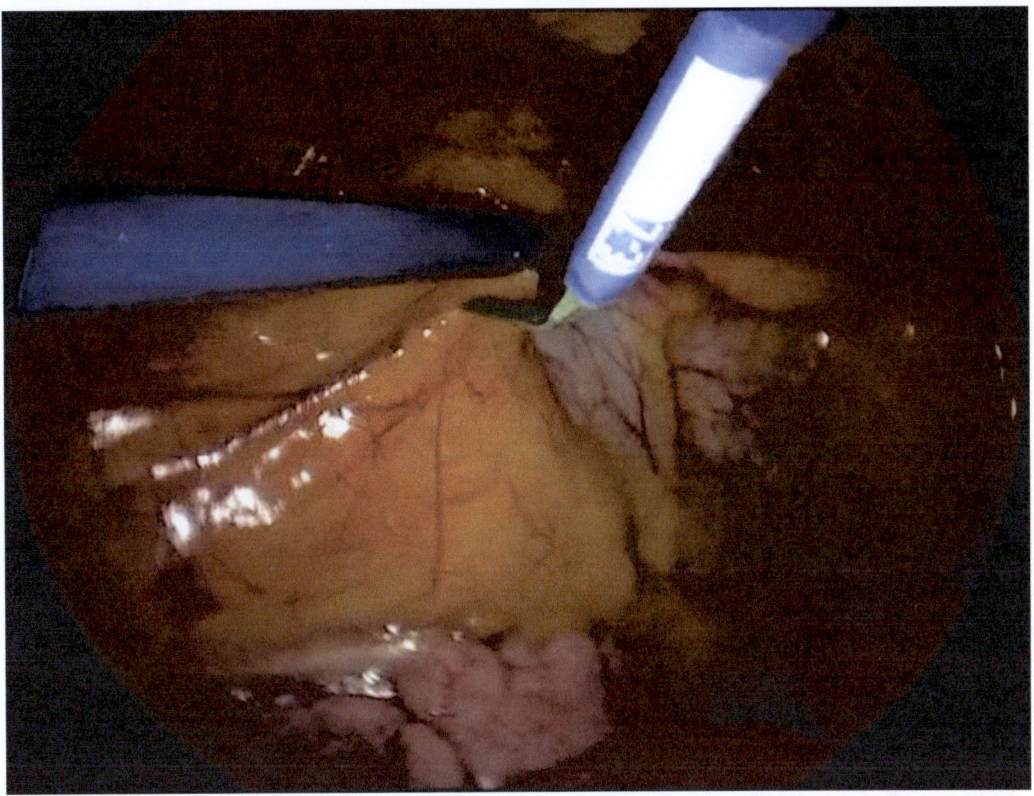

Video 1 A step-by-step video of totally endoscopic coronary artery bypass grafting (▶ https://doi.org/10.1007/000-a8b)

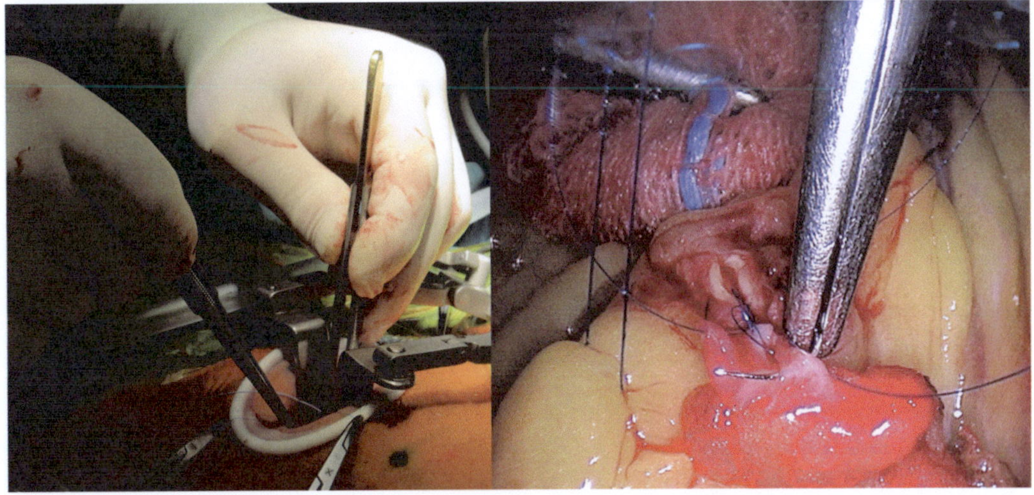

Fig. 15 A normal Castroviejo needle-holder and forceps is used for anastomoses

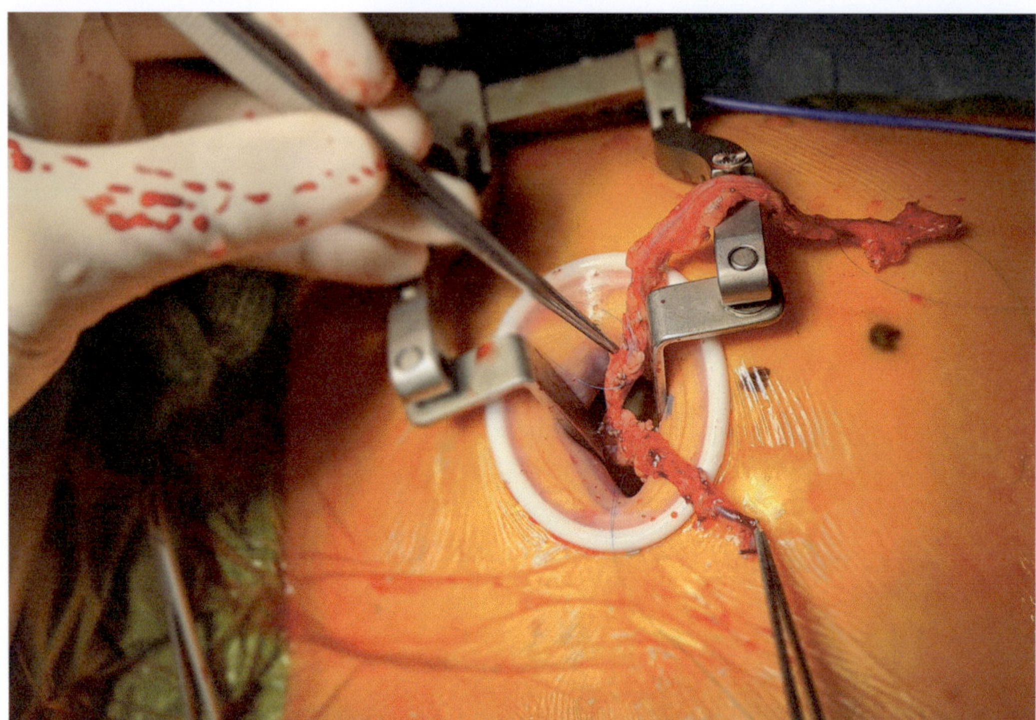

Fig. 16 A Y-graft construction with on top the free RIMA

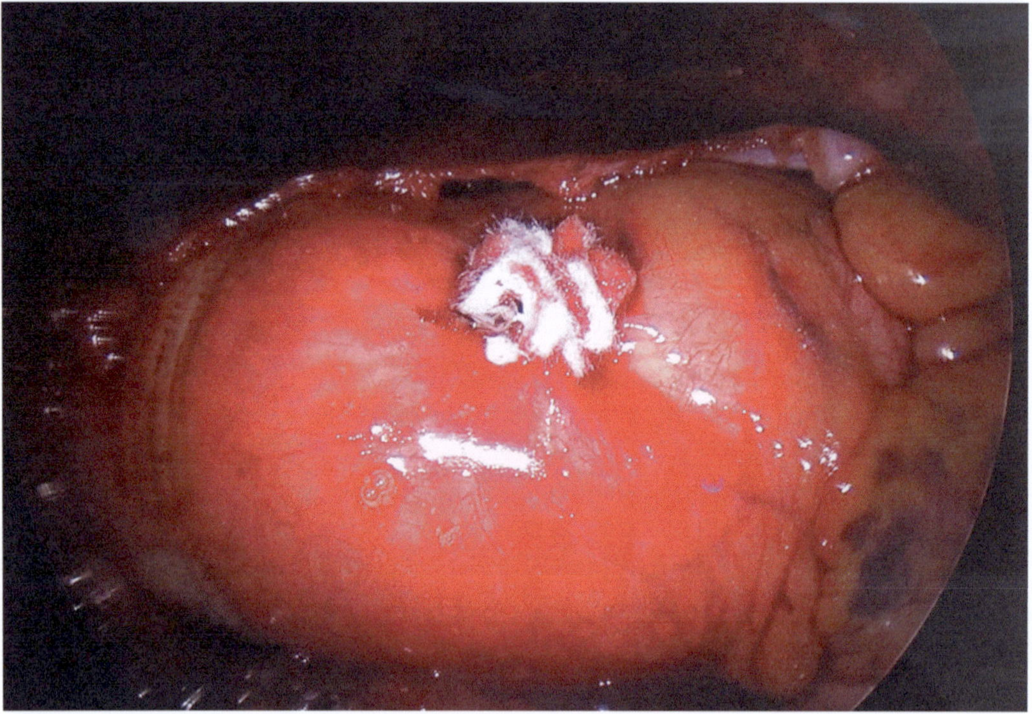

Fig. 17 The aortic clamp is released, the cardioplegia catheter removed, and its suture tied down with an automated knotting device

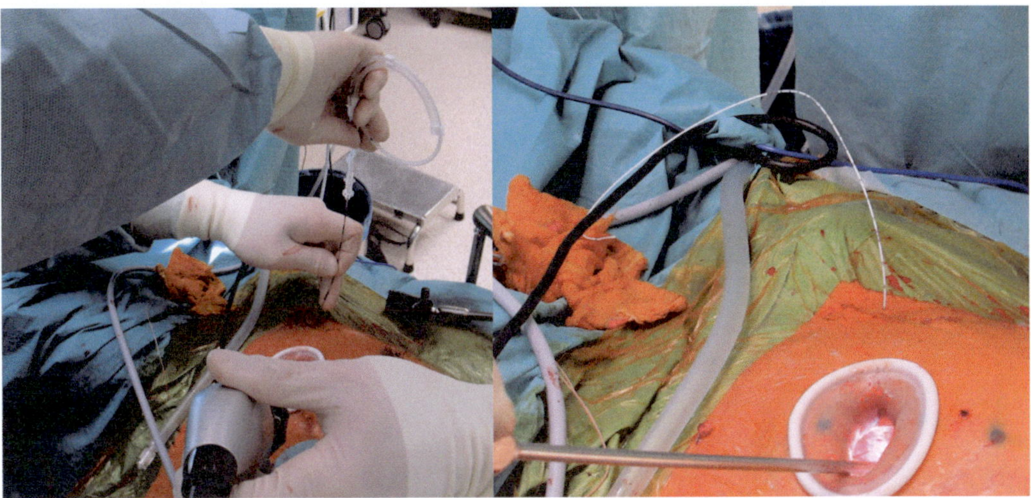

Fig. 18 Pain catheter insertion

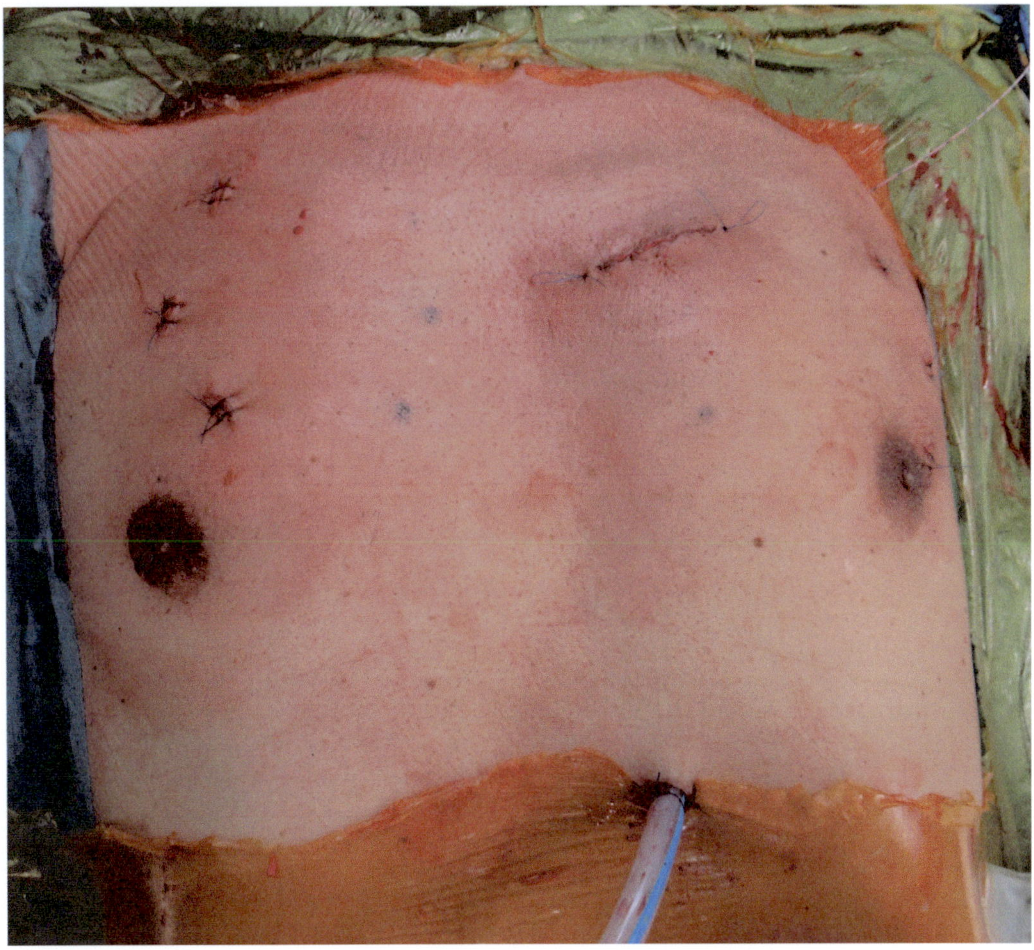

Fig. 19 Final view on surgical wounds

Fig. 20 LIMA-MO and RIMA-LAD anastomoses

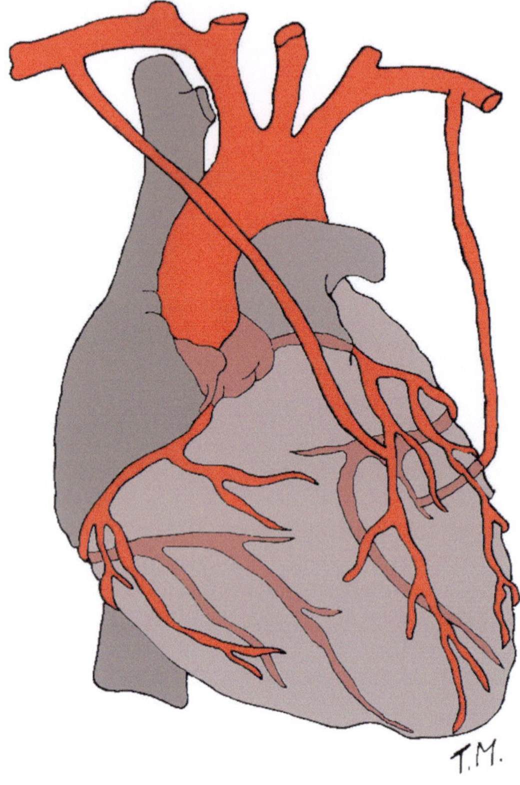

Fig. 21 LIMA-LAD and RIMA-RCA anastomoses

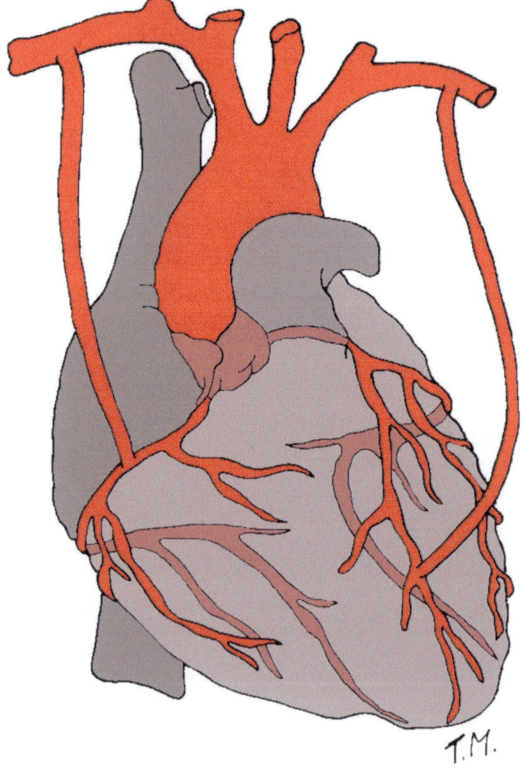

Fig. 22 LIMA-D-LAD and RIMA-MO anastomoses

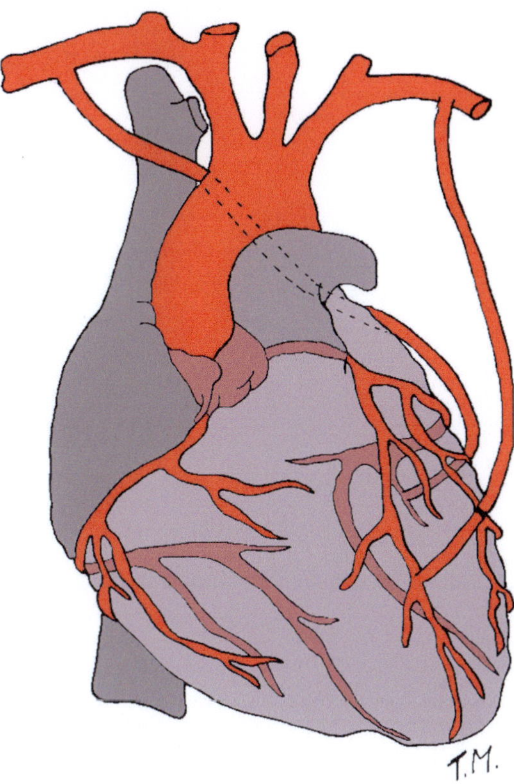

References

1. Head SJ, Kieser TM, Falk V, Huysmans HA, Kappetein AP. Coronary artery bypass grafting: Part 1–the evolution over the first 50 years. Eur Heart J. 2013;34(37):2862–72.
2. Olearchyk AS, Vasilii I. Kolesov. A pioneer of coronary revascularization by internal mammary-coronary artery grafting. J Thorac Cardiovasc Surg. 1988;96(1):13–8
3. Collet C, Capodanno D, Onuma Y, Banning A, Stone GW, Taggart DP, et al. Left main coronary artery disease: pathophysiology, diagnosis, and treatment. Nat Rev Cardiol. 2018;15(6):321–31.
4. Benetti FJ, Ballester C, Sani G, Doonstra P, Grandjean J. Video assisted coronary bypass surgery. J Card Surg. 1995;10(6):620–5.
5. Subramanian VA, McCabe JC, Geller CM. Minimally invasive direct coronary artery bypass grafting: two-year clinical experience. Ann Thorac Surg. 1997;64(6):1648–55.
6. Mack MJ, Acuff TE, Casimir-Ahn H, Lönn UJ, Jansen EW. Video-assisted coronary bypass grafting on the beating heart. Ann Thorac Surg. 1997;63(6 Suppl):S100–S3.
7. Khajuria A. Robotics and surgery: a sustainable relationship? World J Clin Cases. 2015;3(3):265–9.
8. Leonard JR, Rahouma M, Abouarab AA, Schwann AN, Scuderi G, Lau C, et al. Totally endoscopic coronary artery bypass surgery: a meta-analysis of the current evidence. Int J Cardiol. 2018;261:42–6.
9. Yilmaz A, Robic B, Starinieri P, Polus F, Stinkens R, Stessel B. A new viewpoint on endoscopic CABG: technique description and clinical experience. J Cardiol. 2020;S0914–5087(19):30386–7.
10. Starinieri P, Declercq PE, Robic B, Yilmaz A, Van Tornout M, Dubois J, et al. A comparison between minimized extracorporeal circuits and conventional extracorporeal circuits in patients undergoing aortic valve surgery: is 'minimally invasive extracorporeal circulation' just low prime or closed loop perfusion? Perfusion. 2017;32(5):403–8.

Endoscopic Surgery for Cardiac Tumours

Abdelrehman Abdelbar and Joseph Zacharias

Abstract

With increasing experience in endoscopic techniques a sub group of patients who could benefit from this approach are patients presenting with a diagnosis of cardiac tumours. These are often picked up as an incidental finding and once the diagnosis is made early surgery is warranted. These can provide challenges to get a team together but if an institution offers this approach as a routine, then these cases can be dealt with quickly. In this chapter we summarise some of the case series in the literature and present a case to show the pathway followed. We also include a video to capture the key steps.

Keywords

Endoscopic cardiac tumours · Cardiac myxomas · Papillary fibroelastoma

Supplementary Information The online version contains supplementary material available at https://doi.org/10.1007/978-3-031-21104-1_16. The videos can be accessed individually by clicking the DOI link in the accompanying figure caption or by scanning this link with the SN More Media App.

A. Abdelbar · J. Zacharias (✉)
Department of Cardiothoracic Surgery, Lancashire Cardiac Centre, Blackpool, England
e-mail: a.abdelbar@nhs.net

1 Epidemiology and Pathology

Cardiac neoplasms are extremely rare conditions which are represented by a small group of patient population even in large tertiary cardiac surgery centres [1]. Due to the current status of many of these being under diagnosed, it is very difficult to estimate an accurate prevalence in the living population. The disease load is only obtained from post-mortem studies. These studies have shown that primary cardiac tumors are rarer than secondary deposits with an incidence of 0.05% and 1% respectively. This percentage does not reflect the real practice or case load in the cardiac centres. It is likely that cardiac tumors are underdiagnosed in the real world of clinical practice [2]. Despite the advances and the wide use of cardiac imaging modalities, cardiac tumors are rarely symptomatic and most patients have an incidental pick up following on from an imaging study.

Likewise, to any tumour, cardiac tumours are classified into primary and secondary tumours. Primary cardiac tumours are further divided into benign and malignant.

Benign cardiac tumours include Myxoma (represents 50% of all primary cardiac tumours), rhabdomyoma, lipoma, fibroma and angioma. Malignant cardiac tumours are mainly sarcomas (e.g. angiosarcoma and rhabdomyosarcoma) or lymphomas. Secondary cardiac tumours are usually part of a widespread malignancy which is

J. Zacharias (ed.), *Endoscopic Cardiac Surgery*,
https://doi.org/10.1007/978-3-031-21104-1_16

not only limited to the heart. Metastasis to the heart is most commonly linked to lymphoma, leukaemia and melanoma.

Clinical presentation of cardiac tumours is extremely variable. It depends on the location and the size of the tumour. Most of the cases will be asymptomatic, the diagnosis of which is usually post-mortem. When symptomatic, cardiac tumours are usually presented by one of three classic features. This triad is obstruction, embolic phenomena and constitutional symptoms. Depending on the size and position of the tumour, the effects on the haemodynamics and the site of embolisation are determined. For example, a tumour on the right side of the heart will cause pulmonary embolic manifestations while those on the left are more likely to lead to systemic emboli and its effects. Other presentations might be arrhythmia in case of tumours invading the myocardium. A tumour invading the pericardium might cause pericardial effusion and possible cardiac tamponade.

2 Role of Minimally Invasive Surgery

Generally speaking, minimally invasive surgery is still under-performed in cases of cardiac tumours. This is since cardiac tumours themselves are rare in clinical practice. The increased availability and utilisation of cardiac echocardiogram has increased the number of diagnosed cases, yet, the overall case load is still under 1% of the performed cardiac surgery cases in the United Kingdom. The argument for expanding the role of minimally invasive surgery is to obtain both its well-recognised post-operative benefits and, the comparable or even superior tumour clearance.

Post-operative benefits of minimally invasive surgery are well described in the literature [3, 4]. They include faster patient recovery, less blood loss with consequent less blood transfusion, less wound complications, shorter intensive care and overall hospital stays [5, 6]. The morbidity and mortality were found to be less in minimally invasive surgery. Benefits of minimally invasive

surgery will extend to post discharge benefits in terms of shorter rehabilitation requirements and quicker return to work [7, 8]. All these factors are likely to support increased execution of minimally invasive surgery for better patient care and improvements of the wider health care economy.

In terms of tumour clearance, minimally invasive surgery provides better visualisation of the intra-cardiac structures which, in turn, results in more specific excision. The use of high definition and 3D endoscopes has enabled easy navigation in the difficult access areas such as the ventricles through the corresponding atrioventricular valves which can give a wider working area. In contrast, when sternotomy is utilized, ventricles were accessed through aortic and pulmonary valves which gives a narrower field and increases the risk of injury to those fine valves.

So far, the evidence in terms of minimally invasive resection of cardiac tumors is still relying on case reports, case series [9] and fewer meta-analysis papers. Due to the small numbers and the urgent presentation a randomized control trial is unlikely to be carried out and hence high grade evidence will always be lacking [10].

Some case series have shown the results of MICS approach for resection of cardiac tumors to be excellent. For example, our experience [11] reported the results of 20 patients. This case series showed 18 patients with left atrial myxoma and two with left ventricular fibroelastoma. We highlighted the safety of the procedure with no mortality, stroke or conversion to sternotomy. No recurrence of the tumors was reported. Likewise, Deshpande et al. reported more variable tumor pathologies and sites [9]. Their case mix showed right and left atrial myxomas, aortic valve fibroelastoma, tricuspid valve intravenous leiomyoma with inferior vena cava involvement and plexiform tumor of the sinoatrial node. They have reported no post-operative complications with no recurrence in 27 patients for a median follow up for 3.4 ± 2.7 years. Bianchi et al. reported 30 patients who underwent excision of left atrial myxoma via MICS approach with no hospital mortality or stroke. They have experienced no recurrence in a follow up median of 55.6 ± 32.3 months [8].

While the previously mentioned studies lack comparison with MS, some other teams reported their comparative results in both MICS and MS. Lee et al. compared their retrospective results of 143 MS and 63 MICS patients (total 203 patients) [5]. In this study, they have selected only patients with cardiac myxoma and excluded patients with any accompanied cardiac pathologies including valve haemodynamic pathologies. They concluded the superiority of the MICS approach in terms of blood transfusion and postoperative arrythmia. They did not find a significant difference in the post-operative ventilation or hospital stays. They have also reported a longer cardiopulmonary bypass and cross clamp times in the MICS group which did not reflect on the post-operative results. Conversely, Iribarne et al. did not find that CBP and cross clamp times were longer in the MICS than in MS [6]. They argued that MICS excision of cardiac tumors is performed by experienced MICS teams with already a large MICS valve practice. In the same study, which included 36 MS and 38 MICS (total 74 patients), they have also reported a shorter hospital stay and freedom of recurrence for a mean time of 4.8 years. Pineda et al. reported the results of 39 patients (22 MICS and 17 MS) [7]. They have concluded that with similar outcome in terms of post-operative complications, MICS poses better utilization of resources because of the associated shorter ICU and hospital stays in these case series.

Moscarelli et al. performed the first meta-analysis to compare the outcome between MICS and MS in treating cardiac tumours. They analysed 653 procedures, majority of them were cardiac myxoma (601 patients) [4]. They have concluded excellent outcome of the MICS approach comparable to MS approach or even superior despite the longer CBP and cross clamp times. Tumour size did not influence the choice of the surgical approach, but they found some hesitation from some surgeons to perform MICS in case of right atrial tumour to avoid tumour

fragmentation during cannulation. There was also no conversion in the MICS group which signifies the safety of the procedure and the role of surgical experience with MICS before considering it.

3 Case Scenario

In this section, we will show a step wise approach to a straightforward confirmed case of left atrial myxoma in regard to preoperative, intra-operative and post-operative steps.

To make this case more challenging, we picked up a female patient with breast implants.

Preoperative imaging:

To decide the suitability of any patient to the MICS, there are a few multi-modality imaging which would help. Some of them can be done intra-operatively eg TOE and groin US.

Echocardiogram:

- Final confirmation of diagnosis.
- Valvular lesions if any.
- Strategy of myocardial preservation. (Table 1)

Role of intra-operative TOE will be discussed in the intraoperative section.

Contrast enhanced CT scan:

- Exclude extra-cardiac tumors.
- Cannulation strategy:
    - Suitable femoral vessels:
      Good size femoral arteries with acceptable course eg no tortuosity.
      Freedom of any venous abnormality eg thrombosed femoral vein.
    - Healthy aorto-vascular tree:
      No calcifications
    - Ascending aorta:
      Suitable for using Endo-aortic clamp.
- Right pleural pathology/adhesions.
- Freedom from coronary artery flow limiting lesions (if ECG gated CT scan is available).

Table 1 Aortic occlusion options

	No AR	Mild AR	Moderate AR
Endo-ballon clamp	Yes	No	No
External cross clamp	Yes	Yes	No
Beating heart	Yes	Yes	No

Coronary artery angiogram:

- Freedom from flow limiting lesions.
- Can provide an idea about the aorto-vascular tree and the femoral vessels.

Intraoperative:

Anaesthetic consideration:

This going to be discussed in detail in other chapters but to summarise:

- Single lumen endotracheal tube with a bronchial blocker (right bronchus)
- Central venous catheter
- Radial arterial line catheter:
  - In case of using the endo-aortic balloon clamp, both radial arteries should be used to monitor occlusion of the any of the great vessels.

Surgical positioning and set up:

- Supine position with 30-degree tilt towards the left side. This can be achieved using an inflatable bag below the right-side 4th intercostal space.

- Groin and chest US:
  Final check
  - Femoral vessels size and calcifications
  - Distance from the skin
  - Pleural adhesions
- Mark the MS site and label the rib spaces. (see Video)
- Expose both groins and the MS site when patient is draped.

Cannulation:

Detailed cannulation strategy is described in other chapters. So, we will provide tips and tricks for MICS cannulation.

These flow diagrams show the different possibilities that can rise in case of atrial myxomas. (Flow diagram 1 and 2).

Tips and tricks in case of femoral cannulation: (see Video 1).

- Skin incision is better if performed 1 inch above the femoral crease:
  - Less wound complications.
  - Larger caliber of the femoral vessels.
- Expose only the front service of the vessels to avoid wound complications.

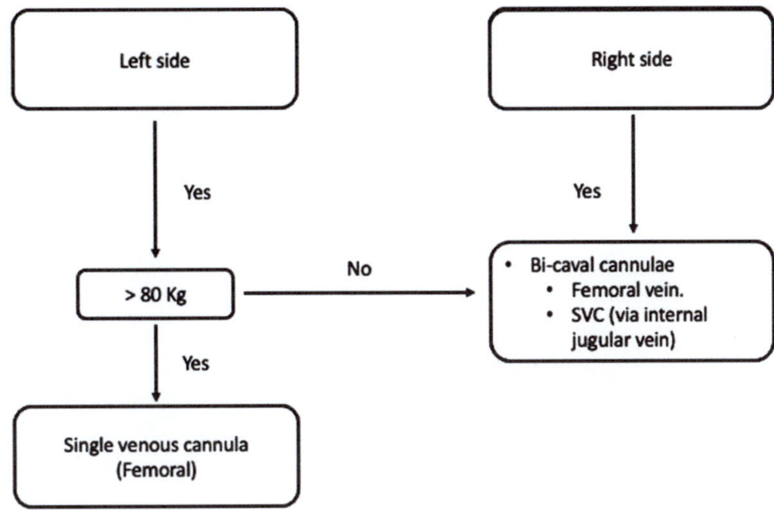

Flow diagram: 1

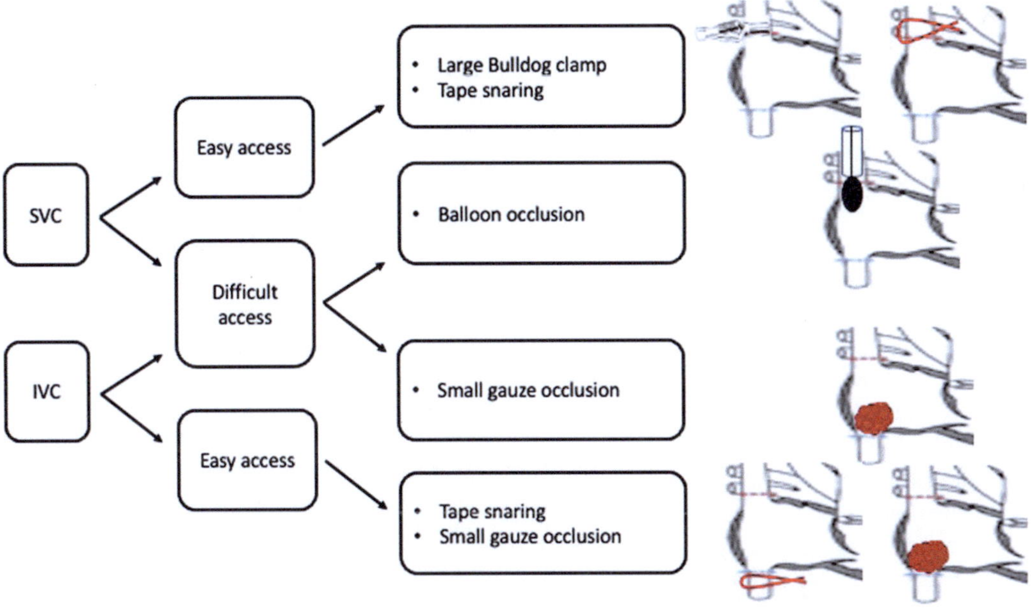

Flow diagram: 2

- Arterial cannulation:
  - Always split the arterial inflow line. In case the contralateral groin cannulation/central cannulation is required.
  - TOE live monitoring of the descending aorta until full flow is achieved.
  - Arterial inflow pressure never to exceed 300 mmHg. If so, bifemoral cannulation.
- Venous cannulation:
  - Live monitoring of the wire and cannula until cannula is in place.
- Generally: never force the guide wires.

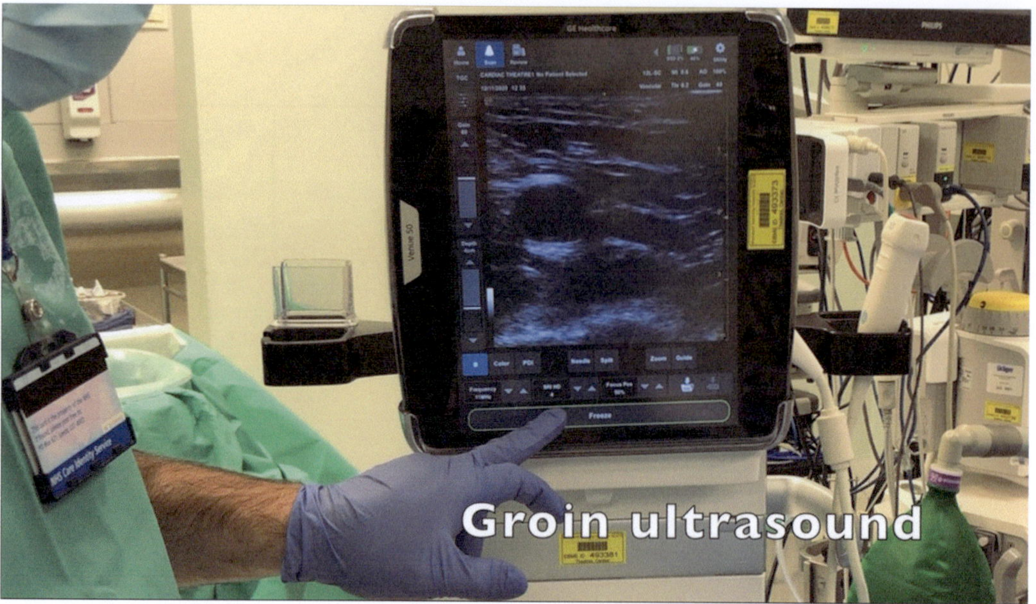

Video 1 Step by step video of a left atrial myxoma excision (▶ https://doi.org/10.1007/000-a8c)

Surgical procedure:

In this section, a step-by-step video will be provided. But we would like to point out a few points:

- Main surgical incision:
  - This can vary from a small peri-areolar incision that enters the chest through the 4th intercostal space in case of endoscopic assisted practice. A larger incision could be utilised at a more lateral position in case of direct vision practice or with pleural adhesions.
  - Better to perform muscle splitting instead of diathermy for less bleeding and better healing.
- Other utility incisions (within the axillary lines):
  - 2nd intercostal space: in case of using an external cross clamp.
  - 3rd intercostal space: 10 mm port for the camera.
  - 5th or 6th intercostal space: for traction and CO_2 line (utility port).
- Better to perform surgical incisions before heparin administration. Wound closure and ports removal should be performed after reversal of heparin.
- Better to use two drains at the end, pericardial and right pleural drains.
- It is favored to perform intercostal blocks before closure. (see video)

Tips, Tricks and Traps:

- In case of right atrial myxoma near the SVC or IVC, cannulae should be withdrawn to a position distal to the cavo-atrial junctions to allow snaring as described before.

- While handling the myxoma, surgeon's concentration should be focused on minimal manipulation of the actual myxoma to fragmentation and embolization. Instead, finding the stalk of the myxoma and using it for manipulation is safer. This can be achieved by using the external suction gently to retract the tumor until the stalk is exposed.

- Large myxomas can be retrieved using a tissue retrieval system to avoid fragmentation with subsequent embolization and seeding.

Post-operative:

Beside the routine post-operative care, a few points are considered in case of the MICS:

- Immediate post-operative chest Xray to check right lung expansion and pleural collection in case of bleeding.
- Drains can be removed as per the local protocol. If there is still high output, pericardial drain to be removed in 24 h and right pleural one to be kept in.
- Look out for damage to the phrenic nerve as post operative atelectasis at the right lower lobe can also present with a raised right hemidiaphragm.
- Despite small incisions the pain around the drain sites can be troublesome so the earlier the drains can come out the better for patient to get involved with Physiotherapy and mobilisation.
- Increasingly we are putting the right sided chest drain on a portable suction device so that patients can mobilise easier with the drains left in.

References

1. Moscarelli M, Rahouma M, Nasso G, Di Bari N, Speziale G, Bartolomucci F, Pepe M, Fattouch K, Lau C, Gaudino M. Minimally invasive approaches to primary cardiac tumors: a systematic review and meta-analysis. J Card Surg. 2021;36(2):483–92.
2. Centofanti P, Di Rosa E, Deorsola L, Dato GM, Patane F, La Torre M, Barbato L, Verzini A, Fortunato G, di Summa M. Primary cardiac tumors: early and late results of surgical treatment in 91 patients. Ann Thorac Surg. 1999;68(4):1236–41.
3. Pineda AM, Santana O, Zamora C, Benjo AM, Lamas GA, Lamelas J. Outcomes of a minimally invasive approach compared with median sternotomy for the excision of benign cardiac masses. Ann Thorac Surg. 2011;91(5):1440–4.
4. Moscarelli M, Casula R, Speziale G, Athanasiou T. Can we use minimally invasive mitral valve surgery as a safe alternative to sternotomy in high-risk patients? Interact Cardiovasc Thorac Surg. 2016;22(1):92–6.
5. Lee HP, Cho WC, Kim JB, Jung SH, Choo SJ, Chung CH, Lee JW. Surgical outcomes of cardiac myxoma: Right minithoracotomy approach versus median sternotomy approach. Korean J Thorac Cardiovasc Surg. 2016;49(5):356.
6. Iribarne A, Easterwood R, Russo MJ, Yang J, Cheema FH, Smith CR, Argenziano M. Long-term outcomes with a minimally invasive approach for resection of cardiac masses. Ann Thorac Surg. 2010;90(4):1251–5.
7. Pineda AM, Santana O, Cortes-Bergoderi M, Lamelas J. Is a minimally invasive approach for resection of benign cardiac masses superior to standard full sternotomy? Interact Cardiovasc Thorac Surg. 2013;16(6):875–9.
8. Bianchi G, Margaryan R, Kallushi E, Cerillo AG, Farneti PA, Pucci A, Solinas M. Outcomes of video-assisted minimally invasive cardiac myxoma resection. Heart Lung Circ. 2019;28(2):327–33.
9. Deshpande RP, Casselman F, Bakir I, Cammu G, Wellens F, De Geest R, Degrieck I, Van Praet F, Vermeulen Y, Vanermen H. Endoscopic cardiac tumor resection. Ann Thorac Surg. 2007;83(6):2142–6.
10. Ravikumar E, Pawar N, Gnanamuthu R, Sundar P, Cherian M, Thomas S. Minimal access approach for surgical management of cardiac tumors. Ann Thorac Surg. 2000;70(3):1077–9.
11. Kenawy A, Abdelbar A, Zacharias J. Minimally invasive resection of benign cardiac tumors. J Thorac Dis. 2021;13(3):1993.

Cannulation Techniques for Cardiopulmonary Bypass in Endoscopic Cardiac Surgery

Karel M. Van Praet, Markus Kofler, and Jörg Kempfert

Abstract

Extracorporeal circulation throughout minimally invasive cardiac surgery (MICS) is often provided by peripheral artery cannulation but is mainly performed through surgical cutdown. Percutaneous placement of cannulas is assisted by vascular closure devices yet their advantages to MICS are still disputed. Hospital stay, operation time and groin complications have been substantially reduced through percutaneous groin cannulation using vascular closure devices for establishing cardiopulmonary bypass in MICS. The outstanding complications, however, are mainly of vascular nature versus wound infection and lymph fistulae with open surgical cutdown. It is of paramount importance to master a variety of cannulation techniques for safe perfusion strategy and operation. The operative techniques for MICS have developed greatly over the past decade to include a wide demographic of patients. Our aim is to describe numerous cannulation strategies and their application and use in different minimally invasive procedures.

Supplementary Information The online version contains supplementary material available at https://doi.org/10.1007/978-3-031-21104-1_17. The videos can be accessed individually by clicking the DOI link in the accompanying figure caption or by scanning this link with the SN More Media App.

K. M. Van Praet (✉) · M. Kofler · J. Kempfert
Deutsches Herzzentrum der Charité (DHZC),
Department of Cardiothoracic and Vascular Surgery,
Augustenburger Platz 1, 13353 Berlin, Germany
e-mail: vanpraet@dhzb.de;
karel.van-praet@dhzc-charite.de;
karel.vanpraet@gmail.com

J. Kempfert
e-mail: kempfert@dhzb.de

K. M. Van Praet · M. Kofler · J. Kempfert
Charité – Universitätsmedizin Berlin, corporate member of Freie Universität Berlin,
Humboldt-Universität zu Berlin, Charitéplatz 1,
10117 Berlin, Germany

DZHK (German Center for Cardiovascular Research), Partner Site Berlin, Berlin, Germany

Keywords

Cardiac surgery · Cannulation · Technique · Open surgical · Percutaneous · Cutdown · Cardiopulmonary bypass · Mitral valve · Tricuspid valve · Minimally invasive surgery · Endoscopic surgery

1 Introduction

There are clear advantages in the adoption of minimally invasive cardiac surgery (MICS); a scaling down in length of stay, usage of blood products, reduction of postoperative pain and neurological deficit all resulting in overall improvement of recovery and outcomes. MIC surgery is a collaboration of innovative surgical techniques performed through a small incision and entails less surgical trauma than full sternotomy conventional cardiac surgery. The limitations of the MICS surgical field elicit essential adaptations of surgical technology, instrumentation, and cannulation strategy. When applying MICS techniques, a deep and comprehensive grasp of various cannulation strategies and their application to a wide spectrum of diseases and patients is required. The appropriate strategy for the necessary cannulation, allowing for optimal exposure and ease of operation, will depend entirely on the surgical approach. MICS procedures are broad and therefore need a wide array of cannulation options as opposed to conventional sternotomy-based surgery that solely uses the central ascending aortic cannulation with right atrial or bicaval cannulation. Typical MICS techniques include performing an upper hemisternotomy, lower hemisternotomy, and a right anterolateral minithoracotomy. Regarding hemisternotomy, some surgeons may choose percutaneous femoral venous cannulation in combination with central arterial cannulation as opposed to the conventional central arterial and venous cannulation. A completely femoral platform may also be implemented. Minithoracotomy-based techniques however often need alternative cannulation strategies.

2 Arterial Cannulation

When a patient is placed on cardiopulmonary bypass (CPB) the initial consideration is not only the cannulation size but also the cannulation site [1]. This is influenced by the presence of disease within the artery, the artery size and the patient's body surface area (BSA). It is preferred to cannulate the femoral artery for peripheral cannulation and select the cannula size based on BSA [1]. For a BSA of <1.7, a 15F arterial perfusion cannula is chosen, and a 17F cannula for a BSA of 1.7 to 2.1 and when the BSA is >2.1, a 19F

cannula is applied [1]. While on CPB, body temperature is maintained at around 34 degrees Celcius. At the authors'institution goal-directed-perfusion with DO_2-guided perfusion is used. This is helpful in regard to optimal venous drainage as it allows the surgeon to safely reduce the pump flow to 70–80% of the calculated flow if required [2]. A 3.2 L flow with a cannula pressure of 350 mmHg can be reached with cannula sizes of 15F, 17F, and 19F and 3.5 L or greater flow rates with a pressure of 350 mmHg, and a 4 L flow rate with pressures of 300 to 350 mmHg, respectively [1]. Notwithstanding these smaller cannula sizes, higher cannula pressures and lower flow rates, there is no proof of any clinical consequences. An alternative cannulation site is sometimes required should there be evidence of significant atherosclerotic disease or a small femoral artery. A computed tomographic angiography (CTA) of the chest, abdomen, and pelvis can reveal such essential information and has become routine in high-volume programs with patients undergoing MICS [3]. The authors believe that CTA should be carried out preoperatively in patients suspected of having aortic and/or peripheral vascular disease [4]. Although the benefits are enormously helpful, the disadvantage of a CTA without contrast is that the subtleties in soft plaque may not be clear and this is an important risk factor to identify prior to peripheral cannulation and retrograde arterial perfusion [2, 5]. An intraoperative finding of grade 4 to 5 atheroma in the descending aorta identified with intraoperative transesophageal echocardiography (TEE) may be a contraindication for retrograde femoral artery perfusion. Safe candidates for peripheral arterial cannulation are those with minimal calcified plaque, thrombus or aneurysmal disease of the aorta [6]. Ipsilateral peripheral arterial access is contraindicated upon confirmation of femoral or iliac dissection or obstructive disease. Should there be any doubt regarding limb ischemia or prolonged cardiopulmonary times, a distal perfusion catheter may be inserted, although this is rarely required.

2.1 Femoral Cannulation

The most prevalent cannulation strategy for MICS procedures, including minithoracotomy, is femoral cannulation and can be achieved either percutaneously or directly via open surgical cutdown [1]. Ultrasound guarantees that the site of cannulation is in the proximal femoral artery regarding percutaneous femoral cannulation and fluoroscopy can also be employed to ensure the cannula is optimally inserted and placed. The puncture site is positioned over the femoral head and access is obtained by puncturing at a point 1/3 of the distance along an oblique line from the pubic tubercle to the anterior superior iliac spine [7]. A Seldinger technique is implemented to pass a guidewire after needle access has been made. A ProGlide system (Abbott Vascular Devices, Santa Clara, CA, USA) is then smoothly moved over the guidewire and is followed by progressive dilatation and finally passage of the arterial cannula. A suture is situated by this device through the anterior wall of the artery which is then tightened following sheath or cannula removal. The Perclose ProGlide device is approved for closure of 5F- to 21F-sized arterial sheaths or cannulas and should therefore only be used on 5 mm or larger vessels. There are other percutaneous closure device options available, including AngioSeal and Manta devices. The Manta device (Teleflex, Morrisville, NC, USA) can close arterial access sites after employing 12F to 25F sheaths. To obtain hemostasis a radiopaque stainless-steel lock and resorbable collagen and anchor are sandwiched into the access site [8]. Conversely a collagen plug is used to seal the arteriotomy in the AngioSeal device (Terumo Medical Corp., Somerset, NJ, USA). This device, however, is not acceptable for sufficient arterial perfusion since it can only be used on 6F or 8F arterial sheaths or cannulas. A safe alternative to percutaneous access is direct (open) cannulation of the femoral artery following cutdown. This direct exposure allows for palpation of the artery and avoidance of excessively atherosclerotic areas as well as allowing for the primary repair of the artery should needs be. This approach, via the right femoral artery, is preferred by the authors

due to the left femoral artery often being used for access during cardiac catheterization. This can result in more difficult left-sided access as well as scarring and hematoma. A 1 to 2 cm vertical skin incision is made above the groin crease, overlying the femoral vessels [9]. The inguinal ligament is then retracted, the vessel exposed proximally on the common femoral artery and a 5–0 Prolene purse-string is then placed. The artery is cannulated through this suture using a Seldinger technique. Should higher flow rates be required, or sufficient perfusion is limited due to the use of an IntraClude endo-aortic balloon occlusion device [10] (Edwards Lifesciences, Irvine, CA, USA), a further arterial cannula can be placed in the contralateral femoral artery (Fig. 1).

Content
1 × 6F Pigtail (Impulse—Boston Scientific)
1 × Amplatz Super Stiff J-Tip 260 cm (Boston Scientific)
Terumo angled guide wire (1 × blue & 1 × brown) 260 cm (Radifocus)
Merit Medical J-Tip Inqwire guide wire 260 cm
1 × Occlusion Balloon Catheter Berenstein (Boston Scientific) + 2 × three-way lock + 2 × 20 mL syringe
4 × Perclose Proglide 6F (Abbott)
1 × Angio-Seal 8F Vascular Closure Device
1 × 6F port

2.2 Axillary Cannulation

Axillary or subclavian arterial access should be followed if significant peripheral vascular disease has been identified, either preoperatively or at the time of femoral cutdown. After a 3 cm skin incision is made 1 cm beneath the clavicle, medial to the deltopectoral groove, the pectoralis muscles are separated or divided and localization is made through finger guidance of the axillary arterial pulse (taking care not to cause injury or excessive traction on the brachial plexus). Flexible vessel loops allow for proximal and distal control of the vessel. The proximal aspect of the artery is clamped with a vascular clamp and the distal loop is retracted. Injury can ensue as the

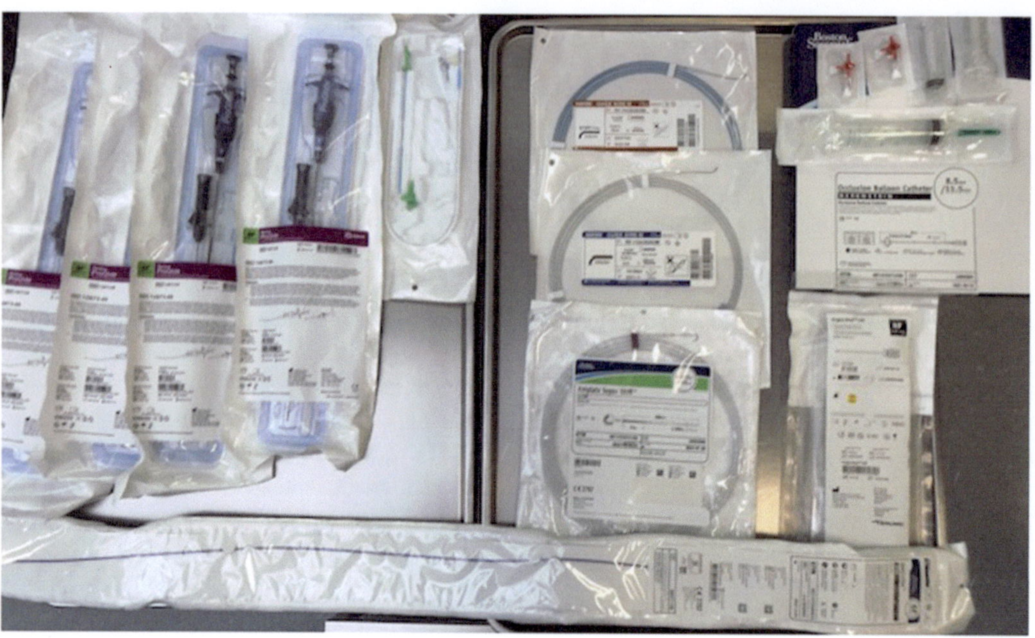

Fig. 1 Standard set at the authors' institution for peripheral percutaneous cannulation

fragile vessel is dilated with a Seldinger technique and so a direct arteriotomy on the vessel is advocated. A guidewire is introduced following the placement of a 6F sheath after the cutdown. Preceding the progression of the cannula through the artery, is necessary to visualize the guidewire with TEE in the ascending or descending aorta. Fluoroscopy can also be used to navigate the guidewire and the cannula. The proper location of, and access to, the cannula can also be performed using intraoperative angiography which can likewise be used to eliminate the presence of atherosclerotic disease. A cannula one size smaller than required for femoral cannulation may be implemented regarding axillary/ subclavian cannulation. Should wire navigation become difficult during axillary/subclavian artery cannulation, the wire is removed from the 6F sheath. In this case, a soft, floppy and slippery glide wire (Terumo Medical Corp., Somerset, NJ, USA) can be used to progress through the tortuous vessels. Fluoroscopic guidance to navigate progression could be used in both cases. As the soft wire reaches the ascending or descending aorta, the sheath is advanced, and the soft wire is replaced with a stiffer wire. Then the sheath is

removed and the cannula advanced. Despite possible interference with standard subclavian/ axillary artery exposure, the patient's arm may be positioned over the head for some MICS procedures. In these circumstances, exposure and cannulation of the axillary artery can be accomplished directly in the axilla. An incision is made in the axilla over the arterial pulse and dissection is followed down to the artery, taking care not to injure and to avoid traction of the brachial plexus. A further cannulation strategy (which also maintains distal arterial perfusion) can include suturing an 10 mm Dacron graft, in an end-to-side fashion, to either the subclavian or axillary artery (Fig. 2).

2.3 Central Aortic Cannulation

The axillary artery is often exempt from serious atherosclerotic disease yet when the artery is too diseased for safe cannulation, central aortic cannulation can be executed. The aorta is identified and, by using pericardial sutures, manipulated toward the operative field. Concentric purse-string sutures are placed and secured with

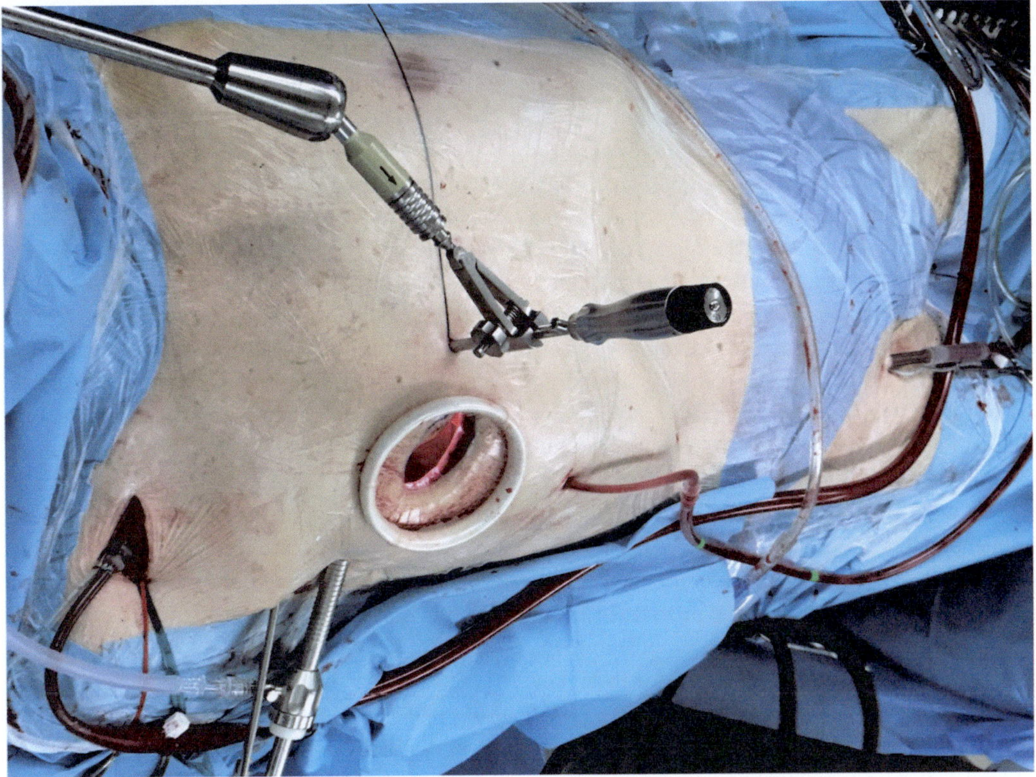

Fig. 2 Axillary cannulation during a minimally invasive surgical mitral valve repair procedure

tourniquets and by using a Seldinger technique the aortic cannulation is concluded through the purse strings. The cannula is secured with the tourniquets and additionally to the skin. Central cannulation is possible via any MICS approach although it could cause the exposure in an already limited field to be further inhibited. Should better exposure and a more convenient procedure be necessary, an upper hemisternotomy could be performed. A further challenge to central cannulation using the minithoracotomy approach is if the aorta is extremely shifted to the left. To establish which approach is most suitable, a CT scan of the chest should be realized. Dissection of the aorta occurs in 0.01 to 0.09% of patients as a complication of central aortic cannulation. Suspicion of such dissection should be aroused when confronted with an aortic bluish hue or a high arterial line pressure post-CPB initiation. An additional TEE assessment for dissection of the ascending aorta is performed after cannulation and decannulation. CPB should be stopped and further assessment of the situation should be made if this is identified in good time.

2.4 Endo-Clamp Occlusion Balloon

For standard-, even complicated and reoperative cases, an endo-aortic balloon clamp, IntraClude (Edwards Lifesciences, Irvine, CA, USA) is highly effective. Under guidance from TEE, the balloon is introduced into the femoral artery or subclavian artery and positioned in the ascending aorta. The balloon is inflated and antegrade cardioplegia can then be delivered and the aortic root can be vented through the cannula tip. Difficulties such as diminished perfusion to the arch vessels can arise should the balloon migrate, thus prompting careful placement and positioning.

3 Venous Cannulation

Optimal cardiac surgery demands sufficient venous drainage and decompression of the heart. Adequate drainage is reached by employing vacuum assistance and the right cannula size. These two components differentiate between conventional sternotomy-based heart surgery and MICS. In conventional sternotomy-based heart surgery the venous drainage is often achieved via gravity and without the assistance of vacuum. Furthermore, the size of the cannula may vary depending on the type of cannula and patient BSA. Regarding the cannula size, the authors prefer to use a 25F femoral venous cannula in most patients regardless of their BSA. A vacuum-assisted device is implemented in almost all modes of MICS venous cannulation to allow for effective drainage and to prevent air entrapment. Vacuum pressures start at -30 mmHg and can go as high as -60 mmHg; gaseous micro-emboli has been related to higher vacuum pressures. Successful use of new minimally invasive CPB circuits on minimally invasive cases has been documented.

3.1 Femoral Cannulation

The most frequently implemented technique for venous drainage in MICS is femoral venous cannulation. Venous access, as with arterial access, is achieved percutaneously or via direct exposure with a femoral surgical cutdown. Apart from cannula positioning, the femoral vein cannulation technique follows that of arterial cannulation. A three-stage cannula is recommended to guarantee sufficient drainage and this is to be positioned, under guidance of TEE, into the superior vena cava (SVC). This achieves a bicaval view at 120° and the essential visualization of the wire as it is inserted through the inferior vena cava (IVC) and into the SVC. Should other lines be present in the SVC, such as a Swan-Ganz catheter or pacemaker, the wire must be distinguishable. When sufficient

visualization is achieved, the cannula is inserted over the wire using a Seldinger technique. TEE guidance is again employed for the visualization of the cannula entering the SVC. Should an open technique be employed, a 5–0 Prolene purse-string is placed prior to cannula insertion, enabling direct closure following decannulation. This direct venous closure is not possible, however, when a percutaneous approach is used. Although many of the available devices for percutaneous arterial closure may be applicable for venous closure, they are not usually employed. A further option is the placing of a large and deep 0 Vicryl U-stitch around the site of percutaneous venous access covering the site of the venous puncture. After decannulation, the suture is tied down, thus closing the track of the cannula and using the patient's native soft tissue to tamponade the venotomy.

3.2 Internal Juglar or Subclavian Venous Cannulation

Further sites for venous cannulation are the internal jugular or subclavian vein. Cannulation at these sites is often performed percutaneously and with a 17F or larger arterial cannula. A Seldinger technique is used to place the cannula and ultrasound guidance used to localize the vein. To ensure the positioning of the cannula is correct, TEE should be employed. These cannulation sites are seldom used individually, but as ancillary sites when venous drainage is not sufficient with femoral venous cannulation alone. Also, left subclavian or internal jugular venous cannulation may be necessary to facilitate sufficient venous drainage should there be anatomic abnormalities as in the presence of a persistent left SVC. It is not always possible to identify these abnormalities preoperatively, requiring the surgeon to change cannulation strategy at the time of surgery in order to ensure safe and sufficient drainage. Likewise, a further femoral cannula may be inserted percutaneously in the opposite femoral vein, internal jugular vein, or via a purse string suture in the SVC directly through the working incision, should insufficient venous drainage be detected.

Venous drainage can be supported by using a low right jugular approach. This is done either by the anesthesiology team or by the surgeon, using a small previously placed sheath [4]. In this case, the venous cannula would only be forged to the IVC-RA junction. Adding an SVC cannula is especially practical in case of tricuspid valve- or ASD-closure procedures [4, 11]. Aternatively, using a single femoral dual-stage cannula would make a complete bypass possible.

3.3 Central Venous Cannulation

In certain MICS procedures it may be necessary to introduce central venous cannulation. For example, during ascending aortic replacement, the surgeon may follow retrograde cerebral perfusion via the SVC. In such cases a further venous canula can be tunneled through the chest tube insertion site and then into the SVC directly through a purse-string suture. When right atrial isolation may be necessary during tricuspid valve or other right atrial procedures, to assist with bicavical cannulation a venous cannula may similarly be placed either through the chest tube site or directly through the incision. Also, MICS aortic procedures may benefit from central venous cannulation as the primary source of venous drainage. In this case, a low-profile venous cannula is inserted into the right atrium directly through the incision. This cannulation strategy is not an option, however, for mitral valve procedures nor MICS coronary artery bypass procedures performed via a left minithoracotomy. It is possible to place a femoral venous cannula into the IVC in many tricuspid valve operations, without encircling and snaring the cavas. It is crucial to use vacuum assistance as more blood may be experienced in the operative field leading to obscured visualization. This technique is extremely useful during reoperative tricuspid surgery.

4 Complications of Cannulation

4.1 General Considerations

Despite femoral cannulation being the pillar of MICS, risks continue to exist. Retrograde dissection, embolization, and limb ischemia have all been correlated with femoral cannulation. One study reported femoral cannulation stroke rate of 1.17% [12]. From the authors' experience, despite the cannulation technique employed, minimally invasive valve surgery has an acceptable stroke rate. For procedures performed without an aortic cross-clamp, to help minimize the incidence of stroke, the techniques for removal of air should not be compromised and should mimic the technique used during standard median sternotomy.

4.2 Arterial Cannulation Site Complications

The order of preference during MICS arterial cannulation is the femoral artery, subclavian artery, axillary artery, and finally central aortic. The patient dictates which arterial cannulation option is most favorable and this depends on the procedure, atherosclerotic load and body habitus. The risks involved with arterial cannulation include limb ischemia, compartment syndrome, retrograde dissection, seroma and hematoma development, lower-extremity neuropathy from femoral nerve injury, femoral or axillary artery stenosis post-cannulation, and stroke. The most feared complication of peripheral cannulation, especially with femoral access, continues to be stroke. LaPietra et al. [13] reviewed 1,501 consecutive patients undergoing a minithoracotomy valve procedure where femoral cannulation was employed in 90.5% of the cases. The incidence of stroke, which was not statistically indicative, from femoral artery and axillary or direct cannulation in total was 1.4% and 2.9%, respectively (P = 0.15). The safety of femoral cannulation in MICS in 2,645 patients, specifically regarding stroke risk, was retrospectively evaluated by

Lamelas et al. [14]. This included patients with a previous history of stroke or peripheral vascular disease. Compared to central cannulation, the study reported a low incidence of stroke at 1.17%, with no increase in complications. Indeed, the stroke rate was lower in the femoral cannulation group (1.17%) compared to axillary or central cannulation (2.6%). Equally low stroke rates were recorded in other evaluated surgeries; Lamelas et al. [15] evaluated 1,018 cases of isolated minimally invasive aortic valve replacement surgeries and 378 cases of minimally invasive aortic valve with concomitant procedures (stroke rate 0.8% and 1.1%, respectively; P = 0.62).

4.3 Venous Cannulation Site Complications

Although vascular complications from venous cannulation performed via a direct cutdown approach are rare, the risk of injuring the femoral artery through percutaneous venous cannulation is present when it lies over the femoral vein. Also, with or without injury to the femoral artery, bleeding with localized hematoma formation can still take place. Perforation of the SVC, IVC, right atrium, and right ventricle remain the foremost potential complications even when using TEE or fluoroscopy.

5 Comment

Kastengren et al. [16] concluded that traditional complications frequently seen with surgical cutdown with no femoral access site seroma and infection can be eliminated through percutaneous femoral artery cannulation using a novel plug-based VCD in minimally invasive mitral valve surgery. This is, however, at the cost of an increased risk of vascular complications. Substantial reduction in groin complications, operation time and hospital stay were concluded by Moschovas et al. [17] with regard to percutaneous groin cannulation using arterial closure devices for establishing CPB in minimally invasive valve surgery. Any outstanding complications are of the vascular type as opposed to wound infection and lymph fistulae with cutdown (Videos 1, 2, and 3).

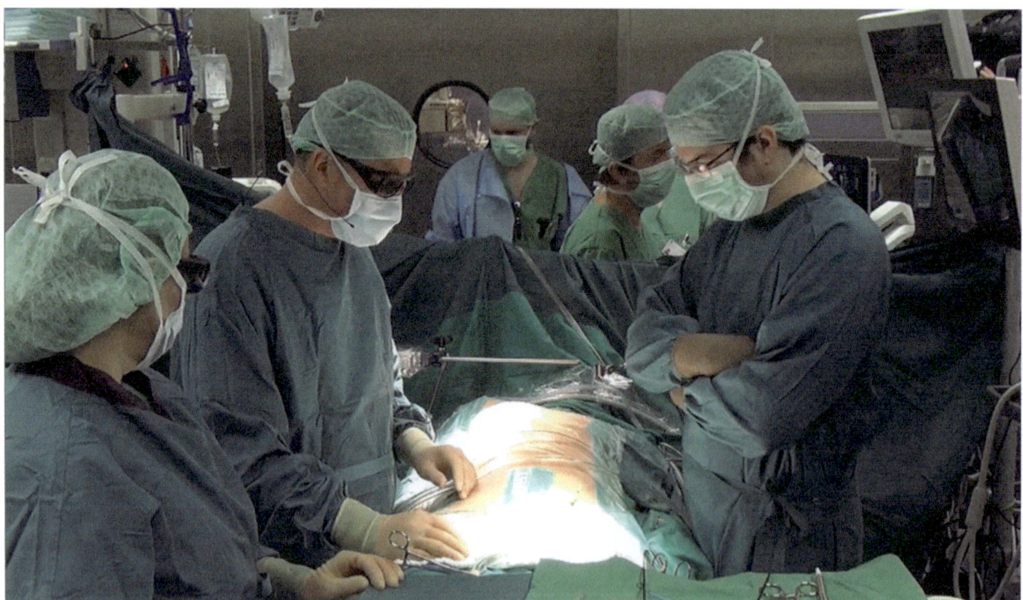

Video 1 Case 01 – Percutaneous cannulation with the 23F endoreturn cannula for MIMVS
(▶ https://doi.org/10.1007/000-a8e)

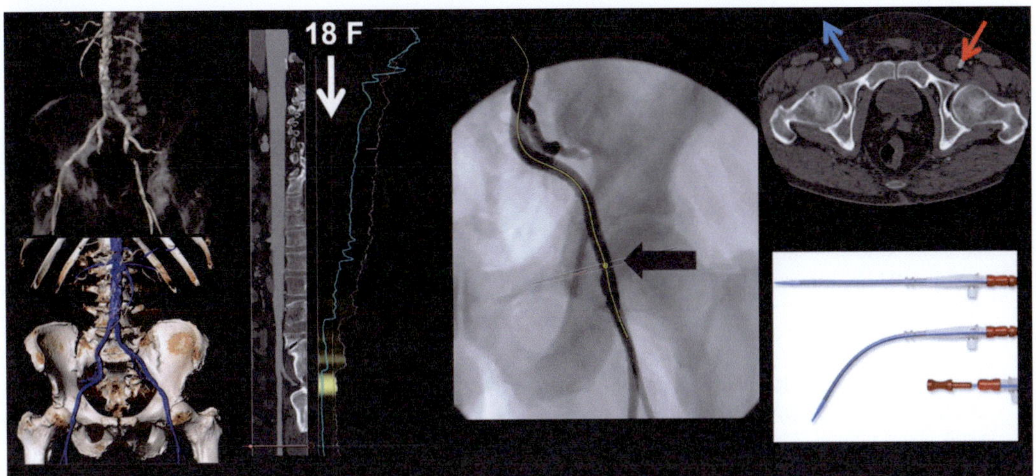

Video 2 Case 02 – Percutaneous cannulation with the FemFlex 18F cannula for MIS SAVR (RALT)
(▶ https://doi.org/10.1007/000-a8d)

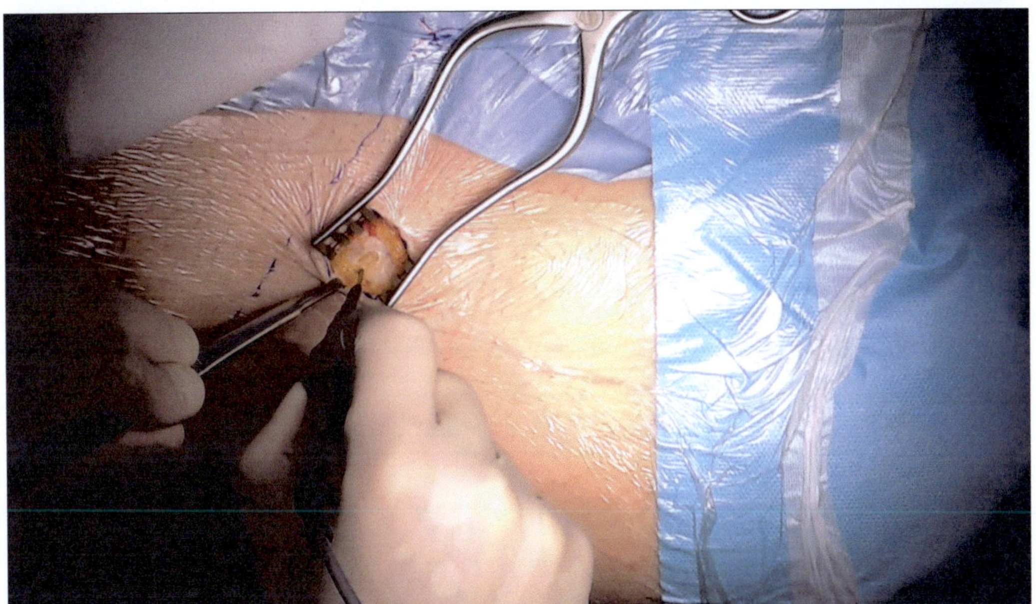

Video 3 Case 03 – Open surgical femoral cutdown with the 23F endoreturn cannula for MIMVS
(▶ https://doi.org/10.1007/000-a8f)

References

1. Lamelas J, Aberle C, Macias AE, Alnajar A. Cannulation strategies for minimally invasive cardiac surgery. Innov Technol Tech Cardiothorac Vasc Surg. 2020;15(3):261–9. https://doi.org/10.1177/1556984520911917.

2. Van Praet KM, van Kampen A, Kofler M, et al. Minimally invasive surgical aortic valve replacement: the RALT approach. J Card Surg. 2020:1–6. https://doi.org/10.1111/jocs.14756

3. Karel M. Van Praet, Antonia Van Kampen, Markus Kofler, Axel Unbehaun, Matthias Hommel, Stephan Jacobs, Volkmar Falk JK. Minimally invasive surgical aortic valve replacement through a right anterolateral thoracotomy. Multimed Man Cardiothorac Surg. doi: 10.15.

4. Van Praet KM, Kofler M, Montagner M, et al. Minimally invasive mitral valve repair using external clamping—pearls and pitfalls. J Vis Surg. 2020;6 (45). https://doi.org/10.21037/jovs-2019-amvis-07

5. Van Praet KM, Kofler M, Unbehaun A, et al. Reply to Del Giglio, Tamagnini, Biondi, and Di Mauro. J Card Surg. 2020:4–7. https://doi.org/10.1111/jocs.14998

6. Van Praet KM, Stamm C, Sündermann SH, et al. Minimally invasive cardiac surgery removal of an interatrial intraseptal bronchogenic cyst through a periareolar approach. Innov (Phila). 13(3):230–2. http://journals.lww.com/innovjournal.

7. Van Praet KM, Stamm C, Sündermann SH, et al. Minimally invasive surgical mitral valve repair: State of the art review. Interv Cardiol Rev. 2018;13(1):14–9. https://doi.org/10.15420/icr.2017:30:1.

8. Van Praet KM, Kofler M, Jacobs S, Falk V, Axel Unbehaun JK. The MANTA vascular closure device for percutaneous femoral vessel cannulation in minimally invasive surgical mitral valve repair. Innov. 2020:1–4. https://doi.org/10.1177/1556984520956300.

9. Van Praet KM, Kempfert J, Jacobs S, et al. Mitral valve surgery: current status and future prospects of the minimally invasive approach. Expert Rev Med Devices. 2021. https://doi.org/10.1080/17434440.2021.1894925.

10. Van Praet KM, Kofler M, Sündermann SH, et al. Minimally invasive approach for infective mitral valve endocarditis. Ann Cardiothorac Surg. 2019;8 (6):702–4. https://doi.org/10.21037/acs.2019.07.01.

11. Van Praet KM, Stamm C, Starck CT, et al. An overview of surgical treatment modalities and emerging transcatheter interventions in the management of tricuspid valve regurgitation. Expert Rev Cardiovasc Ther. 2018;16(2):75–89. https://doi.org/10.1080/14779072.2018.1421068.

12. Crooke G, Schwartz C, Ribakove G. Retrograde arterial perfusion, not incision location, significantly increases the risk of stroke in reoperative mitral valve procedures. Ann Thorac Surg. 2010;89:723–30.

13. LaPietra A, Santana O, Mihos C. Incidence of cerebrovascular accidents in patients undergoing minimally invasive valve surgery. J Thorac Cardiovasc Surg. 2014;148:156–60.

14. Lamelas J, Williams R, Mawad M. Complications associated with femoral cannulation during minimally invasive cardiac surgery. Ann Thorac Surg. 2017;103:1927–32.

15. Lamelas J, Mawad M, Williams R. Isolated and concomitant minimally invasive minithoracotomy aortic valve surgery. J Thorac Cardiovasc Surg. 2018;155:926–36.

16. Kastengren M, Svenarud P, Källner G, Settergren M, Franco-Cereceda A, Dalén M. Percutaneous vascular closure device in minimally invasive mitral valve surgery. Ann Thorac Surg. 2020;110(1):85–91. https://doi.org/10.1016/j.athoracsur.2019.10.038

17. Moschovas A, Amorim PA, Nold M, et al. Percutaneous cannulation for cardiopulmonary bypass in minimally invasive surgery is associated with reduced groin complications. Interact Cardiovasc Thorac Surg. 2017;25(3):377–83. https://doi.org/10.1093/icvts/ivx140.

Endoscopic Mitral Surgery in Cardiogenic Shock

Mario Castillo-Sang

Abstract

Endoscopic mitral surgery is not only limited to elective cases. The technique can be used in more complicated and acute situations involving cardiogenic shock of different etiologies. In this chapter we illustrate our experience and learned best practices in the surgical management of the patient in cardiogenic shock from mitral valve disease. Techniques to treat a mitral valve do not change, but preoperative, intraoperative and postoperative conduct do and are of great importance. Different etiologies of mitral disease in shock have a common denominator in their preoperative management including hemodynamic stabilization, right ventricular protection, metabolic optimization and improvement of coagulopathy.

Keywords

Cardiogenic shock · Endoscopic mitral valve surgery · Acute mitral regurgitation · Secondary mitral regurgitation · Mitral stenosis · Mechanical circulatory support

M. Castillo-Sang (✉)
20 Medical Village Drive, Suite 271, Edgewood, KY 41017, USA
e-mail: mcastillosang@gmail.com

1 Introduction

- **Mitral Valve Emergencies**

True mitral valve emergencies are uncommon and in our experience make up 2–7% of all operations year-to-year performed for the mitral valve at our center. Gammie et al. reported 7.8% of all minimally invasive mitral valve operations recorded in the STS registry between 2004 and 2008 to be other than elective [1].

A mitral valve emergency is better defined in the context of the hemodynamic status of the patient. Most patients with mitral valve disease do not have an acute presentation, but those that do often require inotropic or mechanical support for hemodynamic instability compounding intractable respiratory compromise (pulmonary edema).

We use the SCAI definition for cardiogenic shock as a persistent systolic blood pressure of less than 90 mmHg, mean arterial pressure less than 60 mmHg or a drop of over 30 mmHg from baseline (Table 1). Stage B or early cardiogenic shock includes those presenting with the above criteria without clear signs of hypoperfusion (cardiac index >2.2 and SVO2 >65%). Stage C includes those with pressures below the aforementioned levels requiring inotropic or mechanical support with clear signs of hypoperfusion (cardiac index <2, wedge >15 mmHg,

Table 1 Classification of cardiogenic shock (adapted from SCAI classification) [2]

Stage	Description	Laboratory findings	Hemodynamic values
A—At risk CS	No signs or symptoms of CS, but at risk (AMI, acute on chronic CHF)	Normal lactic acid Normal GFR	Normal SBP; CI ≥ 2.5; CVP <10; SVO2 $\geq 65\%$
B— Early CS	Relative hypotension or tachycardia without organ hypoperfusion	Normal lactate Mildly decreased GFR Elevated BNP	SBP <90 mmHg, MAP <60 mmHg; drop over 30 mmHg from baseline; CI ≥ 2.2 SVO2 $\geq 65\%$
C— Classic CS	Hypotension requiring intervention beyond volume	Lactate ≥ 2 $2\times$ creatinine or >50% drop in GFR Elevated LFT's Elevated BNP	Same blood pressure values as Stage B CI <2.2; SVO2 <65%; Wedge >15; PAPI <1.85; RAP/Wedge ≥ 0.8

Adapted from Baran et al., 2019. *Catheterization and Cardiovascular Interventions*, 94(4), 29–37. AMI = acute myocardial infarction. CHF = congestive heart failure. GFR = glomerular filtration rate. LFT = liver function test. BNP = b-type natriuretic peptide. SBP = systolic blood pressure. CVP = central venous pressure. CI = cardiac index. PAPI = pulmonary artery pressure index. RAP = right atrial pressure. SVO2 = mixed venous saturation

pulmonary artery pressure index <1.85) and require typically inotropic support. Stage D patients are deteriorating and require multiple pressors or additional mechanical circulatory support devices to maintain systemic perfusion. Patients in Stage E are in extremis and are unlikely to survive an attempt at surgical intervention [2] By making the above distinctions one can then clearly categorize the higher acuity presentation of mitral valve disease into acute or 'super-acute' and deploy care appropriately. Figure 1 portrays a practical classification of mitral valve pathologies and their acute presentation with hemodynamic compromise.

It is important to consider those patients that present normotensive, without signs of endo-organ hypoperfusion, but with significant respiratory compromise or in fulminant respiratory failure who fall into the Stage A of the SCAI classification [2, 3]. These are typically patients that may find a level of stability with only mechanical ventilation and/or aggressive diuresis but are at high risk of requiring further hemodynamic assistance.

It is clear that patients in cardiogenic shock from mitral valve disease have a historically high surgical mortality of 20% to 40% and that their management is labor intensive throughout the spectrum of the hospital stay [4–6]. It is well warranted to have a pre-established algorhythm that can expedite diagnostics, triaging, early therapeutics, and advanced therapeutics/surgical approach.

Patients in cardiogenic shock or near cardiogenic shock secondary to or accompanying severe mitral valve disease present to the surgeon in two ways. First are those hemodynamically unstable who undergo an emergent coronary angiogram demonstrating severe coronary artery disease and severe mitral regurgitation perhaps

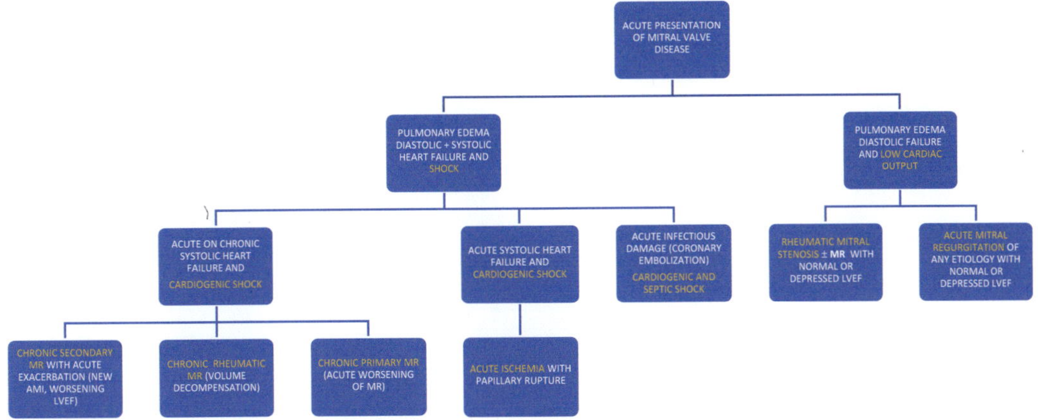

Fig. 1 The acute presentation of mitral valve disease with hemodynamic compromise. LVEF = Left ventricular ejection fraction. AMI = Acute myocardial infarction

on left ventriculogram or immediate transthoracic echocardiogram. If the patient undergoes surgical revascularization the mitral valve is addressed concomitantly. Second are those that have undergone percutaneous coronary revascularization prior to presentation to the surgeon leaving the mitral valve regurgitation therapy pending. This last scenario is common with contemporary PCI/stent management of STEMI [5, 6]. These patients may now have a papillary muscle rupture or acute worsening of chronic ischemic mitral regurgitation and are candidates to a minimally invasive approach.

The objective of this chapter is to describe the acute presentation and endoscopic minimally invasive treatment of the mitral valve patient in cardiogenic shock. In addressing these patients we have to discuss those presenting in acute respiratory failure requiring pharmacological and mechanical support to alleviate cardiac/pulmonary congestion too and those with mixed picture of cardiogenic and septic shock in the setting of endocarditis.

The etiology of cardiogenic shock in the setting of mitral valve disease varies. For the purpose of this chapter and therapeutic considerations, we have divided mitral valve disease with acute presentation into those with predominantly low cardiac output (low forward flow) and those with diastolic heart failure and pulmonary congestion. Both groups of patients

tend to have an inflammatory response component leading to low SVRI [7].

Low cardiac output shock (cardiogenic shock) can also be divided into 'wet' or volume overloaded and 'dry' or euvolemic cardiogenic shock. Invasive hemodynamic monitoring with pulmonary artery catheter is key in differentiating these two situations, finding a high SVRI and low cardiac index in both, but high wedge pressures in the wet cardiogenic shock and low-to-normal in dry cardiogenic shock [2]. Use of pulmonary artery catheter has been shown to improve outcomes in cardiogenic shock and should be instituted as early as possible [8]. Dry cardiogenic shock typically involves the diuretic-responsive patient with chronic heart failure and subacute decompensation representing 28% of cardiogenic shock associated to myocardial infarction and may account to up to 30% of all cardiogenic shock cases [9].

- **Left ventricular versus biventricular failure**

Differentiating between isolated left ventricular failure or biventricular failure is important to select the best inotropic support and/or mechanical circulatory support as well as starting an inhaled pulmonary vasodilator therapy. Right ventricular driven cardiogenic shock is thought to have an incidence of 5.3% [10]. For patient with biventricular failure VA-ECMO is a reliable approach (but does not offload the left ventricle), while those with isolated left ventricular failure can be stabilized with either Impella (Abiomed, Danvers, Massachusetts, USA), IABP or another temporary percutaneous left ventricular assist device.

- **Mitral valve pathology**

The type/etiology of mitral valve pathology is very relevant in the early stages of evaluation of the patient in cardiogenic shock. In general, pathology can be primary (including endocarditis) or secondary mitral valve regurgitation; mitral regurgitation or stenosis; mitral prosthesis malfunction (Table 2).

- **Different forms of minimally invasive mitral valve surgery**

There are different techniques for minimally invasive mitral valve surgery that vary by center and surgeon. In all, in the United States approximately 23–25% of all mitral valve operations are performed minimally invasive with 8% robotic assisted and the rest with other forms of minimally invasive techniques, predominantly right minithoracotomy [11, 12]. In Germany 55% of all mitral valve operations were performed minimally invasive while in Italy up to 71% of all mitral operations were performed minimally invasive based on a multicenter study [13, 14]. In the United Kingdom, based on study including three centers 27% of all mitral valve operations were performed minimally invasive between 2008 and 2016 [15].

- **The endoscopic approach to mitral valve surgery**

We perform our operations endoscopically assisted using a 5 mm 30-degree thoracoscope positioned in the second intercostal space and mid clavicular line allowing us to create a small 1.5–2-inches right chest working incision in the 4th intercostal space lateral to the nipple in men and lateral to the breast in women. We find that

in order to insert mitral prostheses into the chest without undue deformation the minimal size incision is 1.5 inches (Fig. 2A and B). We use a deployable crossclamp (Cygnet clamp, Peters Surgical, Bobigny France) applied through the right minithoracotomy. A 5 mm port in the 4th parasternal space is used for an atrial lift retractor.

- **Contraindications to endoscopic mitral surgery approach in cardiogenic shock**

In the past many have deemed a prior right chest operation as a contraindication to endoscopic minimally invasive heart surgery, but we find that this is relative to the type of previous operation. If the patient had undergone a video assisted lung resection an endoscopic mitral valve surgery is possible within the reasonable time it takes to take down adhesions. We have routinely performed endoscopic mitral valve surgery in patients who underwent right thoracotomies, but the time spent carefully taking down lung adhesions may prove too long in the setting of cardiogenic shock. Patients who had empyema and mechanical or chemical pleurodesis on the right side are true contraindications [12].

We perform the endoscopic mitral operation in patients with systemic or near-systemic pulmonary artery pressures as well as those with a previous open-heart operation as this has been proven to be safe in redo sternotomies and in minimally invasive approaches [16, 17]. One true anatomical contraindication for endoscopic mitral surgery in cardiogenic shock is the presence of severe mitral annular calcification unless there is availability of an off label transcatheter balloon expandible valve with direct surgical implantation into mitral annular calcification (MAC), but we have not experienced this operation in the setting of cardiogenic shock.

- **Our experience**

Our decision-making process in patients presenting with severe mitral stenosis or regurgitation, respiratory failure, on inotropic/pressor

Table 2 Etiology and management of severe mitral pathology in cardiogenic shock

Etiology	Pulmonary vasodilator	Inotropic support	Mechanical support	Transcatheter (TMVr/R)	Surgical therapy
Primary MR	Start if depressed RV and/or PAS $\geq 2/3$ systemic	Implement early (SBP >90 mmHg with elevated lactate, large base deficit or SVO2 <60%)	When 1 high-dose or 2 inotropes with SVO2 <60%	TEER option	Endoscopic option
Infectious MR	Start if depressed RV and/or PAS $\geq 2/3$ systemic	Implement early (SBP >90 mmHg with elevated lactate, large base deficit or SVO2 <60%)	When 1 high-dose or 2 inotropes with SVO2 <60%	No TMVr/R option	Endoscopic option
Secondary MR	Start if depressed RV and/or PAS $\geq 2/3$ systemic	Implement early (SBP >90 mmHg with elevated lactate, large base deficit or SVO2 <60%)	When 1 high-dose or 2 inotropes with SVO2 <60%	TEER option	Endoscopic option
Bioprosthetic valve MR or MS (structural deterioration)	Start if depressed RV and/or PAS $\geq 2/3$ systemic	Implement early (SBP >90 mmHg with elevated lactate, large base deficit or SVO2 <60%)	When 1 high-dose or 2 inotropes with SVO2 <60%	Valve in valve option	Endoscopic option if no TMVR
Mechanical valve MR or MS	Start if depressed RV and/or PAS $\geq 2/3$ systemic	Implement early (SBP >90 mmHg with elevated lactate, large base deficit or SVO2 <60%)	When 1 high-dose or 2 inotropes with SVO2 <60%	No TMVr/R option	Endoscopic option
Rheumatic MS	Start if depressed RV and/or PAS $\geq 2/3$ systemic	Implement early (SBP >90 mmHg with elevated lactate, large base deficit or SVO2 <60%)	When 1 high-dose or 2 inotropes with SVO2 <60%	Primary PTMB if criteria met	Endoscopic option if no PTMB
Rheumatic MR	Start if depressed RV and/or PAS $\geq 2/3$ systemic	Implement early (SBP >90 mmHg with elevated lactate, large base deficit or SVO2 <60%)	When 1 high-dose or 2 inotropes with SVO2 <60%	No TMVr/R option	Endoscopic option

Etiological classification of cardiogenic shock accompanying severe mitral valve disease. TMVr = transcatheter mitral valve repair. TMVR = transcatheter mitral valve replacement. PTMB = percutaneous transcatheter mitral balloon valvuloplasty. MR = mitral regurgitation. MS = mitral stenosis. RV = right ventricle. SVO2 = mixed venous oxygen saturation

support and/or mechanical circulatory support hinges on the viability of the patient, expected quality of life and patient's wishes. A clear and candid conversation with the patient and family about the expected risks and benefits of a mitral valve operation under the above circumstances is paramount.

Our experience in managing mitral valve patients in cardiogenic shock in the last two years is summarized in Table 3. We have encountered patients in different levels of shock, some requiring only an inotrope and/or pressor while others required advanced mechanical support. The etiology behind the mitral valve pathology varied, the most common being ischemic mitral regurgitation (secondary MR) with an acute on chronic presentation due to decompensation. The predominant mechanical support was IABP

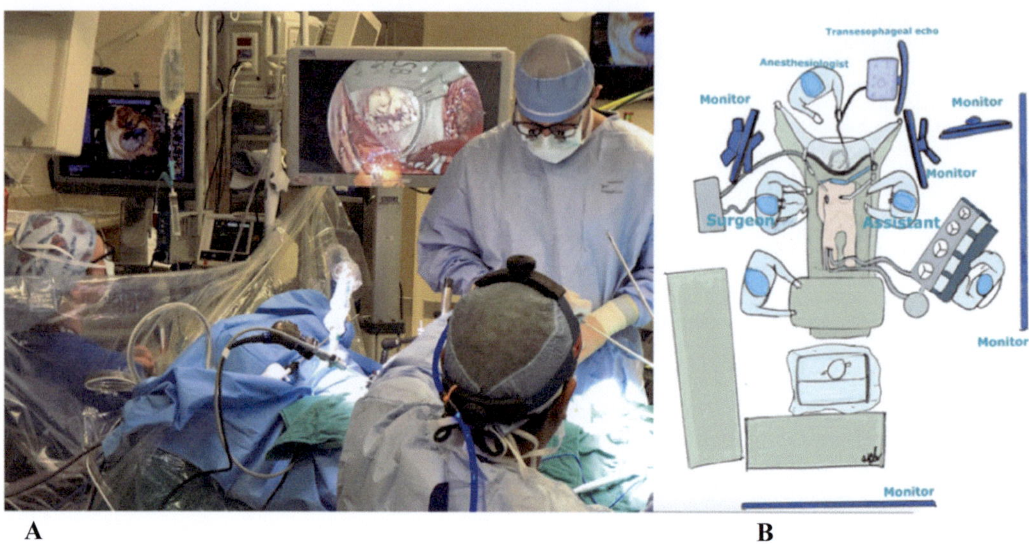

Fig. 2 **A** and **B** Surgeon's view of the operative field using the 5 mm 30-degree angled endoscope

Table 3 Two-year experience of endoscopic mitral valve surgery in cardiogenic shock

Patient	Age	Etiology	Procedure	Pharmacologic support	Mechanical support	Nitric oxide
1	52	Papillary rupture-ischemic MR	MVR	Pressor + Inotrope	Impella VA-ECMO	Yes
2	68	Acute on chronic ischemic MR	MVR	Pressor + Inotrope	Impella	Yes
3	64	Acute on chronic ischemic MR	Redo-MVR	Pressor + Inotrope	Impella	Yes
4	70	Acute presentation of chronic Rheumatic MR	MVR/ TVR	Pressor + Inotrope	IABP	No
5	69	Acute presentation of chronic Rheumatic MR	MVR/ TVR	Pressor + Inotrope	Impella	Yes
6	65	Acute on chronic ischemic MR	MVR/ TVR	Pressor + Inotrope	IABP	Yes
7	27	Endocarditis acute MR	MVR	Pressor + Inotrope	None	Yes
8	31	Endocarditis acute MR	MVR	Pressor + Inotrope	None	Yes
9	57	Acute presentation of Rheumatic MR/MS	MVR	Inotrope	IABP	Yes
10	58	Acute presentation of Rheumatic MS	MVR	Pressor	IABP	Yes
11	50	Papillary rupture non-ischemic	MVr	Pressor + Inotrope	IABP	No
12	62	Endocarditis + chronic primary MR	MVR/ TVr	Pressor + Inotrope	IABP	Yes
13	53	Acute on chronic ischemic MR	MVR/ TVr	Inotrope	IABP	Yes

Unpublished data of endoscopic mitral valve surgeries performed in the setting of cardiogenic shock and mitral valve disease. MR, mitral regurgitation. IABP, intra-aortic balloon pump. MVR, mitral valve replacement. MVr, mitral valve repair. TVR, tricuspid valve repair. ABE, acute bacterial endocarditis. VA ECMO, veno-arterial extra-corporeal membrane oxygenation. MS, mitral stenosis. Impella (Abiomed, Danvers, Massachusetts, USA)

followed by Impella (Abiomed, Danvers, Massachusetts, USA). There were no operative mortalities, and all patients were discharged from the hospital. One patient died at 4 months from recidivism of IVDA, 12 were alive at follow-up up to 1 year. There were no operative strokes and one patient required hemodialysis postoperatively for one month.

2 Operative Considerations

- **Anesthesia considerations**

There are several considerations for the anesthesia team managing the cardiogenic shock patient undergoing endoscopic mitral valve surgery. An important one is whether a double-lumen or single-lumen endotracheal tube will be used. We routinely use single-lumen tubes.

On induction of anesthesia, we focus on right ventricular protection for those without mechanical or with only an IABP. We prevent hypotension and once the patient is orotracheally intubated, or when connected to the anesthesia circuit if previously intubated, the inhaled nitric oxide is started 40 PPM if the systolic pulmonary artery pressure is greater than 2/3 systemic or at 20 PPM between 50% and 2/3 systemic (Fig. 3A and B). This dosing is based on the response we have observed in the operating room in acute settings with active pulmonary edema complicating right ventricular dysfunction.

- **Cannulation strategy**

If we have the advantage of a preoperative CT scan to evaluate the aorto-iliac vasculature we opt to cannulate via the femoral vessels or alternatively via the right axillary artery (for those with prohibitive aorto-iliac disease). Our axillary cannulation consists of a pursestring on the artery and direct cannulation with a 15 or 17 Fr cannula with transesophageal echo guidance to identify the guidewire in the ascending or descending aorta. In cannulating the axillary artery, one must have a left arm arterial line, but we request bilateral arm arterial lines. The venous cannulation is universally via the common femoral vein with a two-stage 23Fr to 27Fr cannula (23Fr for BSA 1.6 m2; 25Fr for 1.6–2.2m2; 2Fr for 2.2m2 or higher) (Fig. 4). We favor the bicaval cannulas such as the Medtronic Bio-Medicus NextGen (Medtronic, Minneapolis, Minnesota, USA). In patients supported with VA-ECMO we convert the cannulation to the cardiopulmonary bypass circuit and at the end of the operation, depending on the myocardial contractility weaning off bypass we decannulate or convert again to VA-ECMO.

The mitral valve replacement is performed with prosthesis selection based on standard EACTS or AHA guidelines. For those patients

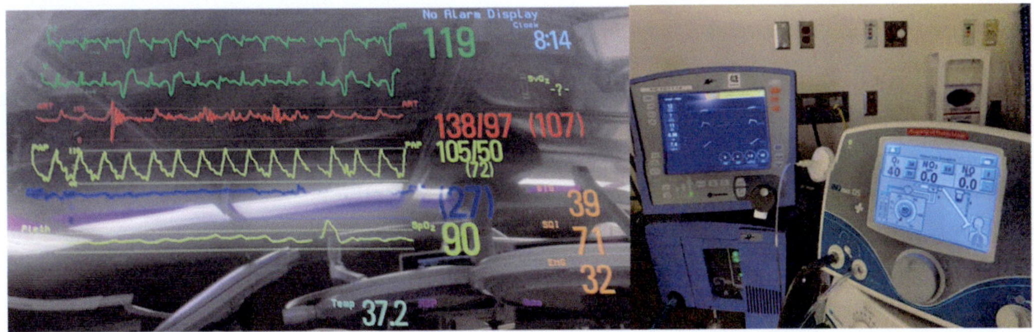

Fig. 3 **A** intraoperative vital signs at the time of induction of a patient supported with inotropes showing systemic pressures preserved, pulmonary artery pressures (105/50 mmHg) over 2/3 systemic and an elevated CVP of 27 mmHg. **B** This patient was supported with an IABP and inhaled nitric oxide

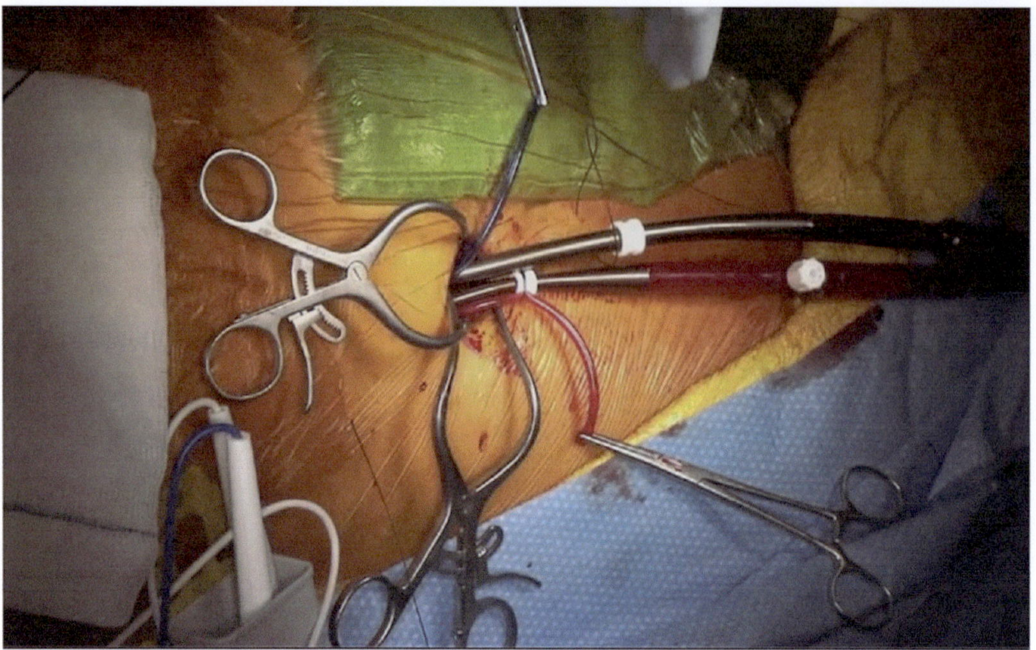

Fig. 4 Femoral canulation strategy

on inotropic or IABP support and less than 60 years old we select a mechanical prosthesis if no contraindications for anticoagulation exist. For those with deeper hemodynamic compromise requiring Impella (Abiomed, Danvers, Massachusetts, USA), VA-ECMO or both, we elect to place a bioprosthesis. The argument for the latter is that with full unloading of the ventricular preload there will be stasis and poor washing of the prosthesis which may lead to thrombosis [18].

- **Cardioplegia**

We exclusively use Del Nido Cardioplegia for all minimally invasive mitral valve operations. In the setting of cardiogenic shock having adequate cardiac protection to minimize myocardial dysfunction is paramount, but it is also important to abbreviate the crossclamp time. Our arresting dose is 1,000 to 1,200 ml and redosing is performed at 60–70 min with 300–500 ml extra if 30 or more minutes of work are required.

Application of the crossclamp can be challenging in cases where there is an indwelling Impella pump (Abiomed, Danvers, Massachusetts, USA). In our experience applying a soft insert crossclamp such as the Cygnet clamp (Peters Surgical, Bobigny France) results in better occlusion of the aorta. One should turn to bypass mode the Impella device and advance it as much as possible into the ventricle so as to crossclamp only the smaller diameter driveline. Alternatively, the Impella can be pulled back into the descending aorta to apply the crossclamp understanding that it will not be reinserted and that a new one or an alternative mechanical support will be needed at the end of the case. In cases where the ascending aorta cannot be clamped and there is no aortic insufficiency fibrillatory arrest with hypothermia is also an acceptable option in the absence of Impella pump.

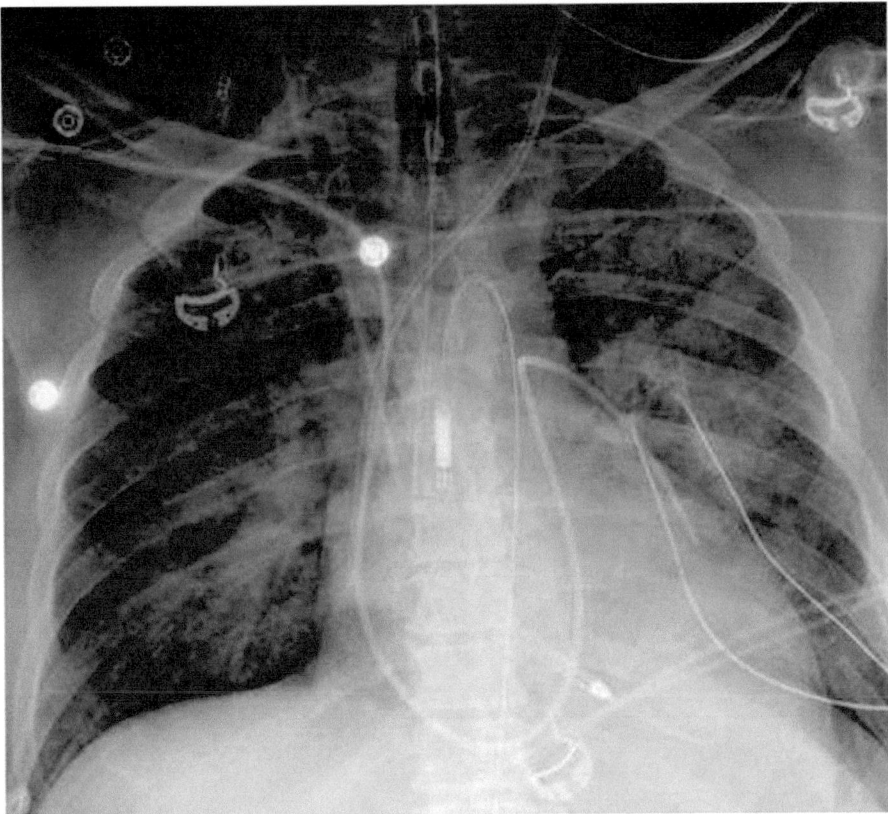

Fig. 5 Preoperative chest X-ray of a patient presenting in cardiogenic shock and acute severe mitral regurgitation secondary to papillary muscle rupture showing pulmonary edema. A pulmonary artery catheter, a percutaneous temporary LVAD and an endotracheal tube are in place

- **Volume and coagulopathy management on cardiopulmonary bypass**

Patients undergoing emergent mitral valve operations in the setting of acute cardiovascular decompensation are volume overloaded (Fig. 5). Managing their volume overload improves pulmonary function, right ventricular recovery as well as hepatic congestion increasing the probability of renal recovery and weaning off inotropic and/or mechanical support. Alleviating hepatic congestion will also improve the coagulation profile and risk of postoperative bleeding. For patients with longer standing heart failure and hepatic congestion with documented coagulopathy and on preoperative anticoagulation we will prime the cardiopulmonary bypass circuit with fresh frozen plasma typically 3–4 units. We also aggressively ultrafiltrate and remove volume from the patient between 2–5 L depending on the preoperative condition.

- **Conduct of replacement**

Mitral valve replacement should be chordal sparing and the choice of valve prosthesis is a result of a discussion with the patient/family and clinical situation. We arrest the heart with antegrade cardioplegia and enter the heart through the interatrial groove. Once the atrial exposure is achieved using the USB Medical HV retractor (USB-Medical, Hatboro, PA, USA) the anterior leaflet of the mitral valve is resected preserving the commissural and all posterior chordae. If the

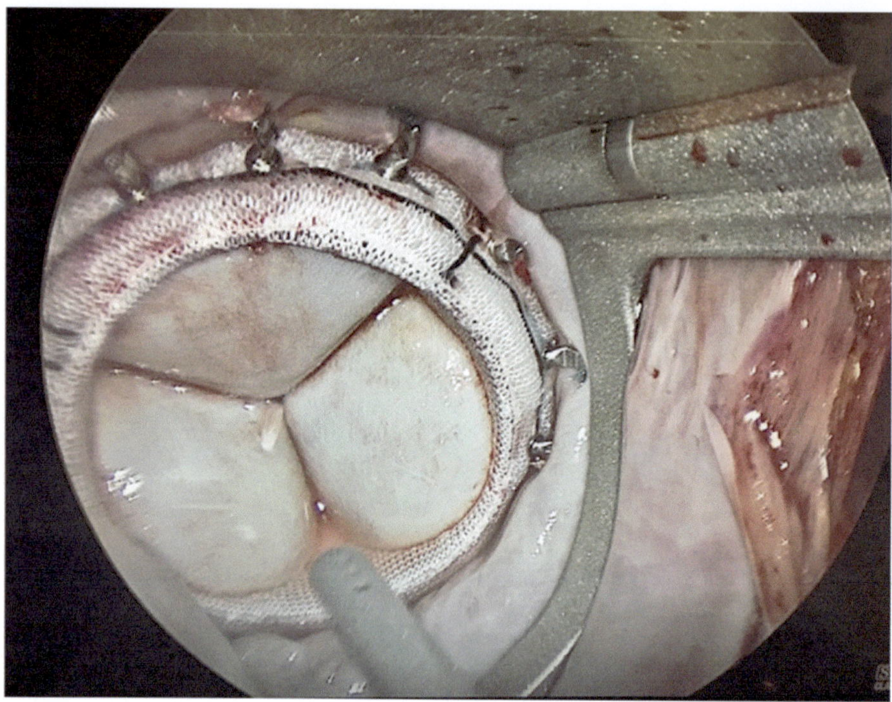

Fig. 6 Implanted bioprosthesis using an endoscopic technique

replacement is performed for an ischemic/ruptured papillary muscle it is important to resect all non-viable tissue and if necessary recreate the chords using ePTFE (Fig. 6). It is important to have appropriate chest and mediastinal drainage postoperatively as pleural and pericardial effusions can be common in the postoperative period. On elective cases we deploy a 24 Fr soft silastic drain in the pericardium through the oblique sinus and a 19 Fr in the right pleural cavity. For emergent cases we use two 24 Fr drains in the pleural cavity and one in the pericardium.

3 Postoperative Management

- **Postoperative inotropic support and fate of the mechanical support**

Once the endoscopic mitral operation is completed, if the patient is not mechanically supported, judicious use of inotropes allows for hemodynamic stability and recovery. For patients with biventricular dysfunction and pulmonary hypertension a combination of epinephrine, milrinone and inhaled nitric oxide are our preferred combination. Patients will be transported to the intensive care unit on inhaled nitric oxide for a wean that will depend on the pulmonary artery pressures and right sided filling pressures. Once the patient is capable of taking oral sildenafil we start it and continue this treatment if the pulmonary artery pressures and right ventricular function dictate it.

For those on mechanical support that can be weaned off onto inotropes alone removal of these devices is important to avoid the need for anticoagulation postoperatively. We universally perform a groin cutdowns to remove devices such as Impella, IABP and VA-ECMO cannulas and are prepared to perform a thrombectomy in all these cases. Our rationale is that attempting a percutaneous approach for removal may lead to complications that can jeopardize a favorable outcome for the patient. In removing mechanical support that requires anticoagulation one also decreases the risk for acute blood loss anemia and transfusions which can perseverate right ventricular dysfunction.

4 Severe Mitral Valve Stenosis

slightly depressed LVEF. We have experienced a systolic function deterioration in these patients perhaps also secondary to a systemic inflammatory response that compounds the diastolic failure and ultimately leads to more advanced hemodynamic support such as Impella

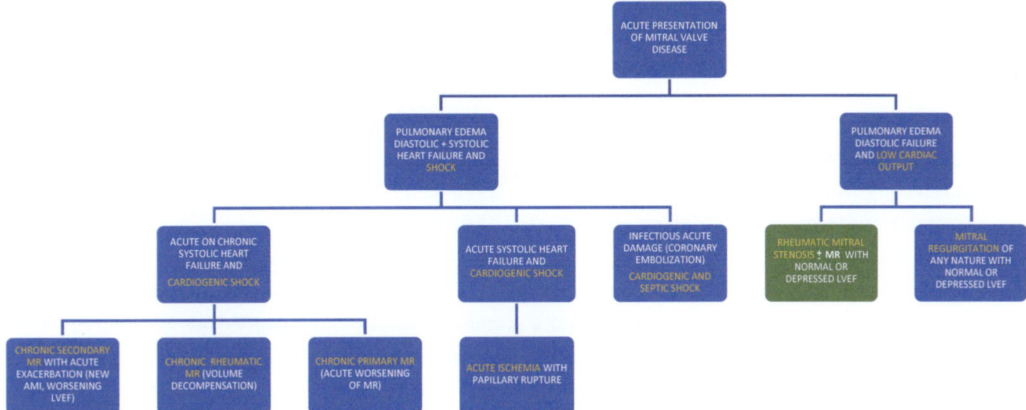

Patients presenting acutely with decompensated severe mitral valve stenosis are typically in diastolic heart failure with pulmonary edema and a degree of low cardiac output state which negates afterload reduction but requires support to improve forward cardiac flow and decrease pulmonary congestion. This often cannot be achieved with pharmacological agents alone and thus needs mechanical support, typically in the form of an intra-aortic counter pulsation balloon. In addition, many of these patients will go into atrial fibrillation which places them in a low cardiac output state despite of preserved or

(Abiomed, Danvers, Massachusetts, USA) and/or VA-ECMO implantation. Others have reported the presentation of severe mitral stenosis as cardiogenic shock with variable outcomes (Fig. 7A–C) [19]. Atrial fibrillation is poorly tolerated in mitral stenosis and leads to further decrement of the cardiac output and use of inotropic drugs often precipitates this circumstance [20]. For this reason, it is important to identify the need and institute mechanical support early to maintain a better hemodynamic state and preserve end organ function. In these situations, early operation is the key to having a favorable outcome.

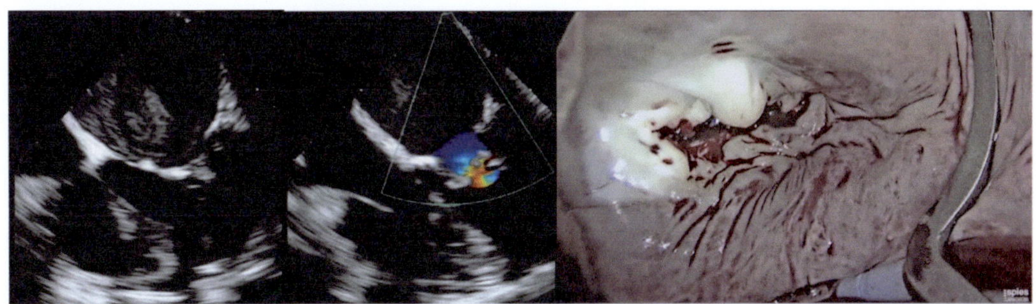

Fig. 7 **A** Intraoperative transesophageal echo showing smoke in the left atrium and a poorly opening mitral valve. **B** Severe mitral stenosis with color flow. **C** Intraoperative picture of the severely stenotic rheumatic mitral valve

Patient with decompensated presentation of mitral stenosis require management in the intensive care unit with invasive monitoring in the form of pulmonary artery catheter, arterial line and foley catheter. Goal directed therapies need to be instituted to maintain adequate cardiac output, minimize pulmonary edema and to preserve the right ventricular function [21, 22]. In doing this end-organ function is preserved in the kidneys and liver. Maintaining mean arterial pressure of at least 65 mmHg, a cardiac index of 2 L/min/m^2 and a central venous pressure below 15 mmHg are important goals. Often times these patients have significant pulmonary hypertension and elevated pulmonary vascular resistance which taxes the right ventricular function and can lead to cardio-renal syndrome. We are relatively liberal in the use of inhaled pulmonary vasodilators such as inhaled iloprost or nitric oxide (for non-intubated patients) or nitric oxide (in intubated patients) to support the right ventricle [23, 24]. We also favor the use of milrinone for pulmonary vasodilation if tolerated by the hemodynamics and cardiac rhythm without inducing vasoplegia or atrial fibrillation. For those with a uremic syndrome and volume overload it is important to institute renal replacement therapy and improve the overall metabolic state of the patient as well as to improve platelet function.

The first-line management of mitral stenosis is percutaneous transcatheter mitral balloon valvuloplasty (PTMB) and this has been used even in the setting of cardiogenic shock [25]. Patients with rheumatic stenosis and accompanying regurgitation or valve calcification are not candidates to PTMB and in these patients our approach for isolated mitral or mitral and tricuspid valve surgery is universally through the right chest endoscopically with a 1.5–2-inch incision at the 4th intercostal space and with a 5 mm 30-degree angled scope in the 2nd intercostal space mid-clavicular line (Fig. 8) with a femoral vessel cutdown of 1–2-inch incision which has been proven to be safe and effective in rheumatic mitral stenosis [26]. This is the case even in emergency operations and reoperations with no sternotomy conversions and an average of 5–7 such operations per year.

We would be remiss not to emphasize that it is paramount that not only the surgeon be comfortable with elective complex endoscopic mitral valve surgery, but also the anesthesia, perfusion and nursing members of the team as many of these operations take place outside of regular work hours and are performed perhaps with less familiarized members of the team. To this end we recommend that everyone in the cardiac team gets experience performing endoscopic valve surgery.

5 Ruptured Papillary Muscle

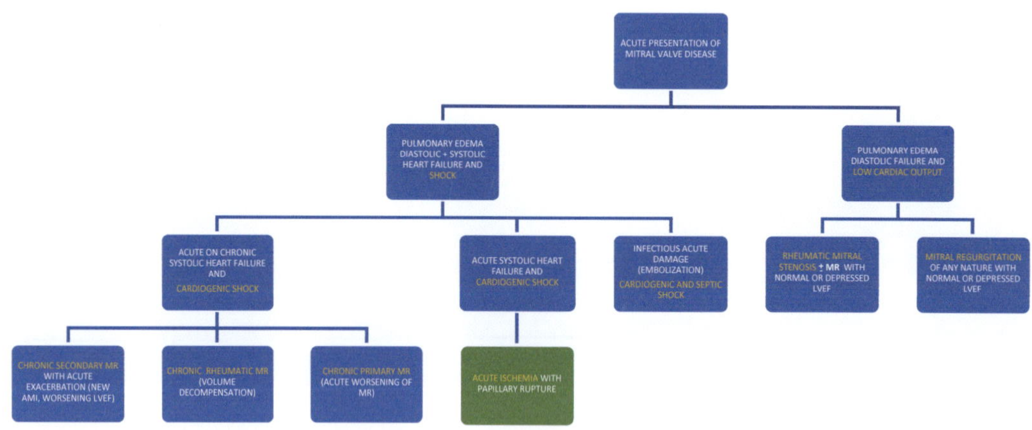

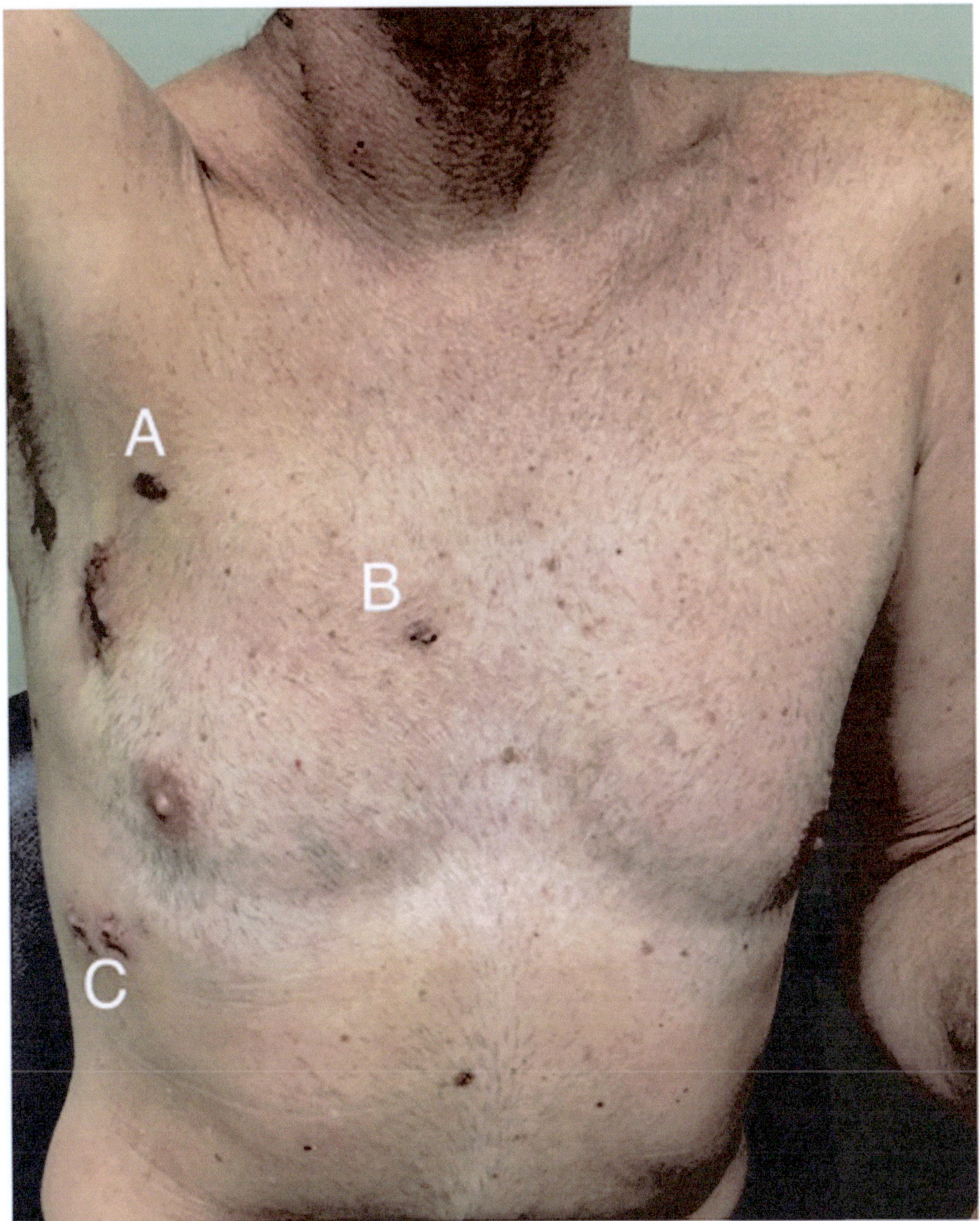

Fig. 8 Postoperative picture 10 days after surgery showing the endoscopic approach. **A** =5 mm 30-degree endoscope. **B** =Atrial lift retractor port. **C** =Chest drain

- **Historical background on therapeutics**

Post myocardial infarction papillary muscle rupture (PMR) has become an uncommon complication in our times with a reported incidence of 1–2% [27, 28]. Kilic et al. recorded a decrease in the number of mitral valve operations performed for papillary muscle rupture from 277 in 2013 to 135 in 2017 [5]. Mitral valve surgery in the setting of cardiogenic shock carries and elevated mortality rate between 20 and 40% [3–6]. The reported 5-year survival of the papillary muscle rupture patients that have undergone MVR is 67% [28]. The posteromedial papillary muscle is known to rupture 6 to 12 times more frequently than the anterolateral muscle. The diagnosis of papillary muscle rupture is usually made between 2 and 7 days after acute myocardial infarction [4].

The majority of the data on the management of this complication is derived from earlier experiences via a median sternotomy [3–6]. Kilic et al. in a report of the STS registry between 2011 and 2018 found that 1,342 patients underwent emergent MVR for PMR with a 20% mortality [5]. In most reports the valve has been replaced, but repairs have also been reported [5, 27, 29–31]. Less frequent but reported etiologies of papillary muscle rupture include Ehlers-Danlos and isolated papillary muscle infarct in the absence of coronary artery disease [29, 30].

There have been reports of minimally invasive approaches in the management of ruptured papillary muscles, but these amount to a handful including a report by Nguyen et al. on postpartum papillary muscle rupture and our own post infarction papillary muscle rupture (Fig. 9A and B) [30, 31]. More recently transcatheter edge-to-edge repair has been used and proposed as the management of papillary muscle rupture [32].

Clearly if these patients present with active, un-revascularized coronary artery disease they will require an approach to satisfy both problems. In our experience the majority of these patients present to our center with revascularized coronaries hours or days prior, a finding that is confirmed by others [6]. The presentation of the patient with an acute papillary muscle is drastic involving cardiogenic shock, pulmonary edema, renal dysfunction and at times liver dysfunction [6, 28]. Those that present for surgical care do so assisted by mechanical circulatory support to

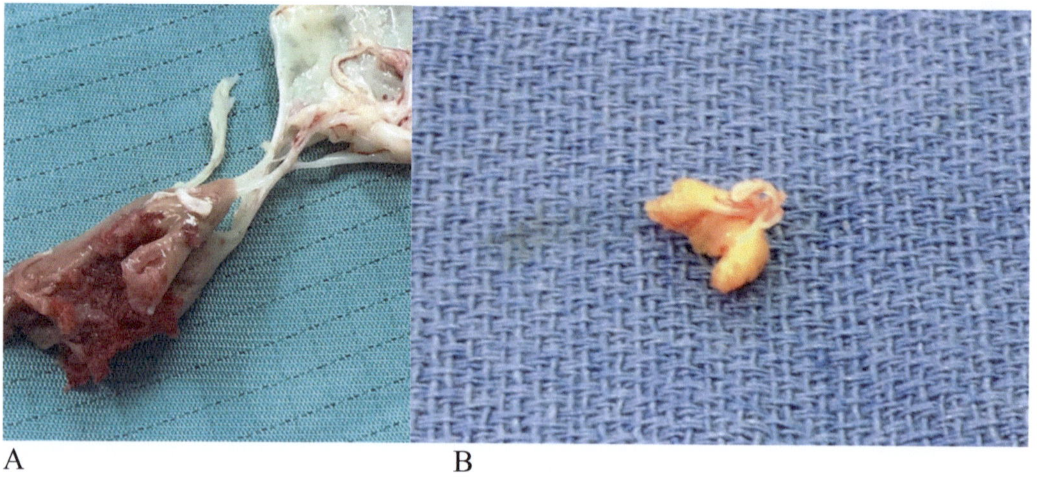

A   B

Fig. 9 **A** Specimen of a papillary muscle rupture from an AMI. **B** Specimen of papillary muscle rupture of a non-ischemic nature

survive the insult of the acute infarction, cardiogenic shock and pulmonary edema that ensues. According to Fujita et al. over 70% of patients with papillary muscle rupture presented in cardiogenic shock and 81% of patients were supported with IABP while 32% were supported with VA-ECMO [6].

From a practical standpoint these patients present after having delayed or recent management of their coronary artery disease. A study of the STS database reported the need for concomitant CABG to be higher with 59.3% than the rate of those percutaneously revascularized [5]. In our experience it is more common that these patients present after having undergone percutaneous revascularization of the culprit vessel. This was confirmed by Fujita et al. who found 31% of patients needed concomitant surgical revascularization while 47% had already undergone PCI [6]. There are important implications for surgery in these circumstances as these patients have been loaded with therapeutic antiplatelet agents and likely therapeutic anticoagulation for mechanical circulatory support which in contemporary experience is most commonly axial temporary percutaneous left ventricular assist devices (Impella, Abiomed, Danvers, Massachusetts, USA) and in more profound shock cases implies veno-arterial extracorporeal membrane oxygenation (VA-ECMO).

- **Patient evaluation**

Evaluation of the patient with severe acute ischemic mitral regurgitation status post percutaneous revascularization and in cardiogenic shock, mechanically and inotropically supported needs to be expedited. Basic workup should include a CXR, but a CT scan of the chest, abdomen and pelvis without IV contrast could prove helpful in directing cannulation strategies. Echocardiogram (surface or transesophageal) are also very important in delineating the original and concomitant valvular pathology as well as LV and RV function. It is important to understand the degree of aortic insufficiency if present in order to tailor cardiac protection, but it is also important to know if the tricuspid valve requires treatment too as this will facilitate right ventricular recovery. Coagulation studies including platelet function, liver function and renal function are paramount in order to have the necessary blood products. It is imperative to have blood products available at the time of surgery. These patients require invasive hemodynamic monitoring including pulmonary artery catheter, arterial line and foley catheter and are commonly being ventilated with moderate to high oxygen and PEEP requirements. In patients on maximal support including VA-ECMO, LV venting with Impella and a modicum of pressors and inotropic medications one should continue to provide ventilatory support and minimize oxygen toxicity relying more on PEEP and tidal volumes. We have found that preoperative use of inhaled nitric oxide therapy around the time of induction of anesthesia in these patients is advantageous in protecting the right ventricle and therefore we institute it early on. A cornerstone to treating these patients is to stop the left ventricular damage and to protect the right ventricle as the existing isolated mechanical right ventricular support options are not ideal.

Patients with this form of acute presentation should be managed in centers that have experience in mitral valve care, advanced heart failure therapies and the capability of deploying all forms of temporary mechanical circulatory support therapeutics and pulmonary vasodilators.

- **Preoperative optimization**

The old adage of 'fools rush in' applies in these decompensated presentations of mitral regurgitation. Specifically, if a patient is already adequately supported with VA-ECMO and Impella for LV decompression one should attempt to optimize variables prior to surgery even if it means delaying the operation for 12–48 h. In their STS report Kilic et al. showed that 64% of patients undergoing emergency surgery for papillary muscle rupture were mechanically supported, with the most common device being the IABP (56.9%), Impella pump (4.1%) and VA-ECMO (3.1%) [5]. Correcting an acid–base imbalance and ruling out catastrophic conditions such as bowel ischemia, profound coagulopathy, hepatic failure, ischemic or hemorrhagic strokes are paramount. Avoiding a futile high-risk operation will avoid submitting a patient to unnecessary suffering.

We have performed these operations in patients with and without prior sternotomies and the principles of preoperative optimization are the same to both. A candid discussion with the patient and/or family decision maker is important. The risks for complications such as death, transfusions, ischemic or hemorrhagic stroke, acute renal failure requiring hemodialysis, prolonged mechanical respiratory support are higher in these cases.

For patients who present with only inotropic and vasopressor medications it is important to establish if they are adequately supported. Goal directed therapies should provide adequate forward flow, so ideally there is a normal or near normal lactate level, the base deficit is corrected, and the mixed venous oxygen saturation is over 55% all while maintaining a mean arterial pressure of at least 65 mmHg. If this is not achieved the decision to institute mechanical circulatory support should be made early. The decision of which form of mechanical support is mandated by the respiratory status, the right ventricular function and contingent on arterial access. For those with profound hypoxia and right ventricular dysfunction VA-ECMO may be prove better than isolated Impella or IABP, at the risk of not venting the left ventricle and creating more pulmonary congestion [33]. Impella device (Abiomed, Danvers, Massachusetts, USA) has been used before as a bridge to intervention in papillary muscle rupture [32].

- **Intraoperative considerations in acute papillary muscle rupture**

Minimally invasive papillary muscle rupture repair in a puerperal woman has been reported before [30] and we have also encountered this in our practice in a young man in whom the muscle was debrided and neochords were anchored at the very base of the muscle for a neochordal reconstruction repair. We have always replaced the mitral valve after acute ischemic events, and this is the most common operation performed for papillary muscle rupture (Fig. 10) [5]. For

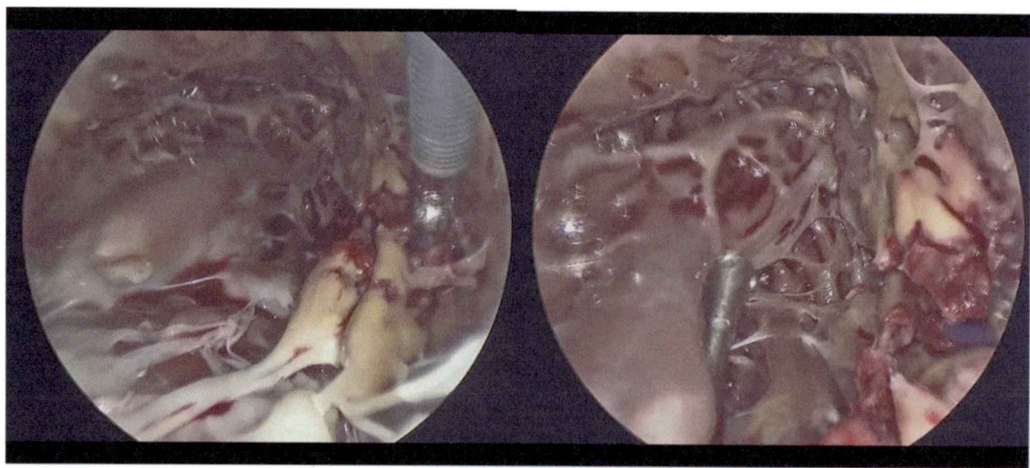

Fig. 10 Posteromedial papillary muscle with ischemia and rupture. Notice the lighter color of the base of the muscle compared to the rest of the darker myocardium. The percutaneous LVAD device is seen in the ventricle

patients on isolated vasoactive drugs for support one needs to consider the insertion of an IABP at the beginning or end of the operation prior to weaning off bypass based on the clinical circumstances. For those with IABP, VA-ECMO or Impella (Abiomed, Danvers, Massachusetts, USA) one has to evaluate the removal of the device at completion of the cardiac operation if hemodynamics and cardiac function permit it which would allow stopping the anticoagulation decreasing the postoperative risk hemorrhage risk. We advocate for surgical removal of Impella and ECMO cannulas to mitigate the risk of vascular complications when using percutaneous closure devices in these critically ill patients.

- **The role of surgery versus transcatheter edge-to-edge in the management of regurgitation in cardiogenic shock**

There are reports of acute papillary muscle rupture managed with percutaneous edge-to-edge repair (Mitraclip, Abbott Park, IL, USA) [32]. The data on transcatheter edge-to-edge repair in the setting of cardiogenic shock is growing [32, 34–38]. This therapeutic option is available in advanced heart centers and in reported cases have proven to be effective in the acute phase, but the long-term durability is still not known, more over it does not address tricuspid valve pathology nor the risk of embolization of the avulsed papillary muscle tip. One must take into account the bias of publication of successful case report and/or series. Percutaneous repair, much like a minimally invasive endoscopic approach requires expertise by the operating team/catheterization lab team. Our structural cardiology colleagues are less used to managing cardiogenic shock in general, leaving most of these patients to be treated by a surgeon. In our experience, for elderly and/or frail patients this therapeutic option may prove advantageous to cardiac surgery.

6 Secondary Mitral Regurgitation and Acute on Chronic Systolic Heart Failure with Shock

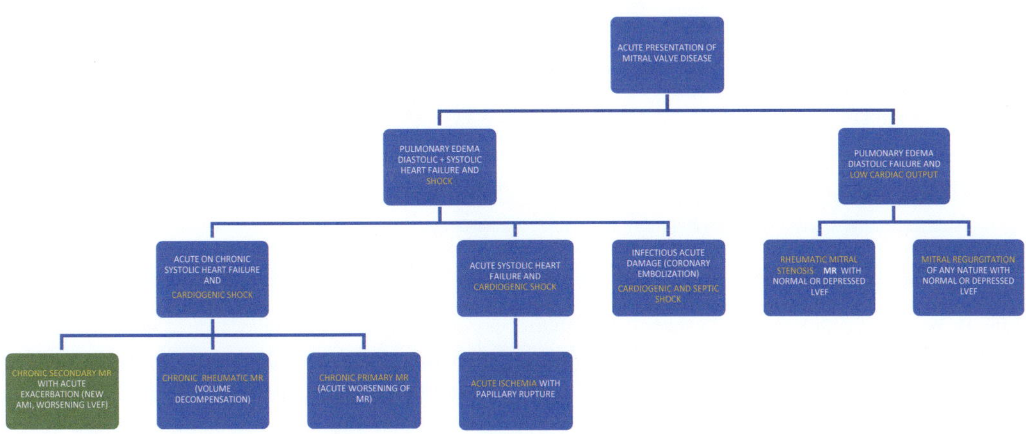

Patients with chronic systolic heart failure can have exacerbation of their heart failure and sometimes present acutely in cardiogenic shock. The most common precipitating factor leading to acute exacerbation of CHF include arrhythmias, uncontrolled hypertension, non-compliance with diet or medications and worsening renal function [39]. In fact, after arrhythmias and acute coronary syndromes valvular disease was the third most common reason for acute exacerbation of chronic CHF [40, 41].

Secondary mitral regurgitation can exacerbate chronic systolic heart failure and present as cardiogenic shock. When it does, typically the patient with profound chronic systolic heart failure and LVEF acutely decompensates due to loading conditions or a new coronary event. Patients that present under these circumstances and have been revascularized percutaneously on presentation are candidates to an endoscopic approach. Hemodynamic support is almost uni-

perfusion and persistent low cardiac output mechanical support should be instituted. For those on mechanical support metabolic optimization should be pursued including establishing renal replacement therapy. Those already on VA-ECMO should have left ventricular venting as left ventricular decompression with Impella pump (Abiomed, Danvers, Massachusetts, USA) or IABP has been shown to improve survival and rates of weaning off ECMO [43, 44].

Once adequate forward flow has been restored one can perform the operation when the best logistical circumstances are available including personnel and equipment to facilitate a good outcome and this usually during daylight hour in most institutions so long as the delay is not more than 12–48 h.

7 Infective Endocarditis of The Mitral Valve

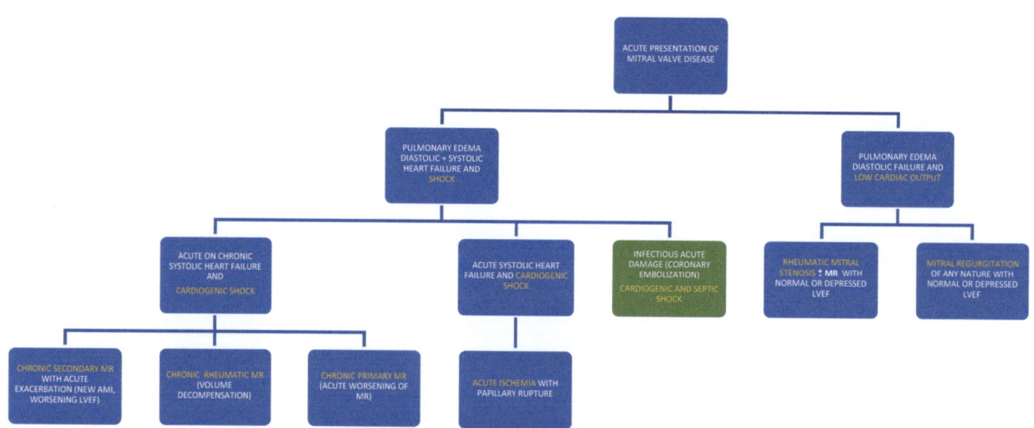

versally with inotropes, pressors and mechanical support. Mechanical support in more recent times has evolved from the IABP to the Impella pump (Abiomed, Danvers, Massachusetts, USA) which can be placed transaxillary for longer duration of support in cardiogenic shock [41, 42].

The previously discussed principles of preoperative optimization, intraoperative and postoperative right and left ventricular protection and support apply. For those on only inotropic/pressor support showing signs of poor

Acute bacterial endocarditis is more prevalent these days in the United States and many countries around the world secondary to the opioid abuse epidemic. Presentation of these patients in cardiogenic shock is not common and when it occurs it is likely secondary to coronary embolization or myocardial depression from sepsis. Septic shock is the most common form of shock in these patients and requires pharmacological support with pressors and inotropes. The role of the cardiac surgeon in these cases is to provide source control, prevent further embolic events, and restore mitral valve function.

The use of mechanical circulatory support in acute bacterial endocarditis outside of an IABP is fraught with risk of furthering the septic shock as well as creating embolic events. We typically maximize pharmacological therapy and perform an early operation as long as the circumstances surrounding the patient are not futile. It is our experience that with adequate resuscitation and correction of acidosis one can separate from cardiopulmonary bypass only on inotropes and pressors, but pulmonary vasodilator may be needed if the right ventricle has been depressed by the disease process and we favor inhaled nitric oxide. In cases of acute bacterial endocarditis, we will typically use inhaled nitric oxide on induction, and this could be weaned off after the bypass run if the patient's oxygenation and right ventricular function are preserved. We most often perform a mitral valve replacement based on the degree of damage of the mitral valve and the need to have a prompt and succinct operation in the setting of shock.

The recovery period for these patients is usually long with an average of 15 days in the hospital and many have had embolic strokes on presentation which makes the rehabilitation more difficult [45]. Old dogma would support delaying surgery for weeks in the setting of acute embolic stroke, but more recent data has supported that there is no increased risk of worsening strokes or hemorrhagic conversions if operated on early [46]. Many of these patients would not survive if their operation is delayed.

8 Conclusion

Endoscopic mitral valve surgery is a viable and safe option for mitral valve surgery in the setting of cardiogenic shock that should be performed at referral centers. Management of these patients is complex and requires infrastructure that is not available in primary or secondary level care. In-

depth understanding of the valvular etiology behind the cardiogenic shock, early recognition of shock and early implementation of stabilization strategies are the cornerstone for a good outcome. Expertise in the surgical team beyond the cardiac surgeon is very important and familiarity with forms of mechanical support such as Impella pump, VA-ECMO and other forms are crucial. Surgical teams should attempt endoscopic mitral valve surgery in the setting of cardiogenic shock only after a high level of comfort with successful elective minimally invasive cases.

References

1. Gammie JS, Zhao Y, Peterson ED, O'Brien SM, Rankin JS, Griffith BP. Less-invasive mitral valve operations: trends and outcomes from the Society of Thoracic Surgeons Adult Cardiac Surgery Database. Ann Thorac Surg. 2010;90(5):1401–10.

2. Baran DA, Grines CL, Bailey S, Burkhoff D, Hall SA, Henry TD, ... & Naidu SS. SCAI clinical expert consensus statement on the classification of cardiogenic shock: this document was endorsed by the American College of Cardiology (ACC), the American Heart Association (AHA), the Society of Critical Care Medicine (SCCM), and the Society of Thoracic Surgeons (STS) in April 2019. Catheter Cardiovasc Interv2019;941)29–37.

3. Menon V, Slater JN, White HD, Sleeper LA, Cocke T, Hochman JS. Acute myocardial infarction complicated by systemic hypoperfusion without hypotension: report of the SHOCK trial registry. Am J Med. 2000;108(5):374–80.

4. Thompson CR, Buller CE, Sleeper LA, Antonelli TA, Webb JG, Jaber WA, ... & Shock Investigators. Cardiogenic shock due to acute severe mitral regurgitation complicating acute myocardial infarction: a report from the SHOCK Trial Registry. J Am Coll Cardiol. 2000;36(3S1):1104–9.

5. Kilic A, Sultan I, Chu D, Wang Y, Gleason TG. Mitral valve surgery for papillary muscle rupture: outcomes in 1342 patients from The Society of Thoracic Surgeons Database. Ann Thorac Surg. 2020;110(6):1975–81.

6. Fujita T, Yamamoto H, Kobayashi J, Fukushima S, Miyata H, Yamashita K, Motomura N. Mitral valve surgery for ischemic papillary muscle rupture: outcomes from the Japan cardiovascular surgery database. Gen Thorac Cardiovasc Surg. 2020;68 (12):1439–46.

7. Kohsaka S, Menon V, Lowe AM, Lange M, Dzavik V, Sleeper LA, Hochman JS. Systemic inflammatory response syndrome after acute myocardial infarction complicated by cardiogenic shock. Arch Intern Med. 2005;165(14):1643–50.

8. Hernandez GA, Lemor A, Blumer V, Rueda CA, Zalawadiya S, Stevenson LW, Lindenfeld J. Trends in utilization and outcomes of pulmonary artery catheterization in heart failure with and without cardiogenic shock. J Cardiac Fail. 2019;25(5):364–71.

9. Menon V, White H, LeJemtel T, Webb JG, Sleeper LA, Hochman JS, & SHOCK Investigators. The clinical profile of patients with suspected cardiogenic shock due to predominant left ventricular failure: a report from the SHOCK Trial Registry. J Am Coll Cardiol. 2000. 36(3S1):1071–6.

10. Jacobs AK, Leopold JA, Bates E, Mendes LA, Sleeper LA, White H, ... & Hochman JS. Cardiogenic shock caused by right ventricular infarction: a report from the SHOCK registry.J Am Coll Cardiol2003;41 (8):1273–9.

11. Gammie, James S., Joanna Chikwe, Vinay Badhwar, Dylan P. Thibault, Sreekanth Vemulapalli, Vinod H. Thourani, Marc Gillinov et al. "Isolated mitral valve surgery: the Society of Thoracic Surgeons adult cardiac surgery database analysis." *The Annals of thoracic surgery* 106, no. 3 (2018): 716–727.

12. Nissen AP, Miller III CC, Thourani VH, Woo YJ, Gammie JS, Ailawadi G, & Nguyen TC. Less invasive mitral surgery versus conventional sternotomy stratified by mitral pathology. Ann Thorac Surg. 2020.

13. Beckmann A, Meyer R, Lewandowski J, Markewitz A, Harringer W. German heart surgery report 2018: the annual updated registry of the German Society for Thoracic and Cardiovascular Surgery. Thorac Cardiovasc Surg. 2019;67(05):331–44.

14. Paparella D, Fattouch K, Moscarelli M, Santarpino G, Nasso G, Guida P, ... & Del Giglio M. Current trends in mitral valve surgery: a multicenter national comparison between full-sternotomy and minimally-invasive approach. Int J Cardiol. 2020;306:147–151.

15. Grant SW, Hickey GL, Modi P, Hunter S, Akowuah E, Zacharias J. Propensity-matched analysis of minimally invasive approach versus sternotomy for mitral valve surgery. Heart. 2019;105 (10):783–9.

16. Castillo-Sang M, Guthrie TJ, Moon MR, Lawton JS, Maniar HS, Damiano RJ Jr, Silvestry SC. Outcomes of repeat mitral valve surgery in patients with pulmonary hypertension. Innovations. 2015;10 (2):120–4.

17. Helmers MR, Kim ST, Altshuler P, Han JJ, Iyengar A, Kelly J, ... & Atluri P. Mitral Valve Surgery in Pulmonary Hypertension Patients: Is Minimally Invasive Surgery Safe? Ann Thorac Surg. 2020.

18. Combes A, Price S, Slutsky AS, Brodie D. Temporary circulatory support for cardiogenic shock. Lancet. 2020;396(10245):199–212.

19. Leon MN, Harrell LC, Simosa HF, Mahdi NA, Pathan A, Lopez-Cuellar J., ... & Palacios IF. Mitral balloon valvotomy for patients with mitral stenosis in atrial fibrillation: immediate and long-term results. J Am Coll Cardiol. 1999;34(4):1145–52.

20. Mohanan Nair KK, Pillai HS, Thajudeen A, Krishnamoorthy KM, Sivasubramonian S, Namboodiri N, ... & Tharakan J. Immediate and long-term results following balloon mitral valvotomy in patients with atrial fibrillation. Clin Cardiol. 2012;35(12):E35–9.

21. Van Diepen S, Katz JN, Albert NM, Henry TD, Jacobs AK, Kapur NK, ... & Cohen MG. Contemporary management of cardiogenic shock: a scientific statement from the American Heart Association. Circulation. 2017;136(16):e232–68.

22. Chioncel O, Parissis J, Mebazaa A, Thiele H, Desch S, Bauersachs J, ... & Seferovic P. Epidemiology, pathophysiology and contemporary management of cardiogenic shock–a position statement from the Heart Failure Association of the European Society of Cardiology. Eur J Heart Fail. 2020;22(8):1315–41.

23. Harjola VP, Mebazaa A, Čelutkienė J, Bettex D, Bueno H, Chioncel O, ... & Konstantinides S. Contemporary management of acute right ventricular failure: a statement from the Heart Failure Association and the Working Group on Pulmonary Circulation and Right Ventricular Function of the European Society of Cardiology. Eur J Heart Fail. 2016;18 (3):226–41.

24. Kline JA, Puskarich MA, Jones AE, Mastouri RA, Hall CL, Perkins A, ... & Lahm T. Inhaled nitric oxide to treat intermediate risk pulmonary embolism: a multicenter randomized controlled trial. Nitric Oxide. 2019;84:60–8.

25. Ananthakrishna Pillai A, Ramasamy C, Kottyath H. Outcomes following balloon mitral valvuloplasty in pregnant females with mitral stenosis and significant sub valve disease with severe decompensated heart failure. J Interv Cardiol. 2018;31(4):525–31.

26. Chernov I, Enginoev S, Koz'min D, Magomedov G, Tarasov D, Sá MPB, ... & Zhigalov K. Minithoracotomy vs. conventional mitral valve surgery for rheumatic mitral valve stenosis: a single-center analysis of 128 patients. Braz J Cardiovasc Surg. 2020;35(2):185–90.

27. Fasol R, Lakew F, Wetter S. Mitral repair in patients with a ruptured papillary muscle. Am Heart J. 2000;139(3):549–54.

28. Russo A, Suri RM, Grigioni F, Roger VL, Oh JK, Mahoney DW, ... & Enriquez-Sarano M. Clinical perspective. Circulation. 2008;118(15):1528–34.

29. Sève P, Dubreuil O, Farhat F, Plauchu H, Touboul P, Broussolle C. Acute mitral regurgitation caused by papillary muscle rupture in the immediate postpartum period revealing Ehlers-Danlos syndrome type IV. J Thorac Cardiovasc Surg. 2005;129(3):680–1.

30. Nguyen S, Umana-Pizano JB, Donepudi R, Dhoble A, Nguyen TC. Minimally invasive mitral valve repair for acute papillary muscle rupture during pregnancy. Ann Thorac Surg. 2019;107(2):e93–5.

31. Castillo-Sang M. Emergent/salvage minimally invasive mitral valve replacement. August 2020. https://doi.org/10.25373/ctsnet.12766133

32. Vandenbriele C, Balthazar T, Wilson J, Adriaenssens T, Davies S, Droogne W, ... & Price S. Left Impella®-device as bridge from cardiogenic shock with acute, severe mitral regurgitation to MitraClip®-procedure: a new option for critically ill patients. Eur Hear Journal Acute Cardiovasc Care. 2020

33. Obadia B, Théron A, Gariboldi V, Collart F. Extracorporeal membrane oxygenation as a bridge to surgery for ischemic papillary muscle rupture. J Thorac Cardiovasc Surg. 2014;147(6):e82–4.

34. McInerney A, Martinez-Gomez E, Triado-Contre G, Nombela-Franco L. 28 Percutaneous mitral valve repair with mitraclip device in hemodynamically unstable patients: a systematic review. 2020.

35. Kovach CP, Bell S, Kataruka A, Reisman M, Don C. Outcomes of urgent/emergent transcatheter mitral valve repair (MitraClip): a single center experience. Catheter Cardiovasc Interv. 2020.

36. Flint K, Brieke A, Wiktor D, Carroll J. Percutaneous edge-to-edge mitral valve repair may rescue select patients in cardiogenic shock: findings from a single center case series. Catheter Cardiovasc Interv. 2019;94(2):E82–7.

37. Jung RG, Simard T, Kovach C, Flint K, Don C, Di Santo P, ... & Hibbert B. Transcatheter mitral valve repair in cardiogenic shock and mitral regurgitation: a patient-level, multicenter analysis. Cardiovasc Interv. 2021;14(1):1–11.

38. Falasconi G, Pannone L, Melillo F, Adamo M, Ronco F, Carrabba N, ... & Agricola E. Use of MitraClip system for severe mitral regurgitation in cardiogenic shock: results from a multicentre observational Italian experience (the MITRA-SHOCK study). Eur Hear J. 2020;41(Supplement_2): ehaa946–2635.

39. Fonarow, G. C., Abraham, W. T., Albert, N. M., Stough, W. G., Gheorghiade, M., Greenberg, B. H., ... & Young, J. B. (2008). Factors identified as precipitating hospital admissions for heart failure and clinical outcomes: findings from OPTIMIZE-HF. Arch Intern Med. 2006;168(8):847–54

40. Nieminen MS, Brutsaert D, Dickstein K, Drexler H, Follath F, Harjola VP, ... & Tavazzi L. EuroHeart Failure Survey II (EHFS II): a survey on hospitalized acute heart failure patients: description of population. Eur Heart J. 2006;27(22):2725–36.

41. Tarabichi S, Ikegami H, Russo MJ, Lee LY, Lemaire A. The role of the axillary Impella 5.0 device on patients with acute cardiogenic shock. J Cardiothorac Surg. 2020;15(1):1–5.

42. Castillo-Sang MA, Prasad SM, Singh J, Ewald GA, Silvestry SC Thirty-five day Impella 5.0 support via right axillary side graft cannulation for acute cardiogenic shock. Innovations;8(4):307–9.

43. Na SJ, Yang JH, Yang JH, Sung K, Choi JO, Hahn JY, ... & Cho YH. Left heart decompression at venoarterial extracorporeal membrane oxygenation initiation in cardiogenic shock: prophylactic versus therapeutic strategy. J Thorac Dis. 2019;11(9):3746.

44. Russo JJ, Aleksova N, Pitcher I, Couture E, Parlow S, Faraz M, ... & Hibbert B. Left ventricular unloading during extracorporeal membrane oxygenation in patients with cardiogenic shock. J Am Coll Cardiol. 2019;73(6):654–62.

45. Misfeld M, Girrbach F, Etz CD, Binner C, Asper KV, Dohmen PM, ... & Mohr FW. Surgery for infective endocarditis complicated by cerebral embolism: a consecutive series of 375 patients J Thorac Cardiovasc Surg. 2014;147(6):1837–46.

46. Sorabella RA, Han SM, Grbic M, Wu YS, Takayama H, Kurlansky P, ... & George I. Early operation for endocarditis complicated by preoperative cerebral emboli is not associated with worsened outcomes. Ann Thorac Surg. 2015;100(2):501–8.

The Role of Simulators in Safe Adoption of Endoscopic Mitral Valve Surgery

Luca Aerts and Peyman Sardari Nia

Abstract

Minimally invasive mitral valve surgery (MIMVS) is one of the most complex and challenging procedures in cardiothoracic surgery. This approach coheres with the continuous trends towards minimally invasive approaches within the surgical field. To this date the learning curve has proven to be challenging. Patient-specific simulation, in combination with mitral valve modelling and three-dimensional printing can help in adaptation of this difficult procedure by enhancing surgical skills and reduce the learning curve. In light of this, we have developed a high-fidelity minimally invasive mitral valve surgery simulator with structural training program for endoscopic mitral valve surgery. In the current chapter we present the promising results of simulation-based training and adaptation of three-dimensional printing for minimally invasive mitral valve surgery.

Supplementary Information The online version contains supplementary material available at https://doi.org/10.1007/978-3-031-21104-1_19. The videos can be accessed individually by clicking the DOI link in the accompanying figure caption or by scanning this link with the SN More Media App.

L. Aerts (✉) · P. Sardari Nia
Department of Cardiothoracic Surgery, Maastricht University Medical Center, Maastricht, The Netherlands
e-mail: luca.aerts@mumc.nl

Keywords

Mitral valve repair · Minimally invasive surgery · Three-dimensional valve modelling · Three-dimensional printing · Simulation · Surgical training

1 Introduction

Minimally invasive mitral valve surgery (MIMVS) is one of the most complex and challenging procedures in cardiothoracic surgery [1, 2]. This approach coheres with the continuous trends towards minimally invasive approaches within the surgical field. Minimally invasive approach requires a different palette of surgical techniques due to the keyhole approach, the use of long-shafted instruments and the use of video assistance. To this date the learning curve has proven to be challenging. Competence and expertise are acquired by surgical volume [3]. Limited data suggest that MIMVS necessitates 75 to 125 operations to overcome its associated learning curve for a surgeon [1].

In the past decades, mitral valve repair has been well established to be superior to replacement for degenerative mitral regurgitation [4, 5]. Moreover, MIMVS has proven to be a safe, effective and a less invasive alternative compared to traditional sternotomy and is widely accepted in multiple centres [6, 7].

Due to the limited working hours and rising development of new techniques, it is necessary to

J. Zacharias (ed.), *Endoscopic Cardiac Surgery*,
https://doi.org/10.1007/978-3-031-21104-1_19

move educational endeavour outside the operative theatre. A concomitant learning platform, which offers simulation-based training for both residents and experienced surgeons, can serve as a training platform to gain proficiency in shorter time without intraoperative trial and error. Furthermore, experienced surgeons can use the simulator to develop and learn new techniques, as well for preoperative planning of the complex procedure.

Simulation-based training is well established in laparoscopic surgery and has also proven effective in reducing the learning curve of in vivo procedures [8]. In cardiac surgery various studies demonstrate the beneficial effect on the learning curve and the improvement of surgical skills by application of simulators, especially in mitral valve surgery [9–11].

In recent years numerous simulators and surgical models have become commercially available. An obstacle that inhibits the realistic experience of these simulators is the lack of high-fidelity feedback systems and structural training [12–14]. It has been shown that feedback is an essential part of learning and specially if this feedback is objective, reproducible, and metric-based [15, 16].

For this reason, we have developed a high-fidelity MIMVS simulator that produces objective, real-time and reproducible feedback. In combination with 3D-mitral valve modelling and printing we can offer near to in-vivo simulation training.

2 Simulation for Mitral Valve Surgery

In recent years, various simulators for mitral valve surgery have been developed to facilitate in training purposes [12–14, 17, 18]. Most of the simulators or training models are low fidelity simulators, which means there is no feedback mechanism and therefor no efficient learning. To this date just two simulators have been proven effective and usable in endoscopic minimally invasive mitral valve surgery [13, 19].

Development of the high-fidelity simulator

In 2012, we developed a high-fidelity minimally invasive mitral valve simulator based on pre-set requirements, acquired by interviewing experienced cardiac surgeons, specialized in mitral valve procedures. Fidelity in simulation is described as "the degree to which the simulator replicates reality" [15]. We choose a high-fidelity simulator to create a learning platform that offers a realistic set up of the procedure. We completed a design which provides objective and reproducible feedback that one could use to train oneself repeatedly.

The thoracic model

We choose a model thoracic torso for the simulator to mimic a lifelike appearance (Fig. 1). In MIMVS an incision is made in the fourth intercostal space to provide endoscopic or robotic access, for this reason a 4-cm access port was added at the same level in our model. This way the resident or surgeon will be trained working with a unique angle of view and limited working space for long shafted instruments. Additionally, a detachable camera with white LED lighting strips was mounted inside the model to provide a realistic on-screen endoscopic view. The simulator was attached to a mobile height-adjustable table, to provide a correct ergonomic position.

There is no model that resembles all mitral regurgitation variations, nor the consequent geometrical change of the left-sided heart structures. Therefore, a model with slightly dilated atria and mitral valve was chosen, characteristic for mitral valve regurgitation. Dimensions were retrieved from the available literature [20–23]. For the atria, ventricles and the mitral valve a silicone-like material was developed. We develop this special silicone to be able to provide a true-to-nature suturing experience and to maintain a distinct level of toughness to prevent it from tearing after suture placement.

Feedback system

As mentioned above, one of the cornerstones of educational endeavour is feedback. There is no

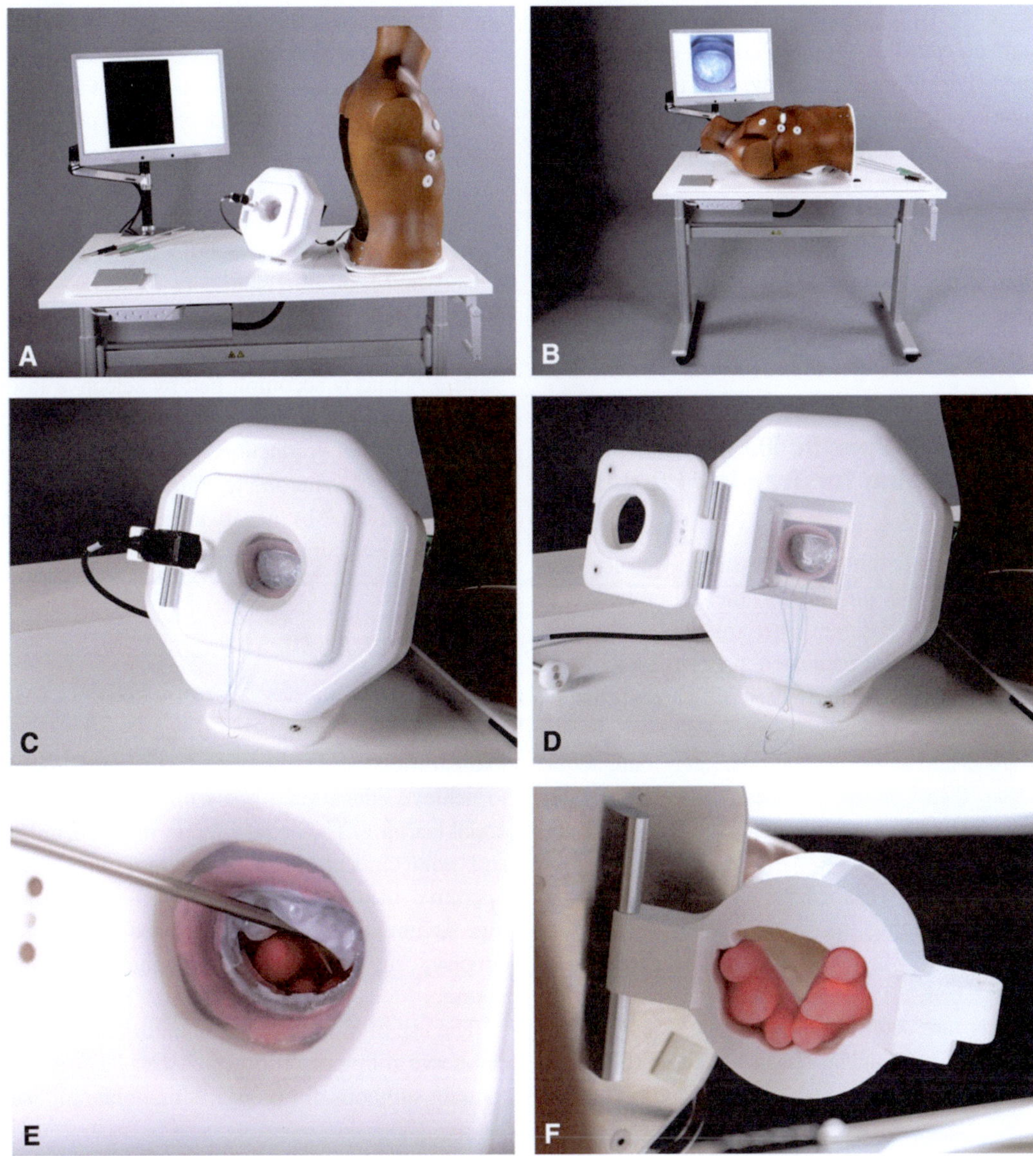

Fig. 1 Final version of the simulator. **A** and **B**, View of the assembled simulator. **C** and **D**, Feedback system. **E** and **F**, Magnetic, papillary muscles mounted in the 3-dimensional–printed ventricle. Reprinted from The Journal of Thoracic and Cardiovascular Surgery, Volume 157, Nia, P. S., Daemen, J. H., & Maessen, J. G, Development of a high-fidelity minimally invasive mitral valve surgery simulator, 1567–1574, 2019, with permission from Elsevier [18]

efficient learning without feedback [16]. To create a learning platform for mitral valve surgery, one should receive objective and reproducible feedback to gain proficiency and become acquainted with the procedural steps. Moreover, procedures as MIMVS are composed of many layers of complexity. Four cameras around the silicone valve and an edge detectable algorithm to calculate the suture width and depth were installed [18]. This way, the simulator provides a metric-based performance feedback about suturing depth and length. The idea behind having feedback about suturing is not to mimic the exact suture depth or width of an actual operation. The objective is to provide a platform on which a surgeon could develop full control over the long-shafted instruments in way that any pre-setted suturing could be realized. Additional to this, the metric-based feedback gives objective scoring for assessments of trainees.

Especially in the beginning, expert feedback is necessary for the most effective use of the simulator. The combination of formative and objective feedback is the basis for long-term knowledge retention.

3 Patient Specific 3D Mitral Valve Modelling for Training Purpose

In the simulation-based training, we use 3D-modelling and printing of the mitral valve to interact with different anatomy and pathology. We developed a dedicated process to replicate any mitral valve pathology in 3D-printed silicone replica from TEE. This process can roughly be divided into six major steps, namely data acquisition, data conversion, mesh refinement, rapid prototyping, negative mould fabrication and casting (Fig. 2).

Mandatory components in 3D-modeling are clinical imaging modalities. Imaging data is obtained by 3D transoesophageal echocardiography (TOE). These high-quality volumetric 3D images are converted into Cartesian Digital Imaging Communications in Medicine (DICOM) format. The mitral valve annulus and the leaflets are reconstructed. Because of technical difficulties it is not yet possible to reconstruct the sub-valvular apparatus. The mitral valve is reconstructed in the mid-systolic phase to reproduce the coaptation defect. The data is exported to a Surface Tessellation Language (STL) file, the standard format for 3D printing.

In the third step, mesh refinements are conducted in MeshLab (Istituto di Scienza e Tecnologie dell' informazione, Pisa, Italy) and subsequently manufactured into a model on 1:1 scale. Printing is accomplished by selective laser stereolithography, which is the golden standard in 3D bio model production. The model is casted in a deformable silicone to mimic true-to-nature suture experience by negative mould fabrication and silicone-casting [19].

4 Clinical Applications

In generic terms, simulation-based training refers to an artificial representation of a realistic process to achieve educational goals throughout experiential learning. The acquisition of many technical and nontechnical skills is moving outside the operative theatre, using simulation-based training. Achieving surgical competence in complex surgery, such as MIMVS, requires surgical volume.

The use of high-fidelity simulators in MIMVS can serve different purposes. It can be used for training surgeons, for preprocedural planning and

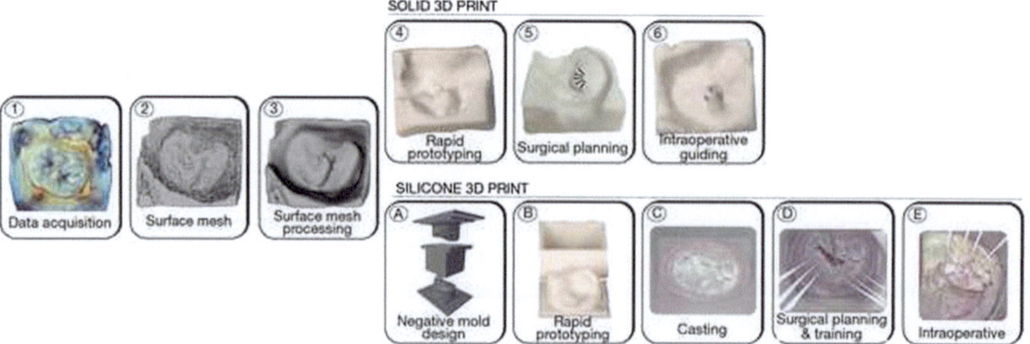

Fig. 2 Step by step process for solid and silicone 3D print fabrication. Reprinted with permission from The Journal of Visualized Surgery, https://doi.org/10.21037/jovs.2019.05.01 [25]

for assessment and certification of skills. Furthermore, the simulator can also be used for product development, testing new instruments, refining, and developing new surgical techniques.

For example, by using the simulator, a suturing map was designed after identifying the most effective suturing sequences and techniques with minimal tissue manipulation and maximal visual experience (Fig. 3). Additionally, it was evaluated successfully in the operating room and used in course to evaluate its teachiblity [24].

Furthermore, we conducted a study to develop a process for modelling and 3D-printing for preoperative planning and procedural simulation by analyzing 10 prospective patients with different mitral valve pathologies. This study demonstrated the additional benefit of the designed and printed models, which can be implanted in the simulator to improve preoperative planning and simulation of complex surgeries for training purposes. The case below is to illustrate the process [19].

Mitral valve repair for posterior leaflet prolapse and annular dilatation

A 63-year-old man presented on the outpatient clinic with severe mitral valve regurgitation based on posterior leaflet prolapse and annular dilatation. The patient was discussed in our multidisciplinary consultation and was found eligible for mitral valve surgery. A normal right and left ventricular function with an end diastolic dimeter of 58 mm was seen on transthoracic echocardiography. Transoesophageal echocardiography showed severe mitral valve regurgitation with an eccentric jet due to P2 prolapse with chordal rupture. Additionally, there was a mild P1 prolapse, a minimal trace of tricuspid valve insufficiency and no signs of aortic insufficiency. Computed tomography showed no contraindications for peripheral cannulation and the patient was accepted for MIMVS. A silicone mitral valve was created by 3D modelling and printing, and eventually mounted in the simulator for in vitro preoperative planning (Fig. 4).

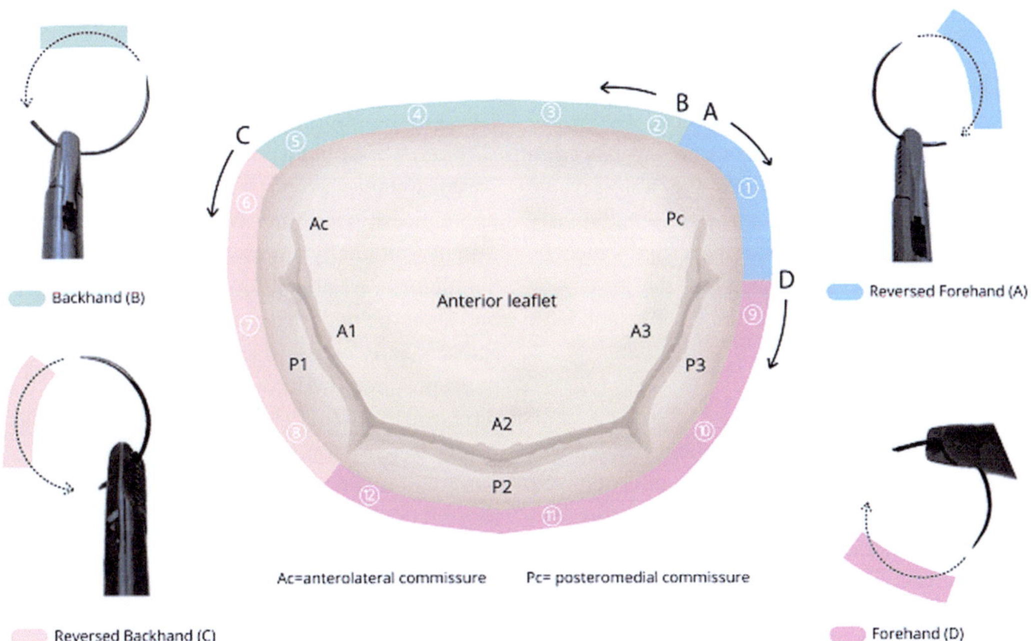

Fig. 3 Suturing map. A: Reversed forehand position, B: Backhand position, C: Reversed backhand position, D: Forehand position. Images provided courtesy of The Multimedia Manual of Cardio-Thoracic Surgery https://mmcts.org/tutorial/1041 [24].

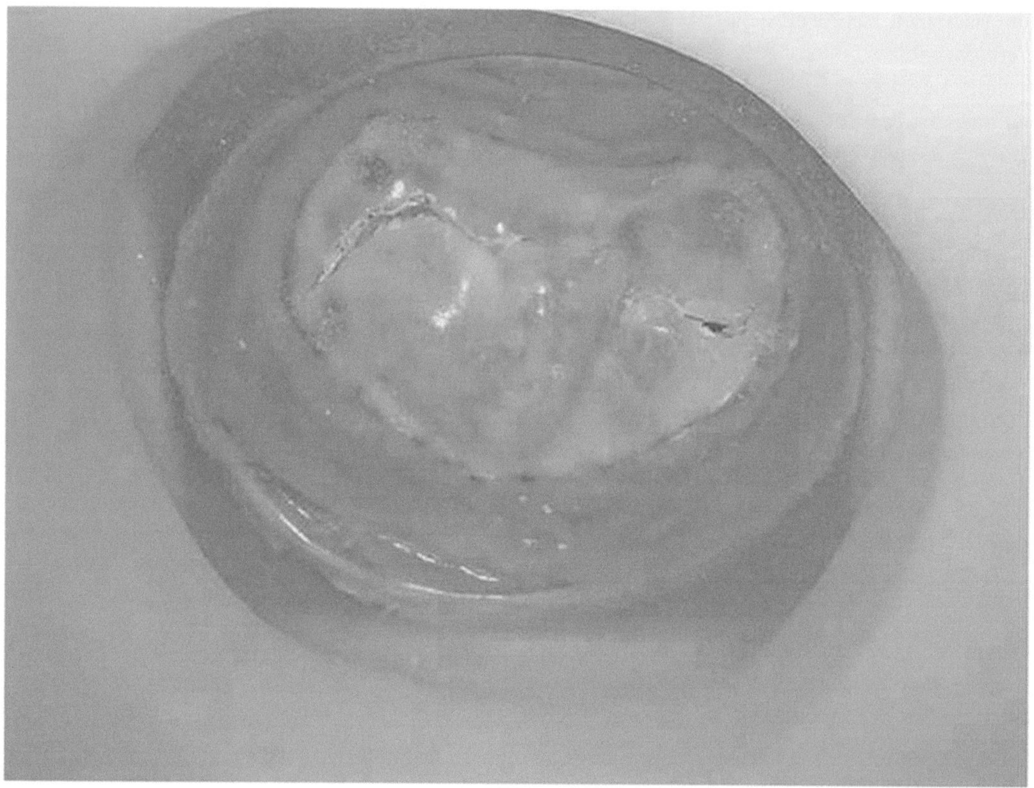

Fig. 4 Silicone model showing posterior leaflet pSilicone model showing rolapse and annular dilatation. Reprinted with permission from The Journal of Visualized Surgery, https://doi.org/10.21037/jovs.2019.05.01 [25]

During the simulation 2 neochordae were placed in the P2 segment. 1 neochord was placed in the P1 segment and another one was placed in the P3 segment. To stabilize the mitral valve annulus and the repair, a semi-rigid annuloplasty ring (size 34) was fitted into place (See Video 1). The patient was than operated the next day simulating the operation done in the simulator with successful result [25].

Structural training

Simulation based training may help residents to achieve proficiency in basic and more complex surgical skills, while practicing surgeons can develop new strategies or learn new techniques more swiftly. This type of education is already implemented in laparoscopic surgery and has been proven to be effective by reducing the learning curve in vivo procedures [8]. The question is no longer if we should practice on simulators but how we should implement simulation-based training.

First, we should acknowledge that simulation-based training is no substitute for traditional apprenticeship training. We showed that the high-fidelity minimally invasive mitral valve surgery simulator is a valuable tool for the development and assessment of endoscopic mitral repair skills. Subsequently we designed an air-pilot training concept, through European Association for Cardiothoracic Surgery (EACTS), Endoscopic Mitral Valve Repair Course. This 2-day course design was based on the following basic learning objectives (Fig. 5).

1. Awareness
2. Acquiring theoretical knowledge
3. Acquiring endoscopic skills.

Firstly, it is important for the participants to get introduced to the mitral valve simulator and

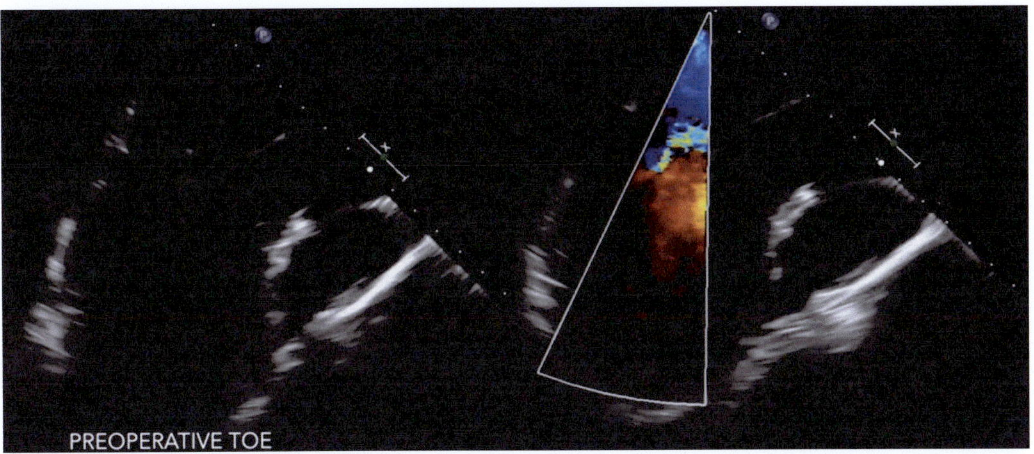

Video 1 Mitral valve repair for posterior leaflet prolapse and annular dilatation. Available online: http://www.asvide.com/article/view/32377. Reprinted with permission from The Journal of Visualized Surgery, https://doi.org/10.21037/jovs.2018.09.07 [26] (▶ https://doi.org/10.1007/000-a8g)

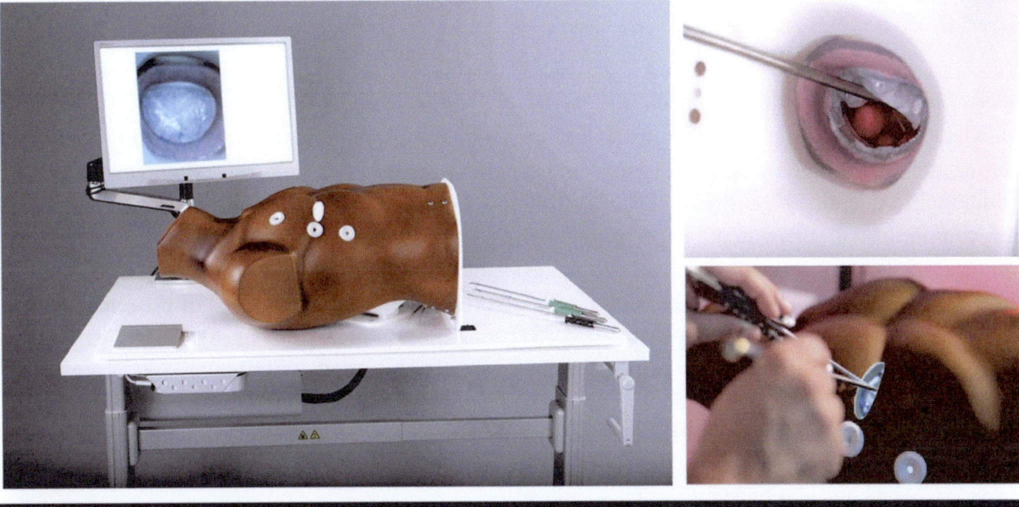

Fig. 5 Overview of the philosophy of simulation based training and its inclusion in the endoscopic mitral valve course in our centre. 3D: three-dimensional. Reprinted from Interactive CardioVascular and Thoracic Surgery, Volume 30, Issue 5, Peyman Sardari Nia, Samuel Heuts, Jean H T Daemen, Jules R Olsthoorn, W Randolph Chitwood, Jr, Jos G Maessen, The EACTS simulation-based training course for endoscopic mitral valve repair: an air-pilot training concept in action, 691–698, 2020, with permission from Elsevier [26].

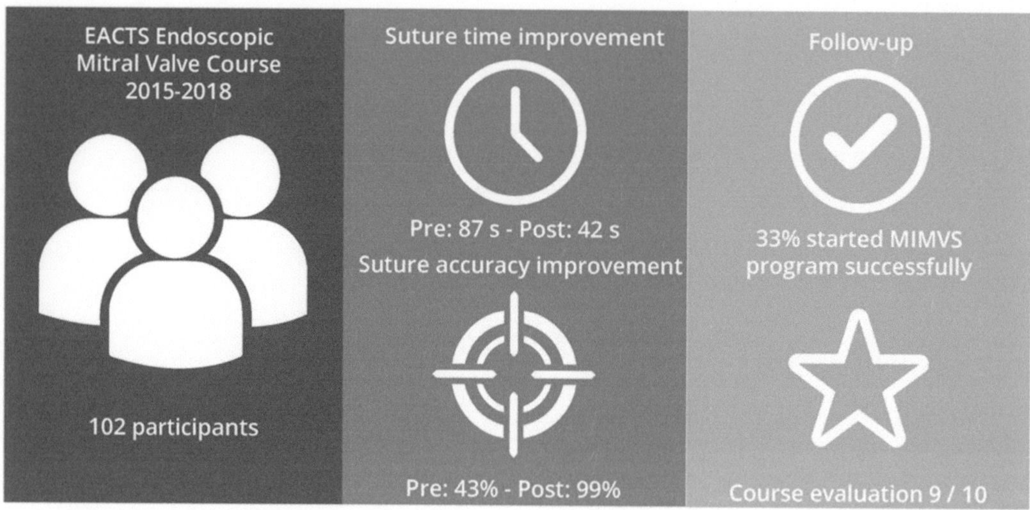

Fig. 6 Simulation based training for endoscopic mitral valve repair: an air-pilot training concept in action. Reprinted from Interactive CardioVascular and Thoracic Surgery, Volume 30, Issue 5, Peyman Sardari Nia, Samuel Heuts, Jean H T Daemen, Jules R Olsthoorn, W Randolph Chitwood, Jr, Jos G Maessen, The EACTS simulation-based training course for endoscopic mitral valve repair: an air-pilot training concept in action, 691–698, 2020, with permission from Elsevier [26]

create awareness for the demanding skills, knowledge, organization and teamwork before starting the endoscopic mitral valve programme. Additional to this, one should focus on acquiring the complemental theoretical knowledge and technical skills (for example the use of long-shafted instruments and the use of video assistance) for simulation-based training on MIMVS.

One hundred two participants completed the full endoscopic mitral valve programme between February 2016 and September 2018. 83 (83.3%) participants were staff/attending surgeons, 12 (11.8%) participants had finished residency and 5 (4.9%) participants were residents.

The course started with theoretical and technical skills pre-assessment on the simulators. During the course formative feedback was provided by an expert on MIMVS and metric-based feedback was provided by the simulator. At the end of the course there was a theoretical and technical skills post-assessment and a course evaluation with follow up.

The study showed significantly higher theoretical knowledge of endoscopic mitral valve surgery after completion of the mitral valve programme compared to before the training

(median score 58% vs. 67%, P < 0.001). Furthermore, participants significantly improved their technical skills on the simulator in terms of accuracy (suture accuracy 43% vs. 99%, P < 0.001) and speed (87 vs. 42 s., P < 0.001) in the pre—and post-assessment of technical skills on the simulator, regardless of the expertise level or trainee's position (Fig. 6). We showed that by practising on the simulator one significantly improves the accuracy and speed of endoscopic suturing on the simulator, independent from the expertise level [26].

5 Future Perspectives

For future, we envision a training trajectory rather than a single course. Successful adaption of a new procedure requires structural and repetitive training. To develop and optimize a MIMVS curricula that incorporates simulation, one should have an air-pilot training concept course and accessibility of simulation models at the institution or at home to continue practicing. During the training one should receive

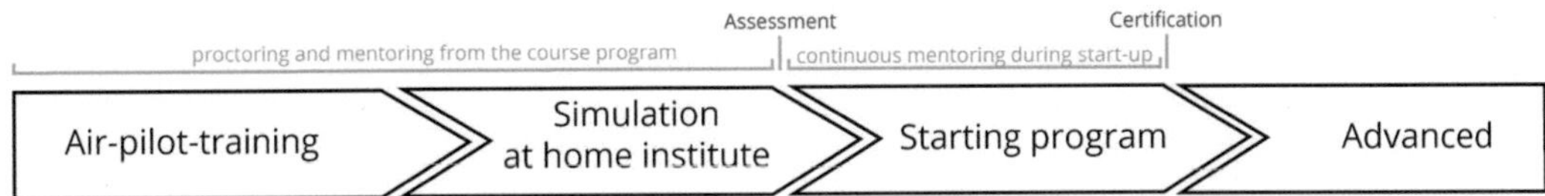

Fig. 7 Timeline of the air-pilot concept programme with inclusion of the training at our course, simulation and proctoring at the participants' home centre and actual start of a self-managed programme. Reprinted from Interactive CardioVascular and Thoracic Surgery, Volume 30, Issue 5, Peyman Sardari Nia, Samuel Heuts, Jean H T Daemen, Jules R Olsthoorn, W Randolph Chitwood, Jr, Jos G Maessen, The EACTS simulation-based training course for endoscopic mitral valve repair: an air-pilot training concept in action, 691–698, 2020, with permission from Elsevier [26]

mentorship and proctorship to gain formative and metric based feedback. Finally, a clinical objective certification may be commissioned (Fig. 7) [24].

References

1. Holzhey DM, Seeburger J, Misfeld M, Borger MA, Mohr FW. Learning minimally invasive mitral valve surgery: a cumulative sum sequential probability analysis of 3895 operations from a single high-volume center. Circulation. 2013;128:483–91.
2. Ng CK, Nesser J, Punzengruber C, Pachinger O, Auer J, Franke H, Hartl P. Valvuloplasty with glutaraldehyde-treated autologous pericardium in patients with complex mitral valve pathology. Ann Thorac Surg. 2001;71:78–85.
3. Bolling SF, Li S, O'Brien SM, Brennan JM, Prager RL, Gammie JS. Predictors of mitral valve repair: clinical and surgeon factors. Ann Thorac Surg. 2010;90:1904–12.
4. Shuhaiber J, Anderson RJ. Meta-analysis of clinical outcomes following surgical mitral valve repair or replacement. Eur J Cardiothorac Surg. 2007;31: 267–75.
5. Galloway AC, Colvin SB, Baumann FG, Grossi EA, Ribakove GH, Harty S, Spencer FC. A comparison of mitral valve reconstruction with mitral valve replacement: intermediate-term results. Ann Thorac Surg. 1989;47:655–62.
6. Modi P, Hassan A, Chitwood WR Jr. Minimally invasive mitral valve surgery: a systematic review and meta-analysis. Eur J Cardiothorac Surg. 2008;34:943–52.
7. Sündermann SH, Sromicki J, Biefer HRC, Seifert B, Holubec T, Falk V, Jacobs S. Mitral valve surgery: right lateral minithoracotomy or sternotomy? A systematic review and meta-analysis. J Thorac Cardiovasc Surg. 2014;148:1989–95.
8. Aggarwal R, Ward J, Balasundaram I, Sains P, Athanasiou T, Darzi A. Proving the effectiveness of virtual reality simulation for training in laparoscopic surgery. Ann Surg. 2007;246:771–9.
9. Carpenter AJ, Yang SC, Uhlig PN, Colson YL. Envisioning simulation in the future of thoracic surgical education. J Thorac Cardiovasc Surg. 2008;135:477–84.
10. Hicks GL, Brown JW, Calhoon JH, Merrill WH. You never know unless you try. J Thorac Cardiovasc Surg. 2008;136:814–5.
11. Feins RH. Expert commentary: cardiothoracic surgical simulation. J Thorac Cardiovasc Surg. 2008;135: 485–6.
12. Joyce DL, Dhillon TS, Caffarelli AD, Joyce DD, Tsirigotis DN, Burdon TA, Fann JI. Simulation and skills training in mitral valve surgery. J Thorac Cardiovasc Surg. 2011;141:107–12.
13. Verberkmoes NJ, Verberkmoes-Broeders EM. A novel low-fidelity simulator for both mitral valve and tricuspid valve surgery: the surgical skills trainer for classic open and minimally invasive techniques. Interact Cardiovasc Thorac Surg. 2013;16:97–101.
14. Hossien A. Low-fidelity simulation of mitral valve surgery: simple and effective trainer. J Surg Educ. 2015;72:904–9.
15. Sardari Nia P. From Bench to Reality: Development of Simulation, 3D Printing, and Air-Pilot-Training Concept Course for Endoscopic Mitral Valve Surgery. April 2019. doi:https://doi.org/10.25373/ctsnet.8035631.
16. Cates CU, Gallagher AG. The future of simulation technologies for complex cardiovascular procedures. Eur Heart J. 2012;33:2127–34.
17. Greenhouse DG, Grossi EA., Dellis S, Park J, Yaffee DW, DeAnda Jr A, ... & Balsam LB. Assessment of a mitral valve replacement skills trainer: a simplified, low-cost approach. J Thorac Cardiovasc Surg. 2013;145:54–9.
18. Nia PS, Daemen JH, Maessen JG. Development of a high-fidelity minimally invasive mitral valve surgery simulator. J Thorac Cardiovasc Surg. 2019;2019 (157):1567–74.
19. Daemen JH, Heuts S, Olsthoorn JR, Maessen JG, Sardari Nia P. Mitral valve modelling and three-dimensional printing for planning and simulation of mitral valve repair. Eur J Cardiothorac Surg. 2019;55:543–51.
20. Khabbaz KR, Mahmood F, Shakil O, Warraich HJ, Gorman III JH, Gorman RC, ... & Hess PE. Dynamic

3-dimensional echocardiographic assessment of mitral annular geometry in patients with functional mitral regurgitation. Ann Thorac Surg. 2013;95:105–10.

21. Maceira AM, Cosín-Sales J, Roughton M, Prasad SK, Pennell DJ. Reference left atrial dimensions and volumes by steady state free precession cardiovascular magnetic resonance. J Cardiovasc Magn Reson. 2010;12:1–10.

22. Lam JHC, Ranganathan N, Wigle ED, Silver MD. Morphology of the human mitral valve: I Chordae tendineae: A new classification. Circulation. 1970;41:449–58.

23. Ryan LP, Jackson BM, Enomoto Y, Parish L, Plappert TJ, John-Sutton MGS, ... & Gorman III JH. Description of regional mitral annular nonplanarity in healthy human subjects: a novel methodology. J Thorac Cardiovasc Surg. 2007;134: 644–8.

24. Sardari Nia P, Olsthoorn J, Heuts S, Maessen J. Suturing map for endoscopic mitral valve repair developed on high-fidelity endoscopic simulator. Multimed Man Cardiothorac Surg. 2018;26:2018. https://doi.org/10.1510/mmcts.2018.038. PMID: 30192451.

25. Olsthoorn JR, Heuts S, Daemen J, Maessen J, Sardari Nia P. Clinical implications of three-dimensional mitral valve modelling, printing and simulation in mitral valve surgery. J Vis Surg. 2019. https://doi.org/10.21037/jovs.2019.05.01.

26. Sardari Nia P, Heuts S, Daemen JHT, Olsthoorn JR, Randolph Chitwood W Jr, Maessen JG. The EACTS simulation-based training course for endoscopic mitral valve repair: an air-pilot training concept in action. Interact Cardiovasc Thorac Surg. 2020;30 (5):691–8. https://doi.org/10.1093/icvts/ivz323.

Trial of Current 3D Imaging Systems

Ludwig Müller

Abstract

The use of an endoscope in surgery is now commonplace in many specialities. Unfortunately for patients its use in cardiac surgery has had a slow uptake. Gradually more surgeons are starting to trial it out and are getting encouraging results. The introduction of 3D endoscopes was originally only as a part of a robotic system but over the past few years more industry partners have started to supply endoscopes capable of three dimensional visualisation. This chapter goes through the advantages and disadvantages of all the systems currently available on the market and also covers reasons to consider the use of these advanced imaging options in cardiac surgery. The final decision will need to be made by the surgeon and his team regarding this technology but we hope this chapter acts as a good introduction for those starting to look at this technology.

Keywords

3D videoendoscopy · Endoscopic cardiac surgery · Human vision · Convergence

L. Müller (✉)
Department of Cardiac Surgery, Medical University Innsbruck, Innsbruck, Austria
e-mail: ludwig.mueller@tirol-kliniken.at

1 Introduction

Endoscopic 3D imaging systems have heavily influenced the practice of minimally invasive mitral valve surgery, isolated as well as in combination with tricuspid, atrial fibrillation ablation and atrial septal surgery including benign atrial tumours [1]. To a lesser extent but very important also endoscopic aortic valve replacement has been made feasible [2]. 3D video endoscopy had originally been limited to robotic systems [3–5] but was made available separately in 2014, i.e. without the extensive high tech and costly features of a surgical robotic system. Interestingly, one of the first 3D video systems using rod lenses and introduced successfully for minimally invasive cardiac surgery was and is still made by the same manufacturer (Schölly Fiberoptic GmbH, 79211 Denzlingen, Germany) as the 3D endoscope of the "Da Vinci SI" Surgical System" (Sunnyvale, CA USA).

In 2021 various 3D video endoscopic systems are on the market and merit an in-depth analysis of function and use in daily practice as well as teaching.

Before the most up to date technology is analyzed it is reasonable to spend a few thoughts on human vison and 3D perception.

First, we have to realize that 3-dimensional vision and binocular or stereoscopic vision is not necessarily the same. Therefore also the term "3D imaging" might be misleading.

As we know from daily experience also single eyed, i.e. monocular vision works well for a 3-dimensional perception of our environment. Single eyed people are perfectly capable of car driving for example. And lots of pseudo 3D images are cheating us, e.g. in street art [6]. This is due to so called "monocular cues" of 3D vision. More on that later.

Second: In addition to monocular cues depth perception is highly facilitated by so-called binocular cues, i.e. stereoscopic vision or stereopsis. Different binocular cues contribute to a 3D image. Here 3D imaging systems come into place. Most interesting and striking news for those not specialized on this topic may be that we can perceive depth even if there is no 3-dimensional structure at all. This was studied intensively by Bela Julesz by construction of so-called random dot stereograms [7]. More on that also below.

Briefly, depth perception can be accomplished by monocular and binocular cues and does not necessarily require a real 3-dimensional structure.

Third: We must apprehend that our eyes are not video cameras which record images or movies, but vision takes place exclusively in the brain. We discern between sensation and perception. Sensation is the process located in the eyes when photons activate receptors in the retina which send electrical signals to the brain. Now the highly complex process of perception, i.e. vision takes place. It involves a number of different brain areas located not just in the visual cortex but distributed widely over the brain. At the end our inner image appears in the frontal cortex including the perception of depth, i.e. 3D vision. And this process is not just complex with many different circuits involved, it is also not unidirectional, that means our final vision is also determined by earlier experience and not limited to the visual sense but strongly determined also by multiple other e.g. tactile inputs. Multiple signals travel from the frontal cortex back to the thalamus and optical cortex thereby influencing the signals from the visual cortex which are sent to the frontal cortex. This complex process is understood today only in part. Seeing without experience of the other sensory organs is not very helpful in daily life. It is demonstrated impressively by the history of Mike May [8] who lost his eye sight by a chemical explosion at the age of three. Although normal eye function was widely restored at the age of 46 by successful surgery, he did not regain normal vision, being unable to grasp three-dimensional vision and to recognize members of his family by their faces alone, as he says. This is of importance also for the understanding of our requirements on a surgical endoscopic video system.

The following is a short overview of the basics of 3D vision which may be important for the surgeon using a 3D imaging system. It is not a summary of actual knowledge on vision in neurophysiology and neuropsychology

Monocular cues for depth perception [9, 10]:
Relative size: familiar objects appear smaller in distance.

Texture gradient: on closer objects more details of surface structure can be seen.

Height in field of view: distant objects tend to appear higher in our field of view than closer ones.

Linear perspective: parallel lines e.g. railway rails appear to converge in the distance.

Aerial (atmospheric) perspective: effect of the atmosphere on the appearance of objects in the distance. They appear bluer.

Light and shadow: are strong indicators as they appear only in three dimensional structures.

Interposition (overlap, occlusion): an object which obstructs the view of something else is closer.

Defocus blur: because the depth of focus of the human eye is limited distant objects appear blurred.

Motion parallax (while the observer moves objects of different distance appear to move at different speed).

Depth from motion is calculated by use of the changing size of an object moving towards or off the observer.

Kinetic depth effect: When a certain object (e.g. a wire cube) is placed in front of a light source and its shadow falls on a translucent screen one will see a two-dimensional pattern of lines on the other side of the screen. If the cube rotates, however, the brain extracts information for perception of the third dimension from the movements of the lines, and a 3-dimensional cube is seen.

Accommodation: When focusing on a distant object the ciliary muscles stretch the eye lens to change the length of focus and kinesthetic sensations of the ciliary muscles are used by the brain to calculate distance by triangulation.

Binocular cues—require two eyes [10, 11]:

Stereopsis is the perception of depth produced by binocular disparity: because our eyes are offset objects in different distance are depicted on different areas of the retina. Two different images are received by the brain and fused to a single "cyclopean" image with perceived depth.

This effect is responsible also for so-called autostereograms. A 3-dimensional image can be seen in a strictly 2-dimensional picture. Like random dot stereograms [7] these are computer generated images of random dots. Two identical images (without any depth cues) are presented, but in one of them a slight shift of a part of the image is made. By viewing each image with one eye by focusing either in front or behind the images finally both images are fused in the brain and a single 3-dimensional image appears [11].

Vergence (convergence): looking at closer objects causes the eyes to converge, therefore these objects are depicted more laterally on the retina than distant ones, which causes the brain to calculate distances.

Different perspective for either eye (each eye sees a slightly different image of a 3-dimensional object).

All these cues lead us two perceive depth (even if there is no depth at all) and are integrated by the brain involving not just the visual cortex in the occipital lobe, but many other brain areas including the lateral geniculate nucleus in the thalamus, the temporal lobes, the frontal lobes and others. The frontal lobe is where the final

perception takes place and provided with emotion and as already mentioned, vision as we experience it, is only possibly by additional information from other sensory systems.

All that is information may be helpful when we use 3D imaging for endoscopic surgery. Becoming a successful endoscopic surgeon is not just a matter of having a high-end 3D endoscope at hand but experience helps not just to become a skilled surgeon but also to develop optimal 3D vision. However, technical issues play an important role.

3D videoendoscopic technology:

3D imaging systems are composed of 4 main components:

Optical system (lenses)
Sensor chips
Processing unit
Display (monitor)

Differing components and composition as well as additional not directly imaging related features make the difference between products.

In general 2 types of endoscopes and 5 types of 3D display systems are available for use in the surgical theater. All of them produce two images, one for the left, one for the right eye. Fusion to a single 3-dimensional image takes place in the brain implying all the cues described above. All systems use stereo displays with dual 2D images and have to be differentiated from 3D displays, which are not available for our purposes so far, but may have an important role in the future.

Stereodisplays and 3D displays [12]:

Real 3D displays display an image in three full dimensions. The most notable difference from stereoscopic displays with only two 2D offset images is that the observer's head and eyes movement will not increase information about the 3-dimensional objects displayed. So it is simply an overstatement to refer to dual 2D images as being "3D".

Stereodisplays:
1. Anaglyph systems: A red filter for the left and a cyan filter for the right eye are used to filter

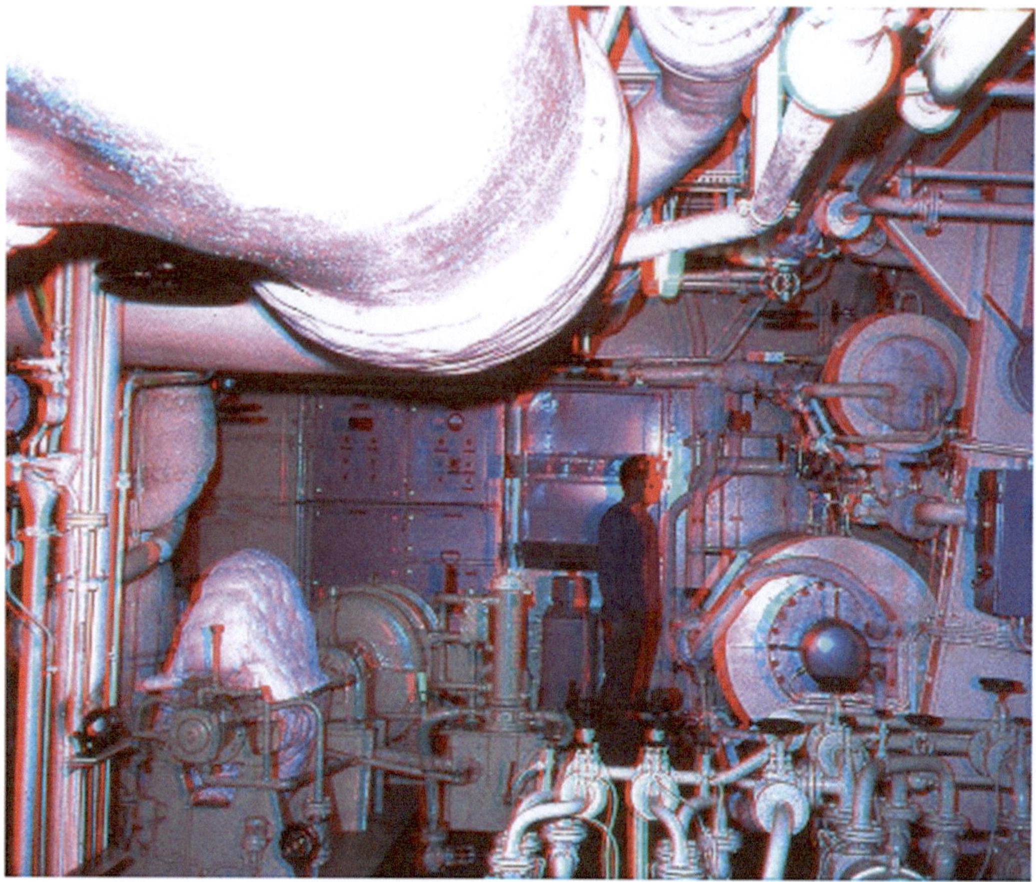

Fig. 1 Anaglyph: Von Heamberg–Eigenes Werk, CC BY-SA 3.0, [13] GNU Free documentation License. https://commons.wikimedia.org/w/index.php?curid=2984751. GNU Free documentation License

out the respective images for either eye (Fig. 1).

2. Polarizing filters: They do the same as they let pass only light of a certain polarization. Two sets of polarized images of the left and right eye image are displayed either by the odd or even lines of the monitor and are viewed with the respective eye by the use of corresponding polarizing glasses. This technology is used in all current surgical 3D video imaging systems.

Further possibilities include:

3. Interference filter technology (e.g. Dolby 3D, Omega 3D/Panavision 3D): Specific wavelengths of red, green, and blue for one eye, and different wavelengths of red, green, and blue for the other eye are used while eyeglasses filter out the very specific wavelengths and the wearer can see a 3D image.

4. Shutter glasses: The monitor projects the left or right eye image in rapid succession and in synchrony with the monitor either the left of the right eye glass is shut. Due to the speed of alternation one single 3-D image is seen. Flickering may occur and the shutter glasses need energy (batteries).

5. Autostereo displays (used in hand held devices). They use either parallax barriers or a lenticular lens system, thereby providing different images to either eye. Due to technical limitations they are not used in medical video displays.

Real 3D Displays:

Volumetric 3D display
Holographic displays
Integral imaging
Compressive light field display

The technology behind these systems and applications are not discussed in this article since they are not employed in surgical imaging system today. As soon as they become available and reliable in clinical use, however, they may again be a major leap forward in surgical imaging. For further reading and more detailed information on the subject refer to [12].

In conclusion each display technology has its limitations, whether the location of the viewer, cumbersome or unsightly equipment or great cost. The display of artifact-free 3D images remains difficult.

In clinical video systems only the polarizing filter technology is used. Two sets of lines (even and uneven) are displayed on the monitor and can be seen after polarization either by the right or left eye. Without polarizing glasses double pictures are seen. If the channels are exchanged (by wrong connection) the image is inverted, i.e. more distant objects appear closer and vice versa. Performing surgery is not possible in this situation.

2 3D Endoscope Practice Test

In Europe Aesculap (Aesculap AG, 78532 Tuttlingen, Germany) Olympus (Olympus Corporation, Shinjuku, Tokyo, Japan) and Karl Storz (Karl Storz SE & Co. KG, 78,532 Tuttlingen, Germany)—in alphabetical order—provide 3D video endoscopes. Aesculap offers the Einstein Vision® system, Olympus the Visera Elite II® and Karl Storz the Image1 S®. The flexible Olympus Endoeye Flex 3D® provides less quality and is not discussed further in this test which applies also to Storz's 4 mm endoscope which is not appropriate for cardiac surgical applications.

In a test series as well as in daily routine four systems were tested. Tests took place between 10/2017 and 07/2021. Olympus and Aesculap have brought no innovations since the original test in 2017, Storz has completely revolutionized its system and provided a test system in 2021. According to recent verbal communication, Aesculap is working on its Einstein 4.0 which will feature 4 K resolution, ICG fluorescence and horizon stabilization in addition to specific features typical for the Einstein system.

3D video endoscopic systems in test:

Aesculap Einstein Vision 2.0®
Aesculap Einstein Vision 3.0® (Fig. 2a).
Olympus: System Visera Elite II Endoeye 3D® (Fig. 2b).
Karl Storz: Tipcam1 Rubina® (Fig. 2c).

Technical features:

All systems come with 0° and 30° endoscopes and share an outer diameter of 10 mm. Features allowing fluorescence imaging in the near infrared (NIR) spectrum with indocyanine green (ICG) dye do not play a role in routine cardiac surgical endoscopic procedures and therefore are not included and evaluated in this test.

All systems use dual channel endoscopes what means that real stereoscopy is possible (in contrast to single channel 3D endoscopes). Olympus and Karl Storz place the sensor chips directly behind the front lens of the endoscope, so called chip-in-the-tip technology. Aesculap uses a rod lens system. In the first case only basic optical technology is required since the sensor sits in the tip of the endoscope and only wires run through the shaft for connection to the camera head and the processing unit. The smaller size of the sensor chips (with theoretically less resolution) could be a disadvantage, while less optical stuff is built in and therefor the endoscopes should be more resistant to wear. The camera head and shaft of the endoscope come in one single unit. In the Einstein Vision systems Aesculap uses rod lenses and the sensor chips sit in the camera head giving more space for bigger

A

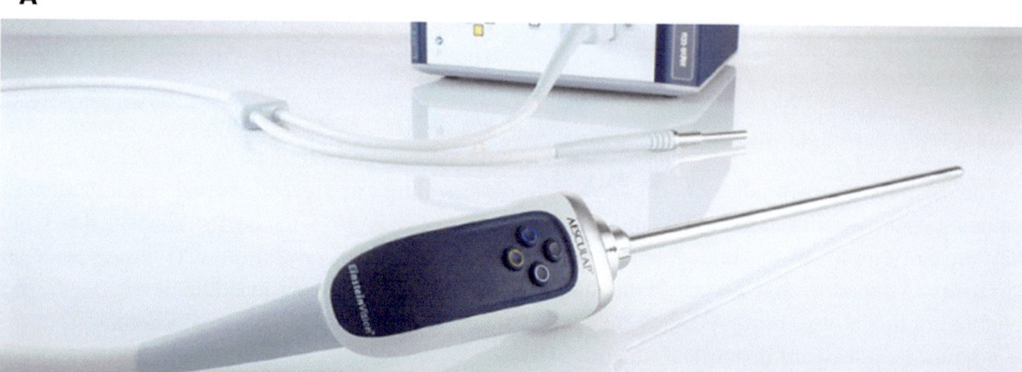

B

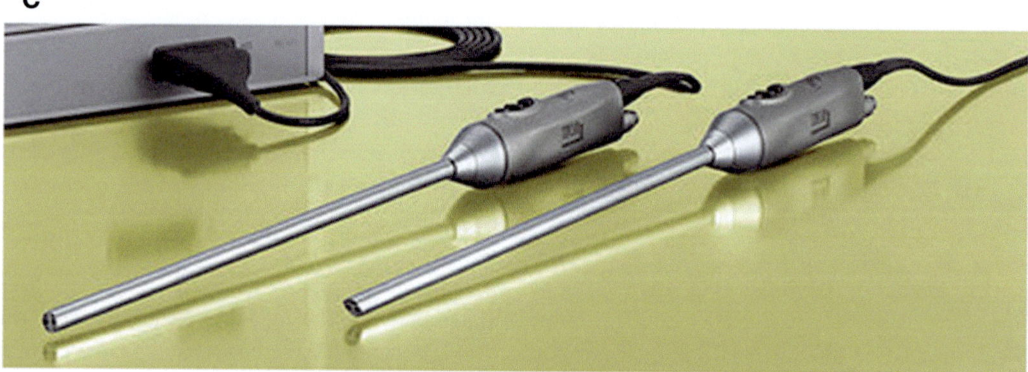

C

Fig. 2 **a** Aesculap: Einstein Vision 3.0, https://www.bbraun.de/content/dam/catalog/bbraun/bbraunProduct Catalog/S/AEM2015/de-de/b4/einsteinvision-30.jpeg.transform/400/image.jpg. **b** Olympus: Endoeye 3D, https://youtu.be/lP9HtTnZ0wg?t=62. **c** Karl Storz: Tipcam 1S, https://www.google.com/imgres?imgurl=https%3A%2F%2Fwww.karlstorz.com%2Fstatic%2Ffile_pics%2Fpic_editorial%2Fde%2FHM_TP%2F3434328_rdax_80.jpg&imgrefurl=https%3A%2F%2Fwww.karlstorz.com%2Fde%2Fde%2Fhighlights-tp.htm&tbnid=h1FgZytEjZtA6M&vet=12ahUKEwi_xN6D15nyAhXIM-wKHaH_Cx8QMygAegUIARDGAQ..i&docid=34DGZqHPYyDaCM&w=800&h=450&q=image%201s&client=safari&ved=2ahUKEwi_xN6D15nyAhXIM-wKHaH_Cx8QMygAegUIARDGAQ

chips. Light for illumination of the surgical field comes in a common cable combining light and electrical wiring in the Aesculap and Olympus systems, Storz uses a separate light cable. Due to inherent features of the dual channel technology rotation of the endoscope also leads to a rotation of the image on the screen. At 180° rotation an image inversion is possible with the normal upside up image on the screen. Storz uses a so-called automatic horizon straightening system. The term is somewhat misleading as the system switches automatically from 3 to 2D when rotation exceeds a predefined angle and then the stereoscopic 3D image is lost until full 180° rotation when the two channels are in a horizontal position again and the image is inverted automatically. This feature has to be chosen from the menu controlled by switches on the camera head. If autorotation is chosen the endoscopic image is not displayed on full screen but has a circular shape. If the endoscope is positioned more than vertically (e.g. to check for bleeding from port sites) autorotation again is activated and leads to an upside-down image. Only the Olympus endoscope allows rotation up to 174° without rotation of the image on the screen (stable horizon). The final basic difference is that Olympus and Storz endoscopes need sterilization between applications. Aesculap in contrast provides a single use drape. This is made from a metal sheet with a front window to cover the endoscope shaft and is connected to a plastic sleeve to cover the camera head and cable. The advantage is immediate reusability of the endoscope after a procedure and potential contaminations during surgery can be solved by easy change of the drape during the procedure. Unavoidable wear associated with sterilization is no issue. In addition the endoscope shaft is protected from mechanical damage by the hard cover. A potential disadvantage may be the theoretical lower infection safety since covering the endoscope is done when the sterile draping of the patient is already completed. Contamination could occur.

A specific feature of the Einstein Vision 3.0 is heating of the endoscope tip to avoid fogging. With chip in tip technology this is not necessary.

All systems were subjected to evaluation by three experienced endoscopic cardiac surgeons. Rating was performed on a scale from 1 to 5 (with 5 being the best grade). Testing occurred according to the following features:

Resolution, 3D effect, correct depth reproduction, depth of focus, brightness of the image on screen. Further factors investigated included the depicted area on the monitor, field of view, viewing angle (angle between observer and monitor required for 3D vison), endoscope diameter, quality and factors of zoom and ease of sterilization. Camera control units, monitors, light sources as well as peripheral devices for documentation or connection to local IT systems were used as provided by the companies but not subjected to separate test and evaluation since these features are offered in multiple configurations and may change quickly. Information on image quality is given according to subjective surgeons' assessment. Respective information from industry was omitted since it often is confusing and used mainly for advertising.

In Tables 1 and 2 comparative results are listed.

In summary three companies sharing the market of 3D video endoscopes have provided test systems. All suffice the requirements of endoscopic cardiac surgery. Image quality is good in all tested systems, but differences are not negligible. With up-to-date sensor technology differences in position of the chips in the endoscope tip or in the camera head and therefore sensor size do not reflect image quality any more. Most important appears the possibility of utilizing a single use sterile drape versus the need for sterilization after use. In departments with 2 or more procedures per day or if the system is shared with other specialties this may be of importance. Also potential damage by sending the video endoscope out from the OR to the sterilization facility, handling by different personnel and the wear due to the sterilization process itself may be important factors. Active and automatic image inversion are specific details differing between systems. Peripheral devices for additional imaging, recording, connection to local networks etc. and finally costs may be

Table 1 Technical features

	Aesculap Einsteinvision 2.0	Aesculap Einsteinvision 3.0	Olympus Visera Elite II Endoeye 3D	Karl Storz Tipcam 1 Rubina
Shaft diameter	10.5 mm (including sterile sheath)	10 mm (including sterile sheath)	10 mm	10 mm
Opening angle (°)	72°	72°	67°	82°
Depth of focus	20–200 mm	20–200 mm	Not provided	30–200 mm
Digital zoom	1.2–1.8×	1.2–1.8×	2×	2×
Endoscope tip heating	No	Yes	No	No
Sterilization required	No	No	Yes	Yes

Table 2 Rating of imaging quality (1 = minimum, 5 = maximum)

	Aesculap Einsteinvision 2.0	Aesculap Einsteinvision 3.0	Olympus Visera Elite II Endoeye 3D	Karl Storz Tipcam 1 Rubina
Resolution	4	5	3	5
3D effect	5	5	2	5
Viewing angle	Wide	Wide	Wide	Narrow
Depth perception	5	5	2	5
Brightness	4	5	5	5
Depth of focus	5	5	2	5

relevant but subject to individual requirements and therefore not included in the evaluation.

3 Conclusion

Aesculap (Aesculap Einstein Vision 3.0®) and Karl Storz (Tipcam1 Rubina®) have provided excellent 3D videoendoscopic systems for practice test.

Both share outstanding quality and are recommendable for endoscopic mitral valve procedures. As they differ in various features the user has the opportunity to choose according to her/his requirements. New developments are to be expected. The older Einstein Vision 2.0 is still produced for markets with pending registration of the 3.0 version and is an excellent tool to perform all endoscopic cardiac surgical procedures.

References

1. Westhofen S, Conradi L, Deuse T, Detter C, Vettorazzi E, Treede H, Reichenspurner H. A matched pairs analysis of non-rib-spreading, fully endoscopic, mini-incision technique versus conventional mini-thoracotomy for mitral valve repair. Eur J Cardiothorac Surg. 2016;50(6):1181–7.
2. Tokoro M, Sawaki S, Ozeki T, Orii M, Kato R, Ito T. Totally Endoscopic Aortic Valve Replacement Using the Three-dimensional Endoscope]. Kyobu Geka. 2020;73(7):510–15. Japanese. PMID: 32641670.
3. Reichenspurner H, Boehm D, Reichart B. Minimally invasive mitral valve surgery using three-dimensional

video and robotic assistance. Semin Thorac Cardiovasc Surg. 1999;11(3):235–43. https://doi.org/10.1016/s1043-0679(99)70064-x. PMID: 10451254.

4. Chitwood WR Jr, Nifong LW. Minimally invasive videoscopic mitral valve surgery: the current role of surgical robotics. J Card Surg. 2000;15(1):61–75. https://doi.org/10.1111/j.1540-8191.2000.tb00445.x. PMID: 11204390.

5. Mohr FW, Onnasch JF, Falk V, Walther T, Diegeler A, Krakor R, Schneider F, Autschbach R. The evolution of minimally invasive valve surgery–2 year experience. Eur J Cardiothorac Surg. 1999;15 (3):233–8; discussion 238–9. https://doi.org/10.1016/s1010-7940(99)00033-0. PMID: 10333015.

6. https://www.google.at/search?q=street+art+3d+illusion&tbm=isch&ved=2ahUKEwis6NyD-Z3wAhVP0RoKHVYZCJ8Q2-cCegQIABAA&oq=street+art+3d&gs_lcp=CgNpbWcQARgAMgIIADICCAAyAggAMgIIADIECAAQHjIECAAQHjIECAAQHjIECAAQHjIECAAQHjIGCAAQBRAeOgQIABBDUMP8AljiiQNgzaMDaABwAHgAgAH6AogBmgWSAQcwLjIuMC4xmAEAoAEBqgELZ3dzLXdpei1pbWfAAQE&sclient=img&ei=FcOHYOwJz6Jr1rKg-Ak&hl=de#imgrc=lZ5ld034kQAtEM.

7. Papathomas TV, Morikawa K, Wade N. Bela Julesz in Depth. Vision (Basel). 2019;3(2):18. https://doi.org/10.3390/vision3020018.PMID:31735819; PMCID:PMC6802775.

8. https://en.wikipedia.org/wiki/Mike_May_(skier).

9. Kalloniatis M and Luu Ch: Perception of depth. https://webvision.med.utah.edu/book/part-viii-psychophysics-of-vision/perception-of-depth/.

10. https://www.youtube.com/watch?v=QGYQgoyJzbU, https://en.wikipedia.org/wiki/Depth_perception.

11. https://www.google.at/search?q=autostereogram&hl=de&sxsrf=ALeKk03gsOXPLnI0vSdieeE8Ggtz6rp7rg:1619514568208&tbm=isch&source=iu&ictx=1&fir=BrnKb4UZdIA8TM%252C2W-QcdXoxLVZQM%252C%252Fm%252F02m6l7&vet=1&usg=AI4_-kQwZy5HdDOpBHR6nqNB_96IZ1Q81Q&sa=X&ved=2ahUKEwimkK_0iZ7wAhVG_aQKHTmUAHUQ_B16BAgeEAE.

12. https://en.wikipedia.org/wiki/Stereo_display.

13. Von Heamberg - Eigenes Werk, CC BY-SA 3.0, https://commons.wikimedia.org/w/index.php?curid=2984751.

MiECC as Support for Endoscopic Cardiac Surgery

Pascal Starinieri

Abstract

Beside the tremendous developments in cardiac surgical procedures, the use of cardiopulmonary bypass (CPB) remains the gold standard to perform cardiac surgery but is associated with detrimental effects (e.g. hemodilution and blood-air interface). Minimally invasive extracorporeal circulation (MiECC) has been designed in attempt to integrate all the advances in cardiopulmonary bypass technology in one closed circuit to minimize these systemic deleterious effects and therefore ideally can be used for cardiopulmonary support in addition to bypass for the adaption of minimal invasive surgical approaches. Due to the complexity and extreme invasiveness of CPB, strict attention needs to be paid to all safety aspects when using these minimized circuits. We want to share our experience in multi-vessel coronary bypass surgery by endoscopic set up and other MICS procedures in combination with the use of a minimal invasive perfusion circuit focusing on the overall safety aspects.

Keywords

MIECC · Endoscopic cardiac surgery bypass · Extracorporeal circulation

1 Introduction

Alongside the tremendous developments in cardiac surgical procedures, the use of cardiopulmonary bypass (CPB) remains the gold standard to perform cardiac surgery but is associated with detrimental effects (e.g. hemodilution and blood-air interface). Avoidance of extracorporeal circulation (ECC) emerged as a valuable alternative for conventional coronary surgery but tend to have significantly lower frequencies of complete revascularization which could lead to repeated procedures and increased mortality besides technical difficulties accompanied. These off-pump techniques apply only to coronary surgery (OPCAB) and could increase the difficulty of the surgical technique when more than one-vessel diseases are treated. Extracorporeal circulation is still necessary for the majority of valve surgery cases or "open-heart" procedures.

The focus on the perfusion is an important pilar of the triangle between surgeon, anesthesiologist and perfusionist. The most important

Supplementary Information The online version contains supplementary material available at https://doi.org/10.1007/978-3-031-21104-1_21. The videos can be accessed individually by clicking the DOI link in the accompanying figure caption or by scanning this link with the SN More Media App.

P. Starinieri (✉)
European Certified Cardiovascular Perfusionist, Hasselt, Belgium
e-mail: pascal.starinieri@jessazh.be

progress in this is to optimize the perfusion strategy or system. Depending on each centers preference, coated tubing, centrifugal pumps, assisted drainage, closed circuits, retrograde autologous priming

(Video 1 to Video 2) and the elimination of shed blood recirculation to the system have been used in a strategy to improve patient outcome. Minimal invasive extracorporeal circulation (MiECC) has been designed in attempt to integrate all these advances in one closed circuit which can be divided in 4 different types depending on which components are used (Fig. 1). Although many benefits of MiECC are shown (less transfusion, shorter hospital stay, lower inflammation,…), only few centers are using this technique mainly due to safety concerns regarding air-handling. Larger prospective multi-centered trials are necessary for expanding the knowledge and taking out the fear of using MiECC.

Our ultimate attempt was to create a closed circuit (Fig. 1, Type III) for coronary surgery or closed heart procedures on the one hand and on the other hand an advanced modular circuit with the advantages of a closed circuit for complex surgery (Fig. 2) providing maximum safety creating a minimal invasive 360° approach.

2 MiECC as Support for Minimal Invasive Cardiac Surgery

Although beating heart approaches are viable and the results promising, the technique itself is difficult. The value of beating heart approaches has not been derived from elimination of an optimized CPB circuit, but rather from the benefits of avoiding the cardioplegic arrest of the heart: exclusion of the aortic cross clamp and prevention of the associated reperfusion injury.

Minimally invasive extra-corporeal circulation can therefore ideally be utilized for cardiopulmonary "support", and as such can be an enabling technology for the adaption of less invasive surgical approaches. The most applicable procedural category in this case today is no-touch aorta "assisted" beating heart surgery. This procedure would combine stabilization with

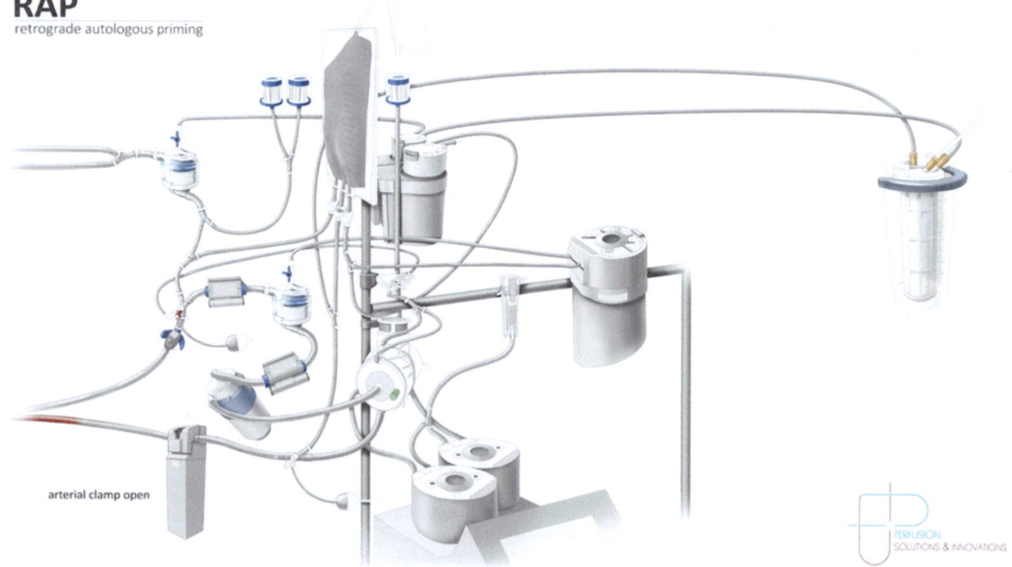

Video 1 Start RAP (▶ https://doi.org/10.1007/000-a90)

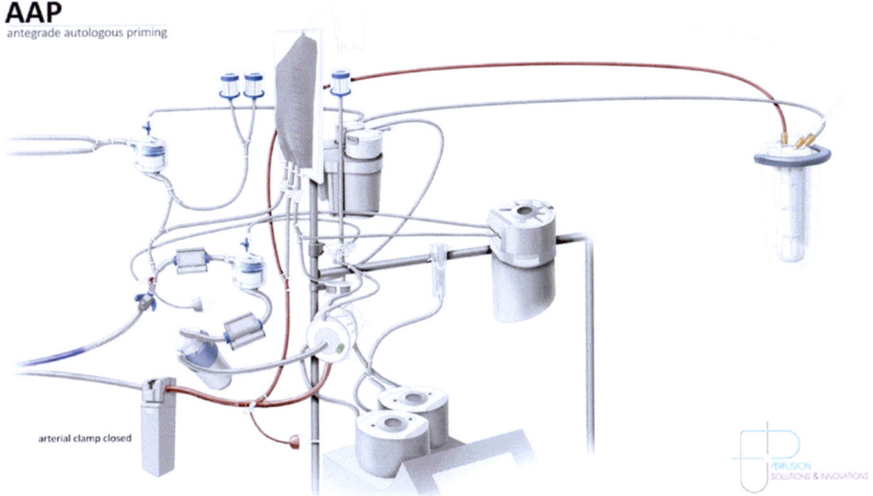

Video 2 Start AAP (▶ https://doi.org/10.1007/000-a8j)

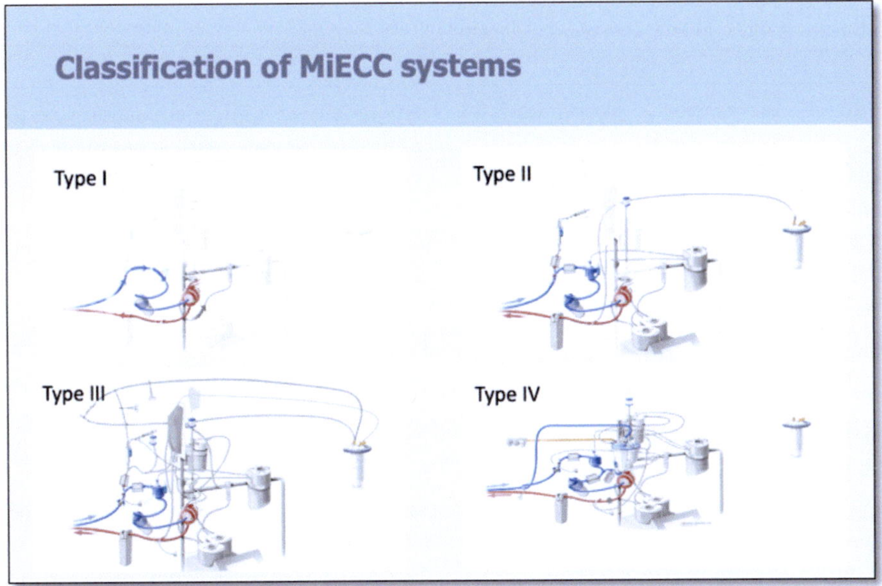

Fig. 1 Classification of MiECC

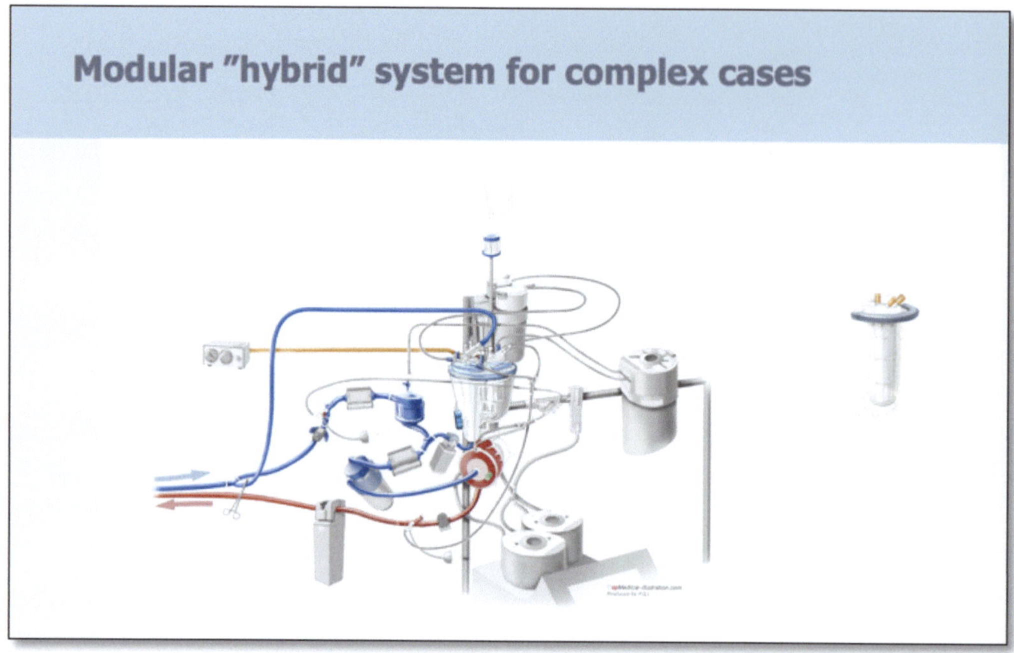

Fig. 2 Advanced modular MiECC for complex surgery

MiECC as an assist device to decompress the heart.

Minimally invasive extracorporeal circulation can seamlessly provide maintenance of hemodynamic stability facilitating the surgeon when manipulating the heart for difficult to reach vessels (lateral or posterior sides of the heart). In this setting, additional grafts can be performed, allowing more complete revascularization. This "hybrid" approach is ideal for the majority of surgeons who wish to provide the benefits of beating-heart surgery without compromising the level of safety associated with stopped heart procedures. Additionally, it can flatten the steep learning curve in minimally invasive cardiac surgery (MICS) by lowering the surgical technical difficulty. MiECC can also facilitate MICS, accompanied with increased CPB and clamping times, by minimizing the side effects of these extended times. We want to share our experience in multi-vessel coronary bypass surgery by endoscopic set up in combination with the use of a minimal invasive perfusion circuit (Video 1 to Video 15) focusing on overall safety aspects.

3 Team Approach

Prior to induction, the patient's physiological parameters are monitored and self-adhesive sensors containing the infrared light source and light detectors are placed on both sides of the forehead. In minimal invasive cardiac surgery as such or in combination with retrograde perfusion, near-infrared spectroscopy (NIRS) is an interesting tool to monitor cerebral oxygen saturation. After induction, a transesophageal echocardiography (TEE) probe is inserted into the oesophagus to provide excellent visualization of the heart and great vessels and to facilitate placement and confirmation of proper positioning of the various cannulas and catheters that are used during CPB.

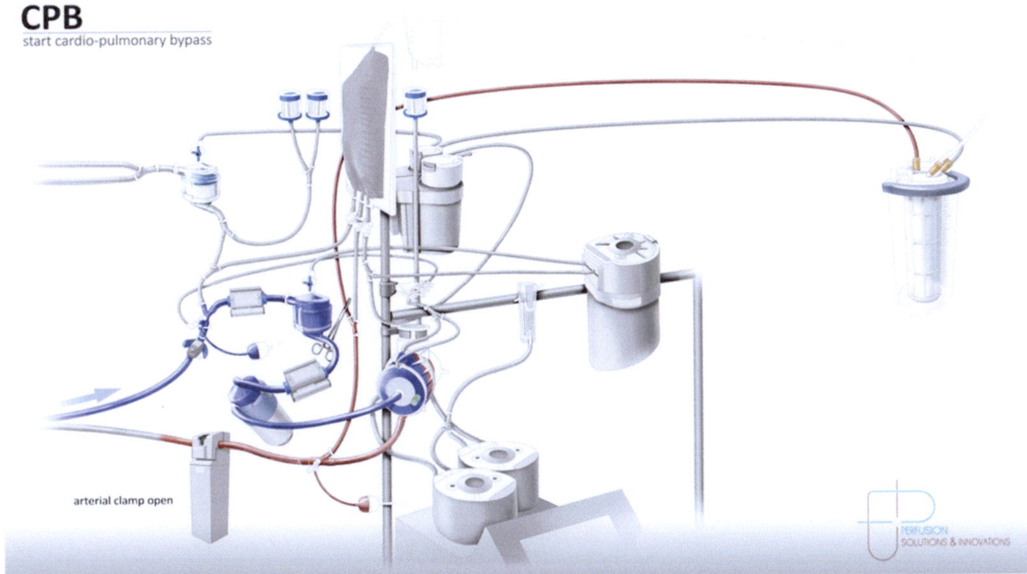

Video 3 Start CPB (▶ https://doi.org/10.1007/000-a8k)

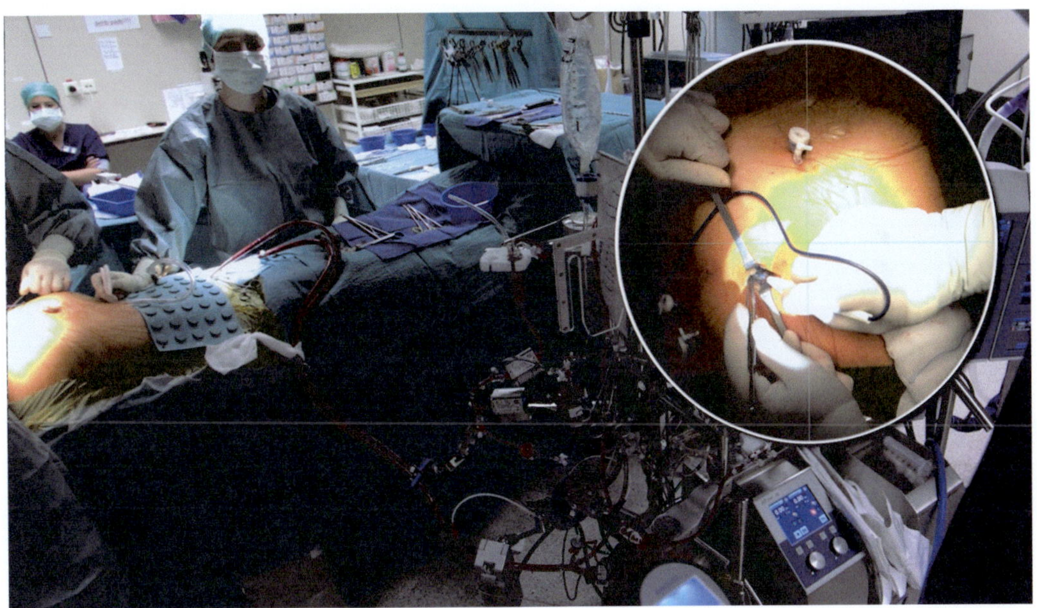

Video 4 Position table (▶ https://doi.org/10.1007/000-a8m)

ADD VOLUME
Excessive Negative Pressure

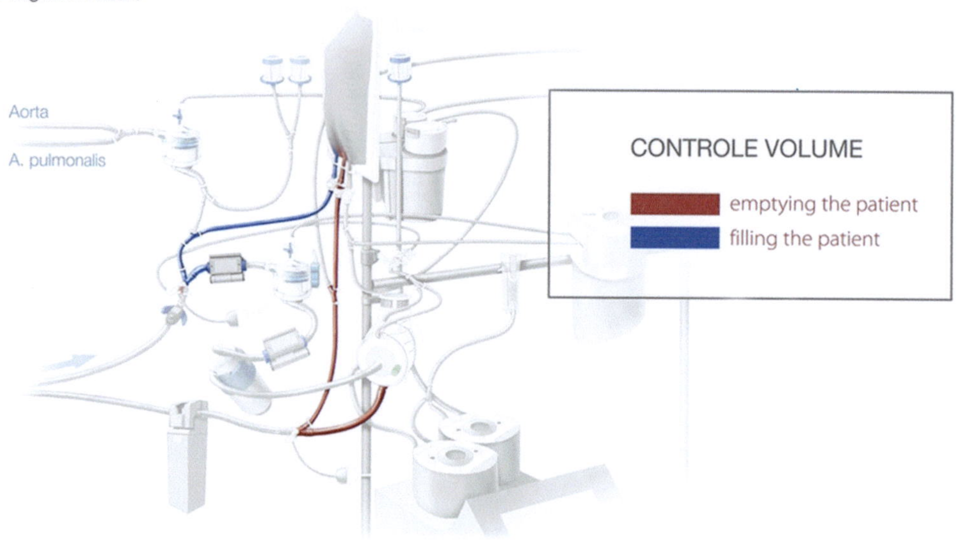

Video 5 Excessive negative pressure (▶ https://doi.org/10.1007/000-a8n)

AIR PURGE CONTROL
start APC to automatically remove air bubble

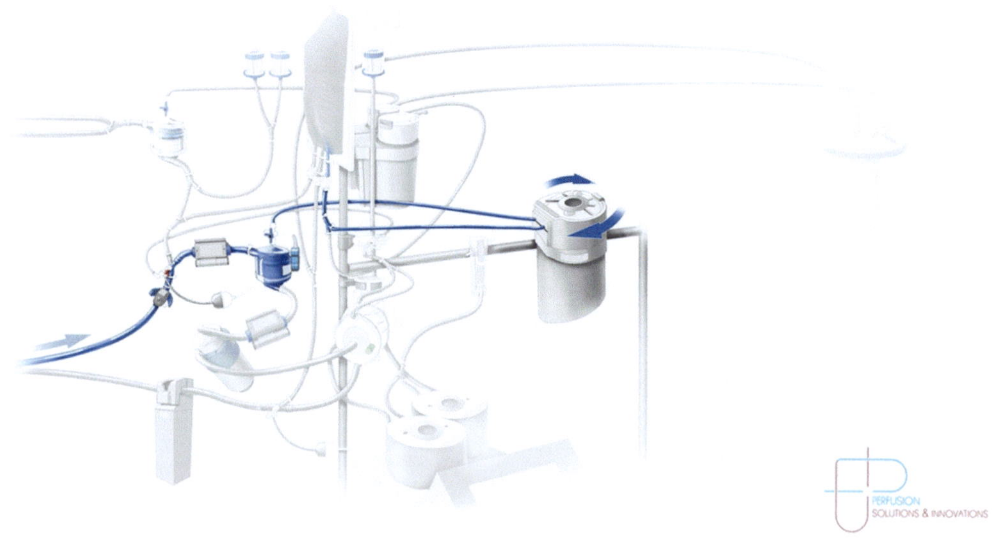

Video 6 Start air purge control (▶ https://doi.org/10.1007/000-a8p)

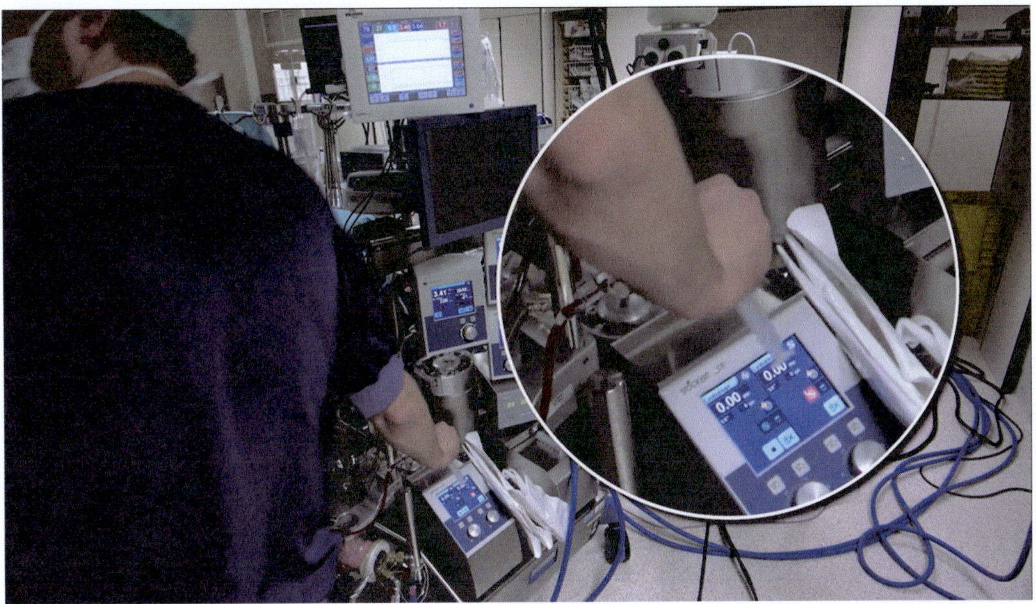

Video 7 Bolus injection medication (▶ https://doi.org/10.1007/000-a8q)

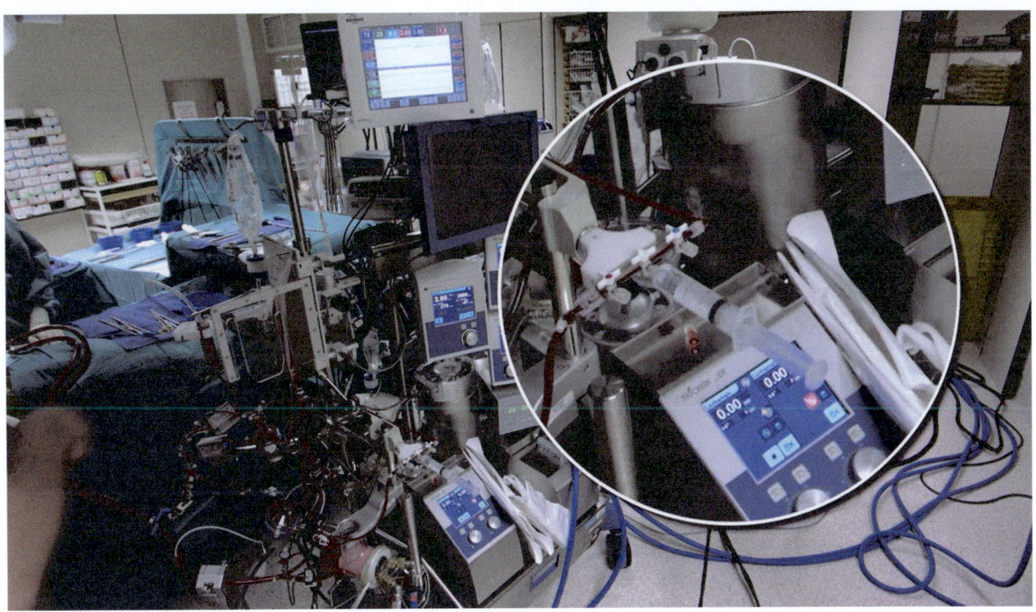

Video 8 Bloodgas sample (▶ https://doi.org/10.1007/000-a8r)

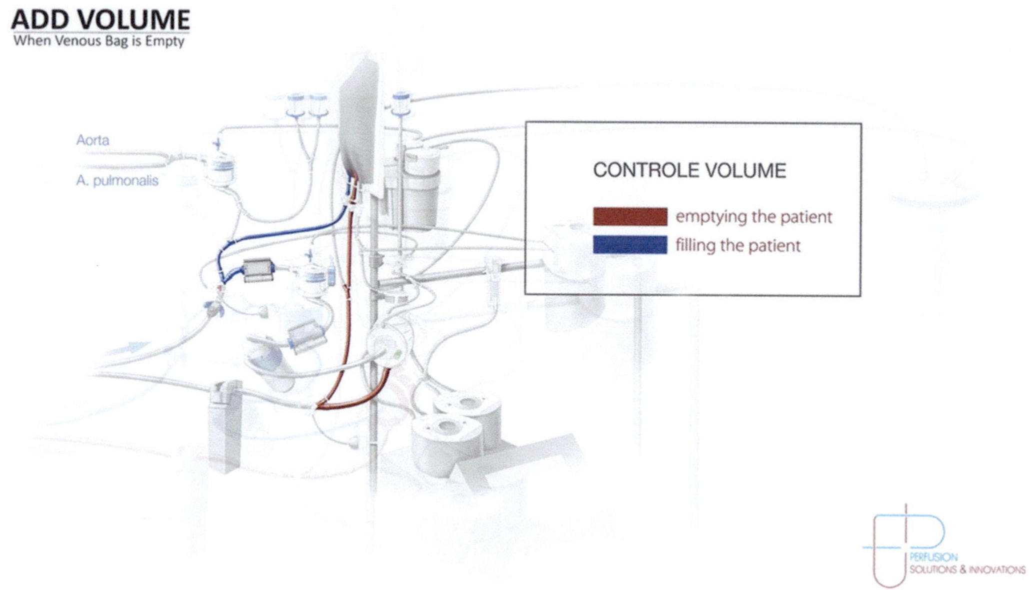

Video 9 Venous bag empty—add volume (▶ https://doi.org/10.1007/000-a8s)

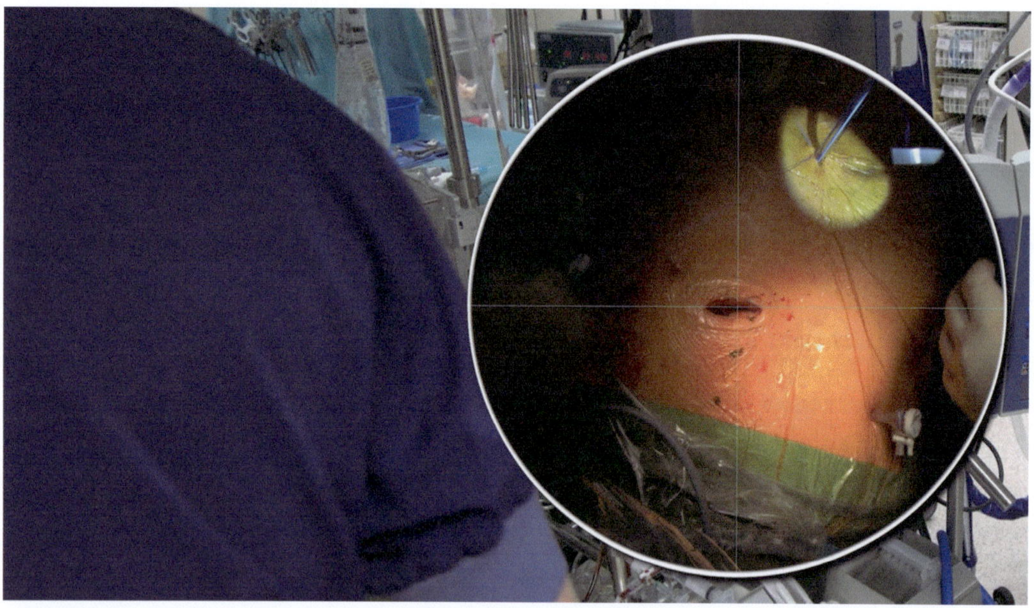

Video 10 Weaning from bypass patient in trendelenburg (▶ https://doi.org/10.1007/000-a8t)

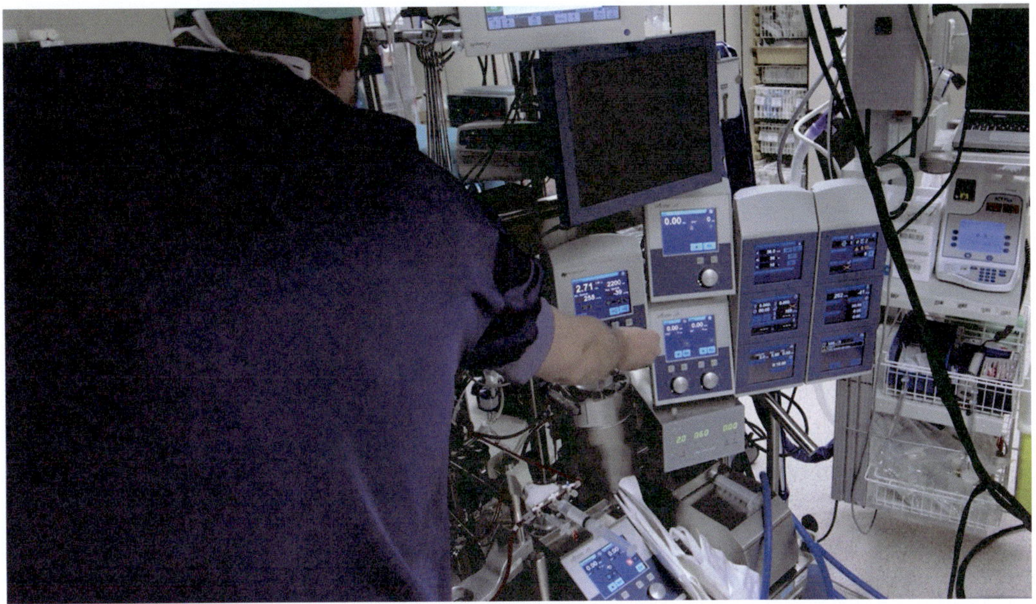

Video 11 Reduce RPM (▶ https://doi.org/10.1007/000-a8v)

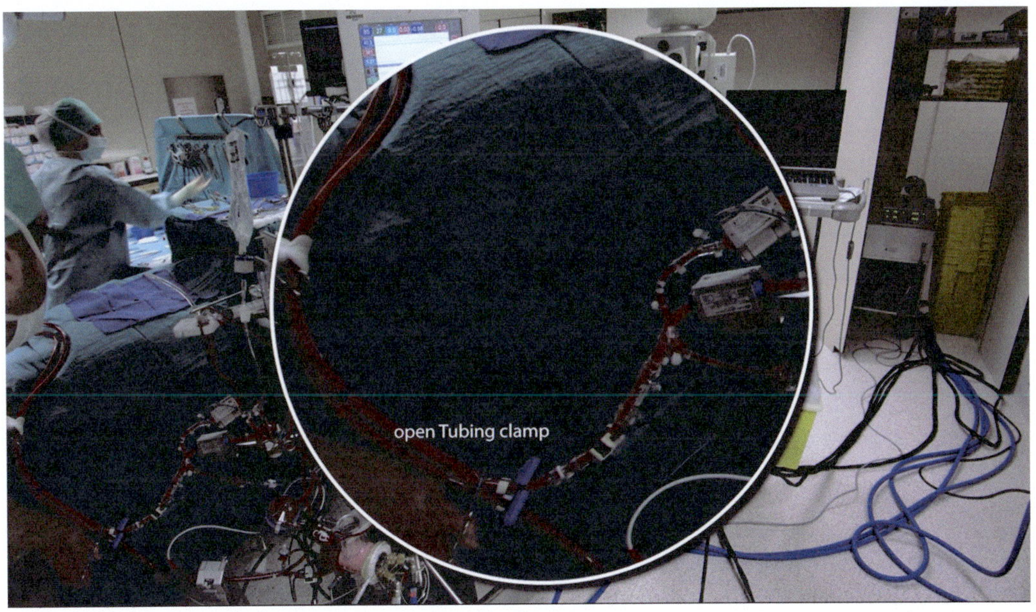

Video 12 Flush venous line (▶ https://doi.org/10.1007/000-a8w)

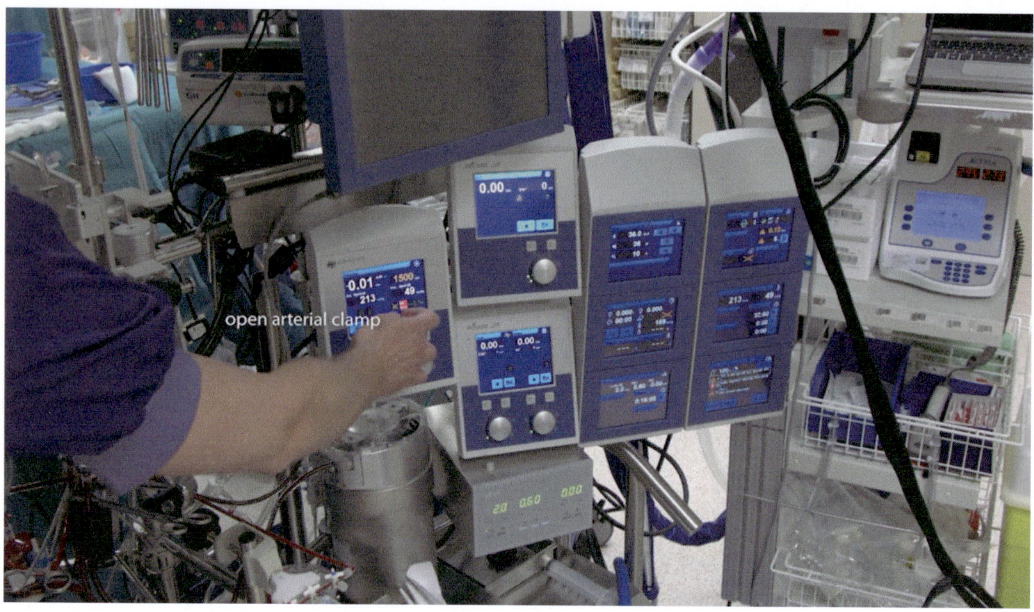

Video 13 Flush antegrade the circuit (▶ https://doi.org/10.1007/000-a8x)

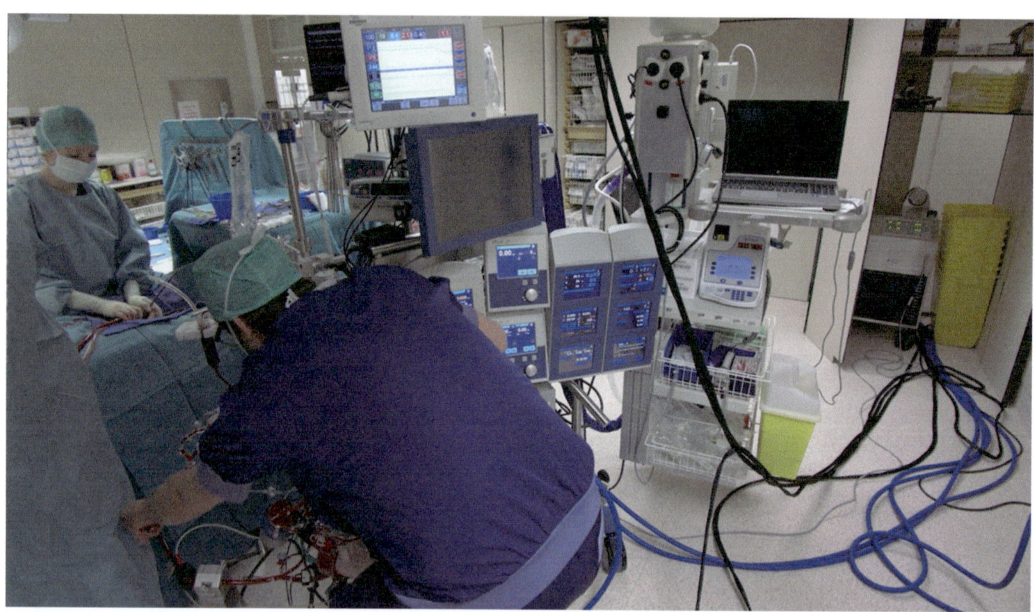

Video 14 Retrieve blood from venous cannula to cellsaver (▶ https://doi.org/10.1007/000-a8y)

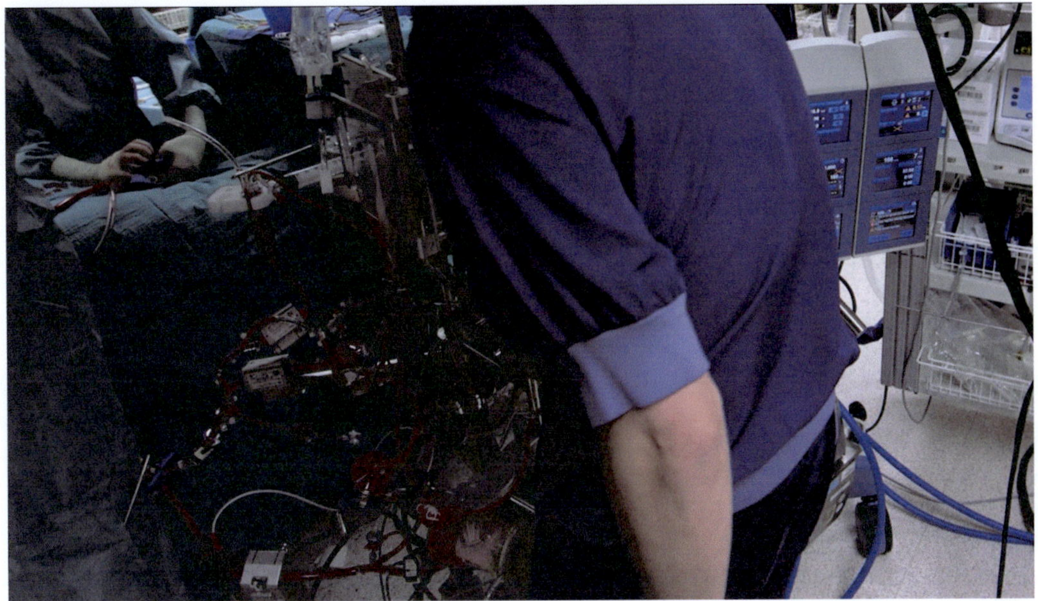

Video 15 Retrieve blood from arterial line to cellsaver (▶ https://doi.org/10.1007/000-a8z)

Proper positioning has become increasingly important with the use of minimally invasive techniques that limit the ability to directly visualize the heart and great vessels.

4 Cannulation

The jugular vein or femoral vessels are acceptable vascular access sites for connection to the heart–lung machine. Vascular access cannulas used for extra thoracic circulatory procedures are typically smaller and longer than standard right atrial cannulas, and some can be inserted percutaneously.

4.1 Venous Cannulation

If the surgical procedure provides access to the right atrium, it may be cannulated directly with a large-bore cannula and drained through gravity siphon. However, many surgeons have found it advantageous, especially in MICS, to utilize the femoral vein to guide an endogenous drainage cannula into the IVC and right atrium. The right

femoral vein is hereby preferred over the left as it provides a straighter path for cannulation passage, which may be done percutaneously or through femoral vein cut down.

The extended length and reduced diameter of extra thoracic venous cannulae increase the resistance of blood return. The issue of inadequate venous return during MICS requires attention of each of the team members. All must recognize the multiple, frequently covert, technical challenges and mishaps-kinked or obstructed catheters, excessive negative pressure on the venous return catheters (Video 5), and/or increased venous capacitance that can lead to inadequate venous return and inadequate oxygen delivery.

Good venous drainage requires more than just a well-designed cannula. The design of the cannula and cannula tip are of great importance and also the correct choice for a certain procedure. Reduced venous drainage can lead to flow reduction. Not only the cannula is responsible for this problem. Improper placement, smaller diameter of the venous cannula, resistance, pressure difference, … all play a role in adequate venous drainage. Poor venous return from the superior vena cava may compromise cerebral blood flow (MAP-CVP = cerebral perfusion pressure) leading to neurologic injuries postoperative.

Although this use of method can create often only partial support for the circulation, total cardiopulmonary support through peripheral cannulas is sometimes difficult to achieve and assisted drainage is needed.

4.2 VAVD-KVAD

In MICS by groin cannulation, gravity-dependent venous drainage mostly initiates partial CPB which indicates the use of assisted venous drainage (AVD). The magnitude of the venous siphon is gradually increased and pressures of -50 to -80 mmHg are usually adequate without causing venous conduit "chatter" or collapse. In contrast to what occurs in conventional CPB, several minutes usually elapse before a steady state of extracorporeal circulation is established. Assisted venous drainage can be proposed for optimal venous drainage by using a vacuum source attached to the reservoir or by the use of an additional centrifugal pump in the venous line.

Using vacuum assisted venous drainage (VAVD), one must try to avoid excessive VAVD negative pressures which limits blood trauma and hemolysis and prevents venous reservoir cracking or implosion. Positive and negative pressure relief valves must be incorporated into the reservoir to prevent both overpressure and underpressure to ensure consistent extracorporeal flow rates. VAVD cannot be applied to closed systems utilizing a (soft-shell) venous reservoir bag.

Using a soft shell venous reservoir, one can use an additional centrifugal pump between the venous cannula and the soft shell reservoir. Kinetic assisted venous drainage (KVAD) uses a kinetic pump to mechanically increase venous drainage. Attention must be made on the fact that this kinetic pump (usually a centrifugal pump) can generate significant negative pressures. MiECC incorporates this assisted venous drainage by using a single centrifugal pump in a closed circuit and is therefore at higher risk for

venous line cavitation and subsequent air entrainment because of the direct connection of a centrifugal pump to the venous cannula. Centrifugal pumps are known to "shred" smaller amounts of air into microbubbles that the downstream components need to handle. Therefore is it important that all air is captured by air handling components (except MiECC Type I) before it can enter the centrifugal pump. Greater diligence must therefore be exercised to prevent air micro-emboli with minimally invasive bypass techniques. Because small bubbles are not very buoyant, they advance readily through the entire perfusion circuit and are expelled through the arterial cannula.

4.3 Arterial Cannulation

Arterial cannulation strategies are dependent upon the surgical procedure, but include aortic cannulation and peripheral vessel cannulation. When surgical exposure allows direct ascending aorta cannulation, it is usually the preferred approach.

The aortic cannula is one of the most critical components of extracorporeal circulation. A high flow rate through the narrow lumen of the tip may lead to a high pressure drop, high local velocities, turbulence and cavitation, and hereby cause hemolysis as well as thrombo-embolic complications by damaging the interior aortic wall. The choice of area of placement is therefore of great importance as well as the size and the direction of the jet flow. The exit flow preferable points not towards the aorta wall where it can potentially generate embolization and consequently postoperative neurologic dysfunction can occur.

When direct ascending aortic cannulation is not possible, peripheral cannulation may be achieved at brachial, axillary, and femoral arterial sites. Femoral cannulation has served as the standard due to ease and cosmetic scarring considerations. Risks of femoral cannulation include embolization due to retrograde aortic flow, femoral or aortic dissections due to vessel manipulation, and femoral vessel injury with hematoma. Retrograde perfusion is therefore not the best option in calcified peripheral vessels and central cannulation is preferred to avoid stroke or cognitive dysfunction.

Besides visualization of proper cannula positioning, TEE is also an excellent means of detecting and locating retained intracardiac air in patients on CPB and contributes to the removal of air before discontinuing CPB and for the detection of interatrial communication. For example, a Patent Foramen ovale (PFO) is of great importance for the perfusionist to choose the proper circuit for a certain operation. If the left heart is opened or an aortatomy is performed in the presence of an existing PFO with single venous cannulation, air can enter the right side and cause problems with venous drainage and air- lock formation in the venous cannula. A MiECC type IV or "hybrid system" to easily convert from MiECC to an incorporated "conventional" system is recommended when a PFO is detected prior to the conduct of bypass providing a safe environment for the team to start the procedure.

4.4 Safety Concerns

Due to the complexity and extreme invasiveness of CPB, strict attention needs to be paid to all aspects of extracorporeal flow, with importance placed on providing a safe environment for both the patient and personnel. Technological advancements, together with an increased understanding of the pathophysiological effects of extracorporeal flow, have made the conduct of CPB both safe and reliable. An essential part of this success has been the development of monitoring devices that measure both physiological and mechanical functions.

One of these functions is the removal of venous air that was suggested in the early nineties for mini-circuits and implemented first in pediatric practice. This system incorporates a separate bubble trap in the venous line before the centrifugal pump with a bubble detector

upstream. With the vent line of the bubble trap connected through a roller pump to a cardiotomy reservoir, cell-salvage device or venous storage bag, the pump can be operated intermittently based on the bubble alarm to "actively" remove entrained air from the circuit (Fig. 3 and Video 6). In case of cannula dislodgement, creating a venous inlet full of air the air handling system will be likely overwhelmed requiring a second safety mechanism to step in. The low level alarm will automatically trigger the arterial clamp (Fig. 4), giving the opportunity to properly de-air the venous line retrogradely.

Air can enter the circuit via different ways: Improper tightening of the venous cannula, direct air injection with medication bolus administration, cavitation or air coming from vent lines.

4.5 Venting

The left ventricle or aorta is vented to remove any air that may accumulate. Besides air, blood may return to the left ventricle through bronchial vessels and through the lungs pulmonary veins even if the venous cannula is removing all blood entering the right atrium. Venting removes blood that may distend the ventricle. Unless the left ventricle is completely decompressed, the heart continues to eject blood which can create an imbalance in oxygenation between upper and lower body part when perfusion is done through groin cannulation.

A vent cannula can therefore be placed directly in the left ventricle or the aorta can be vented through a Y-line off the antegrade cardioplegia cannula when cardioplegia is given antegrade. The venting can also be done through the right superior pulmonary vein, across the mitral valve into the ventricle. Large volumes of continuous air can hereby enter the circuit requiring a system with proper defoamers and de-airing capabilities. These de-airing capabilities, as well as the possibility to convert to a conventional circuit are incorporated in a MiECC type IV or "Hybrid system". One-way suction

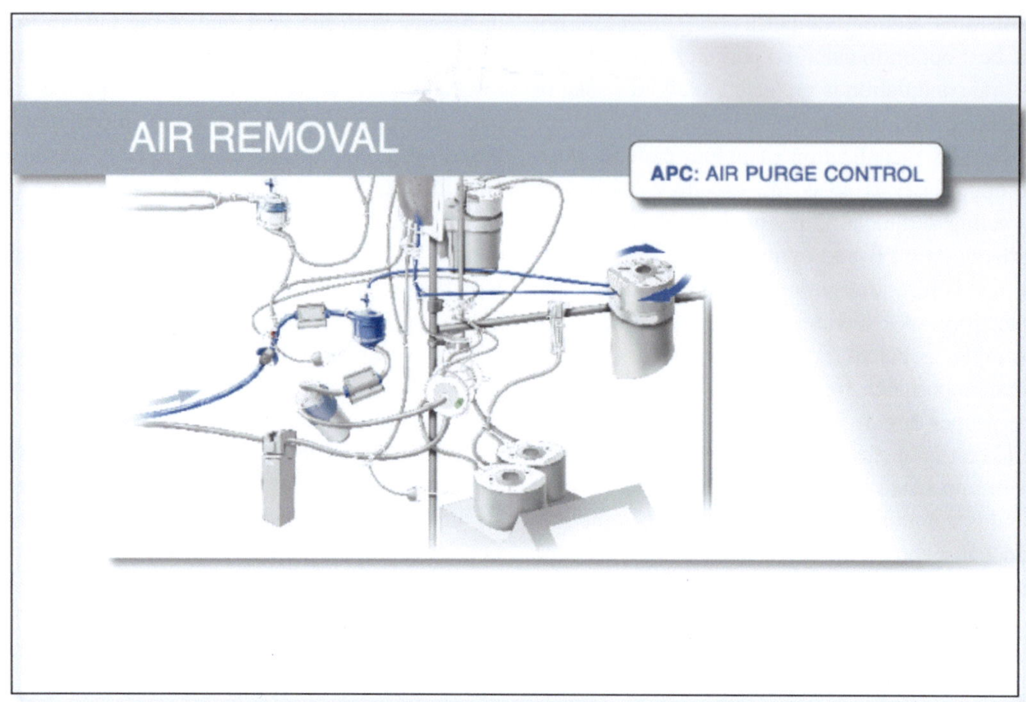

Fig. 3 Air removal device to "actively" evacuate entrained air

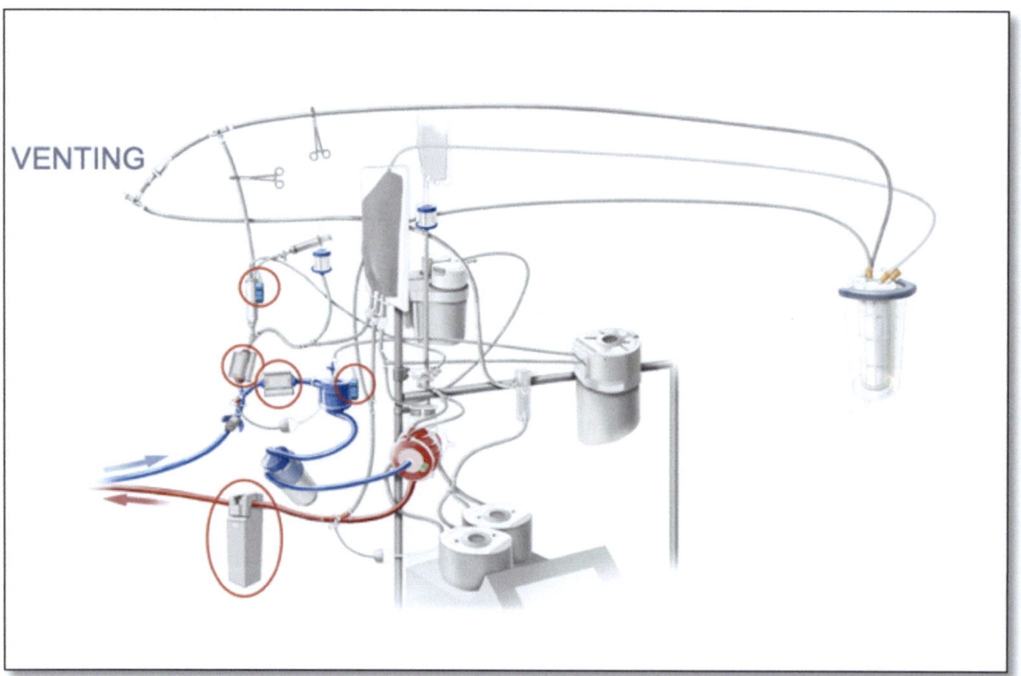

Fig. 4 Safety features in a MiECC circuit

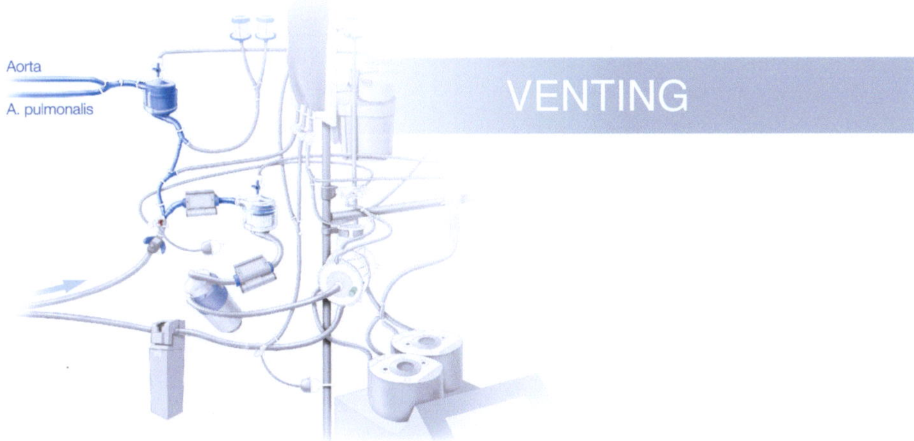

Fig. 5 Venting possibilities using a MiECC circuit

valves prevent excessive suction and accidental introduction of air into the heart. These should be used on all vents running through a roller pump. In some cases it is possible to place a vent in the pulmonary artery (PA) to remove blood going to the lungs and back to the left atrium. Vent return can be initiated for aortic root and pulmonary artery by the use of negative pressure in the venous line. A closed optimized perfusion circuit or MiECC Type II or III can be used when a PA vent is placed (Fig. 5). This closed circuit, MiECC type II or III, is secured by a bubble sensor attached in the vent line before entering the venous line and which is linked to the arterial clamp. When a bubble is detected, the sensor will automatically trigger the arterial clamp, which will close and gives the opportunity to put a tubing clamp below the vent bubble trap. Continuation of the circulation and the possibility to de-air the vent bubble trap through a roller pump towards the cell-salvage device (Fig. 6), is a major advantage.

4.6 Cardioplegia

One of the major concerns of cardiac surgery is protection of the heart during the operation. Whether intracellular solutions with a low sodium degree but a high degree of potassium are used or extracellular solutions with concentrations of sodium higher or equal to 70 mmol/L together with concentrations of potassium from 5 to 3 mmol/L, a well-protected heart that recovers from the arrest period serves as the objective. The repair of the heart is of no use if the heart has not been adequately protected. The surgeon desires a bloodless, motionless heart on which to perform his delicate anastomosis.

The search for this optimal cardioplegic solution, with a quick arrest, prolonged electromechanical silence, minimal damage of ischemia and controlled reperfusion, has resulted in many variations of the solutions. It seems that every institution has a particular prescription that is followed. This solution of preference by each

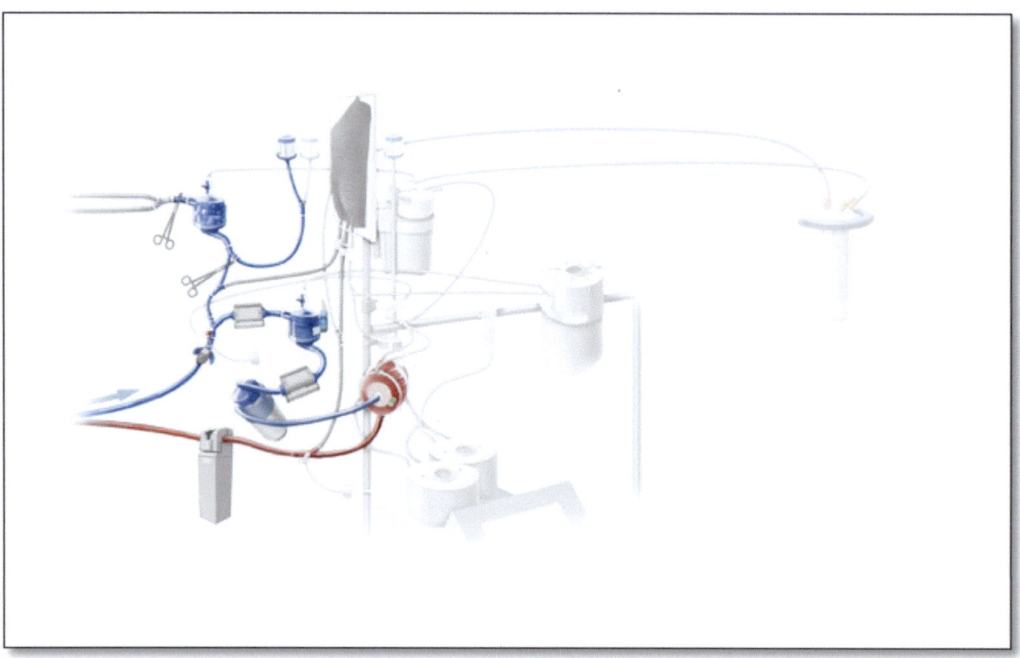

Fig. 6 Properly de-airing the vent bubble trap with continuation of bypass

center is usually accomplished by a single line (cristalloïd) or an arrangement of dual lines (cristalloïd solution mixed with blood) that run through a roller pump together or through two separate roller pumps.

Using MiECC nowadays, variations of the Calafiore method, whereby warm blood is taken from the oxygenator and intermittently injected into the aortic root, with concentrated potassium added by means of a syringe pump, have tremendous popularity.

In MICS procedures, the technique of cardioplegia delivery should ideally be based on a system with minimal surface area and low dilutional volume. A mixture of blood, nourishing the heart muscle, and cristalloïd solution which is administrated with elegant simplicity, minimal added volume and giving a plausible period of time is an ideal method for a MICS approach. (Table 2).

5 MiECC-Experience

The JESSA system Type III was used in a series of 3000 consecutive patients, of whom 540 patients received procedures other than multivessel coronary bypass surgery by endoscopic set up (AVR, SCAR and Bentall operations through mini-sternotomy and previous mentioned procedures in combination with endoscopic coronary bypass surgery).

All patients could be operated on using the minimized closed circuit. Only one patient required flooding of the surgical field due to air entrainment in the venous line by a PFO (patent foramen ovale) created during cannulation. In this minimal invasive surgical approach, it is difficult to close this small iatrogenic PFO. No conversion to open CPB by adding a separate venous reservoir was necessary.

The JESSA modular hybrid system (Type IV) was used in a series of 450 consecutive patients receiving totally endoscopic aortic valve replacement with the use of a pulmonary vein vent or totally endoscopic mitral valve repair whether or not with neo-chordal repair. Five patients with a PFO required a conversion to an open hybrid system (drainage of venous blood will go directly to the venous reservoir instead of going through the venous bubble trap) during closure of the existing PFO. After closing this interatrial communication, the switch was again made to a closed hybrid system (venous blood going through the venous bubble trap instead of going through the reservoir). All five patients received mitral valve surgery.

We observed, with continuation of dual anti-platelet therapy, a need for intra-operative transfusion of 0.45 ± 1.05 units, intraoperative blood loss was 281.45 ± 112.13 mL and 24 h bloodloss was 382.44 ± 169.15 mL. Overall mortality was 1.78%. Based on the feasibility and safety aspects of our system, MiECC provides good clinical results without compromising operative morbidity or mortality.

6 Conclusion

Advances in perfusion technology have been widely implemented in the design of modern cardiopulmonary bypass circuits and systems. Circuits nowadays are getting smaller and systems more advanced [1–3]. When performing MiECC, one is also forced using a certain strategy (separate suction of shed blood, retrograde autologous priming). The circuit itself will not contribute alone to the patients improved outcome but the MiECC strategy will facilitate the surgeon in his minimal invasive approach as well as creating the possibility for the anaesthesiologist to perform ultra-fast track anaesthetic technique. Using the MiECC strategy together with this advanced perfusion technology provides a safe environment for the team to work in (Videos 16 and 17).

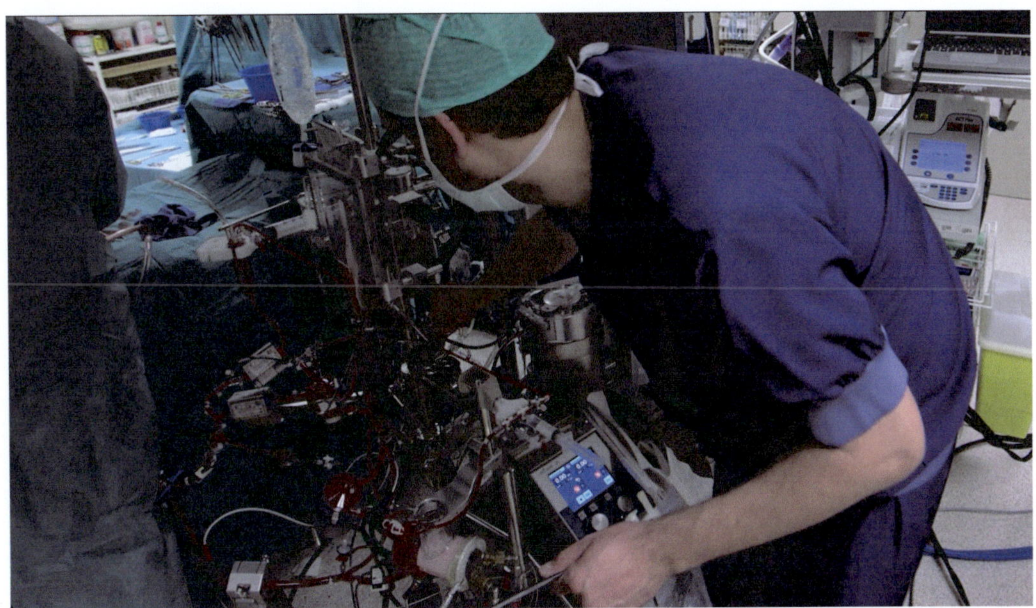

Video 16 Flush circuit to cellsaver to retrieve all red bloodcells (1) (▶ https://doi.org/10.1007/000-a8h)

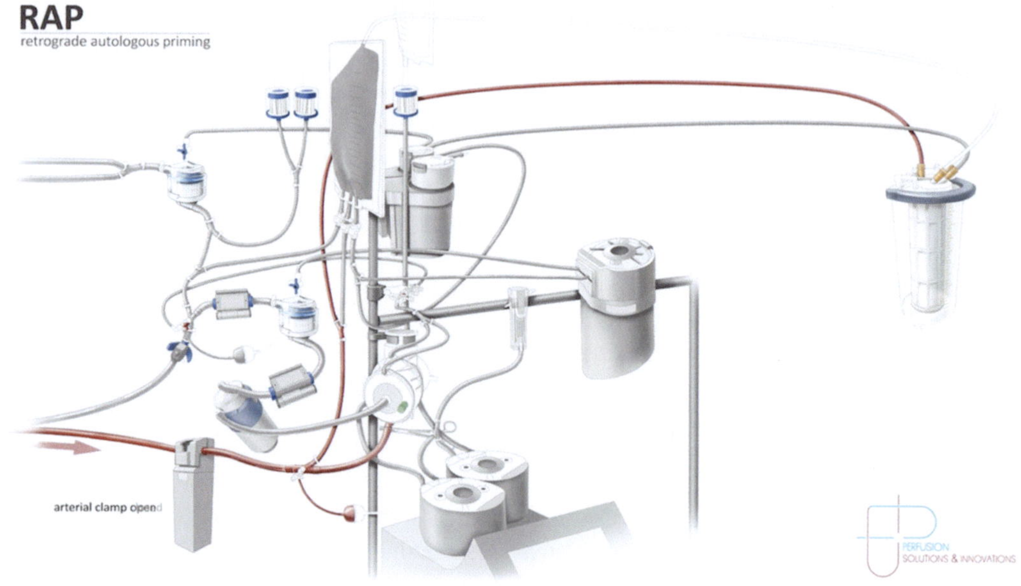

Video 17 Compilation of all chapters (▶ https://doi.org/10.1007/000-a91)

Appendixes

See Figs. 1, 2, 3, 4, 5, 6, Tables 1 and 2.

Table 1 List of videos perfusion

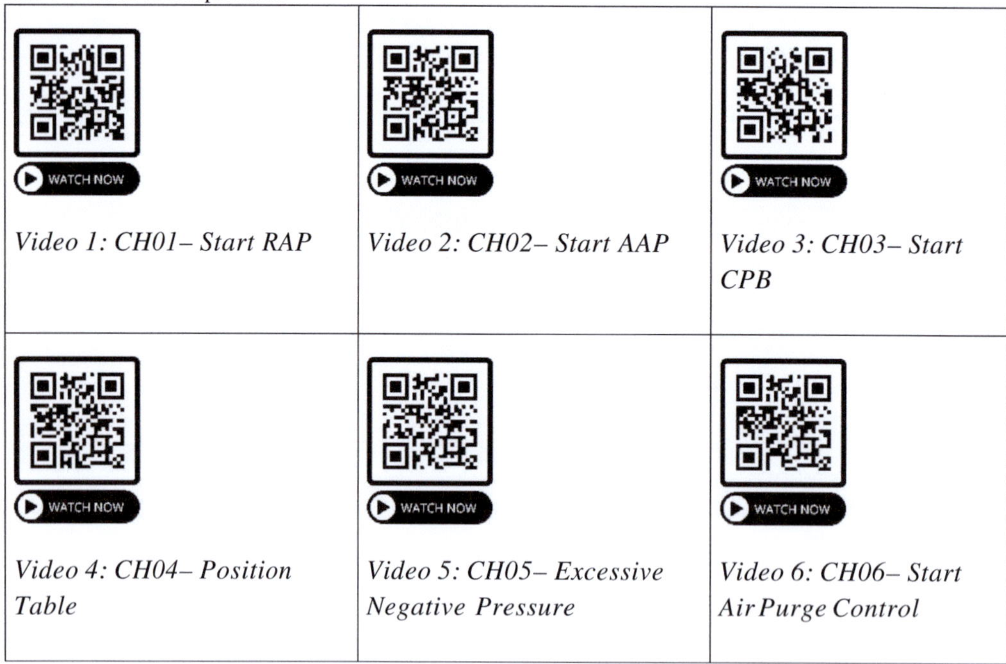

Video 1: CH01– Start RAP	*Video 2: CH02– Start AAP*	*Video 3: CH03– Start CPB*
Video 4: CH04– Position Table	*Video 5: CH05– Excessive Negative Pressure*	*Video 6: CH06– Start Air Purge Control*

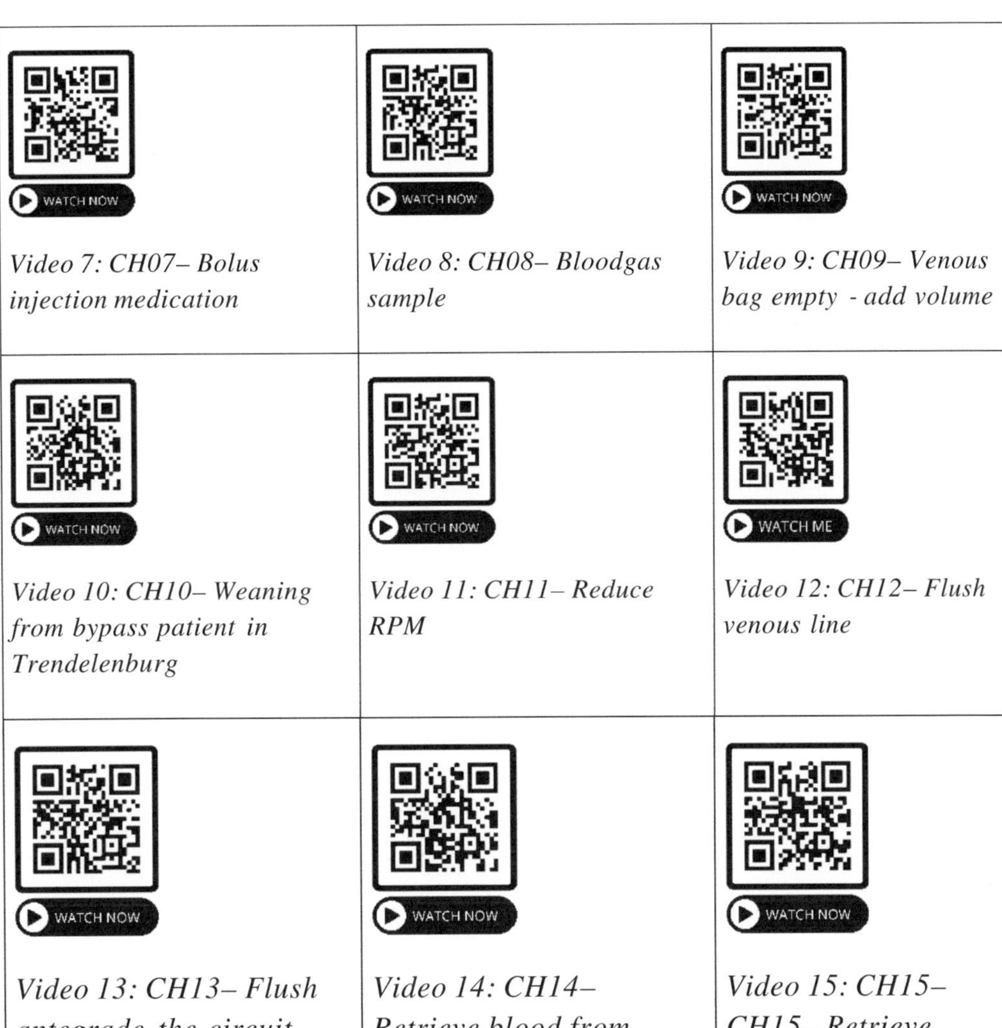

Video 7: CH07– Bolus injection medication	*Video 8: CH08– Bloodgas sample*	*Video 9: CH09– Venous bag empty - add volume*
Video 10: CH10– Weaning from bypass patient in Trendelenburg	*Video 11: CH11– Reduce RPM*	*Video 12: CH12– Flush venous line*
Video 13: CH13– Flush antegrade the circuit	*Video 14: CH14– Retrieve blood from venous cannula to cellsaver*	*Video 15: CH15– CH15– Retrieve blood from arterial line to cellsaver*

 *Video 16: CH16– Flush circuit to cellsaver to retrieve all red bloodcells (1)*	 *Video 17: Compilation of all chapters*	

Table 2 Mixed blood cardioplegia used during MICS procedures

Blood:Crystalloid cardioplegia (3:1)
Sodium 40 mmol/L
Magnesium 76 mmol/L
Chloride 262 mmol/L
Potassium 62 mmol/L
Calcium 1 mmol/L
Procaine 5 mmol/L
Aqua ad 500 mL

References

1. Pramod Reddy Kandakure, FRCS, Mark Batra, DNB, Sandeep Garre, DM, Sai Nagendra Banovath, MD, Farooq Shaikh, MBBS, and Krishna Pani, BSc. Direct cannulation in minimally invasive cardiac surgery with limited resources. Ann Thorac Surg. 2020;109:512–6.

2. De Somer F. Venous drainage—gravity or assisted? Perfusion. 2011;26(S1):15–9.

3. Anastasiadis K, Antonitsis P, Argiriadou H, Deliopoulos A, Grosomanidis V, Tossios P. Modular minimally invasive extracorporeal circulation systems; can they become the standard practice for performing cardiac surgery? Perfusion. 2015;30(3):195–200.

Innovation in Cardiac Surgery: It Takes a Village—Our Team's Story: A Quest for Routine Sternal-Sparing CABG

Jude S. Sauer

Abstract

Innovation is required to further enhance cardiac surgery's benefits for patients by reducing the undesirable factors associated with currently highly invasive procedures. Patients deserve and will demand that routine operations are deliberately designed to minimise postoperative pain, recovery time, complications, and life-altering medications. While tiny bone-sparing minimally invasive or, preferably, microinvasive access sites through soft tissue between the ribs or in the subxiphoid space can offer much less traumatic access to the heart, such small incisions block direct visualisation and obviate traditional tissue manipulation. Innovation toward reliable and affordable customised miniature surgical technology along with facilitative real-time video-assisted endoscopic and augmented imaging can supplant large, injurious surgical access sites to deliver a more gentle, patient-centered paradigm. To provide an example of a cardiac surgery innovation effort, this chapter presents an ongoing coronary revascularisation enhancement project. This R&D effort was undertaken to provide new options toward reliable and ergonomic sternal-sparing microinvasive coronary artery bypass with efficient bilateral internal thoracic artery harvest via subxiphoid access and excellent anastomoses using microthoracotomies. Recent initial clinical results are encouraging. While many dedicated people consider it their privilege to support the innovation of the enabling technology and techniques that will be essential to build this next era, the attitudes and efforts of indomitable heart surgeons regarding this requisite innovation will be the driving force to provide a brighter future for their patients. The fate of heart surgery is in the hands of today's heart surgeons.

Supplementary Information The online version contains supplementary material available at https://doi.org/10.1007/978-3-031-21104-1_22. The videos can be accessed individually by clicking the DOI link in the accompanying figure caption or by scanning this link with the SN More Media App.

J. S. Sauer (✉)
Division of Cardiac Surgery, Department of Surgery, University of Rochester, Rochester, NY, USA
e-mail: jsauer@lsisolutions.com

LSI SOLUTIONS®, Victor, NY, USA

LSI EUROPE™, Düsseldorf, Germany

Keywords

Innovation in cardiac surgery · Minimally invasive surgery · Internal thoracic artery harvest · Subxiphoid ITA harvest · Bilateral ITA · Coronary revascularisation · All-arterial coronary revascularisation

1 Introduction

Good Designs are everywhere;
Great Designs are very rare

Innovation is required to further enhance cardiac surgery's benefits for patients by reducing the undesirable factors associated with currently highly invasive procedures. To remain an acceptable option for today's sophisticated patients, heart surgery must undergo a positive disruption to continue to deliver the best long-term functional results (e.g., optimised prosthetic valves, durable revascularisation, etc.) while also becoming more gentle to the patient (e.g., reduced pain along with a lower risk of protracted recoveries, stroke, death, etc.). Heart surgery must also provide increased value to society.

Patients deserve and will demand that routine operations are deliberately designed to minimise postoperative pain, recovery time, complications, and life-altering medications. The acceptability of procedure access wounds will be judged not compared to the size of a sternotomy, but relative to the invasiveness of endovascular access. Most sternotomies and large thoracotomies must go the way of using a patient's parent for cross-circulation. The next era of heart surgery must transcend the antiquated focus on 30 day mortality rates. Surgical procedures should be expected to be truly minimally invasive, with mortality rates under 1%.

The current dependency on providing the "standard of care" in heart surgery, if interpreted too rigidly, is anti-innovation; this concept, which is mostly of legal, not medical, construct, has a commonly accepted definition: what a reasonable surgeon would do under the same or similar circumstances. Less than 75 years ago, a reasonable surgeon would simply let a patient with heart disease die unmutilated by futile surgery. Standards must evolve. As is now witnessed in more than 25 years of success across all other surgical specialties, much less invasiveness in cardiac surgery will become the only acceptable option.

While tiny bone-sparing microinvasive access sites between the ribs or through the subxiphoid space can offer significantly less traumatic access to the heart, such small incisions block direct visualisation and render traditional tissue manipulation obsolete. Innovation toward reliable and affordable customised miniature surgical technology along with facilitative real-time video endoscopic and augmented imaging can supplant large injurious surgical access sites to deliver a more gentle, patient-centered paradigm. Productive partnerships between surgeons, surgical societies, academia, industry, and inventors are critical to support progress. Additionally, expediting the availability of safe and effective clinical translation systems and convenient training platforms will be crucial.

To provide an example of a cardiac surgery innovation effort, this chapter presents highlights from an ongoing coronary revascularisation enhancement project targeting surgical access only through soft tissue. Since 2016, this team has pursued delivery of a microinvasive coronary artery bypass (μCAB) procedure to realise reliable subxiphoid bilateral internal thoracic artery (ITA) harvest and microthoracotomy (μT) anastomoses. Images from early laboratories in this effort—including a prototype sternal retractor setup, a subxiphoid approach to harvest, and an endoscopic image—are shown in Fig. 1, from this team's January 2021 publication "A Novel Subxiphoid Approach for Bilateral Internal Thoracic Artery Harvesting."

With today's cardiopulmonary bypass outcomes demonstrating much lower risk, and the not infrequent occurrence of off-pump CABG, the two main goals of the μCAB subxiphoid and μT revascularisation approach are:

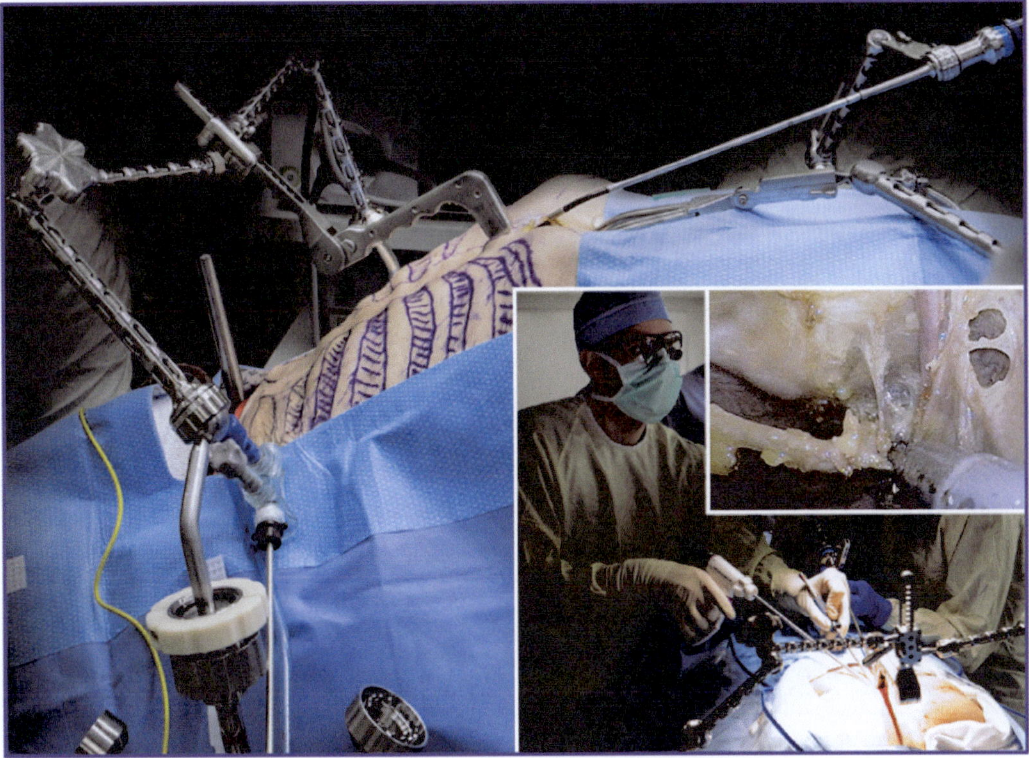

Fig. 1 Images of Dr. Hossein Amirjamshidi conducting a cadaver lab, showing novel sternal retraction system and subxiphoid access to ITA harvest

- Maintain the integrity of the chest wall.
- Retain excellent patency rates for ITA coronary revascularisation grafts.

Nothing that is hard is easy.

2 Rallying to Innovation: Gentle Heart Surgery

Truth passes through three stages:
First, it is ridiculed.
Second, it is violently opposed.
Third, it is accepted as being self-evident.
Arthur Schopenhauer (1788–1860)

Innovation =

The Implementation of Something New

Creativity requires nothing more than thinking about novel concepts. Invention merely requires a new design for a device or process without actual implementation. Meaningful innovation in modern cardiac surgery must *transform* procedures to achieve both improved patient outcomes and enhanced value.

Great Surgery =

Great Outcomes + Great Recovery

To continue its long history of providing optimised benefits to patients, heart surgery must be decoupled from painful, disabling, and protracted postoperative recoveries that have a significant risk of complications and death. Great heart surgery is effective and gentle.

Value = Benefits/Cost

The value of cardiac surgery is measured by the benefits provided over the true total costs to the patient, the patient's family, and society. Today's heart surgeons will be the key determining factor of heart surgery's value across the world during the next few decades. If heart surgeons continue to strive for reduced patient morbidity and mortality caused by potentially avoidable iatrogenic trauma from surgery coupled with affordable care and rapid recovery, heart surgery will retain its enormous value—and stature.

Established Accepted Tradition Versus The Uncertainty of Things New

Humans have a long, rich history of resisting change. Galileo Galilei (1564–1642) died under house arrest for heresy. Anyone can see that the earth is not moving! Ignaz Semmelweis (1818–1865) was driven out of Vienna to an early death for challenging established standards. Why should surgeons wash their hands? Even Joseph Lister (1827–1912) faced fierce resistance for advocating the use of antiseptic agents to sterilise surgical instruments and clean wounds. Maybe that new germ theory of Louis Pasteur (1822–1895) has some validity? If heart surgeons do not accept, and in fact embrace and lead, further progress in heart surgery, who should?

Patient-Centric = Primum non Nocere

The most important way to view heart surgery is from the patient's perspective. After all, it is not the surgeon's operation—it is the patient's. And the patient is "the one who suffers" (from the Latin root *patiens* and similar to the Greek *pēma*, "suffering"). This new, innovative era of heart surgery must be more gentle on the patient, while not compromising therapeutic outcomes, to increase the overall value of the service. Enabling technology and facilitating imaging can enhance the techniques that heart surgeons can offer their patients targeting the optimal therapeutic outcome for the longest duration.

First, Do No Harm. Primum non Nocere: Latin translation of a phrase frequently attributed to the teaching of Hippocrates (c. 460–c. 375 BCE). Gentle surgery also should minimise bleeding, require fewer blood transfusions, and reduce or eliminate complications, such as perivalvular leak or heart block necessitating permanent pacemaker implantation. Gentle surgery can relieve patients of significant postoperative pain,

avoid injury to bones, and leave only tiny scars. Advanced gentle heart surgery can facilitate rapid recovery and a quick return to normalcy without the need for life-altering medications. If surgical operations emerge to also offer less pain and early resumption of the activities of regular living, the well-earned premier status of heart surgeons embracing more gentle techniques will not be eroded by competitive approaches purportedly less invasive but with inferior functionality or unproven durability (e.g., transcatheter replacement valves).

Modernised Efficiency =

Enabling Miniaturised Technology + Facilitative Imaging

There are more than two million routine cardiac surgery operations in the world every year. If surgeons are willing and able to implement innovative minimally invasive cardiac operations that deliberately focus on shorter operative times, thus reducing durations of cardiopulmonary bypass and mechanical ventilator support along with diminished periods requiring intensive care or inpatient hospitalisation, substantial reductions in the many costs currently associated with heart surgery can become a near term reality. Routine operations: smooth is fast, smooth is efficient.

An old persistent criticism of less invasive heart surgery is that operations simply take too long and may compromise patient safety. Surgery should be quick, but not hurried. Patient-centric heart surgery cannot be designed to be slow. For many patients undergoing heart surgery, especially those on cardiopulmonary bypass, protracted surgical procedures are associated with increased morbidity and mortality. Many surgeons are taught that there is no such thing as good, slow surgery. Most surgeons want to complete tasks expeditiously without unnecessary risks and with excellent long term outcomes. More gentle heart surgery must be designed to be faster, safer, and better.

Even if only the most common heart operations in the near term avail themselves to deliberate standardisation, substantial efficiency is achievable. For example, improving the efficiency of only a few of the more common cardiac operations, such as isolated aortic valve replacement, mitral valve P2 repair, and coronary bypass surgery utilising ITA harvesting, could promptly lead to a significant increase in the value of cardiac surgery across the world. As heart surgery becomes less invasive and less expensive, more gentle and more efficient, it should become more readily available to help more patients previously not considered operative candidates or simply unable to afford such life-enhancing care.

μHS = Microinvasive Heart Surgery

The calling of a surgeon is not to put a patient on bypass or suture an anastomosis, but rather to fix complex problems for real people. If developed to its fullest potential, truly microinvasive heart surgery through soft-tissue subxiphoid and μT access can become the standard of care for many patients in need. Research efforts are currently underway to expand μHS offerings in five areas of critical need:

- Revascularisation of coronary arteries
- Replacement of heart valves when indicated
- Repair of heart valves when possible
- Revitalisation (surgical support of heart failure)
- Reharmonisation (stroke reduction and dysrhythmia risk reduction)

Gentle approaches to the heart through small access sites require customised technology, real-time imaging, and a fresh perspective on cardiac surgery. A μT made between ribs can offer surprisingly adequate access to mediastinal structures while sparing the patient's bones (especially the sternum) and reducing bleeding. Advanced real-time intraoperative imaging is critical to establishing user-friendly, reliable, predictable techniques for using tiny incisions.

Most of the surgical devices commonly used in open surgical operations today have not undergone significant innovative changes compared to the surgical forceps, shears, clamps, cannulas, etc., found in the ashes of Mt. Vesuvius (Pompeii, 79 CE). Beyond the heart surgery–specific modern miracles of reliable cardiopulmonary bypass, anticoagulation, cardiac valve prostheses, etc., the two most important advances in surgery over the past century are the use of stainless steel in surgical instruments and the use of endoscopy. The development and deployment of customised surgical technology must deliver novel ergonomic miniature devices that are both robust and precise to ensure dependable accomplishment of the remote tasks encountered in minimally invasive more gentle heart surgery. These new technologies and techniques should also be easy to learn and to teach. They must be affordable and conveniently available to reveal their real value.

Progress = {Technology + Technique}/ {Teaching + Translation}

Reliance upon modest incremental or iterative improvements will not sustain the future of cardiac surgery. Radical technologic and mindset breakthroughs are essential to enable the positive disruption of the not infrequent devastating sequelae associated with the invasiveness of traditional heart surgery. Surgeons should be eager to obsolete their current practices with better procedures; that is certainly a better alternative than to have others do that for you. Too many heart surgeons seem to welcome innovation, as long as it does not involve anything new.

Reinvigorated Teaching Platforms: This digital age accelerates opportunities to improve how knowledge transfer and training occur. To quickly disseminate related information, reliance solely upon more traditional conference presentations and journal publications will not suffice. Online communications will play an ever increasing part of the future of heart surgery training. Live teleconferences and interactive training sessions can become excellent learning platforms.

Cadaver laboratories and in vivo surgical experience will also remain opportunities to become fully prepared prior to initial clinical cases. Academic teaching centres with mentors, industry-sponsored training, and research fellowship programs will likely grow in their contributions. In addition, mobile, customised vehicles equipped with state-of-the-art surgical simulation centers can provide convenient onsite surgical training.

Compelling Clinical Translation: To expedite the next generation of progress in heart surgery, in addition to the quest for advanced technology and technique innovation, there is a clear need for better methods for enhanced clinical translation methodologies to thoroughly, but promptly, evaluate the evolving elements requisite for more gentle heart surgery. Refining or creating reputable programs for the effective translation of new technologies and techniques into surgical enhancement will be a critical consideration for those involved in research and development in this exciting, but potentially perilous, area.

The assurance of low risk for patients in studies along with a high probability of a beneficial clinical outcome are necessary first steps toward the ultimate success for the patient, the advancement under evaluation, and the translation centre itself. The roles of universities, medical centres, government agencies, surgical societies, and industry in clinical translation efforts require development. The availability of trustworthy and cost-effective translational organisations enthusiastic to advance options for heart patients will be pivotal to advancing this worthy cause.

3 Surgical Innovation Team Building—From R&D to Patient

Based in Rochester, New York, LSI SOLUTIONS® was founded by the author during his general surgery internship at the University of Rochester Medical Center (URMC) in 1986. The author still leads the company today and also has a non-clinical appointment in the Division of Cardiac Surgery at URMC. Through NIH Grant Funding, the company initially focused on advancing wound healing; subsequently, research efforts evolved toward minimally invasive surgery, and now microinvasive surgery.

With nearly 400 employees in the United States and Europe, the company strives to be a highly collaborative multifaceted team comprising dedicated people focused on areas ranging from surgical science, R&D, and engineering; to machine shop fabrication, molding, and clean room manufacturing; to regulatory and quality systems, intellectual property protection, and sales consultants working directly with customers.

In 2010, the company expanded from technologies and techniques mostly for pediatric, general, bariatric, gynecologic, and urologic surgery to include R&D and product offerings for heart surgery, where less invasive procedures had yet to gain widespread adoption. The goal was to enable advanced heart surgery through microinvasive approaches and foster widespread adoption of the potential clinical benefits to patients throughout the world. This company's first technology used in open and minimally invasive heart surgery is the COR-KNOT® titanium fastener placed to secure 0, 2-0, and 3-0 suture in lieu of a hand-tied knot, providing enhanced security and reduced operative time. This product line has been well accepted across the world for use in cardiac surgery. More than 11 million fasteners have been placed in nearly 1 million patients in 74 countries, and so far more than 280 peer-reviewed presentations and publications have supported its utility. Figure 2 is a close-up image of a COR-KNOT® titanium fastener next to a smaller fastener, developed as part of the company's μCAB project, to secure the much smaller 6-0, 7-0, and 8-0 suture sizes.

While most of the company's achievements so far are associated with structural heart surgery and cardiac valve replacement and repair (see Additional Resources section), this chapter will highlight efforts over the past five years toward advancing much less invasive surgical coronary revascularisation. These efforts are now coming to clinical fruition. We will also reference our recent related submissions accepted by peer review. Our abstract titled "New Surgical Platform: Subxiphoid Bilateral Internal Thoracic Artery Harvesting for All Arterial Coronary Revascularization" was accepted for podium

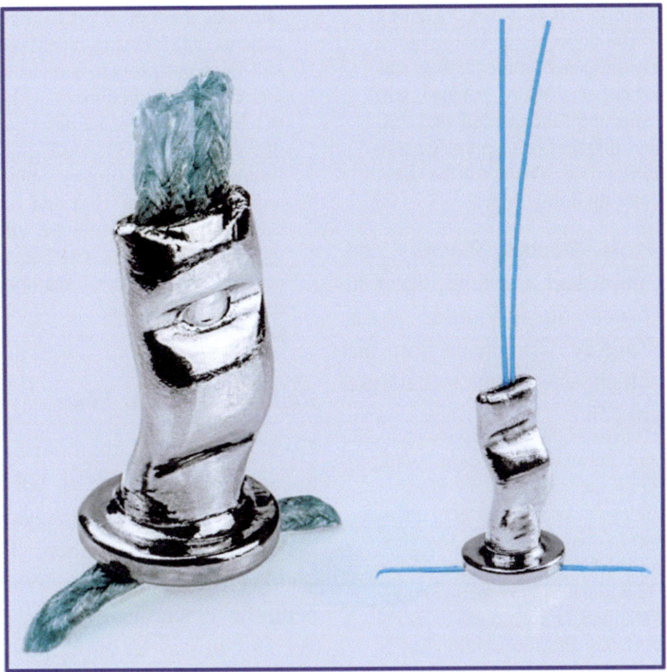

Fig. 2 Close-up of a COR-KNOT® titanium fastener compared to a new, smaller fastener

presentation at the 2020 ISMICS Annual Scientific Meeting. This abstract outlined compelling evidence in support of the innovation the company hoped to spearhead, providing some of the earliest research on our potentially paradigm-shifting technique of less invasive subxiphoid access for remote IMA harvest and all-arterial revascularisation; however, the conference was cancelled due to the pandemic.

This project was further bolstered in early 2021 when *Innovations* published the research manuscript titled "A Novel Subxiphoid Approach for Bilateral Internal Thoracic Artery Harvesting." This more comprehensive look at this new, customised technology for ITA harvesting supplemented the earlier abstract by nearly doubling the experimental size: A total of 50 ITAs were harvested, 36 from 19 pig carcasses and 14 from 7 cadavers. The research conducted in support of this article continued to confirm the innovative benefits that this new technology could offer patients. Subsequently, another 60+ ITAs have been successfully harvested in our pig carcass model.

4 Cardiac Surgery Innovation: Project μCAB

This chapter is meant to be a rallying cry for heart surgeons. The following story of our journey toward meaningful advancement in microinvasive surgical coronary revascularisation is presented to illustrate some of the challenges and triumphs experienced during the first five years and to acknowledge some of the great heart surgeons we have been privileged to learn from and to work with along this exciting path.

Is It Time for Cautious Optimism?

In March 1996, more than a quarter century ago, Dr. Bruce Lytle published a prescient editorial in the *Journal of Thoracic & Cardiovascular Surgery* titled "Minimally Invasive Cardiac Surgery [1]."

> Modern cardiac surgery has been based on cardiopulmonary bypass, myocardial protection, and the median sternotomy … Until now, minimally invasive surgical strategies have not been a major factor in adult cardiac surgery. That is changing … Is a smaller incision worth a longer pump run? …

> Very little compromise in left ITA–LAD grafting can be accepted … The concepts of less invasive surgery will strongly influence adult cardiac surgery over the next decade. Many patients will eventually benefit from the fundamental reexamination of our practices that these concepts demand. Instrumentation will improve. There will be operations that we will end up doing better.

In May 1996, Profs. Stephen Westaby and Federico J. Benetti published a special report in *The Annals of Thoracic Surgery* titled "Less Invasive Coronary Surgery: Consensus from the Oxford Meeting," which was meant to catalyse the start of a new era [2].

> [While] conventional coronary operations with cardiopulmonary bypass are both safe and effective … the aims of less invasive coronary surgery are to reduce perioperative morbidity further and promote earlier hospital discharge. Regardless of the technique … it is important to achieve the long-term aim of curing the patient's problem … Sternotomy carries remarkably little morbidity and is perhaps the least painful surgical incision … Combinations of the so-called less invasive approaches can be used for multiple grafts, but it is difficult to see how these time-consuming incisions are an improvement over median sternotomy.

In May 2021, after reading our paper from January 2021, "A Novel Subxiphoid Approach for Bilateral Internal Thoracic Artery Harvesting" in *Innovations*, Dr. Mark Levinson kindly contacted us about his incredible series of 46 patients, treated from 2005 to 2013, through subxiphoid access using direct visualisation. Dr. Levinson specifically designed his operation to avoid requiring endoscopy assistance since he believed that nondirect imaging would not be well accepted by the practicing surgical community of that era. His initial paper, "Subxiphoid Multi-Arterial OPCAB: Surgical Technique and Initial Case Report," from *The Heart Surgery Forum* in 2005 highlights his perspective and success [3].

> The surgical technique of transsternal coronary artery bypass grafting (CABG) has remained relatively stagnant for the past three decades … cardiac surgery has made very little progress in converting our most common procedure into a minimally invasive alternative … Surgical outcomes have improved despite greater comorbidities in the surgical population … but [this] does not eliminate the fear of open surgery in the minds of patients and referring physicians … Our specialty still does not provide a realistic alternative to the endoluminal procedures … Most of the surgeons practicing today … are unfamiliar (and suspicious) of endoscopically based CABG techniques … The future of cardiac surgery cannot be based on the archaic saphenous vein and full sternotomy procedures of the 1980s, or we will have few patients to operate upon … The solution must rival the non-invasive nature of angioplasty, be cost effective, and "teachable" to any currently practicing heart surgeon.

Right Time, Right Place

Good luck smiled upon our research team during a cadaver laboratory at URMC in the fall of 2016. We were approached by a wonderful congenital heart surgeon, Dr. Joseph Turek, seeking new ideas to avoid sternotomy for pediatric epicardial pacemaker lead placement. We saw this as an opportunity to investigate the intriguing potential subxiphoid access approach to the heart in an upcoming cadaver laboratory. During our dissection under the xiphoid process, the author, along with outstanding cardiac surgery senior resident Dr. Fabio Sagebin (now a heart surgeon in California), unexpectedly but readily observed two bifurcated vascular structures, which Dr. Sagebin promptly identified as the right and left ITAs. Wow—a very pleasant surprise. Figure 3 shows the subxiphoid endoscopic access used at this laboratory.

We immediately recognised that we had stumbled into an opportunity to be part of a potentially important positive disruption to help patients with coronary artery disease. Could subxiphoid access safely provide two "gold standard" arterial inflow grafts with essentially no risk of deep sternal wound infection or dehiscence? The prospect of making a big difference in coronary revascularisation became simply too tempting to resist.

Our first review of the literature revealed only two related publications, both from Japanese sources, regarding subxiphoid access to the ITAs, which are shown below with all of the related literature identified in subsequent searches:

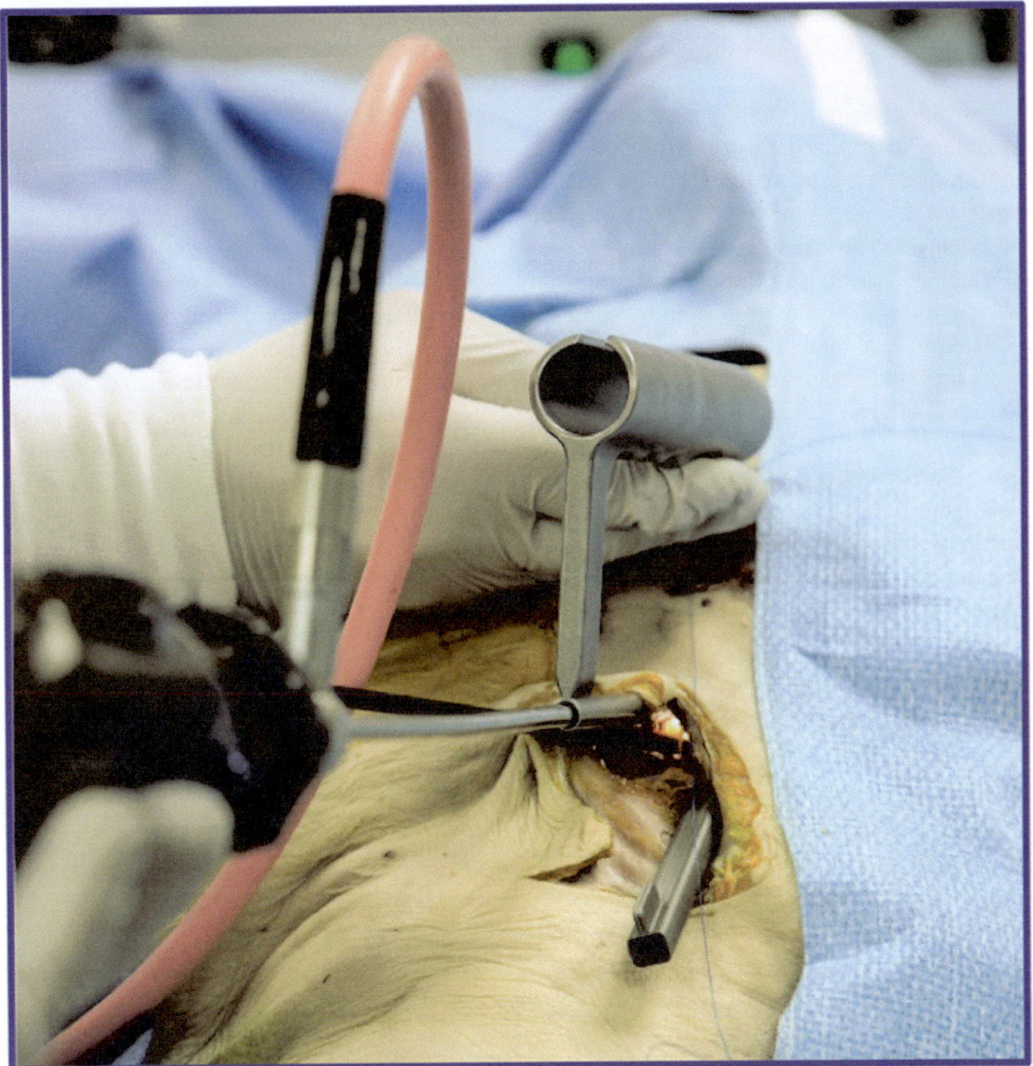

Fig. 3 Close-up of the subxiphoid approach used in the cadaver lab that marked the start of our μCAB project

- Karagoz et al. [4]: Results of 24 patients undergoing ITA-mediated coronary revascularisation via subxiphoid access also including a lower-J ministernotomy without video assistance
- Takata et al. [5]: A case report describing a robotically assisted BITA harvest via subxiphoid approach
- Shimizu et al. [6]: Examination of an ITA harvest technique in an in vivo porcine model using an ultrasonic surgical aspirator and electrothermal bipolar tissue sealing system

via a subxiphoid approach performed with endoscopic imaging with an average harvest time of 45.4 ± 10.9 min for each ITA
- Chakravarthy et al. [7]: Results of 10 patients undergoing CABG surgery via a subxiphoid technique using a commercial retractor and heart stabilisers but without video assistance
- Kiser et al. [8]: Results of 26 patients who underwent attempted transxiphoid CABG, yielding 18 patients who ultimately avoided sternotomy, using a commercial retractor and video imaging, they note "the average

procedure time decreased from 5:37 for the first six cases to 3:54 for the last six cases"

Innovation requires sacrifice and immersion. Innovation in cardiac surgery also requires a network of enthusiastic and insightful heart care physicians sharing common goals. We appreciate and celebrate their vision.

While the above publications have not yet fostered widespread change in routine coronary revascularisation surgery, our ongoing research in this field was encouraged and supported by our heart surgeon colleagues at URMC: Drs. Peter Knight, Sunil Prasad, Igor Gosev, and Bryan Barrus. Drs. Frederick Ling, Christopher Cove, and Karl Schwarz, innovative cardiologists in the heart team at our hospital, also found promise in the potential of sternal-sparing CABG. We hypothesised: If μCAB proved

effective, an estimated 90 patients a year at our center alone might benefit from isolated LITA–LAD bypass over percutaneous coronary intervention (PCI, or coronary stenting). In addition, a collaborative program between heart surgeons and interventional cardiologists potentially providing hybrid revascularisation can offer a win-win-win. The patient could have the best of both worlds: surgical CABG where the literature demonstrates superiority and possible PCI of targets where noninferiority is likely—all without any iatrogenic injuries to bone or cartilage.

In a subsequent cadaver laboratory testing customised devices, Dr. Joseph Zacharias successfully used some of the early-stage technology. An expert in endoscopic saphenous vein takedown and radial artery harvest, Dr. Zacharias was able to use a subxiphoid approach to take down both ITAs. Figure 4 shows Dr. Zacharias

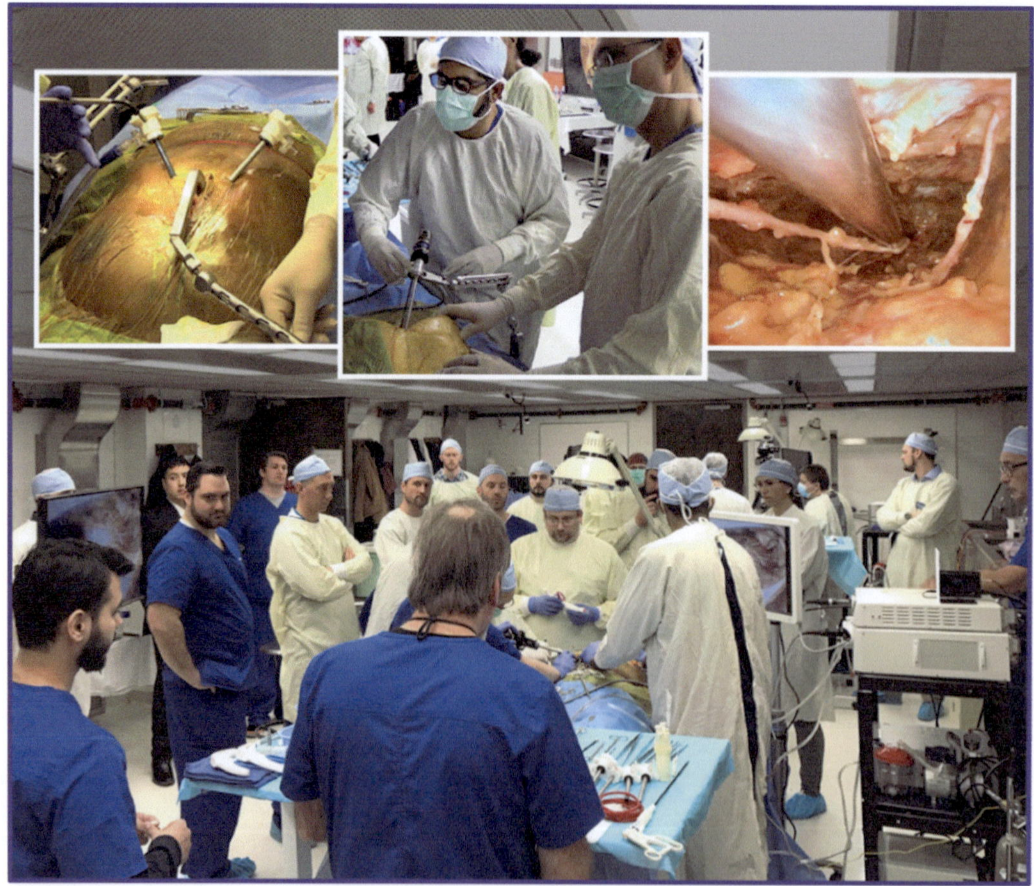

Fig. 4 Composite image from an early cadaver laboratory using customised technology for subxiphoid BITA harvest

(operating) and the team that participated in this laboratory, along with views of subxiphoid access sites and a still image from the endoscope footage from the BITA takedowns. Also at our laboratory, Dr. Boris Robič, an innovator in endoscopic ITA harvest, noted his interest in constructing ITA–coronary artery anastomoses through the subxiphoid access site.

Could we stand on the shoulders of coronary surgery giants to expedite the availability of anaortic, all-arterial, sternal-sparing CABG? Could this new, more gentle approach reliably deliver ITA harvests that were still fast and safe while not increasing the risks of surgically induced target vessel stenosis? Enduring beautiful collaborations developed between our group and world-class heart centers with outstanding leadership by Profs. Günther Laufer, Alfred Kocher, and Martin Andreas in Austria; and by Prof. Victor Costache and Dr. Andreea Costache in Romania. Pioneering heart surgeons, like Drs. Scott Goldman, Charles Mvondo, and Tom Nguyen, visited our facilities and early cadaver labs. Though we learned that the early prototypes were not yet user friendly, enthusiasm grew. Gifted cardiac surgery research fellows Drs. Paul Werner, Hossein Amirjamshidi, Kyle Purrman, and Eric Ndikumana made enormous contributions. For inspiration and affirmation, we visited the less invasive operating rooms of Drs. Francis Sutter and Charles Lutz, to observe robotic ITA takedowns, and Drs. Alaaddin Yilmaz and Boris Robič, to observe endoscopic BITA takedowns. While Drs. Marc Ruel, Piroze Davierwala, Nikolaos Bonaros, and Joerg Kempfert expressed interest in this μCAB research, our plans to work together were suppressed by the pandemic. The interest and active support of Dr. Niv Ad, a trusted innovator and great leader in heart surgery, confirmed that we had a worthy mission. Dr. Ad was the first heart surgeon to use new, smaller titanium fasteners in patients. Over the ensuing half-decade, the potential wonderful impact of this opportunity began to crystallise—momentum grew.

Like the ITAs we had coincidentally identified in that fateful cadaver laboratory, our μCAB coronary revascularisation research program intrinsically bifurcated into two principal surgical objectives: BITA harvest through the subxiphoid approach and reliable anastomoses via left anterior μT access. Both of these main objectives further bifurcated into subordinate technology development projects. Figure 5 shows how the technology research and development bifurcated into the following branches.

For subxiphoid BITA harvest:

- A reusable operating room table–mounted retrosternal retractor system for ergonomic ITA exposure on either side of the sternum
- A single-patient–use device for atraumatic axial soft tissue retraction to aid in remote ITA dissection

For μT anastomoses:

- A specialised pedestal for appropriately holding the "cobra head" end of the ITA graft for suturing next to the target site arteriotomy
- A miniature titanium fastener custom designed for use with 6-0, 7-0 and 8-0 polypropylene suture to enable automatic titanium fastener placement and suture tail trimming of coronary anastomotic suture at even less accessible sites

μCAB: Subxiphoid BITA Harvest: Improved Retrosternal Retractor

Like most things in surgery, if it is worth doing in a patient and worth expending a surgeon's time, it is worth considering customised technology. The prototype table-mounted sternal retraction devices morphed into a more extensive, modular system, including in 2019 a breakthrough "sternal retractor" specific to subxiphoid access. This novel retractor mounts to both sides of an operating room table to create a "bridge" above the patient's chest with a ratcheting mechanism that elevates independent

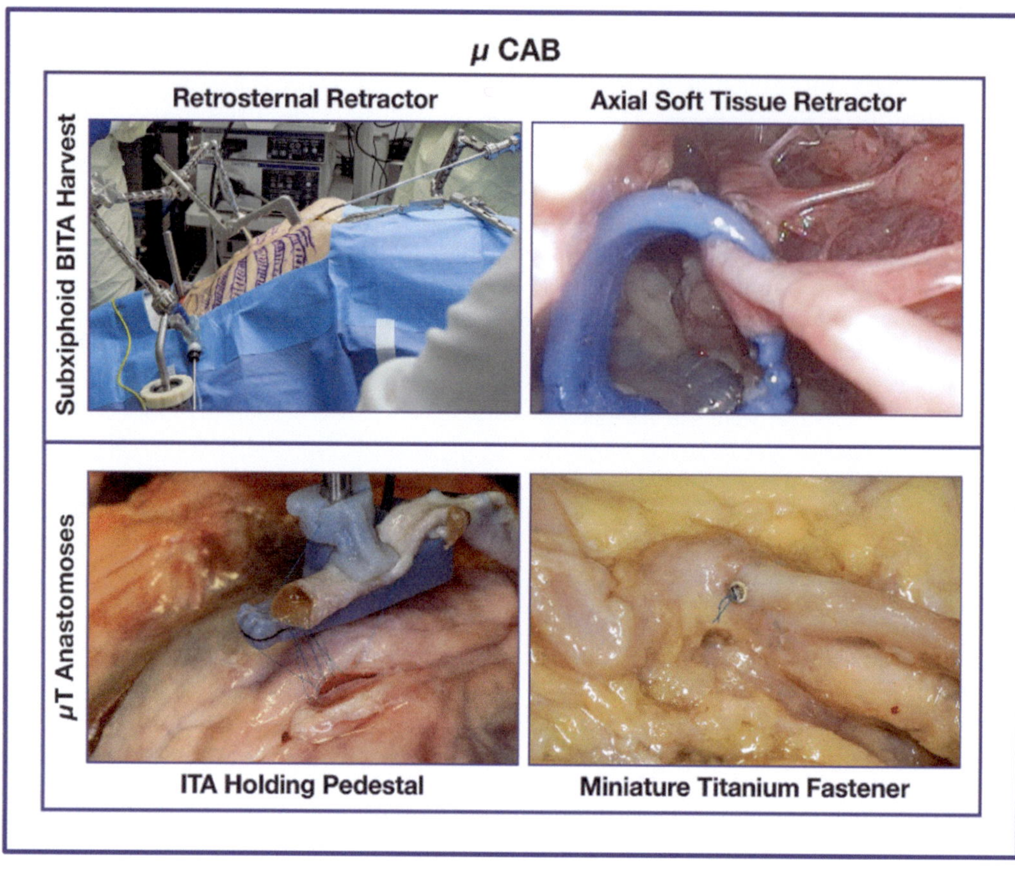

Fig. 5 Highlights from the bifurcated μCAB technology development

retrosternal retractors purpose-built for exposing the LITA or RITA. Figure 6 shows a setup of the sternal retractor system in a porcine carcass model as well as an exploded view of the system's components (Video 1).

μCAB: Subxiphoid BITA Harvest: Axial Soft Tissue Retractor

Since surgeons are traditionally trained to take ITAs via sternotomy, with the direction of their dissection extending medial toward lateral, we recognised that the proposed subxiphoid approach for axial ITA dissection starting distally and progressing toward the proximal origin would require more customised technology if it were to become readily received by most practicing heart surgeons.

In 2019, an atraumatic axial soft tissue retraction device, which functions like a gentle vessel loop, was invented, rapidly prototyped, repeatedly redesigned, and frequently tested in pig carcasses and cadaver labs to enable easier distal to proximal ITA dissection through subxiphoid access. We also designed a custom tool to allow simplified measurement of the dissected ITAs to ensure adequate length to reach the targeted anastomotic site without requiring excessive dissection. Figure 7 shows the iterative development process for this device, starting with early prototypes on the left.

μCAB: μT Access Anastomosis: Custom ITA Holding Pedestal

While a few expert coronary surgeons are able to reliably construct ITA–coronary anastomoses through small thoracotomies, the technique requires exquisite skill and patience. Just as we believe that ITA harvest through the subxiphoid

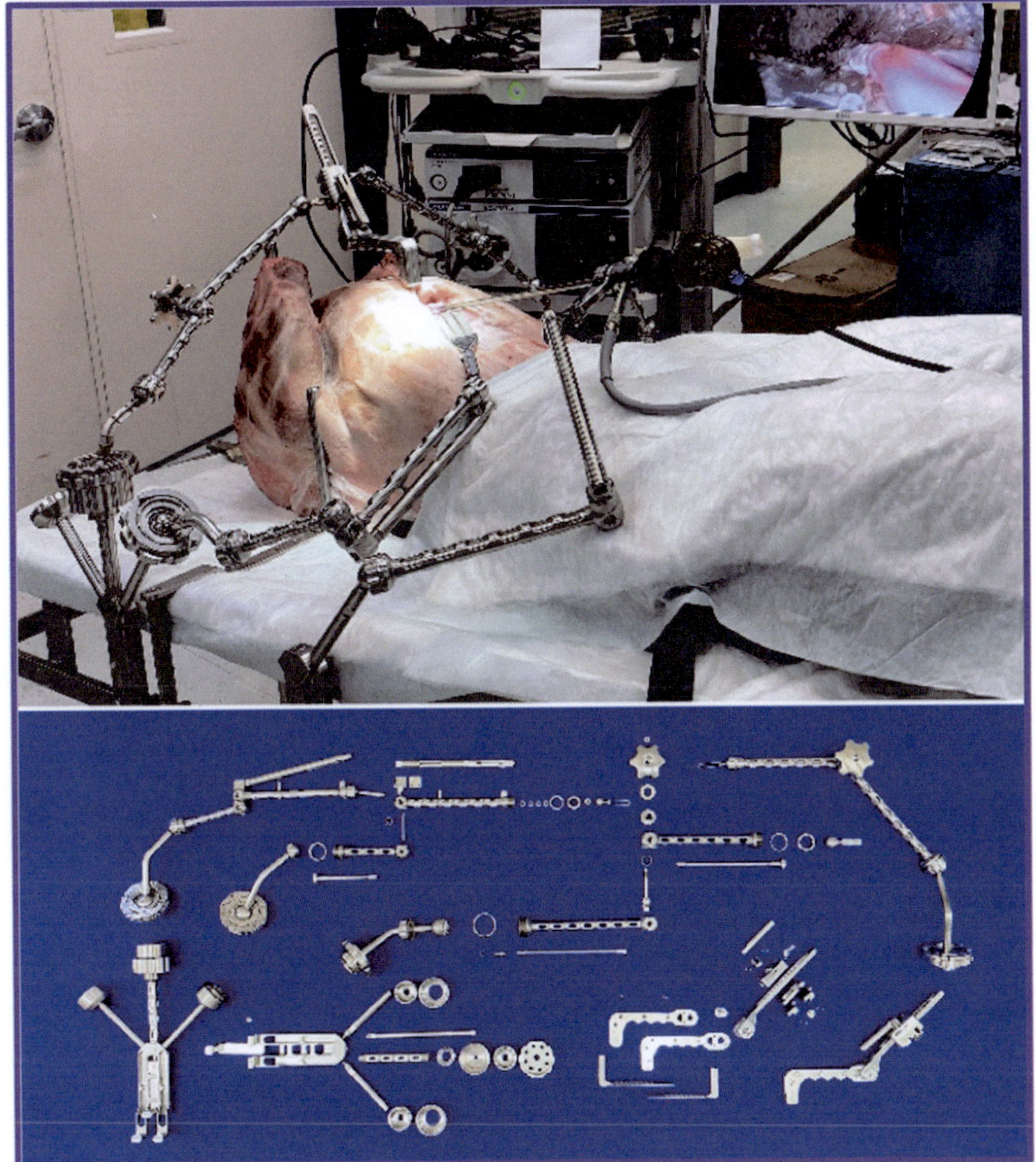

Fig. 6 Sternal retractor setup and view of the components before assembly

space avails itself to innovative techniques and devices, we believe that left anterior µT access can become a viable ergonomic option for surgeons if they are provided with sufficiently enabling technology. To reduce excessive "parachuting" distance of the ITA cobra head (i.e., if positioned too far away from the arteriotomy), we have developed a custom tissue pedestal to hold the mobilised ITA adjacent to the target site and in an orientation that enables more ergonomic anastomotic suturing. Figure 8 displays some of the more recent iterations of this device. While sewing with the tiny 7-0 or 8-0 suture required for distal coronary anastomosis

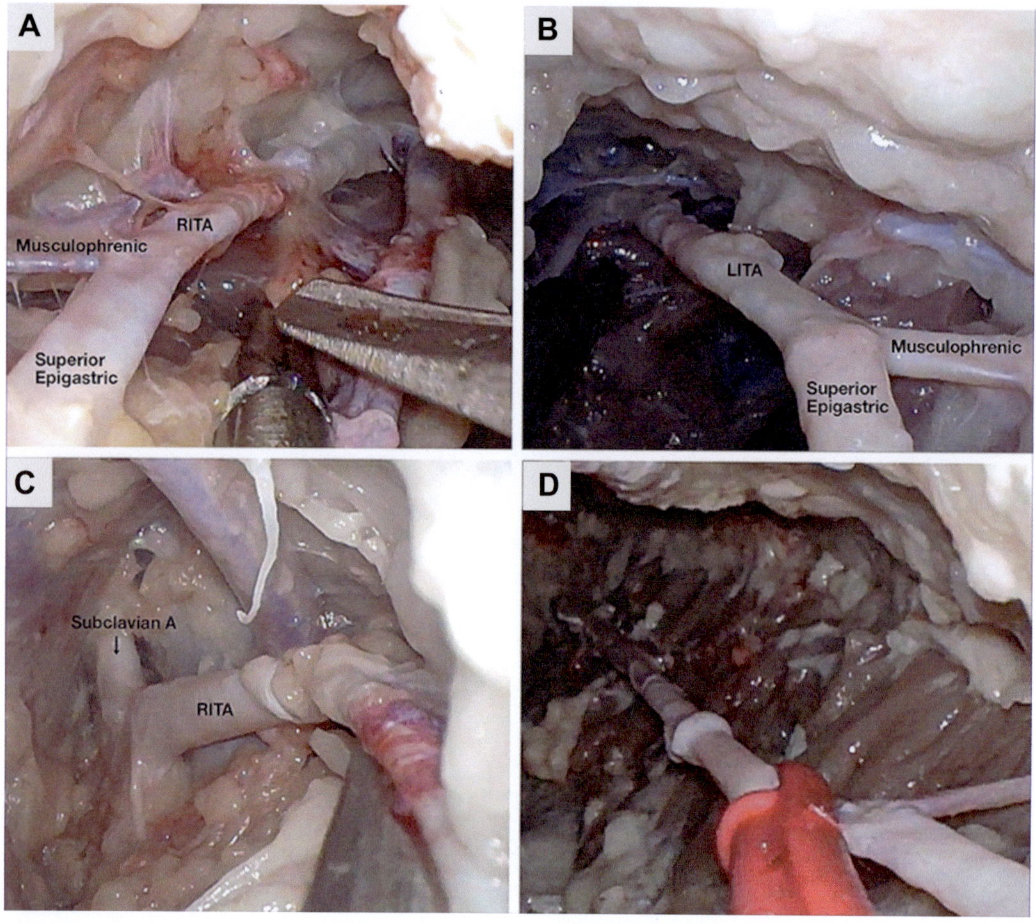

Video 1 Subxiphoid bilateral mammary artery harvest (▶ https://doi.org/10.1007/000-a93)

can be technically daunting, especially without the full access afforded by a traditional sternotomy, this ITA pedestal offers promise to make anastomotic suturing substantially less difficult. Because we appreciate that suturing a durable and accurate coronary anastomosis with 7-0 or 8-0 suture (even with fully open access) remains one of the most impressive skills in all of modern surgery, we recognised that custom accessories are needed to aid in this remote suturing.

The pedestal gently holds the distal ITA inverted near the arteriotomy; it also incorporates other features for suture management and guiding the needles during suturing. Figure 9 is a close-up of the pedestal in position adjacent to the target site with anastomotic suture in place in an ex vivo porcine model. The tissue pedestal is connected to a table-mounted arm that allows its well controlled and stable positioning immediately adjacent to the target site within the µT access site. For an end-to-side (e.g., LITA–LAD) anastomoses, the distal end of the ITA cobra head is rotated ∼180 degrees within the pedestal to enable anastomotic suturing. Recent research regarding use of the pedestal for sequential arterial grafting appears promising (see Fig. 10). The µCAB procedure is intended to enable sternal-sparing all-arterial grafting beyond the single or

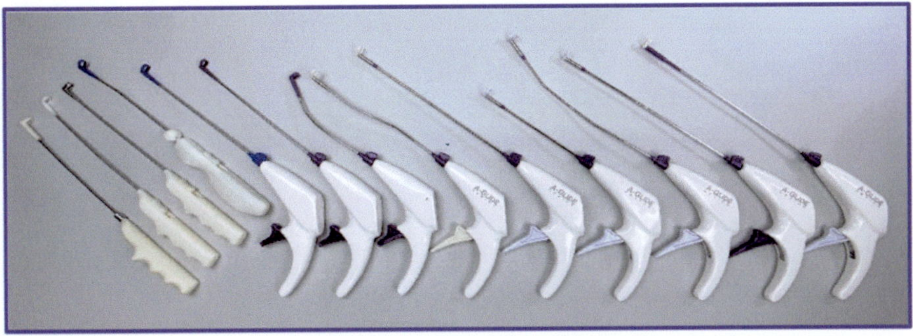

Fig. 7 Progression of soft tissue retraction devices developed for μCAB

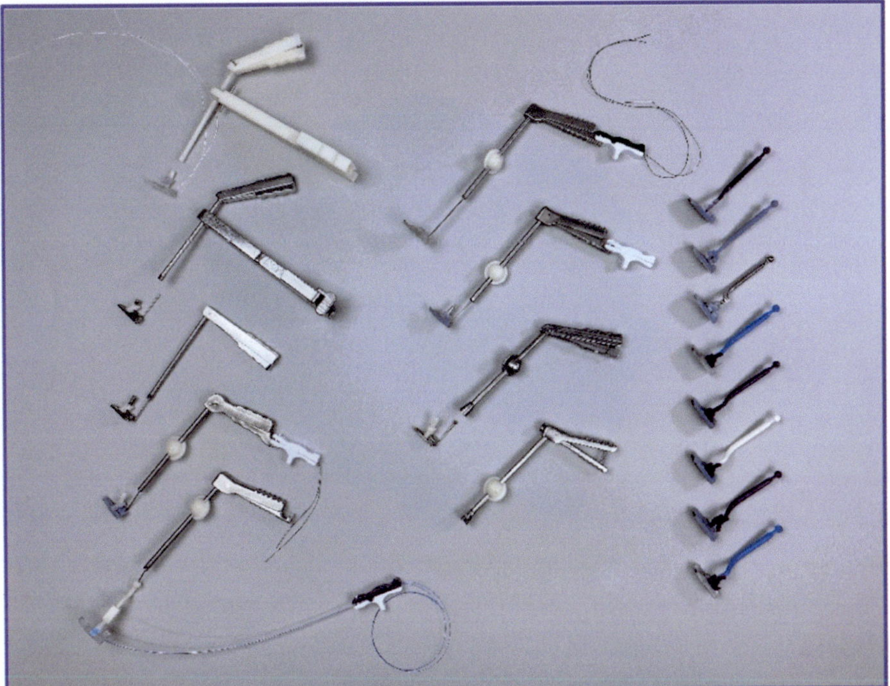

Fig. 8 Tissue pedestal design iterations

double bypass grafts from BITA end-to-side anastomoses alone. Consideration of the use of sequential anastomoses (e.g., skip grafts) and/or additional arterial free grafts (e.g., radial artery or RITA segment Y-graft) expands the potential to surgically treat multivessel disease (Fig. 11).

μCAB: μT Access Anastomosis : Miniature Titanium Fastener

Just as sewing with tiny suture is extremely difficult, manually tying tiny knots through a small, remote access incision can be challenging and unreliable for any surgeon. Based on COR-

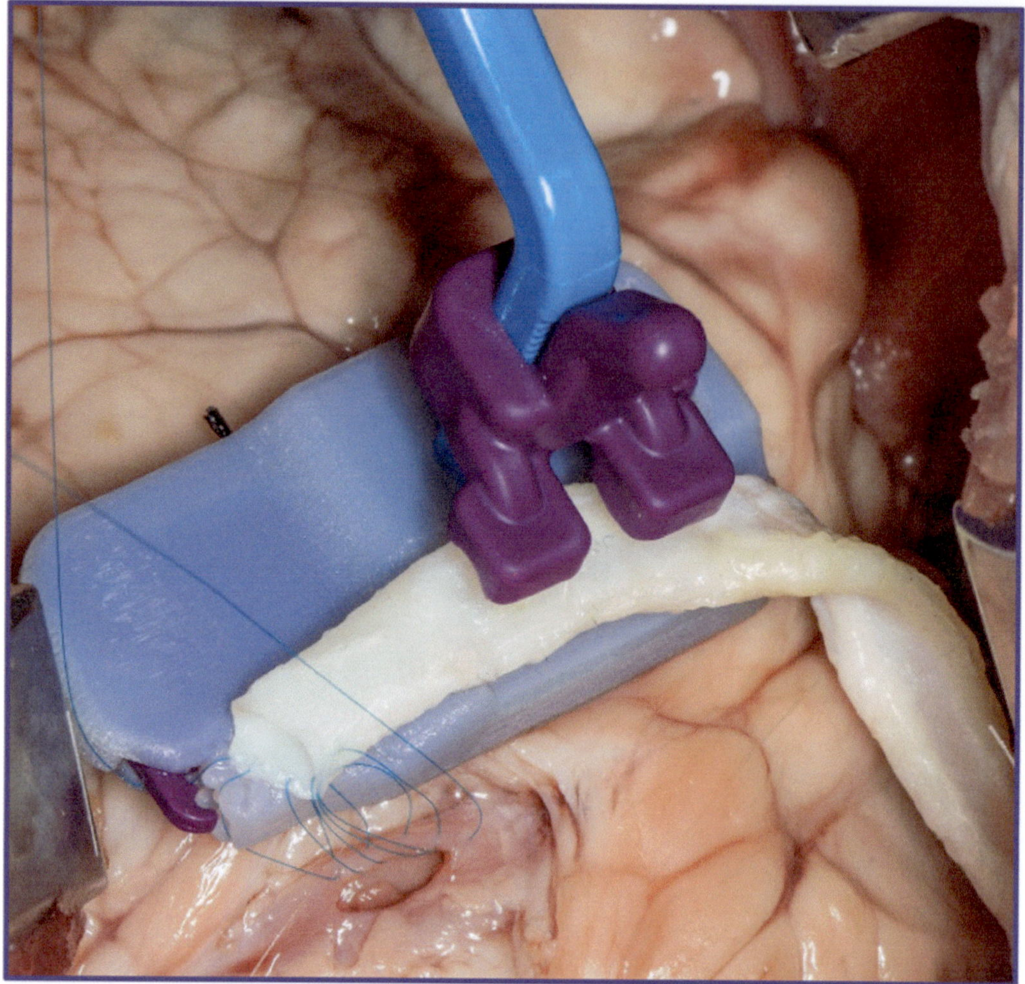

Fig. 9 Tissue pedestal holding graft vessel adjacent to target site

KNOT® technology, a smaller device was developed for the placement of a miniaturised titanium fastener to secure 6-0, 7-0, or 8-0 monofilament polypropylene suture and automatically trim both suture tails (Video 2).

Over the first five years of this project, the miniature titanium fastener technology was put through extensive research, development, and testing in cadaver laboratories and in pig carcasses and in vivo experiments. Figure 10, from left to right, shows the distal tip of the device as applied in a cadaver laboratory to secure a LITA–LAD anastomosis; a miniature titanium fastener as placed to secure and automatically trim the tails of 8-0 suture on an end-to-side anastomosis in a porcine carcass model (note: this anastomosis is the completion of the vessels being sutured in Fig. 9); and two titanium fasteners used to secure two sequential ITA–coronary artery bypass anastomoses in an ex vivo porcine model (Video 2).

After receiving FDA 510(k) clearance in the United States, the COR-KNOT MICRO™ titanium fasteners were first used in CABG patients in July 2021 by Dr. Niv Ad; this technology has subsequently been successfully used by 8 other surgeons in 12 patients receiving coronary revascularisation surgery (Video 3).

Innovation is a lengthy process that often flows in unexpected ways, especially over the

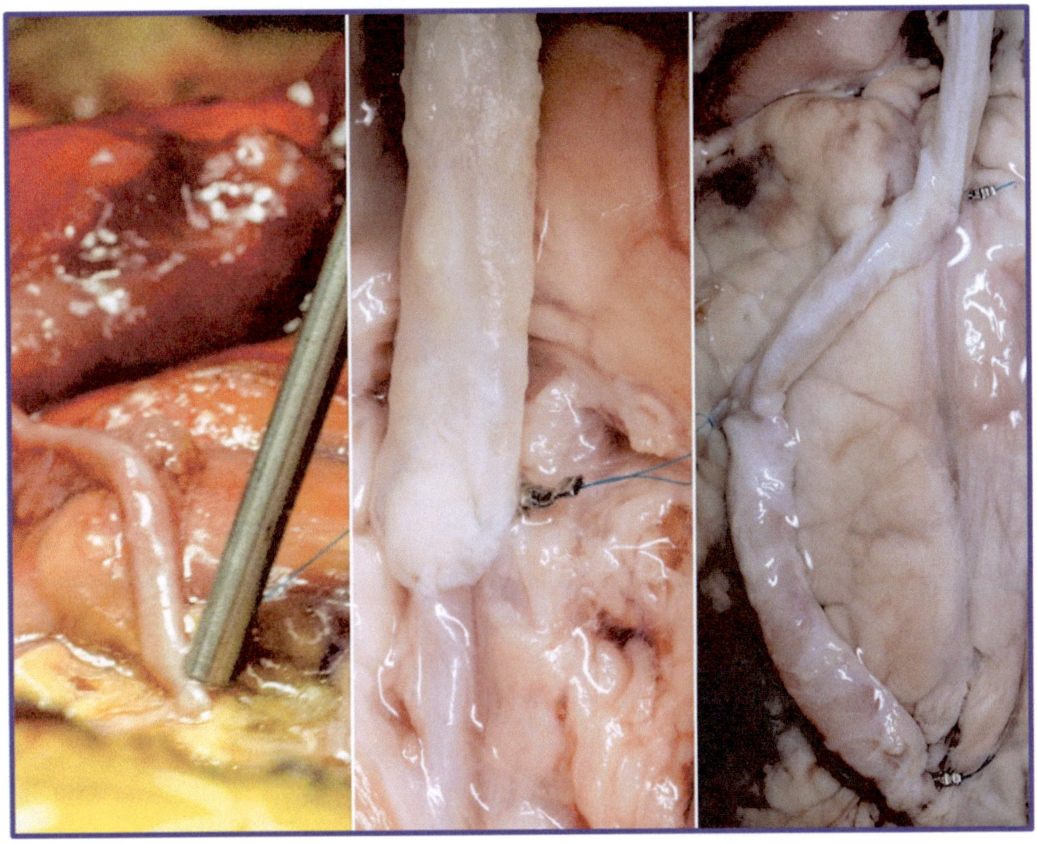

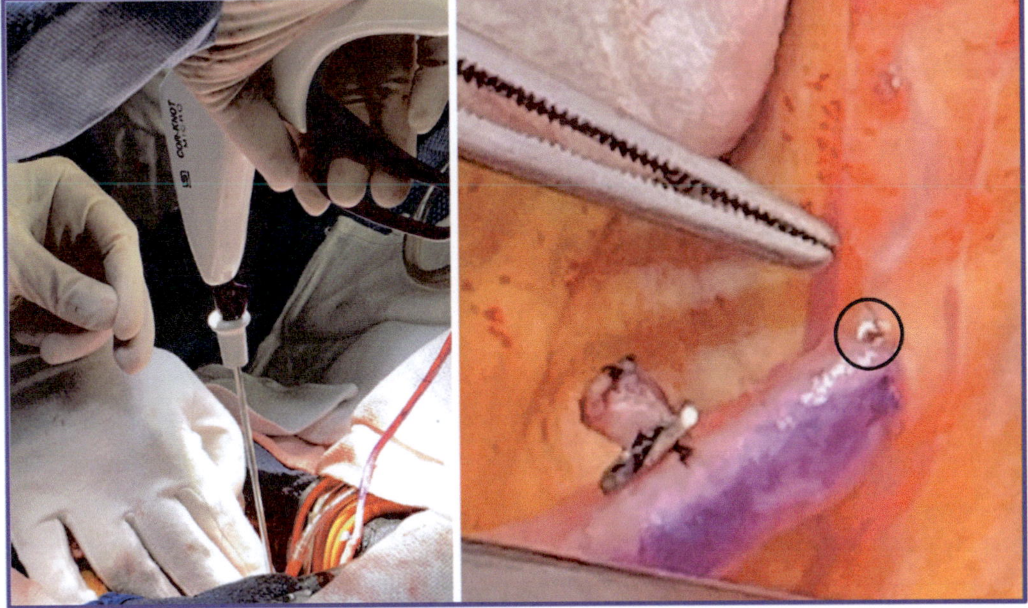

Fig. 10 The miniature titanium fastener deployment device as used in a cadaver laboratory, once on an ITA graft in an ex vivo porcine model, and twice on a sequential graft in an ex vivo porcine model

Fig. 11 Dr. Niv Ad using the COR-KNOT MICRO™ Device for the first time in a patient (left); and a miniature titanium fastener (in circle) securing 7-0 polypropylene suture used in a saphenous vein graft anastomosis

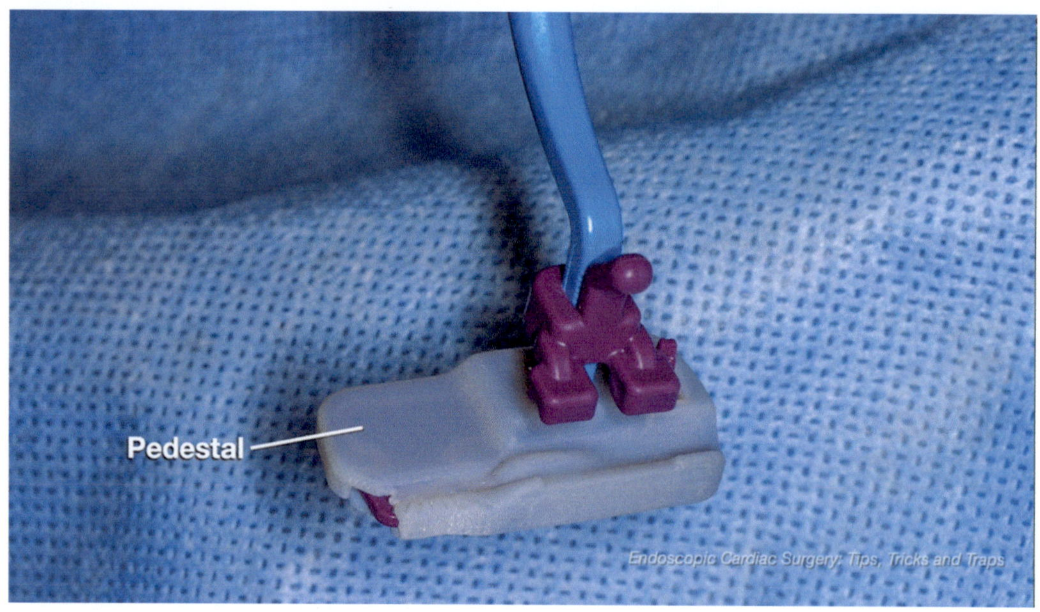

Video 2   Enabling devices for Micro CABG (▶ https://doi.org/10.1007/000-a92)

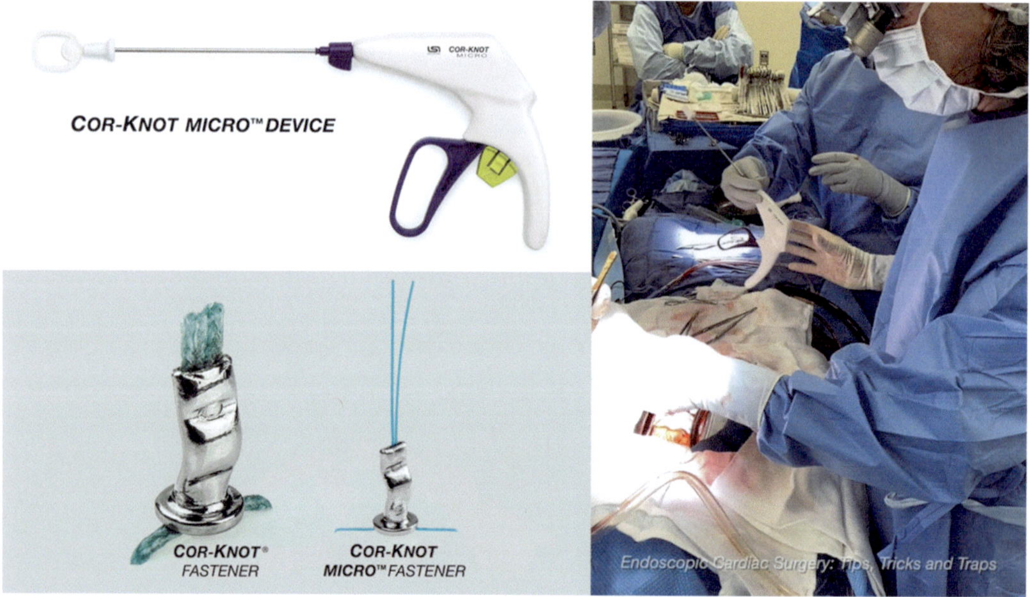

Video 3   CorKnot Micro: First in Human case (▶ https://doi.org/10.1007/000-a94)

course of a long project. Table 1 breaks down the company's µCAB revascularisation initiative by both calendar year and project year, conservatively estimating the amount of time and resources committed to advancing these innovative technologies and techniques. Since 2016, the µCAB initiative has consumed hundreds of thousands of person hours, produced thousands

Table 1 Project μCAB: first five years

Calendar year	2016	2017	2018	2019	2020	2021	Total
Project year	PY1		PY2	PY3	PY4	PY5	
Employee hours	4,080		34,116	34,745	134,136	162,953	370,030
Invention drawings	340		164	40	463	162	1,169
Engineering drawings	7		133	98	86	206	1,365
Pages written	2		1,136	955	1,021	3,660	6,774
Documents completed	1		278	140	169	440	1,028
Components produced	1,344		4,659	4,467	7,902	14,708	33,080
Devices built	24		264	341	649	785	2,063

of pages of documents, required more than 30,000 components plus 2,000 devices, and cost more than $30 million. This focus and energy has been dedicated to enhance heart surgery toward a more gentle patient-centered paradigm.

5 In Conclusion

Innovative thinking is a requirement for the modern cardiac surgeon. This chapter is intended to be a rallying cry to surgeons regarding the need to innovate for the benefit of patients, surgeons, and society at large. Though significant strides have been made toward optimising clinical outcomes since the early days of cardiac surgery, many long-recognised opportunities for innovation have gone unfulfilled. While novel technology and techniques will be essential to advancing cardiac surgery, the attitudes and efforts of cardiac surgeons toward innovation will be the driving force to providing a brighter future for their patients.

There are many opportunities for innovation in developing less invasive ways to operate on the heart. Sternotomies and large thoracotomies must go by the wayside in favor of tiny, microinvasive access sites for the benefit of patients. While nontraditional, less invasive approaches are often thought of as cumbersome and difficult to accept, enabling technology and facilitating imaging can help optimise the widespread adoption of innovations worthy of pursuit by heart surgeons for their patients. Heart surgery must be less traumatic, less risky, more efficient, and less complicated. Collectively, we must strive for a more gentle, patient-centered paradigm.

The demands on the available time of practicing cardiac surgeons are significant. Innovation is often frustrating and draining. The reality of the innovative process is that it is more costly in terms of time, energy, and emotional capital than one might expect. Simple solutions to complex problems are essential, though they are typically the most difficult to develop. We humbly request that heart surgeons remain optimistic, keep a keen eye toward the horizon, and maintain an open mind regarding opportunities

for meaningful innovation. New approaches can and will benefit your patients and our world. Partnership among clinical faculty and experienced industry partners can facilitate this process for the mutual benefit of all involved.

Innovation or obsolescence? It is a great time to be a great heart surgeon. Less invasive heart surgery remains substantially behind relative to the progress of other specialties. The availability of innovative technologies that are customised for remote surgery along with excellent endoscopic imaging can usher in a new golden era of heart surgery. Significant positive disruption can yield enormous positive impact. However, the refinement and utilisation of promising techniques requires heart surgeons to command the destiny of their noble field. Without the insight, enthusiasm, and energy of heart surgeons, this golden opportunity will ultimately fade. Patients have demonstrated their willingness to accept treatments that are potentially inferior in the long term to avoid near-term pain and suffering.

Twenty-five years after a loud plea to advance coronary revascularisation surgery by emphasising less invasive techniques, it still remains unclear whether most heart surgeons will embrace, or even explore, this paradigm.

Great Surgery = Great Outcomes + Great Recovery.

The future of heart surgery is in the hands of today's heart surgeons.

References

1. Lytle B. Minimally invasive cardiac surgery. J Thorac Cardiovasc Surg. 1996;111(3):554–5.
2. Westaby S, Benetti FJ. Less invasive coronary surgery: consensus from the Oxford meeting. Ann Thorac Surg. 1996;62:924–31.
3. Levinson MM. Subxiphoid multi-arterial OPCAB: surgical technique and initial case report. Heart Surg Forum. 2005;8(4):303–10.
4. Karagoz HY, Kurtoglu M, Ozerdem G, Battaloglu B, Korkmaz S, Bayazit K. Minimally invasive coronary artery bypass grafting: the rib cage-lifting technique. J Thorac Cardiovasc Surg. 1998;116(2):354–6.
5. Takata M, Watanabe G, Ushijima T, Ishikawa N. A novel internal thoracic artery harvesting technique via subxiphoid approach—for the least invasive

coronary artery bypass grafting. Interact Cardiovasc Thorac surg. 2009;9:891–2.

6. Shimizu Y, Watanabe G, Tomita S, Matsumoto I, Lino K. A novel technique for harvesting the internal thoracic artery: linear harvesting technique using an ultrasonic surgical aspirator. Interact Cardiovasc Thorac surg. 2011;12:998–1001.

7. Chakravarthy M, Veerappa M, Jawali V, Pandya N, Krishnamoorthy J, Muniraju G, George A, Baishya J. Anesthetic implications of subxiphoid coronary artery bypass surgery. Ann Card Anaesth. 2016;19:433–8.

8. Kiser AC, Nifong W, Elbeery JR, Caranasos TG. Transxiphoid revascularization of the anterior descending coronary artery with the left mammary artery. Innovations. 2021;1–4.

Additional Resources

9. Castillo Sang M, Answini G, Griffin J. Minimally invasive mitral valve repair after endocarditis with bileaflet prolapse using a modification of Leipzig loop technique. CTSNet. 2019. https://doi.org/10.25373/ctsnet.7808774.v1.

10. Fortunato G, Stoger G, Domenech AL, et al. Balloon-expandable transcatheter mitral valve replacement through minimally invasive approach in big MAC. CTSNet. 2020. https://doi.org/10.25373/ctsnet.13242311.v1.

11. Kraev A, Counts S. Robotic left diaphragm plication using automatic (Cor-Knot) device. CTSNet. 2021. https://doi.org/10.25373/ctsnet.13957454.v1.

12. Pitsis A, Nikoloudakis N. Totally endoscopic aortic valve replacement and transaortic mitral valve repair. CTSNet. 2020. https://doi.org/10.25373/ctsnet.11689443.v1.

13. Pitsis A, Nikoloudakis N, Kelpis T, Economopoulos V. Totally endoscopic aortic valve replacement using an automated annular suturing device. CTSNet. 2020. https://doi.org/10.25373/ctsnet.12024627.v1.

14. Pitsis A, Nikoloudakis N, Kelpis T, Economopoulos V. Totally endoscopic aortic valve replacement with a Trifecta GT bovine pericardial valve. CTSNet. 2019. https://doi.org/10.25373/ctsnet.9587900.v1.

15. Pitsis A. Totally endoscopic bileaflet mitral valve repair with preformed chordae loops. CTSNet. 2019. https://doi.org/10.25373/ctsnet.7837853.v1.

16. Pitsis A, Nikoloudakis N, Kelpis T, Economopoulos V. Totally endoscopic mitral valve repair with predetermined length of synthetic chordae. CTSNet. 2019. https://doi.org/10.25373/ctsnet.10070126.v1.

17. Pitsis A, Nikoloudakis N, Economopoulos V, Kelpis T. Totally endoscopic redo tricuspid valve repair. CTSNet. 2019. https://doi.org/10.25373/ctsnet.8199260.v1.

18. Plestis K, Orlov O, Kaleda V. Aortic and mitral valve replacements through J-type partial sternotomy. CTSNct. 2017. https://www.ctsnet.org/article/aortic and-mitral-valve-replacements-through-j-type-partial-sternotomy.

19. Torre T, Theologou T, Franciosi F, Ferrari E, Demertzis S. Modified David with a Valsalva graft. CTSNet. 2020. https://doi.org/10.25373/ctsnet.12857567.v1.

20. Yilmaz A, Dubar E, Dunning J, Revishvili A. Totally Endoscopic Aortic Valve Replacement. CTSNet. 2020. https://doi.org/10.25373/ctsnet.11502975.v1.

Psychological Context, Individual Differences and Adjustment in Relation to Cardiac Surgery Scars

Kate L. Green

Abstract

Cardiac surgery patients around the world typically undergo a sternotomy approach. Advances in cardiac surgery techniques presents patients with potentially increased choice. Factors that impact on adjustment and recovery post cardiac surgery are increasingly generating interest in relation to post-operative outcomes. These include psychological context, individual differences and adjustment in relation to cardiac surgery scars. For a proportion of patients subjective perception of appearance difference (i.e. scars) post cardiac surgery will be an important consideration. The psychological impact of the introduction of non-sternotomy approaches to heart surgery is an emerging field of research that could help to inform clinical decision making and identify groups of patients who are likely to benefit from a minimally invasive cardiac surgery approach.

Keywords

Psychological context · Cardiac surgery · Endoscopic cardiac surgery scars

K. L. Green (✉)
Blackpool Teaching Hospitals NHS Foundation Trust, Blackpool, UK
e-mail: drkategreen@gmail.com

Working as a Clinical Psychologist within a Cardiac Centre, it has been a privilege to learn about the individual experiences of cardiac patients including those awaiting planned cardiac surgery procedures and emergency admissions which allows minimum time, if any, for the patient to prepare for an invasive surgical procedure. The role involves psychological assessment, formulation and intervention at each stage of the patient's cardiac journey. Throughout clinical work in this field, the relevance of historical factors, individual differences (examples include personal characteristics, coping skills, trauma history, social context, pre/post-operative care and support) have been highlighted as important factors in the process of pre and post adjustment from initially receiving a cardiac diagnosis and treatment sequelae including cardiac surgery.

As health professionals, we are in the unique position of both accessing and delivering health care. The range of presentations I have encountered working in cardiac services and breadth of responses from patients prompted me to consider my own experience of adjustment after surgery. During adolescence, I was admitted for an urgent appendectomy. Unfortunately the appendix ruptured into the peritoneum and following an emergency procedure, my primary concern at the time was the size/position of the surgical scar and whether the drain site would ever heal. Postoperatively and as time elapsed, healing took place and I was able to process what happened. Preoccupation with the scar diminished and I was more inclined to think '*I survived.*' This cognitive shift was part of the adjustment process and it is likely the initial concern about the scar was related to my age and stage of development, the lack of prior experience of surgery and possibly a focus away from the unexpected reminder of mortality having only just commenced an undergraduate degree. On reflection, several protective factors including family support and opportunities to vocalise my concerns with individuals who were psychologically aware, assisted my adjustment and enhanced my coping skills to what had been a potentially life-threatening event. More recently, working with patients either preparing for or recovering from cardiac surgery, I have continued to develop a greater understanding about individual differences in factors that influence rehabilitation and recovery.

I have since become aware that it is not uncommon for people to express increased concern about scars on their torso compared to parts of their body that are typically exposed. There is limited understanding about the possible reasons for this but it is plausible to think that scars near areas of the body usually concealed and or associated with an individual's sexual identity could generate increased anxiety and issues relating to body image. Scars on the torso, particularly for women, have been found to have an association with poor adjustment [1]. The strength of relationship between self-rated severity of appearance and associated distress has been documented in relation to skin scarring and evidence suggests no correlations between objective measures (e.g. scar size) and emotional distress [2]. Clinically this has been observed when one patient perceives their sternotomy scar as a positive indicator of 'survival' and something to share almost like a 'badge of honour.' In contrast, another patient feels repulsed by their sternotomy scar and surrounding keloids which negatively affects intimacy with his/her partner, mood, self-confidence and quality of life. Research suggests resilience is an important factor in a person's ability to cope with changes to their appearance and outcome of treatment.

Variance in adjustment to changes in appearance, the potential influence of physiological, developmental, social and cognitive factors and the relevance of subjective severity of appearance difference following cardiac surgery indicates a need for consideration of these in service provision. Meaningful predictors of adjustment could include prior experience of hospitalisation, illness beliefs, length of hospital stay, post cardiac surgery infection, surgical approach and pre/post-operative quality of care.

Focusing on surgical approach, the development of minimally invasive and endoscopic cardiac surgery techniques (non-sternotomy approaches) presents the possibility of a smaller scar compared to the traditional sternotomy. The option of minimally invasive surgery is routinely considered standard of care in other specialities (examples include general surgery, orthopaedics and lung cancer resection). Current literature, in addition to clinical experience, indicates that subjective perception of visible or non-visible difference in appearance post cardiac surgery could have psychological effects that impact on adjustment. The literature also suggests variance in the prevalence of Post Traumatic Stress Disorder (PTSD) of 15–25% in postoperative cardiac patients [3]. Symptoms of PTSD include flashbacks, nightmares, psychological distress and disturbed sleep all of which can significantly impair function, adjustment and quality of life. A younger age group of cardiac patient appears to also be a vulnerability factor for developing PTSD [4]. This highlights the importance of identifying risk factors through comprehensive assessment that incorporates historical information and possible higher risk of post-surgical trauma. Subjective perception of the scar and where clinically appropriate, selection of surgical approach that seeks to optimise recovery both from a physical and psychological perspective is also indicated. It is likely that the reported prevalence of PTSD is among patients who have undergone a sternotomy approach to their cardiac problems. There is emerging evidence that a non-sternotomy, minimal access approach has statistically significant advantages in relation to body image, self-esteem and aesthetic outcomes [5].

At present there is limited knowledge regarding the assessment of surgical scars post cardiac surgery. A recent study from China involving a small number of patients highlights scar assessment as an integral part of assessing the aesthetic outcomes of cardiac surgery. For the SCAR Comesis Assessment and Rating Scale the median sternotomy group scored statistically significantly higher than the non-sternotomy group on the *"overall impression"* and *"patient question"* with higher scores indicating less patient satisfaction [6]. The results in another paper [7], considering the psychological effects of skin incision size in cardiac surgery, highlights significant differences between the non-sternotomy and sternotomy approaches with small incision patients having lower levels of depression and anxiety symptoms and better quality of life. Additionally, mean score differences of scar perception were markedly different with non-sternotomy patients evaluating the scar quality significantly better than sternotomy patients.

According to NHS England and NHS Improvement, mental health difficulties represent the largest cause of disability in the UK, with one in four adults experiencing at least one diagnosable mental health condition in any given year [8]. The current evolving COVID-19 pandemic also has physical, psychological and financial implications for services, patients and their carers. In this context, routine screening of patient's emotional health and trauma histories would assist the multi-disciplinary cardiac team to understand the individual needs of the patient and plan care accordingly both pre and post-surgery. Any assumption that one surgical approach fits all does not account for individual differences, psychological context and potential adjustment issues. The challenge in the complex decision making relevant to any surgical procedure is to consider how patient choice and other factors that could influence adjustment and coping become incorporated in a meaningful, safe and effective way.

The work I have undertaken within the cardiac specialty in addition to my personal experience has helped me to understand that discussions about surgical incisions and the remnant scars warrant attention during the consent process. Patients with a history of psychological and, or physical trauma, those experiencing multiple disadvantage and, or social isolation are likely to be at higher risk of post-operative adjustment difficulties including body image issues, negative scar perception and reduced adherence to medically informed rehabilitation advice. This understanding helps to inform the development of models focused on psychological preparation for cardiac surgery [9]. Endoscopic cardiac surgery incisions may have a role to play in a sub-group of patients particularly where, from a subjective perspective, a smaller scar could reduce potential distress post-surgery. From a clinical perspective, we will only understand this through holistic assessment of individual contexts and risk factors in addition to further research in this area. Psychological adjustment to both traditional surgical approaches and newer endoscopic techniques will be a fertile field for future psychological research. As Salzmann et al. conclude: *"it seems important to treat not only the heart but also the mind as well to improve clinical outcomes after cardiac surgery."* [9].

References

1. Rumsey N, Charlton R, Clarke A, Harcourt D, James H, Jenkinson E et al. Factors associated with distress and positive adjustment in people with disfigurement: evidence from large multi-centered study. In: Rumsey N, Harcourt D, editors. The Oxford handbook of the psychology of appearance. (under review).
2. Brown BC, Moss TP, McGrouther DA, Bayat A. Skin scar preconceptions must be challenged: importance of self-perception in skin scarring. J Plast Reconstr Aesthet Surg. 2010;63(6):1022–9.
3. Ackerman MG, Sharipo PA. Psychological effects of invasive cardiac surgery and cardiac transplantation. In: Alvarenga M, Byrne D, editors. Handbook of psychocardiology. Singapore: Springer;2016. https://doi.org/10.1007/978-981-287-206-7_26.
4. Guler E, Schmid JP, Wiedemar L, Saner H, Schnyder U, von Känel R. Clinical diagnosis of posttraumatic stress disorder after myocardial infarction. Clin Cardiol. 2009;32(3):125–9. https://doi.org/10.1002/clc.20384.PMID:19301284;PMID:PMC6653086.

5. İyigün T, Kaya M, Gülbeyaz SÖ, Fıstıkçı N, Uyanık G, Yılmaz B, Onan B, Erkanlı K. Patient body image, self-esteem, and cosmetic results of minimally invasive robotic cardiac surgery. Int J Surg. 2017;39:88–94. https://doi.org/10.1016/j.ijsu.2017.01.105. Epub 2017 Jan 29 PMID: 28143731.

6. Huang LC, Chen DZ, Chen LW, Xu QC, Zheng ZH, Dai XF. The use of the Scar Cosmesis Assessment and rating scale to evaluate the cosmetic outcomes of totally thoracoscopic cardiac surgery. J Cardiothorac Surg. 2020;15(1):250. Published 2020 Sep 11. https://doi.org/10.1186/s13019-020-01294-w.

7. Piarulli A, Chiariello GA, Bruno P, et al. Psychological effects of skin incision size in minimally invasive valve surgery patients. Innovations. 2020;15(6):532–40.

8. NHS England and NHS Improvement. Adult and older adult mental health. 2020. https://www.england.nhs.uk/mental-health/adults/

9. Salzmann S, Salzmann-Djufri M, Wilhelm M, et al. Psychological preparation for cardiac surgery. Curr Cardiol Rep. 2020;22:172. https://doi.org/10.1007/s11886-020-01424-9.

Leadership, Interpersonal Dynamics and the Adoption of Minimally Invasive Endoscopic Mitral Valve Surgery

Megan Joffe

Abstract

In any field, individuals and teams who implement innovative practices in the workplace face personal, professional, and organizational challenges when they try to encourage widespread adoption of new ways of working. In surgery, where success has historically depended on continuous learning and safe, well-governed adoption, the challenges of introducing disruptive, innovative approaches, are particularly marked. The objectives of this chapter are to explore the challenges faced by a group of early adopters of minimally invasive mini-mitral valve surgery (MIS) in the nationalized health system in the United Kingdom and to outline the lessons learned so that surgical innovators of the future might better prepare their own implementation efforts. It demonstrates that key to understanding the lessons of these innovative practitioners is a recognition of the psychology of behaviour within organisations and how it influences the adoption of new techniques. While training together as a team has been shown to be a key factor in successful implementation (Edmondson et al., Administrative Science Quarterly 46:685–716, 2001) less attention has been paid to the personality of the individual surgeon, and the behaviour of groups of surgeons, and how organizational and collegial politics are navigated to gain support for the implementation of innovative practice. A key finding of this study was that an understanding of psychology rather than a one-dimensional focus on the science, that is on the surgical procedure and its value, would be beneficial to the implementation process. This chapter aims to highlight the contextual, organizational and team issues faced by this group of surgeons and to explore how these link to key concepts in organizational psychology, such as team and organizational dynamics. Individual surgeons' behaviourial reflections are also linked to the concept of learning agility to highlight where lessons can be learned.

Keywords

Innovation · Organizational psychology · Learning agility · Team · Psychological safety

M. Joffe (✉)
Organisational Clinical Psychologist, Edgecumbe Group Limited, Bristol, England
e-mail: megan.joffe@edgecumbe.co.uk

1 Introduction

1.1 Background History of MIS in the United Kingdom

Minimally invasive mitral valve surgery (MIS) was introduced to the United Kingdom National Health Service (NHS) 24 years ago following interest created by American surgeons in the mid-1990s who first experimented with dogs using long instruments to reach the heart through the ribs, rather than the breastbone, before introducing it to humans [1]. Since then, techniques have developed rapidly. Benefits of MIS for patients include less pain, faster recovery, and smaller scars. The advantages for the hospital include shorter length of stay [2], and benefits to patients increase the appeal of the service, and in time, the realization of greater income which may be an incentive in both privatized and nationalized systems. Indeed, there is an economic imperative to adopt new technologies for sustained competitiveness [3] notwithstanding the need to keep up with the latest treatment options. In the UK, many units implemented MIS techniques, following the pioneering US surgeons, but by early 2000 all had reverted to traditional sternotomy surgery, despite MIS gaining traction in Europe [4] and the US [5].

Nevertheless, in the early 2000s, a small number of UK cardiac surgeons, keen to adopt MIS techniques safely, honed their nascent interest in these procedures through independent training and mentoring in Europe. They returned to their units to reintroduce MIS in what was experienced as an unwelcoming, and at times, hostile national and organizational climate. Today there are over 10 units undertaking cardiac MIS, but the approach remains a minority interest and its successes are uncelebrated. Informal figures indicate that MIS mitral valve surgery constitutes approximately 8% of mitral valve cardiac surgery in the UK while in Germany, with a population only slightly larger than the UK, it represents 55% [6]. With the establishment of the British and Irish Society of Minimally Invasive Cardiac Surgery (BISMICS), MIS has achieved a higher profile and there are reportedly signs of support from professional bodies e.g. the Society of Cardio-Thoracic Surgeons (SCTS) and the wider surgical community. Despite the higher profile, there remains a degree of institutional inertia which continues to present a barrier to attracting junior surgeons to the sub-specialty, and to making MIS more widely available to patients, despite individual surgeon experiences being positive with good patient outcomes, and patients reporting high satisfaction with the procedure and outcome.

Surgical innovation typically struggles to report evidence along traditional lines, such as randomized control trials (RCT), and the surgeons in this study struggled in the early stages of the surgical development process, as outlined in the IDEAL framework [7] to produce such evidence. This presented as a significant, but not untypical barrier, to gaining collegial and organizational support. Notwithstanding this, adoption of minimally invasive surgery is well documented in other surgical specialties. Why then has it been a struggle for MIS to gain traction and become as popular a procedure in the UK as it has in Europe or the United States?

This chapter is based on the research outcomes from a qualitative study of the experience of nine surgeons, early adopters of MIS, in the UK. Early adopters are those keen to adopt a new product or technique before the majority [8]. What makes the experience of these nine surgeons unique is that their learning was achieved against a backdrop of intense scrutiny in cardiac surgery, which has low margins for error, and strong collegial skepticism, the latter being typical of most innovation efforts. A small number of the nine reported conditional support from a few colleagues and their organizations but the majority reported active resistance, in the form of public criticism of their ethics and motives; suspicion about outcomes in the absence of RCTs; lack of funding for necessary equipment; resistance to requests to train and form stable operating teams, and lack of curriculum support for training junior surgeons. Although they did not perceive the lack of support and criticism as personal, these factors were significant hurdles. Within this context, introducing MIS mitral surgery has proven a bumpy ride, with some distance yet to go, proving that introducing new, innovative technology into complex organizations is more difficult than expected. A key finding of the study was that an understanding of psychology rather than a one-dimensional focus on the science, that is on the surgical procedure and its value, would be beneficial to the implementation process.

Psychology is defined as the scientific study of the mind and how it dictates and influences our behaviour, from communication and memory to thought and emotion [9]. Broadly speaking, as a group, surgeons are not typically known to have an interest in the psychological aspects of work, although this has been changing with the greater focus on human factors and the role these play in the healthcare system including an interest in a wider range of solutions than checklists, protocols or training [10]. Research has begun to explore the complex relationship between human behaviour and technology, tasks, environment and organization [10].

Human factors support the delivery of patient care by "enhancing clinical performance through an understanding of the effects of teamwork, tasks, equipment, workspace, culture and organisation on human behaviour and abilities and application of that knowledge in clinical settings" [11]. The experiences of the surgeons in this study demonstrate the relevance of understanding how individual, group and organisational behaviour, in other words, psychology, affect the successful introduction of change and implementation of innovative technology. As Edmonson [3] has pointed out, introducing new technology has disrupting effects on relationships AND what she calls "organizational routines", or ways of working. The surgeons in this study reflected that understanding organizational relationships and behaviour, and the politics and power dynamics underlying these, is potentially more important than many innovators acknowledge given that they are often in the thrall of the technology.

This chapter now focuses on a brief description of the national context within which the implementation journey started. It then goes on to describe several features of the nine surgeons' experience and how relevant psychological theory can help to explain those features. Lessons are drawn that it is hoped will help surgeons who wish to introduce innovation in the future.

2   The National Context

The early 2000s in the UK was a time of intense scrutiny of cardiac surgery. The Bristol Inquiry [12] (2001), reporting on the tragic outcomes in paediatric cardiac surgery (1991–1995), together with other tragedies involving individual surgeons with poor patient outcomes, attracted media interest and threatened surgical endeavour that was not fully evidence based. Technically, MIS is a challenging procedure and does not lend itself to the questionable "See one, Do one, Teach one" school of medical training. The development of complex surgical motor skills, perceptual-motor co-ordination and effective motor schemas required in MIS take time to acquire [13] and the misplaced confidence of a few surgeons, after seeing one and then doing one in the early years of MIS in the UK did not serve the MIS cause. The professional and the social context became increasingly skeptical, even hostile to innovation, and systemically risk averse.

The surgeons in this study were members of several systems each embedded in other, larger systems. They were members of the consultant group of surgeons in their hospital; each of the surgeons is also individually affiliated with the Royal College of Surgeons and regulated by the General Medical Council. The hospital in which they each work is part of the larger NHS influenced as it is by the social and political context in which it operates. While it was recognized that the NHS was always going to be cautious in accepting MIS and that, in practice, surgical innovation is not easy even with collegial and managerial support, cardiac surgery's unfortunate history resulted in heightened caution and even mistrust of surgical motivation and innovation.

Personal and professional risk to implementing MIS was increased when, partly because of the Bristol scandal, national scrutiny of cardiac surgeons was introduced in 2005, with systems that reported patient outcomes by individual named surgeons. While this was intended to provide public reassurance, it received a mixed reception. National bodies (e.g. SCTS) championed the initiative [14] but individual surgeons reported being less enthusiastic and even fearful and the process had the unintended consequences [15] of dampening surgical motivation to innovate or to take on higher risk patients, even though the data was risk adjusted.

Funding for innovative cardiac surgery faced (and continues to face) challenges, not least because of competition from industry supported trans-catheter procedures, usually conducted by cardiologists. The suggestion that cardiac surgery in general was being cannibalized (i.e. competed against) and might soon be redundant also made it difficult to persuade others of the value of MIS. Notwithstanding these competitive challenges, evolving research suggests that stents do not confer as long a result as originally expected, compared to coronary surgery [16], and given the increasing demand from patients and the vast need for treatment in the undeveloped world, MIS cardiac surgery is reported to have a bright future if innovation is adopted widely [17].

2.1 Psychology and Lesson

The complexity of these various contextual issues seems to have created a shared mindset that innovation, with its associated risk in cardiac surgery, was not worth the risk. The priority became to reduce risk and perform [18] i.e. to deliver outcomes in the traditionally accepted mode of open surgery rather than to innovate. The personal risk associated with pursuing an interest in MIS against this backdrop was high, with strong potential for being either a hero or a villain. The easier option was, as one surgeon said, to take *"the middle road where you can be assured of a decent life and you won't appear on the front pages of the tabloids"*.

Individual surgeons are unlikely to be able to affect the national context but within this national context is the organizational context in which the surgery takes place. Here there is space for influence.

3 The Organizational Context—The Hospital

Whereas MIS is seen by those offering it, especially in the US and Europe, as an opportunity to offer advanced patient care, attract patients to your hospital and boost organizational reputation and income, in the NHS, interviewees suggested that MIS was often seen as problematic. The political cycle with changing ministers and NHS strategies, coupled with the rapid turnaround of hospital chief executives and shifting commissioner demands, create an unstable climate for innovation. Locally senior and middle management incumbents also change jobs rapidly. Getting senior management support can therefore be difficult given this background. Moreover, many surgeons' typical lack of interest in the financial and operational aspects of organizational functioning that would help create rapport and understanding with management, also presents a challenge. The introduction of professional management in the late 1990s and in early 2000, into the NHS, with its focus on targets and productivity, led to some criticism that management was more important than technical expertise, resulting in surgeons possibly feeling they had less authority. The importance of senior management support [19] in innovation is a key factor in successful implementation as it offers organizational legitimacy for the innovative effort.

MIS procedures proved in this context to be an operational challenge for those who did not join customized units. MIS procedures typically take longer than open access surgery, thereby occupying valuable theatre space; they are not readily standardized making it difficult to train others quickly or delegate to less expensive staff to perform; no tariff changes were made and although some instrumentation was reusable, and manufacturers were helpful, considerable cost and time was added to each case. One surgeon made the point that managers do not see patients in clinic and so cannot readily appreciate the benefits of the surgery, seeing it instead as a costly exercise associated with high risk and disruption. There were also staffing implications, as MIS requires anaesthetic and theatre staff competent and confident to support the specific MIS needs. The surgeons described the challenge of convincing theater management of the need for stable teams when management was promoting the idea of interchangeable and multi-skilled theatre staff in the interests of productivity. From a financial and productivity perspective the organizations were not incentivized to support MIS.

As reported through the interviews, where surgeons adopted a managerial perspective, and worked collaboratively with managers, progress was easier than when they did not. The surgeons in the study recognized that they were not independent operators, but rather worked within a larger system, i.e., the hospital. While they all acknowledged that senior management support was necessary for their project, their experiences of securing that support varied. Those who worked in a custom-built unit or were specifically appointed to lead an MIS program in a larger hospital, were in the good starting position of having organizational legitimacy. Where the surgeon was a lone voice for MIS, skepticism was extremely difficult to overcome, and the individuals had to make a business case requiring collegial endorsement and conduct deft negotiation for which surgeons do not typically have the training, skills, or patience.

Significantly, most of the participants were early in their careers with, what they said was, little *"political clout"* at that early stage so persuading the senior establishment (managerial and surgical) of their cause proved frustrating. For those who could, it proved helpful to secure the support of a senior surgical colleague who could provide an extra voice and be the champion in political and managerial discussions, acting as a *"shield"*. To influence senior management and garner support, another said that he deliberately invited the most senior managers to work with him on the business case, thereby exploring the organisational constraints and consequences together. Another was buoyed by the feeling that he had had the support of the chief executive. A fourth said that he initially resisted productivity pressure to perform more than one case a day so that he and the team could reflect and learn from each case. A fifth reported having to resist pressure from an anaesthetist to work more quickly to finish in time.

3.1 Psychology and Lesson

The instability in the organizational context, described above, makes it all the more important to form a strong local "guiding coalition" [20]—a group of stakeholders in the hospital who champion the innovative effort. The risk of losing an advocate is reduced because the initiative will not be dependent on only individual.

Contextualizing the experiences and examples above through the lens of the Primary Colours Model of Leadership [21] is useful. This model describes the three major capabilities of leadership as being strategic, operational and interpersonal and these overlap with one another with Leadership at the center. The strategic domain is further divided into setting strategic direction, creating alignment, and planning and organizing; the operational domain into planning and organizing, team working and delivering results, and the interpersonal domain into creating alignment, building and sustaining relationships, and team working. While few of the surgeons in this project intentionally focused on accomplishing all three major tasks, the actions they took did fall into these categories, thereby underlining the utility of this model in understanding the different domains of leading innovation. For example, some surgeons through the deliberate engagement of senior management, sometimes with the help of a surgical advocate in the MIS strategy, were setting the strategic direction and creating alignment, some more successfully than others. Planning and organizing was at the center of all the surgeons' activities including a focus on governance, developing their own skill over time and the skills of the team. Delivering results was the outcome which justified the activity and arguably was the most important task, often achieved through deliberately managing the pace, rather than acquiescing to operational (productivity) and individual demands for speed. Results delivery was supported through team and individual critical reflection about the technical aspects of the operation in the interests of seeking greater efficiency and effectiveness during the surgery. The surgeons seemed to pay less attention to the interpersonal domain, from a strategic perspective. For example, although some of the surgeons successfully engaged with managers, for others less attention seems to have been paid to creating alignment with colleagues and with management with their intended direction (MIS) in the run up to implementation, focusing instead on the detailed planning and preparation. Ignoring the challenges from their colleagues (see next section) and ploughing on regardless might, in retrospect, have been in their short-term interests because had they not done so they might not have embarked on MIS. It can be argued that for some, it did not serve their long-term interests either, because they are still struggling, to an extent, to raise the profile of MIS.

The skills of influencing, negotiating, and lobbying are of considerable benefit in creating alignment whether they are held by the individual surgeon or by a colleague who is more skilled in these areas, notwithstanding the guiding coalition. Working as a pair of surgeons co-creating alignment and sharing responsibility can provide reassurance to management that there is more than one person interested in pursuing innovation. The time and effort including the expensive outlay for equipment etc. is mitigated to an extent if there is more than colleague interested in implementing the initiative. It is far easier to champion a widely supported program than one in which one person shows interest. Where the preparation has involved the establishment of a small but influential internal guiding coalition [20] with the necessary political skills and organizational power to champion the initiative and support the implementation this reduces the burden on the individual surgeon who is more often than not focused on the technical aspects of the innovation.

Finally, the leadership aspect of the model provides a unifying force. Leadership is a process in which an individual influences the group to accomplish the common goals and targets and is based in the relationship between the leader and the follower rather than simply in the position. Understanding yourself through actively seeking and receiving feedback; creating the conditions for success, inspiring confidence and trust, focusing efforts on priorities; enabling individuals and groups; and helping people to learn, are all aspects of leadership. Leadership will be discussed further in the sections below *The theatre Team* and *The individual surgeon*.

4 Collegial Support

Strategic rather than purely technical surgical support from your surgical colleagues and other specialties, such as anaesthetists and intensivists, is obviously important and can help or hinder implementation efforts in overt and/or covert ways. A major trap, perhaps due to naivete, or to over-confidence, is to assume others will be as passionate as the innovating surgeon is about innovative practice.

External collegial support seemed easier to come by than internal collegial support for some of the surgeons in this study. Other than in custom-built units where surgeons were specifically employed to develop an MIS program, finding local collegial support proved a challenge. While questions from colleagues were expected, the nature of some of the challenges was not. Examples from this study demonstrate that collegial challenge can take many forms from implied to explicit lack of support and, even threat. This was summed up by one interviewee's comment that *"implied threat is voiced when you are asked if you can do the surgery, and then explicit threat can be assumed when you prove you can because you are then viewed as competition"*. An illustrative example that contributed to the skeptical collegial climate was of experienced surgeons who had attempted MIS unsuccessfully and who then *"rubbished" MIS* as a procedure. Yet another surgeon reported being told by a more senior colleague as he was scrubbing for his first case *"if something goes wrong, I won't support you"*. More insidious sabotaging was evident in the example of a consultant colleague writing to a senior medical manager suggesting the MIS surgeon's work be scrutinized. Challenges also came from supporting consultants (e.g. intensivists) about the length of time operations were taking. Only one interviewee offered that a senior colleague had said to him *"let me know how you are getting on and if you need help"*.

Comments, reported by this small group of surgeons, make it clear that some surgical colleagues felt threatened by this new technique and those who practised it. This is common in those who feel less willing to engage with innovation, often referred to as "late majority" or "laggards" [8]. However, it would be naïve to overlook subtle psychological pressures such as professional jealousy and interpersonal rivalry for patients and for reputations, as these factors are also likely to have affected the willingness of some to offer collegial support.

The potential cost to the patient of even the smallest mistake in MIS, while extremely high, might be mitigated by reverting to open surgery but the surgeons made the point that the associated criticism would not serve the MIS cause. Whereas similarly serious mistakes might occur in open surgery, a mistake in MIS attracted disproportionate criticism and led to comments which confirmed the naysayers' view that mistakes were due to the minimal access and that MIS was dangerous. This is an illustration of the effect of confirmation bias [22] the tendency to use new data and evidence as confirmation of one's extant beliefs, which is a strong barrier to positive support for implementation of innovative practice.

4.1 Psychology and Lesson

Typically, surgeons in the NHS with similar interests are jointly responsible for service delivery but they are not necessarily dependent upon one another to achieve their individual purpose or aspiration. Group members are to a degree reliant on one another for support to have a program of work which allows time for their special interests as well as their other work in support of the wider service. They are potentially more dependent on their multi-disciplinary team to achieve their purpose.

In exploring why the MIS implementers were not offered greater collegial support, notwithstanding the contextual issues, it is useful to consider the competitive nature of surgeons and how this can affect group cohesion and interpersonal dynamics. Cohesion describes the extent to which people are drawn to work in a group and contribute effort to the work it does. Group dynamics are the effects of individual team member's motivations, interests, behaviors and roles on each other and the larger group. These effects are often, but not always, unconscious, and they can combine to provide an unhealthy psychological climate with challenging, tricky interpersonal consequences.

Surgeons are well known for being competitive individuals—simply succeeding through competitive entry into medical school and surgical training requires determination, goal-focus and a competitive spirit. This competitiveness does not simply dissolve in qualified and established surgeons. Competitiveness is one of the psychological and/or behavioral factors which influence the group and its dynamics.

Rivalry, whether public or in the shadows, has the positive potential to increase motivation but also to affect group dynamics by creating interpersonal friction and obstructive behaviour. Whether the rivalry is in the interests of personal reputation, private practice or is located in professional jealousy, it should not be ignored. How the innovating surgeon frames the implementation of the new technology and the way it impacts their own and others' work is important and has the potential to help or hinder its success. When individuals feel excluded or threatened by another colleague's ability to attract patients away from them, particularly if the other colleague is younger than they are or where the younger colleague has not engaged with them, the more experienced colleague might respond by under-mining or even by sabotaging innovation efforts.

Engaging, actively and personally, with surgical colleagues and those in supporting specialties, is essential. Consulting with them on a one-to-one basis exploring their views and specific concerns and acknowledging these suggests that you care not only about yourself and your initiative but about the group. Keeping them updated and communicating as much as possible so that colleagues are not surprised by your activities is time consuming but important. As very likely a younger surgeon, it is important to be aware that one's more recent training in newer procedures might threaten more established surgeons at an advantaged stage in their career and one should take active steps to minimize such a threat. Failing to do so might result in deliberate or unconscious attempts to undermine your personal credibility and that of your initiative. Much goes on in the shadows of teams and while collegial collusion, cliques and competition are almost inevitable in most groups, the more one communicates and is open and transparent the easier it is likely to be to navigate through successfully.

The experience of surgeons who started MIS as a pair appeared to be better than those who started on their own. Based on this research, a buddy system is useful in the initial learning phase to share both the pressure and learning involved in success and/or failure and ensures there are two people who can meet with other colleagues, explain what they plan to do and what governance processes they have in place. The time needed to engage with peers should not be under-estimated. Neither should the time needed to engage and develop the operating theatre team be under-estimated.

5   The Theatre Team

Trust, achieved through shared experience of working together, is essential to the development of interdependence which is important in all surgery, but significantly so in MIS. Given the need to focus on a very narrow field of surgical vision in MIS, situational awareness is the responsibility of the team rather than one single surgeon. How the theatre team works together in MIS was noted by the surgeons, as a significant factor in the success of MIS surgery. The surgeons made much of how they helped the team makes sense of their task. They emphasized that the team was there for the patient and that the surgeon was reliant on them to inform him—*"be my eyes and ears for the sake of the patient"*—rather than that they were simply there to meet the surgeon's ends. Put simply, the team makes a genuine contribution rather than being a set of readily interchangeable cogs there to perform a task. This encourages team cohesion.

The surgeons in this research grappled with whether the MIS procedures should be branded as "special", thereby needing a specially trained team, or whether MIS should be simply another surgical procedure. Ideally, they would have preferred to establish a stable team which trained together and then worked together to develop the necessary trust and interdependence. Trust is necessary for establishing psychological safety i.e. a shared belief held by members of a team that the team is safe for interpersonal risk taking [23]. Psychological safety allows team members the confidence to take on the responsibility of working in an MIS cardiac theatre which includes feeling confident to ask a question and/or voice a concern.

Although most had a stable team for the initial training, they cited the development of a long-term stable team as one of the biggest challenges. Following the initial training, surgeons had in some situations to adapt to working with a wide range of theatre staff and with teams where there was no previous collective learning. This was not the case for those customised units who were lucky enough to have stable teams. Nevertheless, all the surgeons started with a team (anaesthetist, perfusionist and scrub nurse) who accompanied them to be trained by an experienced team. They spoke of instilling pride in these training teams and making each professional feel ownership of their part in the surgery. The training approach reflected the four-step process of enrolment, preparation, trials and reflection [3] for implementing innovation. They reported that to foster ownership and engagement it was necessary to select team members for their skill and not simply because of their availability or seniority. One surgeon said that he chose those he trusted most and who *"wouldn't surprise me"* underlining the importance of trust and predictability but also leading to allegations of racism, sexism, perfectionism, and elitism. Another commented that jealousy increased as the team became successful and his experience at the time was mixed: *"if we had failed it would be bad, but success was also bad"*.

5.1 Psychology and Lesson

Having a joint "aspirational purpose" that draws people together to join a group rather than one which keeps people together for defensive purposes, provides a compelling reason to join the group and an incentive for task ownership. Better patient care and outcomes was the common feature of this compelling purpose in the group studied. It is important in the beginning to train and then work together as a coherent team to construct a new reality and to encourage sense-making of the new technology and develop appropriate norms and behaviours [24].

Clark [25] suggests that "the preparation to perform creates the desire to perform" underlining the importance of training together. However, the theatre team's performance is based not only on their individual skill and training but also on how the surgeon leads the team. Surgeon leadership behaviour contributes a great deal to the development of cohesion and psychological safety. The more traditional, hierarchical approach where the surgeon exercises control

through ensuring that he or she is seen as the resource of knowledge, skill and power while others wait for instruction is increasingly open to question but is especially questionable in MIS. Over-controlling leadership has been shown to correlate negatively with collective efficacy in theatre [26] and associated with weak leadership [25].

Research [27] on surgeon leadership style has differentiated between transactional and transformational styles of leadership each of which contributes in a different way to the interpersonal dynamics. A transactional leadership style is task-focused while a transformational leadership is team-oriented. The former keeps the focus on task performance and is said to promote self-interest. The latter style is described as engaging team members' intrinsic motivation through fostering team identification with the goal. Increased information sharing and encouraging psychological safety behaviours have been associated with successful technology implementation [3].

Cohesive teams exhibit higher levels of performance, effectiveness, job satisfaction, social support and communication. Cohesion arises as a result of the emotional ties that teams develop in interaction with each other such as goal setting, managing conflict and giving feedback [28]. New team members are likely to observe and implicitly learn the behavioural norms. However, it should never be taken for granted that those unfamiliar with the expected ways of working will quickly absorb the norms which are often unspoken in teams familiar with one another.

Expanding the concept of psychological safety and seeing it from a team member's perspective, psychological safety has been described as "a condition in which you feel (i) included, (2) safe to learn, (iii) safe to contribute, and (iv) safe to challenge the status quo—all without fear of being embarrassed, marginalized or punished in some way" [25]. Encouraging a psychologically safe environment is based upon a combination of respecting others' skills and giving them permission to speak. As the leader of the team, it is the surgeon's responsibility to role model openness and create the conditions for psychological safety by spelling out the four conditions. Setting expectations for psychological safety and expectations of the team at the outset of each surgical list, and highlighting those necessary for successful MIS, should be a priority of the surgeon.

6 The Surgeon

Given the highly challenging backdrop of national scrutiny, organizational complexity, peer skepticism and jealousy described in this chapter, our study was interested in identifying the factors, over and above their technical abilities, that enabled these surgeons to succeed. Does their determination in the face of the contextual challenges and lack of obvious support suggest that these nine surgeons possess attributes which differentiate them from other surgeons? The study was based on qualitative group interviews and the completion of a psychometric measure describing Learning Agility. Interesting and somewhat contradictory findings were observed between what the surgeons said about themselves compared to what the psychometric measure reported about them as a group. Nevertheless, the findings offer food for thought for those considering introducing innovation into their workplaces.

Themes from the qualitative interviews of this small group suggested that the common characteristics were (i) curiosity and learning (ii) determination and single-minded focus on the patient; (iii) tolerance for ambiguity and pressure; (iv) confidence and (v) reflection and insight.

The surgeons reported that from an early stage in their surgical career that they could not envisage doing the same thing for the rest of their working lives. This desire for challenge, and curiosity under-pinned by horizon-scanning i.e. checking and anticipating where surgical innovation might take the profession, were important motivating factors in their drive to introduce MIS. They also made much of the need to learn continuously and keep challenging themselves to improve their skills.

The surgeons talked about the need for planning, preparation, and focused concentration before and during the operation. One said his planning and preparation took three years before he performed his first procedure. All repeatedly spoke of the beneficial outcomes of MIS for patients and it was evident how much of a driver this was in their determination to proceed despite the odds and the difficult climate and context.

The reporting of individual surgeon outcomes on a macro-level proved challenging but they also said that scrutiny on a micro level in the hospital and in theatre from immediate colleagues contributed to the pressure of their work. These surgeons were relatively young in age and experience, and it was suggested that it would have been more difficult to tolerate the pressure if they had undertaken the MIS cause at a later stage in their careers, implying that as younger surgeons they were resilient with less life experience and perhaps less appreciation for the difficulties they might encounter. They reported being "comfortable being uncomfortable" and willing to tolerate this feeling even in high-risk situations when they might be faced with a surgical complication they had not encountered before and where there was little collegial support. The MIS surgeons in this study seemed willing to face the risk of collegial opprobrium—perhaps being labelled a 'black sheep' for deviating from the norm and being side lined by the in-group [29] (15) i.e. other cardiac surgeons—the group they are most likely to identify with and risk being 'isolated' from, that is, the establishment. From an ethnicity perspective, only one of the surgeons from this early cohort is White British, four were born in the UK to Asian parents, and the remaining four were immigrants. Thus, they could be viewed as a group that was not typically part of the establishment perhaps with a greater degree of resilience than is typical. This may have emboldened their resilience and determination to implement MIS.

Another commonality was strong self-belief and confidence. All interviewees were aware they might be perceived as arrogant, demanding, and perfectionistic rather than simply confident and diligent. Underneath this confidence was a seemingly paradoxical behaviour described as persistent self-questioning, but which may not be obvious to those who perceive them as arrogant. They spoke about the need for constant critical reflection, continuous improvement and self-awareness exemplified in the following comment: *"When I look back on my proficiency 3 years ago, I can't believe I thought that was good"*.

The psychometric questionnaire results provide some interesting nuances to the above self-reflections. The surgeons completed *The Learning Agility Index* [30]. Learning agility is defined here as the ability to rapidly develop new effective behaviour, based on new experiences, and then to apply this behaviour successfully. It is described in four dimensions: change agility, mental agility, people agility and results agility with one transcending factor, self-awareness, influencing all four dimensions. While this was a small sample, there are some interesting early hypotheses, which both support and contradict the surgeons' views of themselves but which, importantly, offer insights and learning for those wanting to implement new ways of working.

The result analysis suggests strong *Results Agility* describing them as likely to set themselves challenging targets and expectations and to deal well with the stress that achieving these targets entails. *Results Agility* is associated with a driving force to maintain focus under pressure and the desire to perform better than others and better than one has previously performed. *Results Agility* may be what underpins their continuous improvement focus, but on its own does not suggest wider personal development. Rather energy is derived from achieving results and self-reflection is likely driven by a lack of success which directs improvement in results and the desire to prove oneself in the interests of results. *Results Agility* is linked to personality traits associated with being ambitious, self-confident, masterful and goal directed in other words, conscientiousness. Needless to say, these results align with their views of themselves as determined and task focused, terms which are typically descriptive of surgeons in general.

Other *Agility* scores were more variable and lower than *Results Agility*. *Mental Agility,* based on being analytical, comfortable with complexity and open to new ideas was second highest with *People Agility* and *Change Agility* both lower. The low score on *People Agility* implies that the group did not focus on other people's help nor do they believe that others can help them with a better or different analysis, suggesting that firstly they may not access the right people for help in developing their case for change and secondly, that they might not listen as carefully as they need to when others are offering help or questioning them.

Data from the qualitative interviews suggested that the surgeons placed enormous value on their team and encouraged psychological safety. Their narrative indicated that they valued their multidisciplinary team members as people and colleagues. Preliminary data from the *Agility Index* demonstrates that the reasons for psychological safety may be driven more by task necessity than by personal belief or altruism since *People Agility* scores were low.

People Agility suggests one is open to others' opinions, and that one values consulting others to learn from them before forming an opinion. Moreover, one is likely to derive energy and learning from others and from sharing knowledge. If this is the case, then it may explain why their surgical colleagues whose support they wanted, but did not always get, were not committed to their success (notwithstanding fear, jealousy and competition) because the innovating surgeons had not taken sufficient time to engage and consult with them. On the other hand, it could be argued, if they had been influenced by the skepticism and challenges of their colleagues, they may not have got as far as implementation. Whatever the reason, the more an innovating surgeon can influence their peers to support them, the easier the implementation journey is likely to be. Improving their facility for *People Agility* i.e. becoming more emotionally intelligent in the manner in which they influence others and navigate the political realities of organizational life would be beneficial.

As a caveat to their subjective views about their curiosity and open-mindedness, the agility results suggest that while they are determined when implementing their own plans *(high Results Agility)*, they themselves might not enjoy working in a changing environment and are otherwise risk averse *(low Change Agility)*.

7 Conclusions

All surgeons reported awareness of the possible risk to their professional, and consequently personal lives, of pursuing and mastering MIS. There was no definitive science to support the adoption of these procedures and it fell on them to both innovate and create the science to support their patient-centered beliefs.

While this chapter is based on a small and self-selected sample of surgeons it offers interesting insights. The interviewees' experience ranged from 2006 to 2016 demonstrating that this specific innovation did not become easier with time. On reflection these early adopters suggested that the technical challenges were the least of their problems because they were careful to be trained, proctored, and mentored and, in fact, were not the original pioneers but were following those who had broken the ground for them. What was more difficult to manage and understand was the lack of collegial, organisational and systemic support. In retrospect, exploring their own psychology, attempting to understand that of their colleagues, and the psychology of the system, might have made their journey easier. Research [31] suggests that the successful surgeon innovator must be savvy in medicine, technology, and business but this study shows that an understanding of psychology, particularly organizational and interpersonal dynamics, is central too.

References

1. Pompili MF, Stevens JH, Burdon TA, Siegel LC, Peters WS, Ribakove GH, Reitz BA. Port-access mitral valve replacement in dogs. J Thorac Cardiovasc Surg. 1996;112(5):1268–74. https://doi.org/10.1016/S0022-5223(96)70140-X.
2. Grant SW, Hickey GL, Modi P, Hunter S, Akowuah E, Zacharias J. Propensity-matched analysis of minimally invasive approach versus sternotomy for mitral valve surgery. Heart. 2019;105(10):783–789. http://heart.bmj.com/content/105/10/783.info.
3. Edmondson AC, Bohmer RM, Pisano GP. Disrupted routines: team learning and new technology implementation in hospitals. Adm Sci Q. 2001;46:685–716. https://doi.org/10.2307/3094828.
4. Casselman FP, Van Slycke S, Wellens F, De Geest R, Degrieck I, Van Praet F, Vermeulen Y, Vanermen H. Mitral valve surgery can now routinely be performed endoscopically. Circulation. 2003;108 (Suppl 1):II48-54. https://doi.org/10.1161/01.cir.0000087391.49121.ce.
5. Suri RM, Schaff HV, Meyer SR, Hargrove WC 3rd. Thoracoscopic versus open mitral valve repair: a propensity score analysis of early outcomes. Ann Thorac Surg. 2009;88(4):1185–90. https://doi.org/10.1016/j.athoracsur.2009.04.076.
6. Van Praet KM, Stamm C, Sündermann SH, Meyer A, Unbehaun A, Montagner M,Nazari Shafti TZ, Jacobs S, Falk V, Kempfert J. Minimally invasive surgical mitral valve repair: state of the art review. Interv Cardiol. 2018;13(1):14–19. https://doi.org/10.15420/icr.2017:30:1.
7. Altman DR, Campbell WB, Flum DR, Glaziou P, Marshall JC, Nicoll J for Balliol collaboration. No surgical innovation without evaluation: the IDEAL recommendations. Lancet. 2009;374:1105–12. https://doi.org/10.1016/S0140-6736(09)61116-8.
8. Rogers EM. Diffusion of innovations. New York: Free Press;1962/2003.
9. British Psychological Society. https://www.bps.org.uk/public/. Accessed 7 March 2021.
10. Catchpole K, McCullogh M. Human factors in critical care: towards standardized integrated human-centred systems of work. Curr Opin Crit Care. 2010;16(6):618–22. https://doi.org/10.1097/MCC.0b013e32833e9b4b.
11. Catchpole K. Department of Health Human Factors Reference Group Interim Report. 2012. http://www.england.nhs.uk/ourwork/part-rel/nqb/ag-min/.
12. Kennedy I. The Report of the Public Inquiry into children's heart surgery at the Bristol Royal Infirmary 1984–1995. 2001. http://www.wales.nhs.uk/sites3/documents/441/The%20Kennedy%20Report.pdf.
13. Silvennoinen M, Mecklin JP, Saariluoma P, Antikainen T. Expertise and skill in minimally invasive surgery. Scand J Surg. 2009;209–213. https://doi.org/10.1177/145749690909800403.
14. Bridgewater B, Kinsman R, Walton P, Keogh B. Demonstrating quality: the Sixth National Adult Cardiac Surgery database report. Henley-on-Thames, Oxfordshire, United Kingdom: Dendrite Clinical Systems Ltd;2008. https://scts.org/_userfiles/resources/SixthNACSDreport2008withcovers.pdf.
15. Westaby S. Publishing individual surgeons' death rates prompts risk averse behaviour. BMJ. 2014;3499: g5026. https://doi.org/10.1136/bmj.g5026.
16. Head SJ, Milojevic M, Daemen J, Ahn JM, Boersma E, et al. Mortality after coronary artery

bypass grafting versus percutaneous coronary intervention with stenting for coronary artery disease: a pooled analysis of individual patient data. Lancet. 2018;10 391(10124):939–948. https://doi.org/10.1016/S0140-6736(18)30423-9.

17. Zacharias J, Perier P. Seven Habits of Highly Effective Endoscopic Mitral Surgeons. Innov Technol Tech Cardio-Thorac Surg. 2020;15(1):11–16. https://doi.org/10.1177/1556984519888456.

18. Staw BM, Sandelands LE, Dutton, JE. Threat-rigidity effects in organizational behavior: a multilevel analysis. Adm Sci Q. 1981;26:501–24. https://doi.org/10.2307/2392337.

19. Yin RK. Production efficiency versus bureaucratic self-interest: two innovative processes? Policy Sci. 1977;8:381–99. https://doi.org/10.1007/BF01727406.

20. Kotter J. Leading change. Harvard Business Review Press;2012.

21. Pendleton D, Furnham A. The primary colours model. Palgrave MacMillan;2016.

22. Kahneman D. Thinking, fast and slow. London: Allen Lane; 2011.

23. Edmondson AC. Psychological safety and learning behaviour in work teams. Adm Sci Q. 1999. https://doi.org/10.2307/2666999.

24. Edmondson AC. Framing for learning: Lessons in Successful Technology ImplementationCalif Manag Rev. 2003;45(2). https://doi.org/10.2307/41166164.

25. Clark R. The 4 stages of psychological safety: defining the path to inclusion and innovation. US: Berrett-Koehler Publisher Inc;2021.

26. Barling J, Akers A, Beikob D. The impact of positive and negative intraoperative surgeons' leadership behaviors on surgical team performance. Am J Surg. 2018;215(1).

27. Yue-Yung Hu, MD, MPH,1,2, Henrickson Parker S, Lipsitz SR, Arriaga AF et al. Surgeons' leadership styles and team behaviour in the operating room. J Am Coll Surg. 2016;222(1). https://doi.org/10.1016/j.jamcollsurg.2015.09.013.

28. Levi DJ, Askay DA. Group dynamics for teams. Thousand Oaks, California: Sage Publications;2021.

29. Tajfel H, Turner JC. The social identity theory of intergroup behaviour. In: Worchel S, Austin WG, editors. Psychology of intergroup relations. Nelson-Hall;1986.

30. HFMTalentindex—Part of the Assessio Group. https://www.hfmtalentindex.com/en/. Accessed 11 April 2021.

31. Riskin DJ, Longaker MT, Gernert, M and Krummel TM. Innovation in Surgery; a historical perspective. Ann Surg. 2006;244(5). https://doi.org/10.1097/01.sla.0000242706.91771.ce.

Correction to: Endoscopic Cardiac Surgery

Joseph Zacharias

Correction to:
J. Zacharias (ed.), Endoscopic Cardiac Surgery,
https://doi.org/10.1007/978-3-031-21104-1

This book was inadvertently published with the incorrect ESM link and videos for the chapters 1, 2, 3, 5, 6, 9, 11, 14 and 19. This has now been amended in these chapters.

The correction chapters and the book has been updated with these changes.

The updated version of the book can be found at
https://doi.org/10.1007/978-3-031-21104-1

Index

Total arterial Endo grafting, 225
Totally endoscopic, 129, 143, 144, 175, 176, 180, 184, 197–200, 202, 203, 217, 218, 313
Totally endoscopic surgery, 175, 217, 218
Transoesophageal Echocardiography (TOE), 11, 13, 15, 17, 18, 20, 21, 28, 29, 31, 33, 37, 41–43, 45–48, 60, 91, 125, 133, 140, 185, 186, 188, 191, 193, 196, 198–200, 212, 214, 239, 241, 280, 281

Tricuspid Valve (TV), 42, 44, 45, 47, 48, 151–153, 157, 159, 160, 196, 202, 214, 215, 238, 251, 260, 266, 269, 271, 281

V

Valve disease, 3, 4, 20, 151, 175, 184, 196–198, 200–217, 239, 245, 246, 250, 251, 255–260, 268, 278

MIX
Papier aus verantwortungsvollen Quellen
Paper from responsible sources
FSC® C105338

If you have any concerns about our products,
you can contact us on
ProductSafety@springernature.com

In case Publisher is established outside the EU,
the EU authorized representative is:
**Springer Nature Customer Service Center GmbH
Europaplatz 3, 69115 Heidelberg, Germany**

Printed by Libri Plureos GmbH
in Hamburg, Germany